Updates in Hypertension and Cardiovascular Protection

Series Editors
Giuseppe Mancia, Milan, Italy
Enrico Agabiti-Rosei, Brescia, Italy

The aim of this series is to provide informative updates on both the knowledge and the clinical management of a disease that, if uncontrolled, can very seriously damage the human body and is still among the leading causes of death worldwide. Although hypertension is associated mainly with cardiovascular, endocrine, and renal disorders, it is highly relevant to a wide range of medical specialties and fields – from family medicine to physiology, genetics, and pharmacology. The topics addressed by volumes in the series *Updates in Hypertension and Cardiovascular Protection* have been selected for their broad significance and will be of interest to all who are involved with this disease, whether residents, fellows, practitioners, or researchers.

Adel E. Berbari • Giuseppe Mancia
Josep Redon
Editors

Blood Pressure Disorders in Acute and Chronic Kidney Diseases

Springer

Editors
Adel E. Berbari
American University of Beirut
Medical Center
Beirut, Lebanon

Giuseppe Mancia
University Milano-Bicocca
Milano, Italy

Josep Redon
INCLIVA Health Research Institute
University of Valencia
Valencia, Spain

ISSN 2366-4606 ISSN 2366-4614 (electronic)
Updates in Hypertension and Cardiovascular Protection
ISBN 978-3-031-81291-0 ISBN 978-3-031-81292-7 (eBook)
https://doi.org/10.1007/978-3-031-81292-7

This Springer imprint is published by the registered company Springer Nature Switzerland AG
The registered company address is: Gewerbestrasse 11, 6330 Cham, Switzerland

Preface

This book is intended to provide an in-depth and up-to-date information of the various aspects of the association between blood pressure disorders and acute/chronic kidney diseases. In addition, our purpose is to discuss the pathophysiologic mechanisms underlying blood pressure elevation in renal disorders, the cardiorenal relationships and the interaction between the kidney and the extrarenal mechanisms controlling circulation, and the therapeutic approaches in hypertensive nephropathies. The book also includes hypertensive nephropathies infrequently recognized by clinicians, and its spectrum includes glomerulonephritis, nephrolithiasis, polycystic kidney disease, renal artery stenosis, reninomas, drug-related kidney injury, and rarely recognized causes of a blood pressure elevation such as renal embolic disease and blunt renal trauma. Treatment focuses on classical but also new antihypertensive drugs, the very frequently needed drug combinations but also on renal replacement therapy, other surgical approaches, and renal denervation. Kidney disorders in dismetabolic conditions such as diabetes and pregnancy are separately considered.

Co-existence of hypertension and kidney disease is very common. Renal parenchymal diseases represent the most frequent form of secondary hypertensiovn, accounting for over 5% of cases referred to a hypertension clinic. Underlying renal pathology and severity of renal functional impairment are crucial factors in the determination of the degree of blood pressure elevation, with frequently higher blood pressure values in glomerular than in tubulointerstitial nephropathies. In renal disorders, the blood pressure elevation may be so severe as to lead to the clinical picture of malignant hypertension as well as to account for the largest percentage of patients with resistant and refractory hypertension.

This book is divided into a number of sections. Within each section, the chapters have been authored by well-known experts in the Nephrology and Hypertension areas. The editors are deeply grateful to them for their valuable contribution and hope that the book will make a useful updated reading to both general practitioners and specialists.

Beirut, Lebanon — Adel E. Berbari
Milano, Italy — Giuseppe Mancia
Valencia, Spain — Josep Redon

Contents

Part I

Introduction

Definition and Classification of Phenotype of Blood Pressure Disorders in Acute and Chronic Kidney Diseases

1

Adel E. Berbari, Najla A. Daouk, and Majida M. Daouk

1.1 Introduction

Hypertension is a very frequent cardiovascular disorder in both acute and chronic kidney diseases [1]. Most studies have reported more than 60% prevalence rates of hypertension in patients with chronic kidney disease (CKD) [2]. The data of the Chronic Renal Insufficiency Cohort (CRIC) study confirm these findings [3]. The CRIC study included 3612 participants with a racially and ethnically diverse group of adults aged 21–74 years, with a broad spectrum of renal disease severity, an estimated glomerular filtration rate (GFR) of 20–70 mL/min/1.73m^2 [3]. About 90% of the patients had a blood pressure (BP) > 150/90 mmHg [3].

The relationship between hypertension and renal disease was first recognized by Richard Bright in 1836 [4]. Bright noticed a significant association between small contracted granular kidneys, albuminuous urine, and cardiac enlargement [4]. Although no BP measurements were available those days, Bright postulated that the kidneys were responsible for the alteration of chemical composition of blood, causing resistance to outflow from the heart and cardiac hypertrophy [4]. Further, the discovery of renin by Tigerstedt and Bergman in 1898 [5] and the production of experimental hypertension with constriction of one or both renal arteries in the dog by Goldblatt in 1936 led to postulation of the role of the kidneys in BP regulation [6]. However, the modern understanding of the relation between the kidneys and BP regulation was not clarified until the publication of a landmark document by Volhard and Fahr in 1914 [7, 8]. The concepts discussed in this important document formed the basis for the subsequent definition of benign and malignant hypertension and the comprehension of their pathophysiology [7, 8].

A. E. Berbari (✉) · N. A. Daouk · M. M. Daouk
Department of Internal Medicine, American University of Beirut Medical Center, Beirut, Lebanon
e-mail: ab01@aub.edu.lb

A. E. Berbari et al. (eds.), *Blood Pressure Disorders in Acute and Chronic Kidney Diseases*, Updates in Hypertension and Cardiovascular Protection,
https://doi.org/10.1007/978-3-031-81292-7_1

This chapter includes a survey of the classification and definition relevant to the hypertension phenotypes associated with acute and chronic kidney diseases (renal parenchymal diseases).

1.2 Hypertension in Renal Parenchymal Disease

1.2.1 Definition

Renal parenchymal disease represents a serious comorbid condition associated with hypertension and cardiovascular events [9, 10].

Renal parenchymal hypertension is generally defined as BP elevation associated with renal structural and/or vascular lesions [11]. However, the link between renal parenchymal disease and high BP is not always evident [11]. In some patients who exhibit significant constriction of one or both renal arteries, BP elevation is related to the renal vascular lesions [12, 13]. In such patients, surgical correction of the renal artery stenosis leads to improvement or reversal of the hypertension process [12, 13]. Such patients are reported to have renovascular hypertension, an entity which represents a very small minority of the hypertensive population [12, 13]. In contrast, in the great majority of patients with renal parenchymal disease, the renovascular conditions are not evident as the hypertension cannot be cured [13]. Further, many patients with essential hypertension may have coexistent renal disease and are often misclassified as having renal parenchymal hypertension [11].

Renal parenchymal hypertension is the most common form of secondary hypertension, accounting for over 5% of cases in referral hypertension centers [2].

Hypertension secondary to renal parenchymal disease is a phenomenon which occurs with a wide spectrum of acute and chronic glomerular, tubulointerstitial, and renovascular nephropathies [13] (Fig. 1.1).

The expression and clinical aspects of hypertension vary widely with the renal parenchymal diseases [11]. Hypertension is very prevalent in some patients while it is infrequent or even absent in others [11]. It may occur early at the outset or may be delayed until progression to end-stage renal failure of the disease [11]. Further,

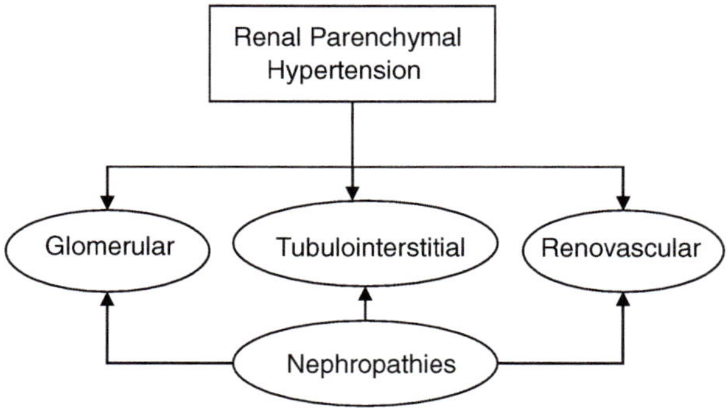

Fig. 1.1 Classification of hypertensive renal parenchymal disorders

hypertension may be mild or severe at the onset, or may increase in severity, with declining renal function [11].

Several factors have been postulated to account for the differences in clinical manifestations of hypertension in the various parenchymal disorders. The most important of these appear to be the type of underlying histopathologic lesion(s) and the degree of impairment of renal function [11, 14–16].

Occurrence and severity of hypertension in various renal disorders may be divided into three groups. In the first group, severe and even malignant hypertension frequently occur in renin-producing tumors of the renal cortex, scleroderma kidney disease, renal infarcts, segmental renal hypoplasia, and in some cases of acute glomerulonephritis [11]. In the second group, in contrast, hypertension is generally mild or even absent in minimal change nephropathy, focal glomerulopathy with benign hematuria, medullary cystic nephronophtisis complex and most of the acute tubulointerstitial kidney disorders [11]. However, progression to end-stage renal failure with fluid and sodium retention often leads to BP elevation in these diseases [11]. In the third and last group, the prevalence and the extent of high BP are variable. These kidney diseases include 1) glomerular diseases with prominent proteinuria (membranous nephropathy), 2) some tubulointerstitial diseases (pyelonephritis, analgesic nephropathy, obstructive uropathy), and 3) cystic kidney disease (polycystic kidney disease, multi-cystic kidney disease) [11].

1.2.2 Classification and Prevalence of Hypertension in Various Renal Diseases

Hypertension is frequently associated with both acute and chronic kidney diseases [2, 17].

1.2.2.1 Acute Kidney Diseases

Several types of acute kidney diseases with or without renal functional impairment are commonly associated with hypertension [15].

In this section, hypertensive forms of acute kidney diseases more frequently encountered clinically will be discussed.

In a retrospective study of 262 patients with acute renal failure, Bomomini et al. reported that 39% of patients had hypertension at some time during the course of their disease [15, 18]. Among the hypertensive patients with acute renal failure, in 73%, hypertension was caused by vascular or glomerular nephropathies, while only in 15% was the hypertension related to acute tubulointerstitial disorders, compared chiefly of acute tubular necrosis [15, 18].

Acute Diffuse Glomerulonephritis

Acute diffuse glomerulonephritis, caused by streptococcal pharyngitis or impetigo, generally occurs in youth, with 70% of patients being younger than 20 years [19]. However, the disease may occur in adults [19].

Clinically, patients present with hematuria, oliguria, edema, and hypertension [19]. Hypertension, which may be severe or even malignant, occurs in over 80% of involved subjects [19]. With remission of the disease, hypertension usually subsides, although it may persist in some subjects.

The acute syndrome may be precipitated also by viral infections, systemic disease, or malignant hypertension [19].

Adult Minimal Change Nephrotic Syndrome (Lipoid Nephrosis)

In adults as in children, minimal change nephrotic syndrome is reported to be a benign renal disease, characterized clinically by edema, normotension and normal renal function, and treatment-induced remission [20, 21]. However, adults with the syndrome are brittle as they are prone to cardiorenal complications [20, 21]. A study of 89 biopsy-proven minimal change nephrotic syndrome evaluated by Nolasco et al. revealed that 50% of nephrotic patients had 10% severe hypertension (diastolic BP >110 mmHg) and significant renal functional impairment at the outset [20]. Treatment induced a remission in two-third of these patients, which is characterized by improvement in renal function and fall in BP [20, 21].

Embolic Renal Disease

Embolic renal disease is a common, generally unrecognized form of ischemic nephropathy [22]. It occurs in elderly subjects, predominantly males, especially those older than 60 years of age, suffering from severe generalized atherosclerotic disease of the abdominal aorta and its major branches [22].

Embolic renal disease is caused by dissemination of cholesterol emboli in large and small arteries in multiple organ systems, but most commonly in the kidneys, in patients undergoing aortic abdominal surgery, invasive cardiovascular procedures, and/or use of anticoagulants [22]. Ulceration or disruption of the abdominal atheromatous plaques exposes the inner surface of the lesion, leading to dissemination of cholesterol emboli, occlusion of the renal vasculature, and ischemic changes [22].

Clinically, the cause of the embolic renal disorder is characterized by sudden onset of acute renal failure, sudden severe BP elevation, worsening renal functional impairment, or worsening existing hypertension [22].

Patients may also present cutaneous and systemic manifestations involving other organs and which may be due to serious underlying pathology [22] adding to the already serious prognosis of the disorder [22].

Prevalence rates of the embolic renal disorder vary widely and depend mainly on differences on treated and untreated patients [22]. In a group of 42 non-operated patients with abdominal aortic aneurysms, embolic renal disease was reported in 31% [22]. Similarly in another group of 38 non-operated patients with severe abdominal aortic atherosclerotic disease and occlusion of the aorta, 18.5% had the embolic renal disorder [22]. In contrast, in 22 patients who died following resection of the abdominal aortic aneurysm, autopsy revealed embolic renal disease in 77% [22]. On the other hand, in 44 cases with minimal atherosclerosis, no embolic renal disease was found [22].

Acute Kidney Injury

Acute kidney injury (AKI) is a serious renal disorder associated with increased mortality, cardiovascular complications, and long-term chronic kidney disease [17, 23, 24]. Acute kidney injury has been reported to be precipitated by pre-renal (volume contraction), renal (intrinsic parenchymal disease), or post-renal (obstructive) factors [17, 24].

Acute kidney injury, defined as a rapid decline in renal function, has been characterized by the development of three stages: (1) persistence of oliguria of more than 6 h (risk stage); (2) an increase in serum creatinine of more than 50% (injury stage); and (3) severe deterioration in renal function (failure stage) [17, 24].

Hypertension is very common in acute kidney injury. In a retrospective analysis of 215 patients with acute kidney injury, Dylewska et al. reported an occurrence rate of hypertension of 70% in AKI with rates of 85% in post-renal cases, 75% in those with intrinsic renal disease, and 30% in those with pre-renal factors [25].

Blunt Renal Trauma-Induced Hypertension

Blunt renal trauma has been reported to cause injury to the kidneys in 1.2% of subjects admitted to the hospital following an accident [23]. The renal injury is characterized by contusion, hematoma, laceration, or vascular injury [23].

Blunt renal trauma has been reported to induce hypertension in 4.5% of involved traumatized subjects [23]. BP elevation is generally moderate but may be severe or even malignant [23]. Renal function is mildly impaired [23]. The hypertensive patients are predominantly young adults, the population most often exposed to accidents [23].

Hypertension generally resolves with antihypertensive therapy, surgery, or spontaneously [23].

In subjects who remain normotensive following the blunt renal trauma, BP should be monitored for several months as hypertension may develop long term [23].

Blood Pressure Disorders in Pregnancy

- Preeclampsia and Eclampsia

  Preeclampsia and eclampsia constitute serious BP disorders in pregnancy, occurring from 20 weeks of gestation to 4–6 weeks postpartum [26, 27]. These are associated with increased risks of maternal/fetal morbidity and mortality [26, 27]. Their incidences vary significantly between different countries [26, 27]. WHO derived an estimated global incidence of 4.6% of preeclampsia and 1.4% of eclampsia from data collected from 40 countries [26, 27].

  Clinically, the affected pregnant women develop either de novo hypertension (140/90 mmHg) or an elevation in BP superimposed on chronic hypertension associated with proteinuria and acute renal functional impairment [26, 27]. Cardio cerebrovascular symptoms and signs including seizures, impaired liver function, and thrombocytopenia may also occur [26, 27].
- Acute Kidney Injury in Pregnancy

- Acute kidney injury in pregnancy constitutes a very serious condition associated with increased maternal and fetal/neonatal mortality and development of acute cortical necrosis [27].

  Acute kidney injury occurs most frequently in the late third trimester of pregnancy and is caused both by hypertensive complications and by the HELP syndrome [27]. Its incidence is variable but is higher in developing countries, with up to 20% [27].

  Acute cortical necrosis, a very dreaded complication in pregnancy, is caused by obstetric complications and disseminated intravascular coagulation [27, 28]. It has been reported in 1.5–2% in developed countries and 3–7% in developing countries. It predisposes to significant morbidity and mortality [27, 29].

Acute Kidney Injury Induced by Non-steroidal Anti-inflammatory Drugs
Nonsteroidal anti-inflammatory drugs (NSAIDs) are among the most prescribed drugs especially for the relief of pain [30].

The use of NSAIDs may cause serious adverse reactions on BP homeostasis and renal function [31, 32].

NSAIDs have been shown to cause BP elevation in both normotensive and hypertensive subjects [33]. The BP elevation is generally mild, in the range of 2–5 mmHg [33]. However, in some individuals, especially the elderly or individuals with comorbid conditions, hypertension can be severe or even malignant [32, 34].

BP levels may be higher in patients receiving beta-blockers, compared to those taking other classes of antihypertensive drugs [35].

NSAIDs-induced AKI occurs mainly in patients with a preexisting compromised renal function [36]. NSAIDs do not appear to alter renal function in healthy individuals [36].

Both traditional and selective COX2 inhibitors can increase the risk of AKI [36]. Further, the concomitant administration of diuretics or RAAS inhibitors can also increase the risk of AKI; this increased risk being of the order of 30–60% [36] reaches its highest levels within 1 month of the administration of both drugs [36].

Selective COX2 inhibitors may have serious outcome in renal function in AKI [36]. In a retrospective cohort study, administration of selective COX2 inhibitors to CKD patients was associated with rapid decline in renal function which was not reversible even after withdrawal of the drug [36].

Antineoplastic Therapy
Novel anticancer therapeutic strategies such as targeted therapies and immunotherapies have improved significantly the therapeutic benefits of several neoplasms [37, 38]. However, in contrast to the traditional cytotoxic chemotherapy, these novel therapeutic antineoplastic agents are associated with significant renovascular toxicity [38].

The introduction of effective and well-tolerated therapies targeting specific genes/proteins and novel immunotherapies has enhanced the occurrence of kidney-related adverse events which include acute kidney injury with proteinuria tubular dysfunction and occasionally CKD [39, 40].

Blood pressure elevation and hypertension occur frequently in untreated and treated cancer patients. The prevalence of hypertension increases from 29% prior to antineoplastic treatment to 39–40% following initiation of newer anticancer modalities [41].

1.2.2.2 Chronic Kidney Disease

Chronic kidney disease (CKD) and hypertension frequently coexist and are associated with a significant enhanced risk of cardiovascular morbidity and mortality [1].

CKD represents a heterogeneous disorder which involves structure and function of the kidneys [42, 43]. CKD is characterized by markers of kidney damage (abnormal urinalysis and sediment, albuminuria, kidney biopsy, and/or radiologic imaging), and/or renal functional impairment persisting for 1 or 3 months [42, 43]. Based on those criteria, it is estimated that 10–15% of individuals worldwide have CKD [42, 43].

Hypertension occurs in 80–85% of CKD patients [2, 3].

The prevalence rates of hypertension are determined by several factors:

- **Severity of Renal Functional Impairment**

  The prevalence of CKD increases as GFR falls from 90 mL/min/1.73 m^2 to 15 mL/min/1.73 m^2 [44]. In a national survey of a representative sample of non-institutionalized adults in USA, it was estimated that hypertension occurs in 23.3% of individuals without CKD, 35.8% of stage 1, 48.1% of stage 2, 59.9% of stage 3, and 84.1% of stages 4–5 CKD patients [45]. Further hypertension is very common in patients on renal replacement therapy. Eighty six percent of patients on dialysis treatment (hemodialysis/peritoneal dialysis) and 70% of renal transplant recipients are hypertensive [45].

- **Underlying Renal Pathology**

  Hypertension is more common in primary glomerular than in chronic tubulointerstitial diseases [46]. Hypertension occurs in 60% of primary glomerulopathies and in 35% of chronic tubulointerstitial nephropathies [47, 48].

- **Causes of Renal Parenchymal Disease**

  The prevalence of hypertension is influenced by the type of renal parenchymal disease and presence of renal insufficiency [49]. In a study of 1921 patients with CKD of various types, the occurrence rates of hypertension were highest in renovascular (93%) and diabetic (87%) nephropathies. Lower rates of hypertension were reported in cases of polycystic kidney disease (72%), in chronic glomerulonephritis (62%) and in chronic pyelonephritis (54%) [49]. In this same group of CKD patients, prevalence of hypertension was higher in those with renal insufficiency (80%) compared to those without (43%) [49].

Chronic Pyelonephritis

Chronic pyelonephritis causes hypertension in over 50% affected individuals only when complicated by renal parenchymal scaring and renal ischemic mechanisms [11, 13]. In contrast, acute pyelonephritis rarely causes hypertension unless it is associated with papillary necrosis, acute renal failure, or obstructive uropathy [11, 13].

Kidney Stone Disease/Nephrolithiasis

Kidney stone disease/nephrolithiasis and hypertension appear to be highly interrelated. On the one hand, hypertension is frequently associated with kidney stone disease (nephrolithiasis), and, on the other hand, the prevalence of kidney stone disease is higher in hypertensives than in normotensives [50]. In a study of 688 male workers of the Olivetti factory, the prevalence of a history of nephrolithiasis was 13.4% in normotensives, 20.3% in untreated hypertensives, and 32.8% in treated hypertensives [50]. In a follow-up of 8 years of the same cohort, the prevalence of kidney stone disease was 16.8% in hypertensives and 8.5% in normotensives [50].

An association between hypertension and kidney stone disease (nephrolithiasis) has been documented also in women [50].

Chronic Glomerulonephritis

Chronic glomerulonephritis is frequently complicated by hypertension [51]. The prevalence of hypertension varied widely depending upon the underlying morphology of the glomerular lesion [51]. A study of 231 patients with biopsy-proven chronic glomerulonephritis and a mean age of 31.6 ± 13.4 years revealed prevalence rates of 97% in those with membranoproliferative glomerulonephritis, 77.3% with membranous glomerulonephritis, 76.3% with focal segmental glomerulosclerosis, and 72% with mesangioproliferative glomerulonephritis [51]. Further, in this group of patients, the frequency of hypertension was higher in those with renal impairment than in those with normal renal function (91.4% vs 72.7%) [51].

Other studies confirmed that frequency of hypertension was influenced by the morphology of the glomerular lesions [52].

IgA Nephropathy

IgA nephropathy which represents the most common form of glomerulonephritis worldwide is complicated by hypertension and end-stage renal disease (ESRD) in 20–30% and 20–40% of patients, respectively [53].

Diabetic Kidney Disease

Hypertension is very common among patients with diabetes mellitus. When diagnosed with type 2 diabetes mellitus, 39% of subjects have hypertension [54]. Further, 40% of type 2 diabetes mellitus eventually develop CKD [55].

Polycystic Kidney Disease

Polycystic kidney disease represents a kidney disorder characterized by a large number of cysts in both kidneys [13].

Hypertension occurs in 60–75% of patients at an early stage when renal function is normal [13]. With the advent of end-stage renal failure, all patients become hypertensive [13].

Renovascular Hypertension

Renovascular hypertension, a potentially curable form of hypertension, has been estimated to occur in 5% of all hypertensive patients, although the prevalence rates may vary between 4 and 53.5% depending upon the evaluated hypertensive population [12, 56]. Higher prevalence rates of renovascular hypertension have been reported in patients with cardiorenal disease [12, 57].

Malignant Hypertension

Malignant hypertension which occurs in about 5% of the hypertension population represents a syndrome of severe BP elevation characterized by markedly elevated BP (DBP > 130 mmHg), multisystem microangiopathy, and rapidly progressive nephropathy and grade III/IV retinopathy [58].

Resistant Hypertension

Resistant hypertension is common in CKD and is a serious risk for increased morbidity and mortality [59].

Resistant hypertension is defined as a syndrome of an elevated BP uncontrolled with adequate doses of three or more antihypertensive agents of different classes, with one agent being a diuretic [59].

The prevalence of resistant hypertension increases with declining renal function [59]. In a study of 10,700 individuals, resistant hypertension was reported in 15.8%, 24.9%, and 33.4% of participants with GFR of >60 mL/min/1.73 m^2, 45–59 mL/min/1.73 m^2, and <45 mL/min/1.73 m^2, respectively [60].

Hypertension in Renal Replacement Therapy

- **Hemodialysis**

  Interdialytic hypertension is highly prevalent in stable patients receiving hemodialysis, with a rate up to 90% [61]. In a cohort of 2535 hemodialysis patients, Argawal et al. found that 86% of patients were hypertensive, with hypertension being defined with a

  BP >150/85 mmHg [61].

  In a recent study, prevalence of interdialytic hypertension was evaluated by a 44 h ambulatory BP in 369 predominantly Afro-American patients receiving hemodialysis [62]. With hypertension being defined as BP ≥135/85 mmHg, the prevalence of hypertension was 82% [62].

- **Peritoneal Dialysis**

  A study performed on 504 patients receiving peritoneal dialysis in 27 peritoneal dialysis centers associated with the Italian Cooperative study group revealed hypertension prevalence of 88.1% [63].

- **Renal Transplant Hypertension**

  Most renal transplant recipients exhibit high BP [64]. Hypertension occurs in more than 70% of transplant recipients [64].

  Several factors predispose to the development of hypertension in renal transplant recipients, including chronic allograft nephropathy, calcineurin and corticosteroid toxicity, recurrence of glomerulopathies, diseased native kidneys, and post-transplant renal artery stenosis [64].

1.3 Conclusion

Renal parenchymal disease, which includes a wide spectrum of renal disorders, represents the most common cause of secondary hypertension. The underlying morphologic renal lesion and the severity of the renal functional impairment determine the range and degree of BP elevation. Hypertension is more common and more severe in glomerulopathies than in tubulointerstitial nephropathies. Nephrolithiasis, embolic renal disease, renal replacement therapy, pregnancy, diabetes, renal artery stenosis, and drugs are frequent causes of renal-induced hypertension. Occurrence of acute kidney injury is associated with serious cardiorenal complications.

References

1. Sica DA. The kidney and hypertension. J Clin Hypertens. 2008;10:541–8.
2. Berglund G, Anderson O, Wilhelmson. Prevalence of primary and secondary hypertension. BMJ. 1976;2:554–6.
3. Lash JP, Go AS, Appel LJ, et al. Chronic Renal Insufficiency Cohort (CRIC) Study: baseline characteristics and associations with kidney function. Clin J Am Soc Nephrol. 2009;4:1302–11.
4. Bright R. Cases and observations, illustrating renal disease accompanied with the secretion of albuminous urine. [Guy's Hospital reports, no. 2]. Med Chir Rev. 1836;25(49):23–35.
5. Tigerstedt R, Bergman PG. Niere Und Kreislauf. Scand Arch Physiol. 1898;8:223–73.
6. Goldblatt H, Lynch J, Hanzal RF, Summerville WW. Studies on experimental hypertension. 1-The production of persistent elevation of systolic blood pressure by means of renal ischemia. J Exp Med. 1934;59:347–79.
7. Volhard F, Fahr T. Die Brightsche Nierenkrankheit. Berlin: Springer; 1914.
8. Whelton PK, Klag MJ. Hypertension as a risk factor for renal disease. Review of clinical and epidemiological evidence. Hypertension. 1989;13(Suppl 5):I19–27.
9. Chobanian AV, Bakris GL, Black HR, et al. Seventh report of the Joint National Committee on Prevention, Detection, Evaluation, and Treatment of High Blood Pressure. Hypertension. 2003;42:1206–52.
10. Rosario RF, Wesson DE. Primary hypertension and nephropathy. Curr Opin Nephrol Hypertens. 2006;15:130–4.
11. Johnson JG, Hunt JC. Hypertension secondary to renal parenchymal disease. In: Amery A, Fagard R, Lijnen P, Staessen J, editors. Hypertensive cardiovascular disease: pathophysiology and treatment. The Hague: Martinus Nijhoff Publishers; 1982. p. 508–25.
12. Kaplan NM, Victor RG. Renovascular hypertension. In: Kaplan's clinical hypertension. 10th ed. Philadelphia: Wolters Kluwer/Lippincott William and Wilkins; 2010. p. 319–38.
13. Guidelines (JSH2009). Secondary hypertension. Hypertens Res. 2009;32:78–90.
14. Coresh J, Astor BC, Greene T, Eknoyan G, Levey AS. Prevalence of chronic kidney disease and decreased kidney function in the adult US population: third national health and nutrition examination survey. Am J Kidney Dis. 2003;41:1–12.

15. Smith MC, Dunn MJ. Hypertension in renal parenchymal disease. In: Laragh JH, Brenner BM, editors. Hypertension: pathophysiology, diagnosis and management. 2nd ed. New York: Raven Press; 1995. p. 2081–102.
16. National Kidney Foundation. K/DOQI clinical practice guidelines on hypertension and antihypertensive agents in chronic kidney disease. Am J Kidney Dis. 2004;43(Suppl 1):S1–290.
17. Kaplan NM, Victor RG. Renal parenchymal hypertension. In: Kaplan's clinical Hypertension. 10th ed. Philadelphia: Wolters Kluwer/Lippincott William and Wilkins; 2010. p. 288–318.
18. Bonomini V, Campieri C, Scolari MP, Vangelista A. Hypertension in acute renal failure. Contrib Nephrol. 1986;54:152–8.
19. Bradley SE, Seegal B. Acute diffuse glomerulonephritis. Am J Med. 1949;7:382–95.
20. Nolasco F, Cameron JS, Heywood EF, Hicks J, Ogg C, Williams DG. Adult-onset minimal change nephrotic syndrome: a long-term follow-up. Kidney Int. 1986;29:1215–23.
21. Dorhout EJ, Roos JC, Boer P, Yoe OH, Simatupang TA. Observations on edema formation in the nephrotic syndrome in adults with minimal lesions. Am J Med. 1979;67:378–84.
22. Vidt DG. Cholesterol emboli: a common cause of renal failure. Annu Rev Med. 1997;48 375–85.
23. Chedid A, Le Coz S, Rossignol P, Bobrie G, Herpin D, Plouin P. Blunt renal trauma-induced hypertension: prevalence, presentation, and outcome. Am J Hypertens. 2006;19:500–4.
24. Chawla LS, Eggers PW, Star RA, Kimmel PL. Acute kidney injury and chronic kidney disease as interconnected síndromes. N Engl J Med. 2014;371:58–66.
25. Dylewska M, Chomicka I, Małyszko J. Hypertension in patients with acute kidney injury. Wiad Lek. 2019;72:2199–201.
26. Hypertension in pregnancy. Report of the American College of Obstetricians and Gynecologists' Task Force on Hypertension in Pregnancy. Obstet Gynecol. 2013;122:1122–31.
27. Bellomo G. Hypertensive disorders of pregnancy. In: Berbari AE, Mancia G, editors. Disorders of blood pressure regulation: phenotypes, mechanisms, therapeutic options. Updates in hypertension and cardiovascular protection. Cham: Springer International Publishing AG; 2018. p. 763–96.
28. Prakash J, Niwas SS, Parekh A, Pandey LK, Sharatchandra L, Arora P, et al. Acute kidney injury in late pregnancy in developing countries. Ren Fail. 2010;32:309–13.
29. Prakash J, Tripathi K, Pandey LK, Sahai S, Usha, Srivastava PK. Spectrum of renal cortical necrosis in acute renal failure in eastern India. Postgrad Med J. 1995;71:208–10.
30. Day RO, Graham GG. Non-steroidal anti-inflammatory drugs (NSAIDs). BMJ. 2013;346:f3195.
31. Davis A, Robson J. The dangers of NSAIDs: look both ways. Br J Gen Pract. 2016;66:172–3.
32. Beilin LJ. Non-steroidal anti-inflammatory drugs and antihypertensive drug therapy. J Hypertens. 2002;20:849–50.
33. Morgan T, Anderson A. The effect of nonsteroidal anti-inflammatory drugs on blood pressure in patients treated with different antihypertensive drugs. J Clin Hypertens (Greenwich). 2003;5:53–7.
34. White WB, Marfatia R, Baker WL. Treating pain and inflammation in hypertension. In: Berbari AE, Mancia G, editors. Special issues in hypertension. Milan: Springer-Verlag Italia; 2012. p. 373–88.
35. Aljadhey H, Tu W, Hansen RA, Blalock SJ, Brater DC, Murray MD. Comparative effects of non-steroidal anti-inflammatory drugs (NSAIDs) on blood pressure in patients with Hypertension. BMC Cardiovasc Disord. 2012;12:93.
36. Klomjit N, Ungprasert P. Acute kidney injury associated with non-steroidal anti-inflammatory drugs. Eur J Intern Med. 2022;101:21–8.
37. García-Carro C, Draibe J, Soler MJ. Onconephrology: update in anticancer drug-related nephrotoxicity. Nephron. 2023;147:65–77.
38. Piscitani L, Sirolli V, Di Liberato L, Morroni M, Bonomini M. Nephrotoxicity associated with novel anticancer agents (Aflibercept, Dasatinib, Nivolumab): case series and nephrological considerations. Int J Mol Sci. 2020;21:4878.
39. Nussbaum EZ, Perazella MA. Update on the nephrotoxicity of novel anticancer agents. Clin Nephrol. 2018;89:149–65.
40. Abbas A, Mirza MM, Ganti AK, Tendulkar K. Renal toxicities of targeted therapies. Target Oncol. 2015;10:487–99.

41. Grossman E, Messerli FH. Secondary hypertension: interfering substances. J Clin Hypertens (Greenwich). 2008;10:556–66.
42. National Kidney Foundation. K/DOQI clinical practice guidelines for chronic kidney disease: evaluation, classification, and stratification. Am J Kidney Dis. 2002;39(Suppl 1):S1–266.
43. Levey AS, Levin A, Kellum JA. Definition and classification of kidney diseases. Am J Kidney Dis. 2013;61:686–8.
44. Borrelli S, De Nicola L, Conte G, Minutolo R. Chronic kidney disease. In: Berbari AE, Mancia G, editors. Disorders of blood pressure regulation. Updates in Hypertension and cardiovascular protection. Cham: Springer International Publishing AG; 2018. p. 325–40.
45. Tedla FM, Brar A, Browne R, Brown C. Hypertension in chronic kidney disease: navigating the evidence. Int J Hypertens. 2011;2011:132405.
46. Brown MA, Whitworth JA. Hypertension in human renal disease. J Hypertens. 1992;10:701–12.
47. Danielsen H, Kornerup HJ, Olsen S, Posborg V. Arterial hypertension in chronic glomerulonephritis. An analysis of 310 cases. Clin Nephrol. 1983;19:284–7.
48. Arze RS, Ramos JM, Owen JP, et al. The natural history of chronic pyelonephritis in the adult. Q J Med. 1982;51:396–410.
49. Ridao N, Luño J, de Vinuesa SG, Gómez F, Tejedor A, Valderrábano F. Prevalence of hypertension in renal disease. Nephrol Dial Transplant. 2001;16(Suppl 1):70–3.
50. Losito A. Calculus renal disease. In: Berbari AE, Mancia G, editors. Disorders of blood pressure regulation: phenotypes, mechanisms, therapeutic options. Updates in Hypertension and cardiovascular protection. Cham: Springer International Publishing AG; 2018. p. 341–50.
51. Martynov S, Kutyrina I. Arterial hypertension in chronic glomerulonephritis P 100. J Hypertens. 2004;22(Suppl 1):S37.
52. Rodicio JL, Alcazar JM. Hypertension in chronic renal failure. In: Gajkowska J, editor. European Society of Hypertension clinical practice newsletters. Update 2011. Gdansk: Via Medica; 2011. p. 7–8.
53. Julian BA, Novak J. IgA nephropathy: an update. Curr Opin Nephrol Hypertens. 2004;13:171–9.
54. Hypertension in Diabetes Study (HDS): I. Prevalence of hypertension in newly presenting type 2 diabetic patients and the association with risk factors for cardiovascular and diabetic complications. J Hypertens. 1993;11:309–17.
55. Saran R, Robinson B, Abbott KC, et al. US Renal Data System 2019 annual data report: epidemiology of kidney disease in the United States. Am J Kidney Dis. 2020;75(Suppl 1):A6–7.
56. Elliott WJ. Renovascular hypertension: an update. J Clin Hypertens (Greenwich). 2008;10:522–33.
57. de Mast Q, Beutler JJ. The prevalence of atherosclerotic renal artery stenosis in risk groups: a systematic literature review. J Hypertens. 2009;27:1333–40.
58. Shantsila A, Lip GYH. Accelerated/malignant hypertension. In: Berbari AE, Mancia G, editors. Disorders of blood pressure regulation. Updates in Hypertension and cardiovascular protection. Cham: Springer International Publishing AG; 2018. p. 653–62.
59. Calhoun DA, Jones D, Textor S, et al. Resistant hypertension: diagnosis, evaluation, and treatment. A scientific statement from the American Heart Association Professional Education Committee of the Council for High Blood Pressure Research. Hypertension. 2008;51:1403–19.
60. Webster AC, Nagler EV, Morton RL, Philip Masson P. Chronic kidney disease. Lancet. 2017;389:1238–52.
61. Santos SFF, Peixoto AJ. Hypertension in dialysis. Curr Opin Nephrol Hypertens. 2005;14:111–8.
62. Agarwal R. Epidemiology of interdialytic ambulatory hypertension and the role of volume excess. Am J Nephrol. 2011;34:381–90.
63. Cocchi R, Esposti ED, Fabbri A, et al. Prevalence of hypertension in patients on peritoneal dialysis: results of an Italian multicentre study. Nephrol Dial Transplant. 1999;14:1536–40.
64. Tedla F, Hayashi R, McFarlane SI, Salifu MO. Hypertension after renal transplant. J Clin Hypertens (Greenwich). 2007;9:538–45.

Part II

Renal Parenchymal Disease as a Cause of Hypertension

Hypertension in Acute Kidney Injury

2

Kavitha Vellanki and Karen A. Griffin

2.1 Introduction

Hypertension (HTN) and renal parenchymal disorders are closely interrelated making it difficult to delineate whether HTN is a consequence of the renal parenchymal injury or the cause of the renal injury [1]. In acute kidney injury (AKI), renal parenchymal-induced HTN is predominant in the initial stages; the precise pathogenic mechanisms are yet to be elucidated. Additionally, an episode of AKI is an independent risk factor for subsequent development of HTN among a previously normotensive population, of both children and adults [2, 3]. While there is an abundance of literature on HTN and chronic kidney disease (CKD), the data on HTN in acute renal parenchymal diseases is relatively sparse. Similarly, there is an abundance of literature regarding the target blood pressure (BP) to be achieved in AKI with sepsis, but the goal BP in AKI from other etiologies is yet to be established. In clinical practice, as the mean arterial pressure (MAP) of >65 mmHg derived for AKI in sepsis is widely applied to other critically ill ICU patients, the BP target for CKD in chronic glomerulopathies is applied to AKI in acute glomerulopathies. The wide variety of etiologies and disease course of AKI, as well as the choice of therapeutic interventions and response to those interventions, pose a significant challenge in having a uniform BP target for the management of HTN in AKI.

K. Vellanki
Edward Hines Jr. VA Hospital, Hines, IL, USA
e-mail: kpotluri@lumc.edu, Kavitha.Vellanki@Va.gov

K. A. Griffin (✉)
Edward Hines Jr. VA Hospital, Hines, IL, USA

Loyola University Medical Center, Maywood, IL, USA
e-mail: Kgriffi@lumc.edu, Karen.Griffin2@Va.gov

A. E. Berbari et al. (eds.), *Blood Pressure Disorders in Acute and Chronic Kidney Diseases*, Updates in Hypertension and Cardiovascular Protection,
https://doi.org/10.1007/978-3-031-81292-7_2

In this chapter, we summarize the epidemiology, proposed pathogenic mechanisms, and available treatment options for HTN in AKI from glomerulopathies, obstructive uropathy/renal calculus disease, and acute renovascular diseases like scleroderma.

2.2 HTN in Glomerulopathies

Glomerulopathies encompass a broad range of disorders related to glomerular structure and function arising as a part of a multi-system or multi-organ involvement (secondary glomerulopathies) or conditions in which the glomerulus is the predominant or sole structure involved (primary glomerulopathies) [4]. They can present as a variety of clinical syndromes, ranging from acute glomerulonephritis (GN), nephrotic syndrome, rapidly progressive glomerulonephritis (RPGN), asymptomatic hematuria or proteinuria, and chronic GN. The underlying pathogenic mechanisms may vary, but immunological disturbances leading to inflammation is a common final pathway in most of the primary glomerulopathies. All these syndromes can present clinically with a variable degree of HTN, hematuria, proteinuria, and glomerular filtration rate (GFR) [5]. Kidney biopsy is generally required to identify the morphological abnormalities that are in turn used for classification of disease processes, prognostication, and therapeutic management. In this chapter, the focus will be on HTN in acute presentations of primary nephritic and nephrotic syndromes.

2.2.1 Epidemiology

BP in acute glomerulopathies can range from normal to extremely high levels, with persistent arterial HTN being more frequent in acute GN when compared to nephrotic syndromes and in some instances even presenting as hypertensive emergency or posterior reversible encephalopathy syndrome (PRES). The reported prevalence of HTN in acute GN and nephrotic syndromes varies widely depending on the BP cut-offs used to define HTN, underlying etiology, patient population studied, stage of disease activity, agents used for management of the underlying disease processes, and medications used to treat BP [6]. Available data is predominantly retrospective observational data, thus lacking a comprehensive review of the associated factors that could affect BP at either disease presentation or during the chronic phase of the clinical course.

In children, reported prevalence ranges from 13% to 95% in minimal change disease, 43.8% in focal segmental glomerulosclerosis, and 72–80% in acute post streptococcal GN [7–9]. A high prevalence of nighttime HTN and nocturnal non-dipping on ambulatory BP monitoring (ABPM) is reported in children with primary nephrotic syndromes [10]. While HTN is more prominent in the initial edematous phase of nephrotic syndrome, it persists in 25–30% of children even after achieving a complete or partial remission [7]. Similar trends are reported in adults with acute glomerulopathies, be it prevalence of HTN, nighttime HTN, or nocturnal non-dipping [11] as well as persistence of HTN despite partial or complete remission of the underlying disease process. In adults with lupus nephritis, when correlated with kidney biopsy findings on presentation, those with hypertensive renal vascular changes had the highest incidence of AKI (67%) [12]. This establishes the functional significance of HTN even at early stages of GN and emphasizes the importance of aiming for good BP control early in the disease process. HTN is indeed an independent risk factor for progressive CKD in glomerulopathies and thus should not be considered simply as a surrogate marker of glomerular injury and/or inflammation [13, 14].

2.2.2 Pathogenesis

Despite changes in vascular reactivity, abnormal pathological sodium retention has long been identified as the predominant etiology of HTN irrespective of GFR on presentation [15, 16]. While historically, two major mechanisms were proposed predominantly for nephrotic syndromes with the "under fill" mechanism being one of them, evolving evidence points to intrinsic defects in renal tubular handling of sodium in the distal nephron segments as being the major culprit leading to sodium retention and HTN in acute glomerulopathies [17]. The cortical collecting duct (CCD) appears to be the primary locus, followed by the medullary collecting duct with increased Na^+/K^+ ATPase activity being the primary mechanism for sodium retention. In experimental animal models, increased Na^+/K^+ ATPase activity in the CCD was noticed within 7 days of inducing nephritis [18], with pump activity correlating inversely with urinary sodium excretion [19].

The increased Na^+/K^+ ATPase activity can be from primary stimulation of the enzyme itself or secondary to activation of epithelial sodium channels (ENaC) as in Liddle's syndrome [16]. There is conflicting evidence as to which factors lead to primary activation of Na^+/K^+ ATPase. Glomerular injury leading to an imbalance between various vasodilators (nitric oxide (NO), atrial natriuretic peptide (ANP), kallikrein-kinin-system, prostaglandins), and vasoconstrictors (sympathetic nervous system, renin-angiotensin-aldosterone system [RAAS]) is thought to be the predominant feature (Fig. 2.1). The collective role of all these factors remains elusive to date. In experimental GN, transient high concentrations of angiotensinogen were noted even prior to the development of proteinuria [20]. As GN evolves, signs of fluid overload predominate suppressing the RAAS, but it is postulated that angiotensin II (Ang II) levels can still be relatively high. Rapid control of moderate-to-severe HTN and subsequent maintenance of BP control with captopril in humans with acute GN [21] and the absence of HTN and proteinuria in an anti-GBM strain of mice that were Ang II receptor deficient despite similar glomerular injury in mice with the receptors [22] support the plausibility of this hypothesis. It is worth noting that results of RAAS activation in animal models were not consistently similar and varied with the animal model used.

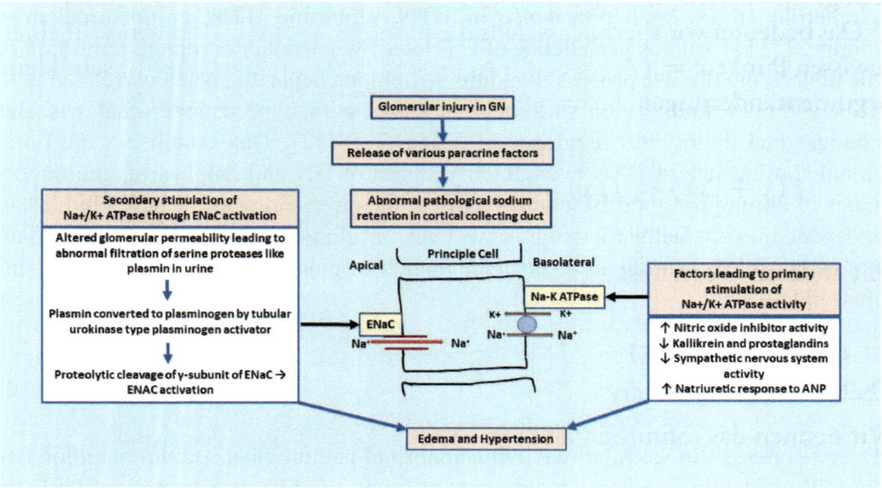

Fig. 2.1 Proposed mechanisms of sodium retention in glomerulopathies

ENaC activation by aberrantly filtered serine proteases through damaged glomeruli is postulated to be one of the primary mechanisms responsible for salt retention in nephrotic syndromes. Experimental evidence, from both animal models and humans, supports proteolytic cleavage of the γ-subunit of ENaC being the predominant pathogenic mechanism. Contradictory data exist on identifying the culprit serine protease that instigates the proteolytic cleavage. Urinary plasminogen, prostasin, cathepsin B, and factor VII activating protease are some of the serine proteases implicated in various studies [23]. The most dominant of the serine proteases in nephrotic urine that activates ENaC is urinary plasmin. Proteolytic activation of plasminogen in nephrotic urine by tubular urokinase-type plasminogen activator (uPA) generates plasmin, which in turn activates ENAC via proteolytic cleavage of its γ-subunit [24]. In children with nephrotic syndrome, urine plasmin was significantly higher in the edematous phase when compared to remission [25]. Similarly, in adults with nephrotic syndrome, urinary plasminogen-plasmin/creatinine ratio was an independent risk factor for edema and correlated positively with fractional excretion of potassium to fractional excretion of sodium, the latter used as a surrogate marker of ENaC activation [26]. However, at the present time, quantitative assays of specific types of urine serine proteases are not at a stage to be employed in clinical trials.

2.2.3 Management

While there is consensus on treating HTN in acute glomerulopathies, the target goal BP to be achieved is not known. There is a paucity of randomized control trials, as most of the glomerulopathies are relatively rare disorders. Existing data is from chronic glomerulopathies. Nevertheless, the 2021 Kidney Disease: Improving Global Outcomes (KDIGO) Clinical Practice Guideline for the Management of

Glomerular Diseases suggests a target systolic BP of <120 mmHg in all adults and a target 24-hour MAP of ≤50th percentile for age, sex, and height by ambulatory BP monitoring in children regardless of etiology [27]. The guidelines do not differentiate between acute and chronic glomerulopathies. Angiotensin-converting enzyme inhibitors (ACEi) or angiotensin II receptor blockers (ARBs) are recommended at maximally tolerated doses as first-line in treating GN patients with both hypertension and proteinuria. The guidelines recommend avoiding use of an ACEi or ARB if kidney function is rapidly changing, which is generally the case in most of the acute glomerulopathies. Dietary sodium restriction is required as well as diuretics for HTN management. Close monitoring of BP, electrolytes, and signs of volume depletion is recommended. Patients should be educated on dietary sodium restriction and daily home BP and weight monitoring with parameters in place to titrate medications accordingly.

Despite extensive research on the pathophysiology of sodium retention and available data from experimental models, the appropriate diuretic strategy in acute glomerulopathies remains a therapeutic challenge. There are no existing recommendations on the specific combination of diuretics. Loop diuretics are the traditional first-line agents with thiazides and mineralocorticoid receptors used for diuretic synergism. Since both loop and thiazide diuretics are highly protein bound, delivery to their respective site of action in the tubules is compromised, both from hypoalbuminemia and reduced GFR [28]. Emerging evidence (limited to case reports and observational studies) supports the use of ENaC blockers, amiloride, and triamterene in resistant cases. Amiloride also inhibits uPA. Short-term non-randomized interventional studies report improvement in BP (average reduction of 6–12 mmHg) in treatment-resistant HTN in both primary and secondary glomerulopathies [29, 30]. However, results have not been consistent. Similarly, the role of sodium-glucose cotransporter-2 inhibitors (SGLT-2i) in acute GN is yet to be explored. SGLT-2i seems to be an attractive option with promising results from non-diabetic CKD, but the risk of infectious complications with concomitant immunosuppression in acute glomerulopathies needs to be studied prior to routine clinical use. The Dapagliflozin and Prevention of Adverse Outcomes in CKD Trial (DAPA-CKD) excluded all patients receiving immunotherapy 6 months prior to enrollment [31]. The Empagliflozin in Patients with Chronic Kidney Disease trial (EMPA-KIDNEY) excluded patients who received any intravenous immunosuppression therapy within 3 months or anyone on >45 mg prednisolone or equivalent at the time of enrollment [32]. The initial protocol excluded patients on ≥10 mg of prednisolone, but this was modified on a subsequent protocol revision [33].

2.3 HTN in Obstructive Uropathy and Renal Calculus Disease

Obstructive uropathy accounts for 5–10% of AKI and as high as 22% in the elderly. It is broadly defined as a functional or structural impediment to urinary flow resulting in renal parenchymal injury, termed by some as "obstructive nephropathy" [34]. It is further characterized as acute or chronic depending on the duration. There is no definite time frame differentiating the two with the terms being loosely used as "acute" when obstruction occurs for a short period of time with perceived reversible renal parenchymal injury and "chronic" when it is present for days to weeks leading to irreversible damage. Clinical manifestations also vary depending on whether it is a unilateral or bilateral, partial, or complete with an intrinsic or extrinsic etiology of obstruction. Most of the available literature comes from complete acute obstructive uropathy including the post-obstructive diuretic phase that follows reversal of complete obstruction [35]. In neonates and children, congenital abnormalities of the urinary tract are the most common causes of obstructive uropathy with ureteropelvic junction obstruction (UPJO) being the most common cause of fetal hydronephrosis [36]. About 10% of children with UPJO are reported to have HTN. The general recommendations from pediatric societies are to rule out UPJO in children presenting with HTN. Renal calculus disease is a common intrinsic cause of obstruction although epidemiological data on associated AKI is very limited. Renal calculus disease is cited as a cause for AKI in up to 30% of obstructive uropathy in children and 10–20% in adults [37].

2.3.1 Epidemiology

Secondary HTN due to obstructive uropathy is reported in both experimental animal models and humans with either unilateral or bilateral hydronephrosis. Unilateral hydronephrosis, even in the presence of a functional second kidney, is sufficient to lead to persistent HTN. Data on the incidence and prevalence of HTN in obstructive uropathy as well as variations in the risk with type, level, or site of obstruction are scarce. In one series of 26 patients, the incidence of HTN was 28.5% in the unilateral and 50% in bilateral hydronephrosis [38]. In an animal study of unilateral partial ureteral obstruction in 3-week-old Sprague-Dawley rats, severity of HTN and salt sensitivity were proportional to the degree of hydronephrosis [39]. In a retrospective study of hospitalized patients with AKI from Poland, the prevalence of HTN was highest in post-renal AKI (85%), followed by renal parenchymal (75%) and prerenal causes (30%) [40]. Whether this holds true in other populations is yet to be studied.

In contrast, there is an abundance of literature in humans suggesting a positive association of renal calculus disease and HTN. The prevalence of renal calculus disease is reported to be 30–79% higher in hypertensives than normotensives, calcium-based stones being most common followed by uric acid stones [41]. HTN was also found to be an independent predictive risk factor for recurrent kidney stones. More importantly, renal calculus disease is associated with a greater risk of developing incident HTN even after adjusting for age, body mass index, and dietary habits, with a 29% higher risk of incident HTN reported in men with renal calculus disease than those without [42]. Comparable results are reported across various populations, including women. On the contrary, hypertensive men or women did not have an increased risk of incident renal calculus disease. In essence, while renal calculus disease appears to precede the development of arterial HTN, the latter does not seem to increase the risk of incident renal calculus disease [43]. The reasons for such observations are poorly understood.

2.3.2 Pathogenesis

The pathogenesis of secondary HTN varies depending on the chronicity, laterality, and severity of obstructive uropathy. Yet, this aspect has not been well explored; probably the main reason for conflicting data from animal and human studies relates to the role of RAAS activation. Sodium retention, increased tubule-glomerular feedback (TGF) activity, and RAAS activation play a predominant role in HTN from acute obstructive uropathy. In bilateral hydronephrosis or hydronephrosis with a solitary kidney, the hypertensive state is primarily maintained by abnormal salt and water retention [44]. Normal renin levels have been reported in hydronephrosis with a solitary kidney and some with bilateral hydronephrosis with BP improving post reversal of obstruction or removal of the obstructed kidney [38]. In experimental animal models of unilateral partial ureteral obstruction where BP was measured by telemetry in conscious animals, BP displayed salt sensitivity the degree to which correlated with the severity of the hydronephrosis. BP was highest in rats with severe hydronephrosis and a high salt diet [39]. Heightened TGF activity due to a reduction in NO availability in the hydronephrotic kidney may ameliorate the deleterious effects of high pressure from obstructive uropathy in the renal pelvis but leads to salt and water retention, contributing to salt-sensitive HTN. While HTN progresses slowly over time, this time-dependent progression was independent of a high-salt diet pointing toward possible intrinsic renal mechanisms playing a predominant role in the setting of persistent obstruction. This is further supported by studies in animal models of unilateral obstruction where increased interstitial volume was reported at 3–7 days and interstitial fibrosis with tubular basement thickening by 16 days of onset of obstruction [45]. In various human and animal studies, activation of RAAS has been shown to be influenced by the duration of obstruction, presence or absence of normal contralateral kidney and dietary salt content. High renin levels are reported in the peripheral blood or in the renal vein of the obstructed kidney with selective renal vein sampling in unilateral hydronephrosis [46]. Evidence of lateralization of renin production has been proposed to have prognostic significance on the effect of surgical intervention on HTN. In a study conducted on patients with unilateral hydronephrosis, nephrectomy normalized BP in all patients (four out of the eight studied) that had hydronephrotic/contralateral kidney renin ratios of >1.5 and ratios between the contralateral kidney and peripheral blood of <1.2. Postoperative changes in BP correlated with changes in peripheral renin levels. Yet, normal renin levels are reported in chronic unilateral hydronephrosis, both in animals and humans [44]. This suggests renin release is possibly transient and plays a predominant role in HTN related to acute obstructive uropathy in unilateral hydronephrosis when pressure natriuresis occurring in the contralateral kidney is unable to compensate completely. The mechanisms leading to high renin secretion during ureteral obstruction are poorly understood and are variably attributed to ischemia, altered TGF activity, and renal parenchymal compression.

In renal calculus disease, various possible hypotheses have been postulated for potential factors contributing to HTN, ranging from hypercalciuria, insulin resistance in metabolic syndrome, unidentified genetic factors, oxidative stress, and underlying CKD [43]. Whether these are random associations or actual causative factors have yet to be resolved. In calcium stone formers, increased calcium excretion in hypertensive men and women is reported when compared to normotensives [41]. High dietary salt intake plays a predominant role in calcium stone formers as enhanced distal sodium delivery leads to decreased calcium reabsorption as sodium and calcium compete for distal tubular absorption [47]. Other studies reported increased uric acid and decreased citrate excretion in hypertensive stone formers compared to normotensives [48]. Insulin resistance in metabolic syndrome is thought to be the contributing factor in maintaining a low urinary pH and predisposing to uric acid stones. Animal studies indicate insulin has a direct effect on renal ammonia genesis from L-glutamine in the proximal tubules. Insulin also activates Na^+/H^+ exchanger in the proximal tubule, which is critical for NH_4^+ transport into the urinary lumen. However, when adjusted for insulin resistance and obesity, uric acid stone formers had excessively low urine pH, suggesting the possibility of additional unidentified factors playing a role [49].

2.3.3 Treatment

Prompt decompression of the urinary tract is the most effective way of achieving BP control in acute obstructive uropathy. There are no large, randomized control trials addressing BP control in obstructive uropathy. In children, both retrospective and prospective data report reduction in systolic, diastolic, and mean 24 h BP monitoring with surgical correction of obstructive uropathy [50]. In a retrospective study that looked at the need for BP medications, BP was normalized without any need for medications in 11 of the 12 patients studied [51]. There are strong proponents for surgical management of partial UPJO in children with the aim of decreasing the risk of HTN and its consequences even if renal function is preserved [52]. Similar BP reductions are reported with surgical intervention of unilateral obstruction in adults. No correlation was observed between BP reduction and split renal function of the obstructed kidney before or after the procedure [53]. In those with persistent HTN despite relief of acute obstructive uropathy, there is no specific drug of choice. RAAS inhibitors should be used with caution as hyperkalemia is frequently seen in obstructive uropathy. Alpha-1 adrenergic receptor antagonists are a good option for patients with benign prostatic hyperplasia or urolithiasis as they induce smooth muscle relaxation and can improve ureteral and urethral flow [35].

There is significant overlap in the therapeutic management of HTN and renal calculus disease (Table 2.1), be it the dietary interventions and/or medications. Yet, there is a paucity of data on the combined effects of these interventions on both disorders. A low-salt diet is the cornerstone of dietary interventions for both HTN and renal calculus disease. The BP reduction effect of the Dietary Approaches to Stop Hypertension (DASH) diet is well documented, and observational studies report similar effects in renal calculus disease. In a large prospective study, a DASH-style diet high in fruits and vegetables, moderate in low-fat dairy products, and low in animal protein reduced the risk of incident kidney stones in both age-adjusted and

Table 2.1 Effects of common dietary interventions and BP medications on urine composition/renal calculus disease

1. Dietary Interventions:	
Low salt diet	Low urinary calcium
DASH diet	High urinary citrate
2. Thiazide diuretics	Low urinary calcium
3. Loop diuretics	High urinary calcium
4. Angiotensin receptor blockers	Uricosuric
5. ACE-inhibitors	High urinary calcium (plausible)
6. Calcium channel blockers	High urinary calcium
7. SGLT-2 inhibitors	High urinary citrate, high urine calcium
8. Special mention: Acetazolamide (mainly used for diuretic effects)	Marked reduction in urinary citrate

multivariate models [54]. The combined effect of the DASH diet on HTN and renal calculus disease is yet to be studied. Thiazide diuretics are first-line agents for hypercalciuric renal calculus disease and HTN, but the combined effects of thiazides on HTN and renal calculus disease in prospective studies are yet to be reported The doses of thiazide diuretics for prevention of recurrent stone disease are higher than those used for HTN. Available evidence suggests the use of indapamide at 2.5 mg/day, chlorthalidone at 25–50 mg daily, or HCTZ 25 mg twice a day or 50 mg daily for recurrent stone disease [55]. Losartan, an angiotensin II receptor blocker, is known for its unique uricosuric effect [56]. Calcium channel blockers (CCBs) are reported to increase uric acid and calcium excretion [57]. The combined effects of CCBs and Losartan on HTN and renal calculus disease are not known. Retrospective observational data correlating the occurrence of kidney stones with anti-hypertensive medication prescriptions suggest decreased risk in adults >65 years old with thiazide diuretics and no association with ACE inhibitors or CCBs [58]. Emerging data suggests a possible role for SGLT-2i in decreasing the risk of renal calculus disease [59], and the combined effect on HTN and renal calculus disease is yet to be explored.

2.4 Acute Renal Vascular Disease (Scleroderma)

Acute renal vascular diseases are a broad spectrum of disease processes characterized by primary blood vessel involvement and can lead to AKI [60]. Typically classified by the size of the blood vessel involved, HTN associated with AKI is a common feature of acute renal vascular diseases regardless of the primary pathogenic mechanisms or the size of the involved vessels. For this discussion, we concentrate on acute renal vascular disease involving the small blood vessels, scleroderma, or systemic sclerosis (SSc) in specific detail. SSc is a rare inflammatory connective tissue disorder of the skin and subcutaneous tissues and predominantly occurs in women of childbearing age. Ninety-five percent of the patients with SSc have autoantibodies against one or more antigens; topoisomerase-1 or Scl-70, centromere, RNA polymerase 3, and ribonucleoproteins U/U3 being the predominant ones identified to date [61]. Yet, whether autoantibodies play a primary or secondary role in the causation of SSc is unknown. Clinical manifestations vary widely depending on internal organs involved, renal involvement being long recognized as one of the most devastating complications since the initial report of "The Kidney of Scleroderma" [62]. Estimates of renal involvement in SSc vary widely, reported to be as high as 50% if AKI, HTN, and proteinuria are considered together as early renal manifestations and 80% if renal pathological findings on autopsies are considered [63]. Scleroderma renal crisis (SRC) in essence is a renal thrombotic microangiopathy. There is significant heterogenicity in the presentation with 40 different definitions of SRC posing significant challenges to further research. As a result, the Scleroderma Clinical Trials Consortium (SCTC) SRC Working Group was formed to develop a consensus classification criteria for SRC. The proposed criteria (Table 2.2) are currently being validated in real-world patients [64]. SRC is a

Table 2.2 Proposed classification criteria for Scleroderma Renal Crisis

BP—measured twice separated by a 5 min interval	Acute rise in BP to ≥140/90 mm Hg Increase in systolic BP ≥30 mm Hg above normal. Increase in diastolic BP ≥20 mm Hg above normal.
Acute kidney injury defined as:	Increase in serum creatinine of ≥26.5 μmol/L (≥0.3 mg/dL) within 48 h Increase in serum creatinine to ≥1.5 times baseline, which is known or presumed to have occurred within the prior 7 days Urine volume <0.5 mL/kg/h for 6 h
Microangiopathic hemolytic anemia and thrombocytopenia	New or worsening anemia not due to other causes Schistocytes or other red blood cell fragments on blood smear Thrombocytopenia = 100,000 platelets/mm^3, confirmed by manual smear Laboratory evidence of hemolysis, including elevated lactate dehydrogenase, reticulocytosis, and/or low or absent haptoglobin A negative direct antiglobulin test
Evidence of target organ dysfunction	Hypertensive retinopathy (not attributable to other causes), confirmed by an ophthalmologist. Hypertensive encephalopathy not attributable to other causes Acute heart failure Acute pericarditis
Renal histopathology: Non-specific findings and should be correlated with clinical and serological data	Small vessel (arcuate and interlobular arteries) changes that predominate glomerular alterations, thrombotic microangiopathic changes can be present in the later. Early vascular abnormalities include intimal accumulation of myxoid material, thrombosis, fibrinoid necrosis, and fragmented red blood cells, sometimes resulting in cortical necrosis. Late changes are manifested by intimal thickening and proliferation (which lead to characteristic vascular "onion-skin" lesions), glomerulosclerosis, and interstitial fibrosis. Nonspecific tubular changes may also occur, including acute tubular injury in the early stage of injury, and later interstitial fibrosis and tubular atrophy.

Kidney biopsy not required for definitive diagnosis
Adapted from Scleroderma Clinical Trials Consortium—SRC Working Group Consensus (Reproduced from Ref. [64] with permission)

medical emergency with the disease being fatal prior to the introduction of ACEi (up to 80% mortality). Mortality in SRC remains at 10–20% despite widespread use of ACEi [65].

2.4.1 Epidemiology

That systemic HTN is common in SSc is widely accepted, but available data is scarce. HTN is reported in 26–42% of patients with SSc and is often thought to herald renal impairment [66] The 5-year risk of incident HTN in SSc is reported to be 20% with age >45 years, pulmonary fibrosis, and increased inflammatory markers associated with increased risk [67]. SSc patients with HTN at the onset are more prone to develop proteinuria and decline in kidney function at 5 years than those without.

With the limitations of lack of uniform criteria for the diagnosis of SRC, the reported prevalence varies across the globe with the risk following the prevalence patterns of specific antibody associations. The risk is higher in SSc patients with anti-RNA polymerase III autoantibodies (associated with diffuse SSc) and lowest with those that have anticentromere antibodies (associated with limited cutaneous SSc) [68]. Those with rapidly progressive diffuse cutaneous SSc within 5 years of disease onset in the presence of joint involvement, anemia, or heart failure and usage of high-dose glucocorticoid therapy (equivalent to >5 mg/day dose of prednisone) have the highest risk of SRC. Whether high steroid use is reflective of the severity of the disease or an independent risk factor is debated. Accelerated HTN and AKI with or without microangiopathic hemolytic anemia or thrombocytopenia are the hallmark of the disease with 90% of patients with SRC having HTN on presentation [69]. Malignant hypertension is frequent and reported in up to 58% of the patients presenting with SRC in some cohorts [70]. Presenting manifestations of headache, blurred vision, seizures, and heart failure may all be related to the degree of HTN on presentation. While 10% of the patients can be "normotensive" on presentation, presenting BP could be significantly higher than their baseline BP (or "normotension" could reflect more severe disease). This is supported by autopsy findings in SSc, where only half of the patients with renal pathology findings suggestive of malignant hypertension were reported to be hypertensive [71]. Importantly, in hypertensives, the degree of renal damage noted in the autopsies was more extensive than would have been expected from the degree of BP elevation; however, these data originated from an era where severity of HTN was classified differently from the current.

2.4.2 Pathogenesis

Microvascular disease remains to be the hallmark feature and the main pathogenic contributing factor for organ-specific manifestations of SSc. However, emerging evidence raises the possibility of atherosclerosis and functional impairment of large and smaller arteries leading to arterial stiffness playing a contributory role [72]. An imbalance between regulatory, inflammatory, and autoimmune mechanisms contributing to direct damage of the endothelial cell lining of small- and medium-sized blood vessels causing obliterative vascular disease from uncontrolled and excessive collagen production remains the predominant pathogenic mechanism in SSc [63]. The inciting events leading to such an imbalance are poorly understood. Inflammatory cytokines, impaired systemic vascular function, increased oxidative stress, and altered hemodynamics have all been cited as possible pathogenic mechanisms for arterial HTN in SSc.

In SRC, ischemic injury is the predominant lesion, similar to acute renal vascular diseases like malignant hypertension and other thrombotic microangiopathies. In the classic description of renal pathological findings on autopsy by Moore and Sheehan [62], renal lesions had obvious analogies to benign and malignant hypertension. Vascular abnormalities affecting the small interlobular and arcuate arteries lead to intimal hyperplasia, fibrinoid necrosis, and downstream ischemic atrophy of large portions of renal cortex supplied by the related arteries. Damage of elastic lamina leads to migration of collagen-producing cells into the intima, media, and further into the perivascular interstitium and is thought to give rise to the characteristic "onion skin" appearance. In contrast to other connective tissue diseases like lupus, there is no cellular infiltration or active glomerular involvement. The findings of glomerular basement membrane wrinkling and glomerulosclerosis are primarily consistent with ischemic glomerular injury. Spasm of intrarenal arterioles causes ischemia of the juxtaglomerular apparatus, stimulating renin release which in turn causes further vasoconstriction, thus resulting in a vicious cycle leading to death in 1–3 months [63] if not promptly treated. What triggers these events even in those that are thought to be at high risk is poorly understood.

2.4.3 Treatment

The mainstay of therapy is effective and prompt BP control. There are no studies establishing the goal BP to be achieved in SSC or SRC, but it is reasonable to aim for a normal BP target of <120/80 mmHg. SRC is treated as a hypertensive emergency, and it is recommended that BP be reduced gradually with no more than a 25% reduction in the first 24 h. ACEi are the standard of care for all patients with SRC unless there is a definite contraindication such as angioedema. Since the disease has a predilection for women of child-bearing age, SRC during early pregnancy can pose challenges and needs extensive counselling. Teratogenic potential of ACEi in such instances is outweighed by life-threatening circumstances to the mother by SRC if left untreated. Captopril is the preferred choice in SRC; other ACEI could be as effective too, but data are lacking. In pregnancy, captopril remains the drug of choice due to a lower risk of fetal complications. There are some concerns about a cumulative effect of the sulfhydryl component of D-penicillamine and captopril, the former used in some patients with SSc. Thus, in patients receiving D-penicillamine, ACEi other than Captopril are preferred. The mortality benefit of ACEi is well established, but their use for the prevention of SRC has conflicting data and is highly debated. Observational data suggest an increased risk of developing SRC with the use of ACE inhibitors [73], and in those presenting with SRC, exposure to ACEi prior to the onset of SRC increased the risk of death [74]. Whether it is the disease or the drug or other factors contributing to these observations is unknown, but expert opinion recommends against the use of ACEi for the prevention of SRC and to avoid ACEi and high-dose glucocorticoid use in SSc patients that are at high risk of developing SRC. Calcium channel blockers (CCB) remain first-line agents for the treatment of Raynaud's phenomenon in SSc and are often used for HTN management as well. Observational data suggest CCBs decrease the risk of developing SRC [75] by counteracting the vasoconstrictor effect of angiotensin. More data are needed to support the routine use of CCBs in clinical practice to prevent SRC. Diuretics should be considered if BP remains uncontrolled and in patients with obvious signs of fluid overload. There are theoretical concerns of diuretics contributing to a high renin state in SRC (but whether this significantly contributes to SRC is unknown). The role of complement inhibitors and vasodilators such as endothelin receptor antagonists and phosphodiesterase-5 inhibitors in the prevention or treatment of SRC remains exploratory and is yet to be established.

2.5 Conclusion

Hypertension is widely acknowledged as a common clinical manifestation of AKI, the intensity and duration of renal injury determining the severity of BP at presentation. Despite this wide acknowledgment, there is a dearth of data on an objective target BP threshold to be achieved in AKI. Pathological retention of sodium and activation of RAAS have long been implicated as playing a predominant role in the pathogenesis of HTN in acute glomerulopathies, obstructive uropathy, and scleroderma renal crisis. Diuretics along with RAAS inhibitors are the drugs of choice for BP control in acute glomerulopathies with ENaC blockers used as alternatives in diuretic resistant states. Prompt decompression is the treatment for HTN in obstructive uropathy with alpha 1 agonist receptors, a good option for persistent HTN in those with benign prostatic hyperplasia or renal calculus disease. Scleroderma renal crisis is a hypertensive emergency with angiotensin-converting enzyme inhibitors being the standard of care for effective BP control to prevent the perpetuation of further ischemic renal injury. Additional research with well-designed clinical trials is currently warranted to better define the true impact of HTN in AKI on patient and renal outcomes, derive targets for goal BP control, and establish therapeutic agents of choice for the management of HTN determined by the underlying etiopathogenesis of AKI.

References

1. Jain M. Hypertensive renal disease: histological aspects, clinical queries. Nephrology. 2013;2:23–8.
2. Askenazi DJ, Feig DI, Graham NM, Hui-Stickle S, Goldstein SL. 3–5-year longitudinal follow-up of pediatric patients after acute renal failure. Kidney Int. 2006;69:184–9.

3. Hsu CY, Hsu RK, Yang J, Ordonez JD, Zheng S, Go AS. Elevated BP after AKI. J Am Soc Nephrol. 2015;27:914–23.
4. Glassock RJ, Cohen AH. The primary glomerulopathies. Dis Mon. 1996;42:329–83.
5. Sethi S, De Vriese AS, Fervenza FC. Acute glomerulonephritis. Lancet. 2022;399:1646–63.
6. Shatat IF, Becton LJ, Woroniecki RP. Hypertension in childhood nephrotic syndrome. Front Pediatr. 2019;7:287.
7. Küster S, Mehls O, Seidel C, Ritz E. Blood pressure in minimal change and other types of nephrotic syndrome. Am J Nephrol. 1990;10:76–80.
8. Sarkissian A, Papazian M, Azatian G, Arikiants N, Babloyan A, Leumann E. An epidemic of acute postinfectious glomerulonephritis in Armenia. Arch Dis Child. 1997;77:342–4.
9. Bhalla K, Gupta A, Nanda S, Mehra S. Epidemiology and clinical outcomes of acute glomerulonephritis in a teaching hospital in North India. J Family Med Prim Care. 2019;8:934–7.
10. Sarkar S, Sinha A, Lakshmy R, et al. Ambulatory blood pressure monitoring in frequently relapsing nephrotic syndrome. Indian J Pediatr. 2017;84:31–5.
11. Haruhara K, Tsuboi N, Koike K, et al. Circadian blood pressure abnormalities in patients with primary nephrotic syndrome. Clin Exp Hypertens. 2017;39:155–9.
12. Naiker IP, Chrystal V, Randeree IG, Seedat YK. The significance of arterial hypertension at the onset of clinical lupus nephritis. Postgrad Med J. 1997;73:230–3.
13. Ward MM, Studenski S. Clinical prognostic factors in lupus nephritis. The importance of hypertension and smoking. Arch Intern Med. 1992;152:2082–8.
14. D'Amico G, Vendemia F. Hypertension in IgA nephropathy. Contrib Nephrol. 1987;54:113–8.
15. Ichikawa I, Rennke HG, Hoyer JR, et al. Role for intrarenal mechanisms in the impaired salt excretion of experimental nephrotic syndrome. J Clin Invest. 1983;71:91–103.
16. Juncos LI. Intrarenal mechanisms of salt and water retention in the nephritic syndrome. Kidney Int. 2002;61:1182–95.
17. Ray EC, Rondon-Berrios H, Boyd CR, Kleyman TR. Sodium retention and volume expansion in nephrotic syndrome: implications for hypertension. Adv Chronic Kidney Dis. 2015;22:179–84.
18. Féraille E, Vogt B, Rousselot M, et al. Mechanism of enhanced Na-K-ATPase activity in cortical collecting duct from rats with nephrotic syndrome. J Clin Invest. 1993;91:1295–300.
19. Deschenes G, Doucet A. Collecting duct Na+/K+-ATPase activity is correlated with urinary sodium excretion in rat nephrotic syndromes. J Am Soc Nephrol. 2000;11:604–15.
20. Yayama K, Konishi K, Ohta A, et al. Elevation of plasma angiotensin in rats with experimentally induced nephrosis. Nephron. 1993;63:89–93.
21. Parra G, Rodríguez-Iturbe B, Colina-Chourio J, García R. Short-term treatment with captopril in hypertension due to acute glomerulonephritis. Clin Nephrol. 1988;29:58–62.
22. Hisada Y, Sugaya T, Yamanouchi M, et al. Angiotensin II plays a pathogenic role in immune-mediated renal injury in mice. J Clin Invest. 1999;103:627–35.
23. Hinrichs GR, Jensen BL, Svenningsen P. Mechanisms of sodium retention in nephrotic syndrome. Curr Opin Nephrol Hypertens. 2020;29:207–12.
24. Svenningsen P, Bistrup C, Friis UG, et al. Plasmin in nephrotic urine activates the epithelial sodium channel. J Am Soc Nephrol. 2008;20:299–310.
25. Andersen RF, Buhl KB, Jensen BL, et al. Remission of nephrotic syndrome diminishes urinary plasmin content and abolishes activation of ENaC. Pediatr Nephrol. 2013;28:1227–34.
26. Chen JL, Wang L, Yao XM, et al. Association of urinary plasminogen-plasmin with edema and wpithelial Sodium channel activation in patients with nephrotic syndrome. Am J Nephrol. 2019;50:92–104.
27. Rovin BH, Adler SG, Barratt J, et al. Executive summary of the KDIGO 2021 Guideline for the management of glomerular diseases. Kidney Int. 2021;2021(100):753–79.
28. Hoorn EJ, Ellison DH. Diuretic resistance. Am J Kidney Dis. 2017;69:136–42.
29. Oxlund CS, Buhl KB, Jacobsen IA, et al. Amiloride lowers blood pressure and attenuates urine plasminogen activation in patients with treatment-resistant hypertension. J Am Soc Hypertens. 2014;8:872–81.

30. Shen W, Alshehri M, Desale S, Wilcox C. The effect of amiloride on proteinuria in patients with proteinuric kidney disease. Am J Nephrol. 2021;52:368–77.
31. Heerspink HJL, Stefánsson BV, Correa-Rotter R, et al. Dapagliflozin in patients with chronic kidney disease. N Engl J Med. 2020;383:1436–46.
32. Herrington WG, Staplin N, Wanner C, et al. Empagliflozin in patients with chronic kidney disease. N Engl J Med. 2023;38:117–27.
33. EMPA-KIDNEY Collaborative Group. Design, recruitment, and baseline characteristics of the EMPA-KIDNEY trial. Nephrol Dial Transplant. 2022;37:1317–29.
34. Yaxley J, Yaxley W. Obstructive uropathy - acute and chronic medical management. World J Nephrol. 2023;12:1–9.
35. Molitoris BA. Low-flow acute kidney injury: the pathophysiology of prerenal azotemia, abdominal compartment syndrome, and obstructive uropathy. Clin J Am Soc Nephrol. 2022;17:1039–49.
36. Lee RS, Cendron M, Kinnamon DD, Nguyen HT. Antenatal hydronephrosis as a predictor of postnatal outcome: a meta-analysis. Pediatrics. 2006;118(2):586–93.
37. Tang X, Lieske JC. Acute and chronic kidney injury in nephrolithiasis. Curr Opin Nephrol Hypertens. 2014;23:385–90.
38. Ezzat M. The pattern of plasma renin activity and aldosterone system in patients with sustained hydronephrosis. Int Urol Nephrol. 1987;19:55–63.
39. Carlström M, Wåhlin N, Sällström J, Skøtt O, Brown R, Persson AE. Hydronephrosis causes salt-sensitive hypertension in rats. J Hypertens. 2006;24:1437–43.
40. Dylewska M, Chomicka I, Malyszko J. Hypertension in patients with acute kidney injury. Wiad Lek. 2019;72:2199–201.
41. Borghi L, Meschi T, Guerra A, et al. Essential arterial hypertension and stone disease. Kidney Int. 1999;55:2397–406.
42. Madore F, Stampfer MJ, Rimm EB, Curhan GC. Nephrolithiasis and risk of hypertension. Am J Hypertens. 1998;11:46–53.
43. Cupisti A, D'Alessandro C, Samoni S, Meola M, Egidi MF. Nephrolithiasis and hypertension: possible links and clinical implications. J Nephrol. 2014;27:477–82
44. Vaughan ED, Bühler FR, Laragh JH. Normal renin secretion in hypertensive patients with primarily unilateral chronic hydronephrosis. J Urol. 1974;112:153–6.
45. Klahr S, Pukerson ML. The pathophysiology of obstructive nephropathy: the role of vasoactive compounds in the hemodynamic and structural abnormalities of the obstructed kidney. Am J Kidney Dis. 1994;23:219–23.
46. Weidmann P, Berretta-Piccoli C, Hirsch D, Reubi F, Massry S. Curable hypertension with unilateral hydronephrosis. Studies on the role of circulating renin. Ann Intern Med. 1977;87:437–40.
47. Nouvenne A, Meschi T, Prati B, et al. Effects of a low-salt diet on idiopathic hypercalciuria in calcium-oxalate stone formers: a 3-mo randomized controlled trial. Am J Clin Nutr. 2010;91:565–70.
48. Taylor EN, Mount DB, Forman JP, Curhan GC. Association of prevalent hypertension with 24-hour urinary excretion of calcium, citrate, and other factors. Am J Kidney Dis. 2006;47:780–9.
49. Abate N, Chandalia M, Cabo-Chan AV Jr, Moe OW, Sakhaee K. The metabolic syndrome and uric acid nephrolithiasis: novel features of renal manifestation of insulin resistance. Kidney Int. 2004;65:386–92.
50. Al-Mashhadi A, Checa A, Wåhlin N, et al. Changes in arterial pressure and markers of nitric oxide homeostasis and oxidative stress following surgical correction of hydronephrosis in children. Pediatr Nephrol. 2018;33:639–49.
51. de Waard D, Dik P, Lilien MR, Kok ET, de Jong TPVM. Hypertension is an indication for surgery in children with ureteropelvic junction obstruction. J Urol. 2008;179:1976–8.
52. Carlström M. Hydronephrosis and risk of later development of hypertension. Acta Paediatr. 2019;108:50–7.

53. Al-Mashhadi A, Häggman M, Läckgren G, et al. Changes of arterial pressure following relief of obstruction in adults with hydronephrosis. Ups J Med Sci. 2018;123:216–24.
54. Taylor EN, Fung TT, Curhan GC. DASH-style diet associates with reduced risk for kidney stones. J Am Soc Nephrol. 2009;20:2253–9.
55. Reilly RF, Peixoto AJ, Desir GV. The evidence-based use of thiazide diuretics in hypertension and nephrolithiasis. Clin J Am Soc Nephrol. 2010;5:1893–903.
56. Hamada T, Ichida K, Hosoyamada M, et al. Uricosuric action of losartan via the inhibition of urate transporter 1 (URAT 1) in hypertensive patients. Am J Hypertens. 2008;21:1157–62.
57. Schmitz A. Acute renal effects of oral felodipine in normal man. Eur J Clin Pharmacol. 1987;32:17–22.
58. Alexander RT, McArthur E, Jandoc R, et al. Antihypertensive medications and the risk of kidney stones in older adults: a retrospective cohort study. Hypertens Res. 2017;40:837–42.
59. Balasubramanian P, Wanner C, Ferreira JP, et al. Empagliflozin and decreased risk of nephrolithiasis: a potential new role for SGLT2 inhibition? J Clin Endocrinol Metab. 2022;107:e3003–7.
60. Pourcine F, Petit-Hoang C, Audard V. Insuffisance rénale aiguë d'origine vasculaire [Acute kidney injury related to acute vascular disorders]. Rev Prat. 2018;68:166–9.
61. Reveille JD, Solomon DH, American College of Rheumatology Ad Hoc Committee of Immunologic Testing Guidelines. Evidence-based guidelines for the use of immunologic tests: anticentromere, Scl-70, and nucleolar antibodies. Arthritis Rheum. 2003;49:399–412.
62. Moore HC, Sheehan HL. The kidney of scleroderma. Lancet. 1952;1:68–70.
63. Donohoe JF. Scleroderma and the kidney. Kidney Int. 1992;41:462–77.
64. Butler EA, Baron M, Fogo AB, et al. Scleroderma Clinical Trials Consortium Scleroderma Renal Crisis Working Group. Generation of a core set of items to develop classification criteria for scleroderma renal crisis using consensus methodology. Arthritis Rheumatol. 2019;71:964–71.
65. Turk M, Pope JE. The frequency of scleroderma renal crisis over time: a metaanalysis. J Rheumatol. 2016;43:1350–5.
66. Wielosz E, Dryglewska M, Górak A, Łyś E, Majdan M. Arterial hypertension in systemic sclerosis. Postepy Dermatol Alergol. 2022;39:865–71.
67. Kuryata OV, Lysunets TK, Semenov VV. Risk and predictors of arterial hypertension in patients with systemic sclerosis. Hypertension. 2022;3:17–22.
68. Cole A, Ong VH, Denton CP. Renal disease and systemic sclerosis: an update on scleroderma renal crisis. Clin Rev Allergy Immunol. 2023;64:378–91.
69. Batal I, Domsic RT, Medsger TA, Bastacky S. Scleroderma renal crisis: a pathology perspective. Int J Rheumatol. 2010;2010:543704.
70. Guillevin L, Bérezné A, Seror R, et al. Scleroderma renal crisis: a retrospective multicentre study on 91 patients and 427 controls. Rheumatology. 2012;51:460–7.
71. D'Angelo WA, Fries JF, Masi AT, Shulman LE. Pathologic observations in systemic sclerosis (scleroderma). A study of fifty-eight autopsy cases and fifty-eight matched controls. Am J Med. 1969;46:428–40.
72. Bartoloni E, Pucci G, Cannarile F, et al. Central hemodynamics and arterial stiffness in systemic sclerosis. Hypertension. 2016;68:1504–11.
73. Bütikofer L, Varisco PA, Distler O, et al. EUSTAR Collaborators. ACE inhibitors in SSc patients display a risk factor for scleroderma renal crisis-a EUSTAR analysis. Arthritis Res Ther. 2020;22:59.
74. Hudson M, Baron M, Tatibouet S, Furst DE, Khanna D, International Scleroderma Renal Crisis Study Investigators. Exposure to ACE inhibitors prior to the onset of scleroderma renal crisis-results from the International Scleroderma Renal Crisis Survey. Semin Arthritis Rheum. 2014;43:666–72.
75. Montanelli G, Beretta L, Santaniello A, Scorza R. Effect of dihydropyridine calcium channel blockers and glucocorticoids on the prevention and development of scleroderma renal crisis in an Italian case series. Clin Exp Rheumatol. 2013;2(Suppl 76):135–9.

Hypertension in People with Diabetic and Chronic Kidney Disease, Obesity, and Renin Secreting Tumors

3

Sarah H. Khan and Matthew R. Weir

3.1 Introduction

Hypertension is a known major risk factor for cardiovascular disease, and clinical trials have proven that lower BP improves and lowers this risk [1, 2].

Hypertension is currently defined as a blood pressure (BP) >130 mmHg systolic BP and or >80 mmHg diastolic BP.

This is adapted from the 2017 American College of Cardiology/American Heart Association (ACC/AHA)—high BP guidelines [3]. The prevalence of high blood pressure in the United States is 45.4% based on 2017–2018 data. The prevalence in men is 51% and in women 39.7% before age 60 years, but becomes more prevalent, as age increases, to 74.5% in adults over the age of 60 years [4].

Hypertension is more common in patients with diabetes, compared to the general population. About 74% of adults' patients with diabetes have a systolic blood pressure >140 mmHg or diastolic blood pressure >90 mmHg [5]. Additionally, they may be on prescription medication for high blood pressure. The combination of diabetes and hypertension increases the risk of cardiovascular disease, mortality, and complications such as nephropathy and retinopathy. The controlling of hypertension is critically important in patients with diabetes to mitigate these risks.

Hypertension is more prevalent in Black adults compared to white adults across all ages and is also more common in men than in women. Using the data from the US National Health and Nutrition Examination Survey (NHANES) 2013–2016, approximately 121.5 million US adults >20 years of age have hypertension [6]. Over the last decade, mortality from hypertension has been rising to 57%;

S. H. Khan · M. R. Weir (✉)
Division of Nephrology, Department of Medicine, University of Maryland School of Medicine, Baltimore, MD, USA
e-mail: mweir@som.umaryland.edu

A. E. Berbari et al. (eds.), *Blood Pressure Disorders in Acute and Chronic Kidney Diseases*, Updates in Hypertension and Cardiovascular Protection,
https://doi.org/10.1007/978-3-031-81292-7_3

additionally, morbidity associated with hypertension, cost of treatment, and long-term care is substantial.

Globally, using data from 135 population-based studies, in 90 countries, 31.1% of the world adult population has hypertension in 2010. This amounts to 1.39 billion adults, with 31.5% prevalence in low- and middle-income countries and 28.5% in high-income countries [7].

The prevalence of HTN has since been increasing substantially, estimated to be 874 million with SBP >140 mmHg in 2015. In 2019, data from the National Center for Diabetes Risk Factor Collaboration—estimates 626 million women (95%CI, 584–668), and 652 million men (95%CI, 604–698) have hypertension, defined by a systolic BP >140 mmHg and a DBP >90 mmHg. This signifies a doubling of the burden of hypertension since 1990, mostly centered in low- and middle-income countries [8].

The estimated number of deaths is 7.834 million in 2015, due to hypertension with systolic BP >140 mmHg [9], particularly in low- and middle-income countries.

Hypertension is prevalent in chronic kidney disease (CKD), especially in those patients with advanced kidney disease, and contributes to high cardiovascular disease risk and mortality and to the progression of chronic kidney disease.

This review will examine the pathophysiology and treatment considerations of patients with hypertension and diabetic kidney disease (DKD), obesity, and renin-secreting tumors.

The terminology of kidney disease associated with diabetes has evolved over time. The initial description by Paul Kimmelstiel and Clifford Wilson in 1936 was "inter-capillary glomerulosclerosis" [10]. This included progressive renal failure, hypertension, edema, and retinal changes with long-standing diabetes—following at least a 10-year duration with diabetes and the classic nodular Kimmelsteil-Wilson nodules found in kidney biopsy [11]. Later arteriosclerosis and arteriolar sclerosis were added to further describe diabetic nephropathy. The term "diabetic kidney disease" (DKD) was described by Mogensen et al. [12] in 1983. DKD represents the form of CKD mainly due to the diabetic milieu, with stages of early nephropathy, mainly as albuminuria, followed by overt nephropathy. This includes proteinuria or non-proteinuria with decrease in renal function.

3.2 Prevalence of Diabetic Kidney Disease

The worldwide incidence and prevalence of diabetes mellitus have increased exponentially, mainly due to an increase in type 2 diabetes (T2DM). In 2021, approximately 537 million people worldwide had diabetes [13] which is 11% of the global population. This number is expected to rise to 783 million (12%) by 2045 [13].

This increase in T2DM is strongly associated with the obesity pandemic. The rise in the use of processed foods, decreased physical activity, and sedentary behavior have contributed to the obesity surge. This is often linked to modern urban lifestyle and technological development.

One of the severest and most common long-term complications of diabetes is diabetic kidney disease (DKD). DKD is defined as chronic kidney disease in an individual with diabetes. About 20–50% patients with T2DM will eventually develop DKD. The leading cause of chronic kidney disease and end-stage renal disease globally is DKD and accounts for 50% of cases [14]. DKD is associated with high cardiovascular morbidity and mortality and impacts on the patients' quality of life.

The rising prevalence of T2DM is also associated with aging, with patients living longer as health care improves [13]. Despite this, these individuals have a nearly double mortality risk from any cause compared to individuals without diabetes and a life expectancy six to seven times shorter than the rest of the population [15].

The prevalence of diabetes in 2021 was the same in men and women but has increased with advancing age. It is higher in urban (12%) versus rural (8%) areas and higher in high- and middle-income countries (11%) versus low-income countries (6%). The highest rates of T2DM were noted in the Indigenous populations of the United States, Australia, and New Zealand [13]. China has more people now with diabetes than any other country with 92 million people affected, a ratio of almost one in ten adults. The highest relative risk of increase in prevalence from 2021 to 2045 is expected in middle-income countries, especially in Africa.

The worldwide pattern of T2DM is steadily changing. It is emerging now with increasing prevalence in younger adults, adolescents, and children, whereas it was previously known better as a chronic disease in middle-aged and older adults [16, 17].

3.3 Diagnosis of CKD in People with Diabetes

The Kidney Disease Improving Global Outcomes (KDIGO) clinical practice guidelines of 2020 and 2022 and the 2022 American Diabetes Associate (ADA)/KDIGO consensus report recommend regular screening of DKD using spot urine albumin-creatinine ratio (UACR) and estimated GFR (eGFR) laboratory values yearly in patients with type 1 diabetes mellitus. This should be started 5 years after diagnosis. In patients with T2DM, this screening should start at the time of diagnosis.

The diagnosis of DKD is based on persistently elevated UACR >30 mg/dL and/or eGFR <60 mL/min per 1.73 m^2 using the race-free 2021 (CKD-EPI) equation [18]. An alternate option to evaluate eGFR is the, 2021 CKD-EPI cystatin C and creatinine-based equation [19]. Once the diagnosis DKD is established, evidence-based therapies should be implemented to reduce CKD progression and improve cardiovascular outcomes (Fig. 3.1).

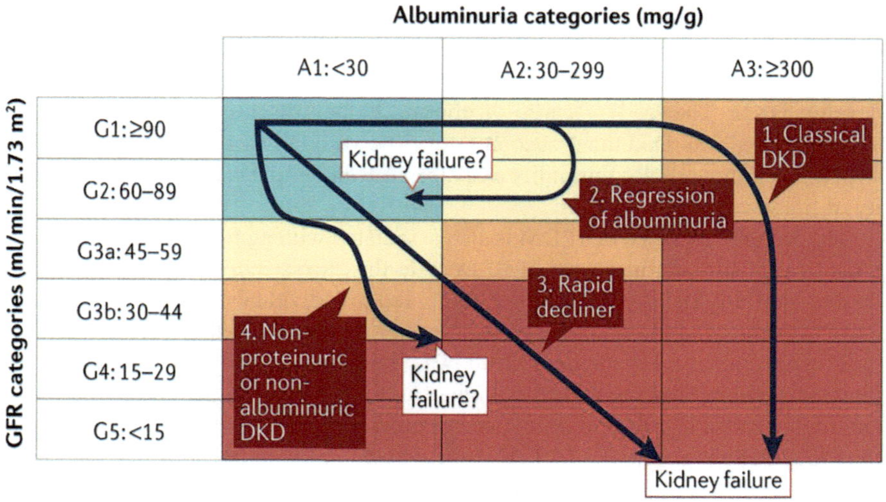

Fig. 3.1 Progression of DKD with early to late nephropathy and associated decline in renal function over time overlaying the KDIGO heat map

3.4 Cardiovascular Risk in Diabetes and CKD

About 10% of people with diabetes and CKD will eventually progress to kidney failure or end-stage kidney disease (ESKD). About 90% of patients will suffer an early premature death from cardiovascular complication, prior to reaching ESKD [20].

In patients with diabetes and CKD, the rate of hospitalizations from cardiovascular disease is fairly common. This is further exemplified by the results of a large clinical trial (15,108 patients) study of platelet inhibition and patient outcomes which investigated antiplatelets for the secondary prevention of cardiovascular disease end points. The results were a 21% multivariate-adjusted risk at 1 year for the end points of cardiovascular death, myocardial infarction, and stroke in patient with diabetes and CKD compared to 7% in those patients who had neither [21].

3.5 Histology of the Kidney in Type 1 and Type 2 Diabetes

The pathology of diabetes and non-diabetes-related causes of CKD in a diabetic individual can only be evaluated by a kidney biopsy. It is often suggested that a kidney biopsy is underutilized and is important in evaluating a non-diabetic cause in CKD patients with diabetes and provides prognostic information.

The histology seen in patients with diabetic nephropathy mainly are glomerular changes consisting of thickened basement membrane and mesangial matrix expansion often with the presence of Kimmelstiel-Wilson nodules seen usually in advanced disease and most often in type 1 diabetes. However, depending on the eGFR and level of albuminuria, about a third of T2DM have minimal glomerular changes but more significantly, tubulointerstitial and vascular changes. These similar changes are also seen in people with type 2 diabetes presenting with low eGFR <60 mL/min/1.73 m^2 in the presence of normal albuminuria. Individuals with diabetes and hypertension, at any given eGFR level, had more advanced glomerulosclerosis, interstitial fibrosis, and tubular atrophy versus those with diabetes but without hypertension [22].

The research on biopsies performed mainly on patients with Type 1 diabetes reveals a high degree of correlation with worsening albuminuria and glomerular basement thickening. An eGFR decline was more closely correlated with mesangial expansion and a loss of glomerular filtration surface area [23].

Data from >118,000 kidney biopsies worldwide regarding safety concerns, from the Kidney Precision Medicine Project, revealed that bleeding post renal biopsy requiring blood transfusion occurred in 1.6% of cases and death was extremely rare, occurring in 0.06% of cases [24].

CKD in patients with diabetes mellitus may be due to diabetic and/or nondiabetic causes and is only revealed by kidney biopsy. The progression of (diabetic) kidney disease may include several pathophysiologic events that eventually lead to ESKD [25].

3.6 Pathophysiologic Mechanisms of DKD

Microvascular damage occurs in the kidney with diabetes. The pathophysiologic mechanism in developing DKD includes hemodynamic and metabolic factors and the effects of inflammation and fibrosis [26]. Additionally, genetic and sex differences also play a role [27]. Understanding these pathways has helped in the discovery of new and innovative therapies.

3.6.1 Hyperglycemia

Hyperglycemia can result in hyperfiltration. GFR can range from 90 to 175 mL/min/1.73 m^2 compared to an age-matched healthy person. This can occur in disease process that includes metabolic syndrome, obesity, diabetes mellitus, sleep apnea, sickle cell disease, and cancer [28]. Glomerular hyperfiltration is seen in the early phase of 10–67% patients with type 1 diabetes and 6–73% patients with type 2 diabetes [29]. The hyperglycemic milieu causes an increase in the presence of vasoactive mediators and the inhibition of tubulo-glomerular feedback mechanism, resulting in an increased activation of the RAAS—renin-angiotensin-aldosterone system. This results in decreased arteriolar afferent resistance and vasodilation with increased efferent arteriolar vasoconstriction.

Hyperglycemia causes an increase in glucose and sodium reabsorption in proximal tubules via the sodium-glucose cotransporter 2 (SGLT2) and SGLT1 systems, leading to decreased sodium delivery to the distal nephron and a reduced juxtaglomerular feedback mechanism, resulting in increased intraglomerular pressures and increased GFR in the single nephron. This eventually results over time with the development of microalbuminuria, overt proteinuria, and a decrease in renal function [30–32]. Renoprotection can be achieved with treatments that address these pathways [33–37].

3.6.2 Oxidative Stress and Inflammation

There is a level of low-grade inflammation chronically and oxidative stress in patients with DKD. This phenomenon leads to apoptosis of unwanted cells and autophagy of cellular elements. The result is loss of podocytes, development of albuminuria, and eventually damage to tubules and kidney injury. Low-grade inflammation can lead to production and release of cytokines such as IL-1, Il-6, and TGFR-B [26]. Understanding these mechanisms helps in developing new treatment modalities [38].

3.6.3 Biomarkers of DKD

Estimated glomerular filtration rate (eGFR) and albuminuria are the main biomarkers to diagnose and manage individuals with DKD. These two biomarkers however have limitations, as disease progression varies in patients with proteinuria and non-proteinuria. Cystatin C is shown to correlate better, in patients with decreased renal function and albuminuria. It is a protein that is produced in nearly all cells in the body and is found in various bodily fluids. It functions as a cysteine proteinase inhibitor, as it helps in the breakdown of other proteins. The kidneys filter cystatin C from the blood. Its production and breakdown occurs at a relatively constant rate. The level of cystatin C in the blood can be used as an indicator of kidney function [39]. Unlike creatinine, cystatin C levels are not influenced by muscle mass, physical activity, or protein intake, which makes it a more reliable marker in these conditions. Cystatin C has been used to predict disease progression and is especially useful in early DKD [40, 41]. Figure 3.2 depicts potential novel DKD biomarkers during hyperglycemia, oxidative stress, hypertension, and inflammation [42].

3.6.4 Pathophysiology of Hypertension in Diabetic Kidney Disease

Blood pressure management in DKD involves primary and secondary prevention. The prevention and occurrence of DKD in individuals with diabetes mellitus is of foremost concern and is considered primary prevention. Reduction in propagation and progression of DKD in patients with diagnosed DKD is secondary prevention.

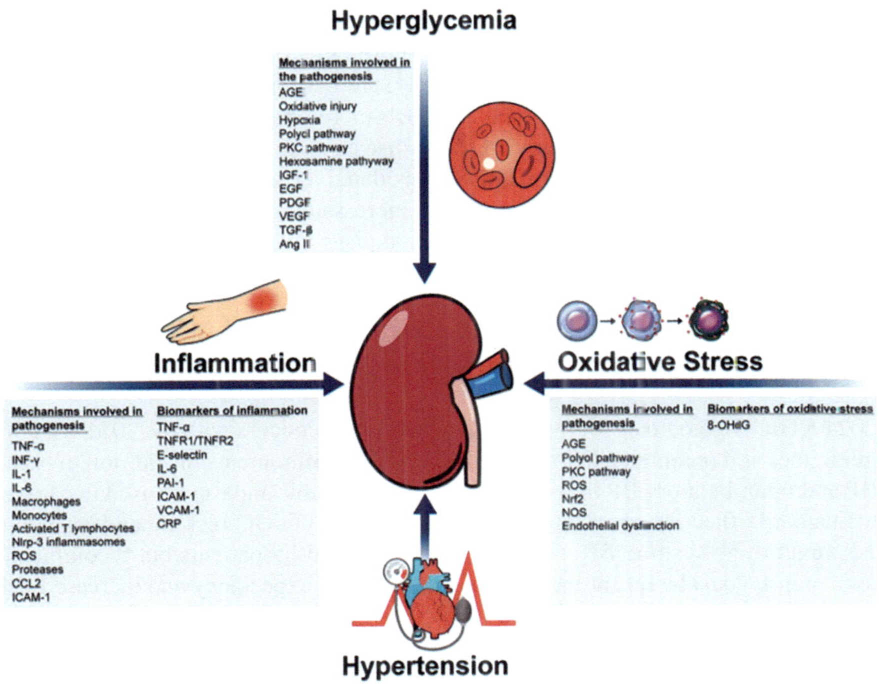

Fig. 3.2 Potentially novel biomarkers of DKD defined by their pathophysiologic pathways. *AGE* advanced glycation end product, *Ang II* angiotensin II, *CCL2* C-C motif chemokine 2, *CRP* C-reactive protein, *EGF* epidermal growth factor, *ICAM-1* intercellular adhesion molecule 1, *IGF-1* insulin-like growth factor-1, *INF-g* interferon-g, *Nlrp3* nod-like receptor protein-3, *NOS* nitric oxide synthase, *Nrf2* nuclear factor erythroid 2-related factor, *8-OHdG* 8-hydroxy-2'-deoxyguanosine, *PAI-1* plasminogen activator inhibitor 1, *PDGF* platelet-derived growth factor, *PKC* protein kinase C, *ROS* reactive oxygen species, *TNFR1* tissue necrosis factor receptor 1, *TNFR2* tissue necrosis factor receptor 2, *VCAM-1* vascular cell adhesion protein-1, *VEGF* vascular endothelial growth factor. Reprinted from ref. [42] with permission

The management and control of hypertension can prevent micro- and macrovascular complications in patients with newly diagnosed diabetes [43].

Several factors are responsible for the development of hypertension in patients with chronic kidney disease. Extracellular volume expansion secondary to salt and fluid retention, activation of RAAS and sympathetic nervous systems and the vasoconstrictive effects of endothelin, all play a role. Additionally, asymmetric dimethylarginine (ADMA), a naturally occurring chemical found in blood plasma, is known to interfere with the production of nitrous oxide (NO). Nitrous oxide is crucial for normal endothelial and cardiovascular health. In patients with chronic kidney disease, ADMA is a strong risk factor for decreased kidney function and progression to end-stage renal disease [44].

The absence of "non-dipping" blood pressure decrease during sleep, increases as CKD worsens from 15% in normal subjects to 75% in those with CKD stage 5 [45].

This is often cited as a risk factor for hypertensive complications along with cardiovascular events, development of albuminuria, progression of CKD, and development of Left ventricular hypertrophy (LVH). In a small study of CKD patients including those with diabetes, ambulatory BP monitoring (ABPM) more strongly predicted death and progression of kidney disease than outpatient blood pressure monitoring (OBP) [46]. Diabetes is also considered a risk factor in the pathophysiology of hypertension as is associated with increased arterial stiffness and accelerated atherosclerosis, a consequence of inadequate glycemic control and protein glycation [47, 48].

3.7 The Blood Pressure Targets in Diabetic Kidney Disease

2024 KDIGO guidelines for managing hypertension concurs with the 2021 KDIGO guidelines and recommends following office BP measurements in addition to home BP and/or ambulatory BP measurements as most reliable and can be used in parallel to standard office BP recording. Additionally, 2024 KDIGO recommends standard BP target to be systolic BP <120 mmHg as tolerated by patients but recommends less intense goals be set for those with decreased life expectancy and increased risk of falls and fractures and those who may develop postural hypotension [49]. The American Diabetes Association (ADA) Standard of Medical Care in Diabetes recommends all patients with diabetes and BP >140/90 mmHg should be considered hypertensive patients with confirmation using several BP readings including home BP monitoring. The ADA recommends BP targets, in patients with diabetes and hypertension, based on the patient's degree of cardiovascular risk. This is defined as the 10-year atherosclerotic cardiovascular risk (ASCVD).

In patients with a higher ASCVD risk of >15%, BP should be targeted to a level of 130/80 mmHg or lower. In individuals with lower ASCVD risk of <15%, <140/90 mmHg target is recommended [50].

The prevalence of hypertension in diabetic patients is known to increase from 36% in CKD stage 1 to 84% in CKD stages 4 and 5 [51].

When treating hypertension in diabetic patients with chronic kidney disease, clinicians should ask what the target blood pressure and which pharmaceutical agents can be used to achieve these blood pressure goals.

The IDNT [51] and RENAAL [52] trials show a strong association between a decrease in progression of chronic kidney disease and tighter blood pressure control. The post hoc analysis of the RENAAL trial demonstrated a 10-mmHg rise in systolic blood pressure increased the risk for end-stage kidney disease (ESKD) or death by 6.7%.

The caveat to this practice is the higher risk of and potential harm from hypotension while aiming for lower blood pressure, and hence, there remains disagreement in deciding on a specific blood pressure goal in this population.

Hence a practical approach is to customize blood pressure goals as best tolerated by the individual patient using available medication and correct tools. While several antihypertensive medications are available for use to manage hypertension in the diabetic population, those that provide additional benefit beyond BP control can be considered. Management of the pathologic sequence in the causation of hypertension is also an important part of lowering blood pressure [53].

Several studies have investigated the frequently asked question of whether intense blood pressure treatment would be more beneficial to control and to decrease cardiovascular risk.

Meta-analyses of several studies were synthesized and noted the effects of a more aggressive approach to blood pressure control lowered the progression to CKD as well as the risk of death [54, 55]. An aggressive approach to lowering blood pressure reduces the risk of CKD progression among patients with proteinuria but not among patients without proteinuria. Proteinuria was defined in these studies as protein/creatine ratio of >0.22 g/g or 24-h protein excretion of more than 300 mg. Additionally, a more aggressive approach to BP control reduces all-cause mortality both in patients with proteinuric CKD and those with non-proteinuria CKD.

The MDRD study noted for each 1 g/day reduction in protein excretion during the first 4 months, the rate of decline in GFR fell by 0.9–1.3 mL/min/year [56]. The fall in proteinuria was related to the blood pressure, being more prominent in those with more aggressive blood pressure control [53].

However, the REIN and AASK did not show an appreciable difference in progression to ESRD between the groups with intensive BP control versus usual BP control. The only exception may be in patients with proteinuria (more than 1 g/day) [57, 58].

(The Action to Control Cardiovascular Risk in Diabetes) trial which is the largest trial was a goal to BP trial. The results showed no benefit in the more intensively treated group, i.e., systolic BP <120 mmHg as compared to systolic BP <140 mmHg. A difference of 53% relative reduction in the risk of stroke was seen [56]. In the ACCORD trial, patients were also randomized to be in either an intensive or standard glycemic control group. In the standard glycemic control group, the more intensive blood pressure group of patients had fewer cardiovascular events [59].

In addition to ACCORD, meta-analyses of other trials suggest that diabetic patients with more aggressive BP lowering generally have decreased the risk of cardiovascular events and that in patients whose baseline systolic pressure is <140 mmHg, further lowering of the BP can prevent stroke and retinopathy [60, 61].

The SPRINT study excluded patients with diabetes. Nine thousand three hundred sixty-one persons with a systolic BP of 130 mmHg or higher with increased cardiovascular risk were randomized to a target BP goal of <120 mmHg versus 140 mmHg. The mean pre-intervention BP was 139.7 mmHg in both treatment arms. At 1 year, the mean BP was 121.4/68 mmHg (versus the usual care group 136.2/76.3 mmHg) in the two groups [1, 62]. During the follow-up period, the mean number of BP medications was 2.8 in the intensive treatment group and 1.8 in the standard treatment group, with an average difference in BP of 13.1 mmHg.

The primary outcome, a composite of myocardial infarction, acute coronary syndrome, stroke, heart failure, or cardiovascular death, was less frequent in the intensive goal group (2.7 vs. 3.2%), and this was consistent with data from the entire SPRINT population. Despite the lack of people with diabetes in SPRINT, most experts agree that people with diabetes mellitus should have the same intensive blood pressure targets as non-diabetic patients.

There was no difference in the incidence of ESRD or a 50% or greater decline in eGFR. Notably, the intense BP control group had an increase in the risk of 30% or more in the decline of eGFR. This decline occurred in the first 6 months of the trial, suggesting acute hemodynamic effects of the lowered BP. After 6 months the difference in the rate of decline between the intensive and standard groups was only minor (annual decline of 0.47 vs. 0.32 mL/min/1.73 m^2 in the intensive and standard groups, respectively) [63].

Despite the results of the SPRINT study indicating the benefits of lower BP goals, clinical decisions about target BP goals need to be individualized. A recent report from the American Diabetes Association (ADA) consensus conference in DKD pointed out the importance of considering adverse safety signals in clinical trials when diastolic BP is lowered to <70 mmHg, and particularly to <60 mmHg in older populations [64]. The ADA consensus panel also noted findings from the Kidney Early Evaluation Program that suggest higher incident rates of ESRD in patients with CKD stage 3 and a diastolic BP of <60 mmHg [65].

Since there are no randomized, multicenter, controlled trials available to address optimal BP targets in patients with DKD, the recommended target BP for patients with diabetes is commonly used as an alternate consideration. The ADA consensus panel points to the relevance of 24-h ambulatory BP monitoring, to identify higher risk groups with diabetes, especially those with masked HTN and nocturnal non-dippers. This group has an increased risk for CKD progression and increased CV morbidity and mortality [66].

The global diabetes epidemic is growing and is attributable to the rising incidence of obesity. Moreover, the rising incidence of obesity is driving the higher prevalence of hypertension and kidney disease that contributes to a growing risk of cardiovascular morbidity and mortality among those with diabetes.

Although incident rates for end-stage renal disease (ESRD) may have stabilized over the past few years [67, 68], the prevalence rates for cardiovascular mortality attributable to diabetic kidney disease (DKD) have not [68]. In this regard, more intensive management of hypertension in this high-risk population contributes significantly to the reduction of the cardiovascular disease (CVD) burden in DKD [33, 43].

3.7.1 Approach to Therapy

The emphasis on treatment of hypertension in patients with DKD should include strategies that address multifactorial risk factor reduction and include pharmacotherapy, lifestyle modification, and patient education to improve self-management of these complex risk factors. Such strategies often require team-based approaches involving primary care providers, endocrinologists, nephrologists, nutritionists, pharmacists, nurse educators, mid-level providers, and mental health professionals (Fig. 3.3).

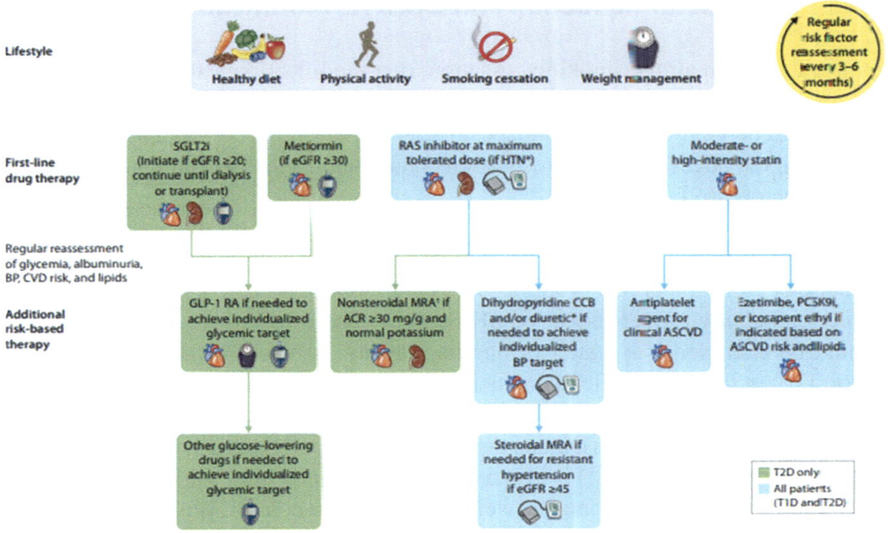

Fig. 3.3 Holistic approach for improving outcomes in patients with diabetes and chronic kidney disease (CKD). Icons presented indicate the following benefits: blood pressure (BP) cuff, BP-lowering; glucometer, glucose-lowering; heart, cardio-protection; kidney, kidney protection; scale, weight management. Estimated glomerular filtration rate (eGFR) is presented in units of mL/min/1.73 m^2. *Angiotensin-converting enzyme inhibitor (ACEi) or angiotensin II receptor blocker (ARB) (at maximal tolerated doses) should be first-line therapy for hypertension (HTN) when albuminuria is present. Otherwise, dihydropyridine calcium channel blocker (CCB) or diuretic can also be considered; all three classes are often needed to attain BP targets. †Finerenone is currently the only nonsteroidal mineralocorticoid receptor antagonist (nsMRA) with proven clinical kidney and cardiovascular benefits. *ACR* albumin-to-creatinine ratio, *ASCVD* atherosclerotic cardiovascular disease, *CVD* cardiovascular disease, *GLP-1 RA* GLP-1 receptor agonist, *MRA* mineralocorticoid receptor antagonist, *PCSK9i* proprotein convertase subtilisin/kexin type 9 inhibitor, *RAS* renin-angiotensin system, *SGLT2i* sodium-glucose cotransporter-2 inhibitor, *T1D* type 1 diabetes, *T2D* type 2 diabetes

Multi-modal risk reduction strategies have been demonstrated to be effective in people with diabetes in reducing CV events. Steno-2 investigators observed reduced risks of cardiovascular events, and progression to ESRD, retinopathy, and autonomic neuropathy in the intensive treatment arm, in which BP averaged ~135/72 mmHg over a 13-year period compared to the conventional treatment arm, which averaged ~145/78 mmHg. In addition, they provided lifestyle modification and intensive treatment of diabetes and lipids.

Integrated healthcare delivery systems, patient-centered medical homes, and accountable care organizations may provide the organizational structure to provide such multidisciplinary team-based care.

3.7.2 Risk Factor Reduction and Lifestyle Modification

Strategies should aim at smoking cessation, diet modification, exercise, and weight loss, with the aim of reducing both CVD risk and DKD progression. The double-blind, placebo-controlled, randomized crossover trial called Low SALT CKD Phase 1 assessed the effect of sodium restriction on ambulatory BP and other cardiovascular risk factors [69].

Investigators observed that dietary sodium restriction significantly decreased ambulatory BP by 10/4 mmHg over the 24-h period [69]. In addition, considerable reductions in extracellular volume and albuminuria occurred, and albuminuria reduction occurred independent of BP changes. The level to which sodium intake should be restricted is a matter of ongoing debate. A recent Institute of Medicine report [70] indicated insufficient evidence for lowering sodium intake to <2.3 g/day with respect to reducing CVD. The possibility of hyperkalemia secondary to high potassium intake in DASH (Dietary Approaches to Stop Hypertension)-type diets in patients with late-stage CKD is also a consideration in people with diabetes.

Moderation of alcohol intake, weight loss, and increased physical activity as recommended by the current ADA standards of care are all beneficial for management of hypertension in patients with DKD [71].

The ADA and KDIGO guidelines both recommend individualized and balanced diets, high in vegetables, fruits, and whole grains, and low in refined carbohydrates and beverages sweetened by sugar. The ADA and KDIGO guidelines also recommend dietary protein intake of 0.8 g/kg/day. The ADA and KDIGO additionally advise moderate to intense or vigorous physical activity of more than 150 min/week and to avoid a sedentary lifestyle [72, 73]. Though specific evidence level is low, smoking cessation is also encouraged.

If a patient has end-organ injury such as left ventricular hypertrophy and albuminuria, then lifestyle modification and antihypertensive pharmacotherapy should be initiated at the initial visit. In the absence of end-organ injury, a trial of 1–2 months of lifestyle modification alone, especially focusing on sodium intake reduction, should be tried. If goal BP is not reached through nonpharmacological approaches, then pharmacotherapy should be considered.

3.7.3 Treatment Targets and Pharmacotherapy: Glycemic Control

Both the ADA and KDIGO recommend twice-yearly assessment of glycated hemoglobin (HbA1c) for stable patients who are meeting their treatment goals and quarterly for those who require intense and close management for those patients whose therapy changed and for those whose treatment goals are not met.

While HbA1c is used as the main tool for assessing long-term glycemic control, both guidelines acknowledge the limitations associated with its accuracy and precision as an indirect metric of glycemic status. This is particularly important to consider in advanced CKD (i.e., CKD stages G4 and G5 without kidney replacement therapy [KRT]) and kidney failure treated by dialysis.

HbA1c does not adequately capture the glycemic variability and hypoglycemic events. The concurrent use of HbA1c use is based on randomized controlled trials (RCT) data, continuous glucose monitoring especially in patients at risk for hypoglycemia and to assess glycemic control when HgA1c is inaccurate, and finally self-monitoring of blood glucose to guide medication adjustment, especially patients treated with insulin [74].

As will be discussed, preferred anti-hyperglycemic agents including the SGLT2 inhibitors and the GLP-1 RA offer the opportunity for not only treating diabetes, but also lowering blood pressure and reducing cardiorenal events.

3.7.4 Treatment Targets and Pharmacotherapy: Blood Pressure Management

Hypertension management is universally accepted as a critical goal for prevention of CKD progression, atherosclerotic cardiovascular disease (ASCVD), and heart failure (HF).

There is uniform consensus that a RAS inhibitor be used as first-line therapy. ACEI or ARB should be initiated in patients with concomitant diabetes, hypertension, and albuminuria with titration to the highest tolerable dose. This is based on RCTs where findings show a decreased risk of progression in patients with DKD and ACR >300 mg/g using a maximally dosed RAS inhibitor versus placebo or an active but comparable antihypertensive drug [33, 75]. Occasionally, patients with albuminuria have normal BP, and evidence to treat with RAAS inhibition is less strong.

Patients with kidney insufficiency have an increased risk of cardiovascular disease. The HOPE study reported improved cardiovascular outcomes in patients with diabetes at high cardiovascular risk when treated with an ACEi versus placebo, even in those patients without a diagnosis of hypertension, and independent of the BP effect [76]. Renin-angiotensin-aldosterone inhibitors (RAASi) blockade should be used at the highest approved tolerated dose as proven benefits were achieved using these doses in trials. Changes were expected in blood pressure, serum creatinine, and serum potassium levels, after the initiation or increase in dosage of these drugs. Therefore, a regular checkup of BP, serum creatinine, and potassium should be performed within 2–4 weeks of any change in medication [77, 78]

Hyperkalemia associated with the use of RAASi can be managed with serum potassium-lowering strategies rather than decreasing the dose of or stopping RAASi. These include dietary potassium restriction, discontinuation of potassium supplements, and certain salt substitutes. Addition of potassium-wasting diuretics and adding oral potassium binders, such as patiromer and sodium zirconium cyclosilicate, can be useful in patients with mild hyperkalemia without EKG changes [79, 80].

Historically, there have been concerns about the residual risk for progression of DKD and cardiovascular outcomes despite maximally dosed ACE inhibitors or ARBs. In the past decade, several investigators have attempted to show benefit of combined use of ACEI and ARB. Data showed a lack of benefit and increased risk of injury and harm by increased incidence of AKI and hyperkalemia. This use of combination of ACEI and ARB is therefore not recommended. This was noted in the VA NEPHRON-D study which involved ACEI and ARB combination treatment in patients with established DKD [81].

3.7.5 Mineralocorticoid Receptor (MRA) Blockers

The combined use of ACEi and ARBs is not recommended, but additional blockade of RAS system can be achieved by the addition of mineralocorticoid receptor inhibitors. Nonspecific MRAs such as spironolactone, eplerenone, and drospirenone are steroidal in nature. They bind and directly block the mineralocorticoid receptor, preventing its activation by aldosterone or 11-deocycortisterone. They also inhibit receptors that are stimulated by testosterone and dihydrotestosterone, leading to side effects such as gynecomastia, breast tenderness, and feminization. However, specific MRAs are non-steroidal and designed to minimize these side effects. The drugs in this class are finerenone and esaxerenone.

In the FIDELIO-DKD study, patients with CKD and type 2 diabetes mellitus were randomized to finerenone or placebo [82]. Finerenone showed a modest change in mean systolic blood pressure but a significant improvement in the composite outcome of renal failure, a 40% decrease in eGFR, or death from renal causes. This study provided the first evidence that mineralocorticoid receptor antagonist was effective in preventing the progression of kidney disease in diabetic patients rather than simply following proteinuria, as a surrogate outcome, as in previous studies [82, 83].

The non-steroidal MRA finerenone is recommended in patients with chronic kidney disease and albuminuria if eGFR is at least 25 mL/min/1.73 m^2. This is a class I recommendation with an "A" level of evidence [84].

Dose interruption as well as the use of potassium binders can be considered if hyperkalemia occurs.

3.7.6 Calcium Channel Blockers

Non-dihydropyridine calcium channel blockers (CCBs), including diltiazem and verapamil, are useful for the treatment of hypertensive patients with DKD. They may be used as first-line therapy in patients intolerant of ACE inhibitors and ARBs or as second-line agents in combination with an ACE inhibitor or ARB [85]. Dihydropyridine CCBs such as amlodipine and nifedipine are effective antihypertensive agents but do not reduce proteinuria and cause dose-dependent peripheral edema as a side effect. They should only be used in conjunction with an RAAS blocker because they do provide benefits in this setting [52]. The incidence of peripheral edema may be reduced by using dihydropyridine CCBs in combination with an ACE inhibitor.

3.7.7 Diuretics

Thiazide or thiazide-like diuretics (e.g., chlorthalidone and indapamide) have an important role in the management of hypertension in patients with diabetes [14, 86]. Although diuretics once were considered initial therapy, recent guidelines now include them with three other drug classes (i.e., ACE inhibitors, ARBs, and CCBs), any of which may be used to initiate BP-lowering therapy.

The important point to understand is volume status in individuals with DKD, because not all patients have volume issues. These agents primarily act through vasodilatation and natriuresis. Thus, they are effective alone or in combination with other antihypertensive agents. Moreover, in advanced CKD (eGFR >30 mL/min/1.73 m^2), chlorthalidone and indapamide have the most significant BP-lowering effect [87].

Combination preparations containing thiazide diuretics with an ACE inhibitor or ARB may be beneficial in reducing the risk of hyperkalemia, as well as patients' pill burden. Long-acting loop diuretics (e.g., torsemide) are effective at an eGFR <30 mL/min/1.73 m^2 and helpful in volume management [88].

3.7.8 Other Antihypertensive Medication Classes

These medications are not associated with unique cardiorenal protective benefits in patients with hypertension and diabetic kidney disease but are helpful in facilitating better control of blood pressure depending on the clinical situation.

Beta-blockers may also be considered particularly in patients with heart failure and reduced ejection fraction, angina pectoris, or hypertrophic cardiomyopathy. They also have an important role in heart rate regulation in patients with atrial arrhythmia. However, they may reduce exercise tolerance, and be associated with fatigue and weight gain. They should be used cautiously in older individuals.

Alpha-blockers may also be a consideration. They are helpful in males to relieve prostatic hypertrophy and will help facilitate blood pressure reduction with other preferred medications such as RAS inhibitors, CCBs, and diuretics. Direct-acting vasodilators such as hydralazine or minoxidil almost always require a boost in the diuretic support. Short-acting alpha antagonists such as clonidine may also be useful for nighttime dosing in patients with recumbent hypertension.

3.7.9 Sodium–Glucose Co-transporter 2 Inhibitors (SGLT2i)

Though prescribed as glucose-lowering medication with proven cardiovascular benefits, sodium-glucose co-transporter 2 inhibitors have demonstrated positive effects on blood pressure control. The EMPA-REG OUTCOME and CANVAS trials demonstrated blood pressure reduction in treatment groups, though the cause of this effect has been subjected to debate and research [53, 89, 90]. The mechanism of this blood pressure-lowering effect is thought to be due to natriuresis and osmotic diuresis via the local RAAS inhibition. The reduction of BP was noted to be between 3.4 mmHg and 4.2 mmHg, respectively, using either 10 mg or 25 mg empagliflozin (95% CI –4.78 to −2.09; $p < 0.001$) [91].

In the most recent guideline for hypertension, SGLT2i and non-steroidal MRAs together have mild to moderate antihypertensive effects when compared to classical anti-hypertensive medication with the additional benefit of improved cardiovascular and renal outcomes. The 2023 European Society of Hypertension suggests adding SGLT2i in addition to standard recommendation of ACEI and ARB in treating patients with diabetic and non-diabetic CKD if eGFR is at least 20 mL/min/1.73 m^2.

In the ADA-KDIGO joint statement for the management of diabetes in patients with CKD, non-steroidal MRAs are recommended as additional risk-based therapy with SGLT2i as first-line add-on medication in patients with persistent albuminuria despite maximum dose of RAAS inhibitors [63].

Not all patients will be able to tolerate SGLT2i in addition to ACEI or ARB. These patients should be considered for non-steroidal MRA use if they meet indication and lab qualifications. Additionally, there is some evidence suggesting that chronic hypoxia may be the main pathophysiologic cause of diabetic kidney disease and CKD, in addition to other causes. Compromised oxygen balance occurs by diabetes mellitus, with impaired oxygen delivery due to hyperglycemic-induced microvascular damage and increased oxygen demand caused by increased sodium reabsorption because of SGLT upregulation and glomerular hyperfiltration. The addition of SGLT2i may decrease hypoxia-inducible factor-1alfha (HIF-1alpha) in the kidney, resulting in less tissue hypoxia [92]. Further research is required regarding kidney hypoxia and its amelioration.

3.7.10 GLP-I Receptor Antagonists

As will be discussed later, this class of mediators has modest anti-hypertensive effects. This therapy can be ideal for diabetic patients who need improvement in diabetic control. The weight loss associated with these drugs can facilitate BP reductions and they possess both cardiovascular and renal protective benefits.

3.7.11 Obesity: A Risk Factor for Diabetic Kidney Disease

Obesity or excessive adipose tissue is a disease that is a major contributor to declining health in many countries globally [93].

Obesity is defined as a body mass index (BMI) of 30 or greater. It affects more than 800 million people globally [94]. In the US population, 42% of adults have obesity [95]. Obesity is associated with increased rates of type 2 diabetes, hypertension, cardiovascular disease, sleep disorders, osteoarthritis, and premature death.

Obesity-related costs are at $173 billion annually [96]. The prevalence of obesity increased worldwide between 1975 and 2014 from 3.2% to 10.8% in men and from 6.4% to 14.9% in women [97]. By 2025, it is anticipated that 18% men and 21% of women worldwide will be obese [97]. In the United States, it is anticipated that by 2030, 48.9% of US adults will be obese and that racial differences in the rates of obesity will increase [93].

Obesity is considered a chronic disease defined by an excess amount of adipose tissue deposition resulting in increased risk of co-morbidities and early mortality [93, 98]. Weight loss improves glucose, lipids blood pressure, and obesity-related co-morbidities. Several effective weight loss therapies can be offered by physicians [99–101].

The connection between obesity and chronic kidney disease includes several common pathways between both diseases. These include oxidative stress, chronic inflammation and high insulin levels, and common risk factors including, hypertension, insulin resistance, and hyperlipidemia [102] (Fig. 3.4).

3.7.12 Pathophysiology of Obesity

Obesity is influenced by our genetic imprint; energy homeostasis is dependent on feedback given by the central nervous system and circulating neuropeptide hormones [103, 104]. The gut-brain axis responds to signals from the GI tract, adipose tissue, and circulating hormones. These signals provide feedback to either stimulate or stop central neurons, based on hunger or satiety [105]. In obesity, there is a disconnect in this feedback system leading to increased feeling of hunger and decreased satiety [106]. Leptin and ghrelin are hormones implicated in this process [107].

3.7.12.1 Adipose Tissue, Energy Homeostasis, and Pathophysiology of Obesity

Obesity can be further defined by white and brown adipose tissue (WAT, BAT).

WAT and BAT

WAT is the main constituent of total body fat and is an endocrine organ system. White fat cells produce adipokines, a group of metabolically active factors that play a major role in the pathogenesis of obesity and regulation of energy balance [107].

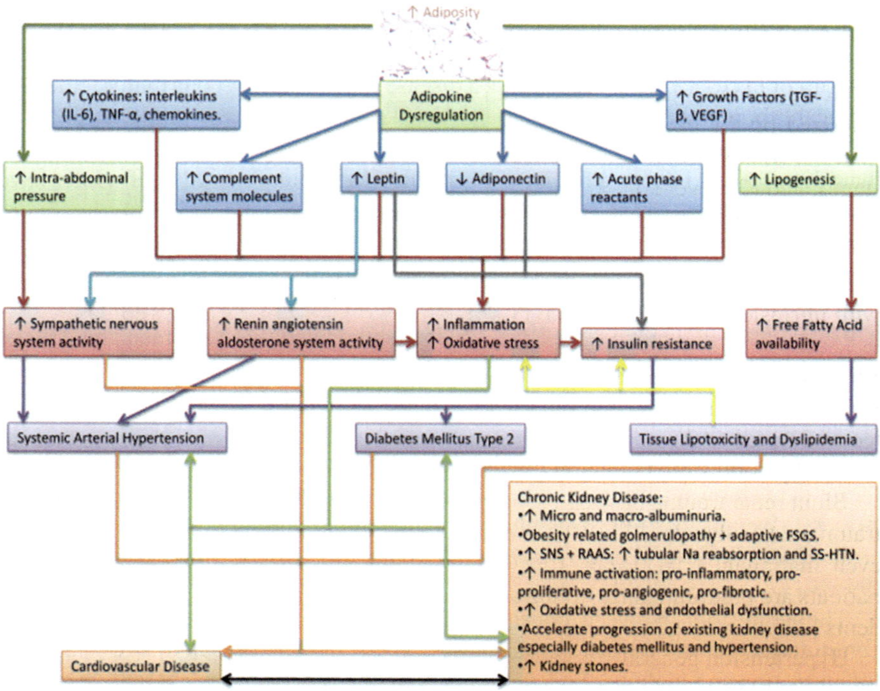

Fig. 3.4 Many of the multiple mechanisms and interactions that can lead to the development of chronic kidney disease and cardiovascular disease [102]

BAT is more prominent at birth and is important in neonatal homeostasis. There is a decline in BAT with age but remains active throughout life. The volume of BAT is inversely proportional to the BMI [108].

WAT dysfunction occurs in obesity. This results in pro-inflammatory reactions, and a disconnection between energy balance, metabolic homeostasis, and results in organ damage at multiple levels [109].

3.7.12.2 Leptin

Leptin is a protein hormone regulating appetite and food intake as well as energy homeostasis and, hence, affects the volume of body fat. It aids to enhance energy expenditure via stimulating anorexigenic hypothalamic receptors. It helps weight loss under normal physiologic conditions [110]. The WAT-leptin system becomes dysfunctional in obesity and its response to sympathetic nervous system (SNS) is blunted. WAT-leptin production and secretion are downregulated by fasting and SNS activation and upregulated with SNS inhibition [110]. The plasma concentrations of leptin are directly proportional to the degree of adiposity, and higher levels are seen in obese people. Leptin is also associated with proinflammatory, proangiogenic, pro-proliferative, and profibrotic actions.

3.7.12.3 Adiponectin

Adiponectin is a protein hormone that promotes glucose metabolism and fatty acid oxidation [111, 112]. Obesity has been associated with a decrease in circulating adiponectin in plasma. This downregulation is associated with deranged glucose metabolism and insulin resistance [113, 114]. Additionally, an association is found between downregulated adiponectin levels and fatty acid metabolism, and ectopic fat accumulation and an increase in oxidative stress. Hence, adiponectin deficiency in obese individuals is linked to a pro-inflammatory state when left unchecked [115].

3.7.12.4 Micro-Ribonucleic Acids

Micro RNAs are short nucleotide sequences that are non-coding but play an important role in regulating gene expression. There are studies to show they serve as biomarkers as well as therapeutic targets in obesity and other metabolic diseases. Micro RNAs play an important role in stimulation and inhibiting of adipose differentiation, in chronic inflammation, diabetic kidney disease, and lipid metabolism [116, 117].

3.7.12.5 Chronic Inflammation

Obesity is associated with chronic subclinical inflammation. There are many reports that point to high levels of circulating proinflammatory mediators in obesity. These are leptin, TNF-alpha, and IL6. Pre-adipocytes are shown to have immune characteristics, resembling the same in macrophages. White adipocytes can trigger ischemia and hypoxia through stimulation of inflammation and vasoconstriction [118–120].

3.7.13 Pathophysiology of Obesity-Related CKD Pathways

Obesity-related hyperleptinemia and leptin resistance set up a series of pathways and, combined with adiponectin deficiency, lead to insulin resistance, hyperinsulinemia, and hyperaldosteronism which result in increased systemic arterial blood pressure, volume expansion, and eventually renal fibrosis. The observations are supported by experimental adiponectin-knockout mice with adiponectin deficiency. In the experimental modal, there is increased urine protein excretion and abnormal podocyte function. Supplementation of adiponectin in cultured podocytes decreased albuminuria and enhanced podocyte function [121].

3.7.14 Obesity-Related Glomerulopathy

Increased body mass from increased adiposity results in chronic structural and functional changes at the nephron level. Obesity-related glomerulopathy is a major clinical manifestation. Central obesity as measured by waist-to-hip ratio (WHR), often used with BMI to measure central visceral obesity, is associated with a decrease in eGFR measured by I-iothalamate clearance, and a decrease in effective renal plasma flow eRPF and glomerular hyperfiltration. This is noted by an increased filtration fraction FF = eGFR/eRPF despite adjustment for BMI [122].

Additional changes noted are podocyte dysfunction, with decreased podocyte density and volume and podocyte hypertrophy [123]. Glomerular capillary hypertension and glomerular hypertrophy are the long-term sequelae heralding secondary adaptive FSGS. The combination of glomerulopathy and FSGS defines obesity-related glomerulopathy (ORG) [123, 124]. The major clinical and pathophysiologic result is sub-nephrotic proteinuria. Other mechanisms are also implicated in obesity impacting the nephron that result in proteinuria in obese patients.

3.7.15 Diagnosis and Classification of Obesity

BMI is used most frequently to describe obesity, defined as weight in kilograms divided by height in meters squared. The WHO describes overweight BMI (25–29.9), class 1 obesity (30–34.99), class II obesity (35–39.99), and class III obesity (>40). Waist hip ratio, a marker for visceral adiposity, is associated with cardiometabolic risk [125]. In men, a waist circumference more than 102 cm and in women more than 88 cm is associated with obesity in patients with associated BMI of 25–34.9, requires risk stratification [126].

3.7.16 Weight Loss Goals

Weight loss personal goals if set up can help achieve at least 10% weight loss over the span of 12 months, especially when compared to those individuals who don't set a weight loss goal (68.2% vs. 31.8% in a study of 24,447 patients with obesity) [127]. A decrease in systolic and diastolic blood pressure of 3 mmHg and 2 mmHg can occur with a 5% reduction in weight loss. Hemoglobin A1C can decrease by 0.6–1.0% among those with diabetes mellitus type 2 if weight loss of 5–10% occurs. Individuals who get bariatric surgery and have associated weight loss of more than 15% have lower risk of all-cause mortality [98, 128].

3.7.17 Anti-Obesity Medications

Several medications are now available approved by the American Food and Drug administration. Individuals who did not benefit from lifestyle modifications and remain overweight or obese (BMI >27), are non-pregnant, and have weight-related comorbidities have the opportunity now to benefit from weight loss medications [93, 100, 101].

In patients with diabetes and who are overweight, a GLP-1 receptor agonist will help improve blood sugar control and help with weight loss. These drugs are usually recommended in association with lifestyle modification and often require lifetime use as weight gain can occur on cessation of these medications [129].

3.8 GLP-1 Receptor Agonists (Liraglutide, Semaglutide, and Tirzepatide)

GLP-1 acts on the hypothalamus to suppress appetite. It delays gastric emptying, increases pancreatic B cell growth, decreases glucagon secretion, and increases glucose-dependent insulin release [130]. Semaglutide given subcutaneously received FDA approval in 2021 and is given once per week. The efficacy of semaglutide was examined in the STEP trials. STEP 1 and STEP 3 trials examined and included individuals with obesity but without diabetes (mean BMI 38) [130, 131]. The mean weight loss at 68 weeks was 14.9% (placebo, 2.4%; difference, 12.4%; 95% CI, 11.5–13.4%) and 16.0% (placebo, 5.7%; difference, 10.3%; 95% CI, 8.6–12.0%) [131, 132].

In a prospective clinical trial of 3731 obese patients, 3.0 mg of liraglutide per week liraglutide was approved for the treatment of type 2 diabetes in 2014. When given subcutaneously, liraglutide achieved a mean loss of 8.0% at 56 weeks compared to placebo (difference, 5.4%; 95% CI, 5.8–5.0%) [133].

Tirzepatide is a synthetic peptide with double agonist action acting agonistically on the GLP-1 receptor, like semaglutide, and at the glucose-dependent insulinogenic receptor. It is dosed subcutaneously once weekly. In a phase 3 randomized controlled trial, 2539 obese adults were randomized in a 1:1:1:1 ratio to receive 1 week 5 mg, 10 mg, 15 mg or placebo for 72 weeks. The mean reduction in weight was −15.0%, −19.5%, −20.9% and −3.1% respectively [134].

3.8.1 Phentermine Topiramate

Combined oral phentermine-topiramate was FDA-approved in 2012 for obesity. Phentermine reduces appetite and affects food intake via increasing norepinephrine release and blocking NE reuptake.

In the recent study on the effects of semaglutide on patient with obesity-related heart failure with preserved ejection fraction and type 2 diabetes, it was noted that semaglutide led to larger reductions in heart failure-related symptoms, greater weight loss than placebo, and improvement in physical limitations related to obesity [135].

Patients with type 2 diabetes and chronic kidney disease are known to have a higher risk for kidney failure, cardiovascular disease, and death. Semaglutide treatment for these patients was studied to evaluate the mitigation of these risks. Semaglutide 1.0 mg/week was noted to reduce the risk of adverse kidney outcomes and death from cardiovascular causes in patients with type 2 diabetes and chronic kidney disease [136].

3.8.2 Perspective

Over the past decade, there has been an explosion of new therapies for patients with hypertension, obesity, and diabetic kidney disease. These new therapeutic options have been associated with important improvement in cardiorenal outcomes. The mechanisms of benefit remain unknown. But what is clear is that they are often associated with improvement in blood pressure, diabetes control, and weight loss. Patients will continue to require earlier identification of cardiorenal risk with screening for UACR and eGFR in addition to traditional measures of BP, cholesterol, and glucose. The earlier opportunity to employ these newer therapies may have a sizable impact on primary prevention of cardiorenal disease. Moreover, we need to provide more intensified effort to control all traditional CV risk factors, as well as learn more about the mechanistic benefits of the many new therapeutic options that are available today.

3.8.3 RENIN-Secreting Tumors or Reninoma

A reninoma is a tumor arising from the afferent juxtaglomerular cells that secrete renin. This leads to hyperactivation of the renin-angiotensin-aldosterone system, causing secondary hyperaldosteronism, resulting in severe hypertension and hypokalemia. These tumor cells are mostly benign.

Since first reported in 1967, about 100 cases have been published. They are mostly diagnosed in adolescents and young adults. The signs and symptoms include severe hypertension, headaches, malaise, and failure to thrive in younger children. Since symptoms are nonspecific, there is usually a delay in diagnosis [137, 138].

High aldosterone levels stimulate the sodium–potassium exchange mechanism, resulting in excessive potassium loss from the principal cells of the collecting duct. This results in hypokalemia and metabolic alkalosis.

The management and treatment for patients with reninomas are RAAS blockers. This is the treatment of choice. They work at multiple levels. Mineralocorticoid receptor antagonists, like spironolactone and eplerenone, and the renin inhibitor aliskiren can also be used. The monitoring of serum electrolytes should ideally be measured before any intervention is initiated. Renin and aldosterone levels need to be monitored as well. High renin with high aldosterone levels with a normal renin/aldosterone ratio suggests excessive secretion of both hormones. This occurs in renal causes of hypertension (renal artery stenosis, renal parenchymal disease, and reninoma). A high aldosterone level with a suppressed renin level suggests an adrenal tumor or hyperplasia. Both renin and aldosterone levels are influenced by the state of hydration, salt intake, postural changes, and use of medications [139].

A renal ultrasound can miss a small reninoma. A contrast CT scan and magnetic resonance imaging of the kidneys are imaging modalities of choice that can lead to the correct diagnosis. CT angiography is reported to have a 100% sensitivity, even with small reninomas [140]. Renal vein renin sampling with lateralization can aid in identifying the site of excessive renin production. Surgical removal and cure are the optimal treatment strategies as it eliminates the need for lifelong medical treatment [141].

3.9 Conclusions

The control of blood pressure to an appropriate target earlier in the course of life is a preferred consideration for the primary prevention of atherosclerotic cardiovascular and kidney disease. This will require earlier identification and education of patients. The adoption of a healthier lifestyle coupled with appropriate choices of pharmacotherapy targeting underlying medical comorbidities, such as diabetes, chronic kidney disease, obesity, and renin-secreting tumors, will assist in minimizing the risk of interval cardiorenal events. Each chronic therapy needs carefully individual based on the therapeutic index over the long-term course of treatment.

References

1. Lewis CE, Fine LJ, Beddhu S, et al. Final report of a trial of intensive versus standard blood-pressure control. N Engl J Med. 2021;384(20):1921–30.
2. Thomopoulos C, Parati G, Zanchetti A. Effects of blood pressure-lowering treatment on cardiovascular outcomes and mortality: 13 - benefits and adverse events in older and younger patients with hypertension: overview, meta-analyses and meta-regression analyses of randomized trials. J Hypertens. 2018;36(8):1622–36.
3. Whelton PK, Carey RM, Aronow WS, et al. 2017 ACC/AHA/AAPA/ABC/ACPM/AGS/APhA/ASH/ASPC/NMA/PCNA guideline for the prevention, detection, evaluation, and management of high blood pressure in adults: executive summary: a report of the American College of Cardiology/American Heart Association Task Force on Clinical Practice Guidelines. Hypertension. 2018;71(6):1269–324.
4. Ostchega Y, Fryar CD, Nwankwo T, Nguyen DT. Hypertension prevalence among adults aged 18 and over: United States, 2017–2018. NCHS Data Brief. 2020;364:1–8.
5. Passarella P, Kiseleva TA, Valeeva FV, Gosmanov AR. Hypertension management in diabetes: 2018 update. Diabetes Spectr. 2018;31(3):218–24.
6. Virani SS, Alonso A, Aparicio HJ, et al. Heart disease and stroke statistics-2021 update: a report from the American Heart Association. Circulation. 2021;143(8):e254–743.
7. Mills KT, Bundy JD, Kelly TN, et al. Global disparities of hypertension prevalence and control: a systematic analysis of population-based studies from 90 countries. Circulation. 2016;134(6):441–50.
8. Worldwide trends in hypertension prevalence and progress in treatment and control from 1990 to 2019: a pooled analysis of 1201 population-representative studies with 104 million participants. Lancet. 2021;398(10304):957–80.
9. Forouzanfar MH, Liu P, Roth GA, et al. Global burden of hypertension and systolic blood pressure of at least 110 to 115 mm Hg, 1990–2015. JAMA. 2017;317(2):165–82.
10. Kimmelstiel P, Wilson C. Intercapillary lesions in the glomeruli of the kidney. Am J Pathol. 1936;12(1):83–98.7.
11. Gauld WR, Sta Lker AL, Lyall A. Renal complications in diabetes mellitus with special reference to the Kimmelstiel-Wilson lesion. Br Med J. 1948;2(4568):194–200.
12. Mogensen CE, Christensen CK, Vittinghus E. The stages in diabetic renal disease. With emphasis on the stage of incipient diabetic nephropathy. Diabetes. 1983;32(Suppl 2):64–78.

13. Sun H, Saeedi P, Karuranga S, et al. IDF diabetes atlas: global, regional and country-level diabetes prevalence estimates for 2021 and projections for 2045. Diabetes Res Clin Pract. 2022;183:109119.
14. Tuttle KR, Bakris GL, Bilous RW, et al. Diabetic kidney disease: a report from an ADA consensus conference. Diabetes Care. 2014;37(10):2864–83.
15. Chen L, Islam RM, Wang J, et al. A systematic review of trends in all-cause mortality among people with diabetes. Diabetologia. 2020;63(9):1718–35.
16. Chen L, Magliano DJ, Zimmet PZ. The worldwide epidemiology of type 2 diabetes mellitus--present and future perspectives. Nat Rev Endocrinol. 2011;8(4):228–36.
17. Magliano DJ, Islam RM, Barr ELM, et al. Trends in incidence of total or type 2 diabetes: systematic review. BMJ. 2019;366:l5003.
18. Delgado C, Baweja M, Crews DC, et al. A unifying approach for GFR estimation: recommendations of the NKF-ASN task force on reassessing the inclusion of race in diagnosing kidney disease. J Am Soc Nephrol. 2021;32(12):2994–3015.
19. Inker LA, Eneanya ND, Coresh J, et al. New creatinine- and cystatin C-based equations to estimate GFR without race. N Engl J Med. 2021;385(19):1737–49.
20. Tuttle KR, Wong L, St Peter W, et al. Moving from evidence to implementation of breakthrough therapies for diabetic kidney disease. Clin J Am Soc Nephrol. 2022;17(7):1092–103.
21. Franchi F, James SK, Ghukasyan Lakic T, et al. Impact of diabetes mellitus and chronic kidney disease on cardiovascular outcomes and platelet P2Y(12) receptor antagonist effects in patients with acute coronary syndromes: insights from the PLATO trial. J Am Heart Assoc. 2019;8(6):e011139.
22. Quinn GZ, Abedini A, Liu H, et al. Renal histologic analysis provides complementary information to kidney function measurement for patients with early diabetic or hypertensive disease. J Am Soc Nephrol. 2021;32(11):2863–76.
23. Di Vincenzo A, Bettini S, Russo L, Mazzocut S, Mauer M, Fioretto P. Renal structure in type 2 diabetes: facts and misconceptions. J Nephrol. 2020;33(5):901–7.
24. Poggio ED, McClelland RL, Blank KN, et al. Systematic review and meta-analysis of native kidney biopsy complications. Clin J Am Soc Nephrol. 2020;15(11):1595–602.
25. Anders HJ, Huber TB, Isermann B, Schiffer M. CKD in diabetes: diabetic kidney disease versus nondiabetic kidney disease. Nat Rev Nephrol. 2018;14(6):361–77.
26. Tuttle KR, Agarwal R, Alpers CE, et al. Molecular mechanisms and therapeutic targets for diabetic kidney disease. Kidney Int. 2022;102(2):248–60.
27. Piani F, Melena I, Tommerdahl KL, et al. Sex-related differences in diabetic kidney disease: a review on the mechanisms and potential therapeutic implications. J Diabetes Complicat. 2021;35(4):107841.
28. National Kidney Foundation Research Roundtable Work Group on behalf of the National Kidney Foundation. Research priorities for kidney-related research-an agenda to advance kidney care: a position statement from the National Kidney Foundation. Am J Kidney Dis. 2022;79(2):141–52.
29. Helal I, Fick-Brosnahan GM, Reed-Gitomer B, Schrier RW. Glomerular hyperfiltration: definitions, mechanisms and clinical implications. Nat Rev Nephrol. 2012;8(5):293–300.
30. Brenner BM, Lawler EV, Mackenzie HS. The hyperfiltration theory: a paradigm shift in nephrology. Kidney Int. 1996;49(6):1774–7.
31. Cortinovis M, Perico N, Ruggenenti P, Remuzzi A, Remuzzi G. Glomerular hyperfiltration. Nat Rev Nephrol. 2022;18(7):435–51.
32. Tonneijck L, Muskiet MH, Smits MM, et al. Glomerular hyperfiltration in diabetes: mechanisms, clinical significance, and treatment. J Am Soc Nephrol. 2017;28(4):1023–39.
33. Brenner BM, Cooper ME, de Zeeuw D, et al. Effects of losartan on renal and cardiovascular outcomes in patients with type 2 diabetes and nephropathy. N Engl J Med. 2001;345(12):861–9.
34. Heerspink HJL, Stefánsson BV, Correa-Rotter R, et al. Dapagliflozin in patients with chronic kidney disease. N Engl J Med. 2020;383(15):1436–46.

35. Lewis EJ, Hunsicker LG, Bain RP, Rohde RD. The effect of angiotensin-converting-enzyme inhibition on diabetic nephropathy. The Collaborative Study Group. N Engl J Med. 1993;329(20):1456–62.
36. Perkovic V, Jardine MJ, Neal B, et al. Canagliflozin and renal outcomes in type 2 diabetes and nephropathy. N Engl J Med. 2019;380(24):2295–306.
37. Wanner C, Inzucchi SE, Lachin JM, et al. Empagliflozin and progression of kidney disease in type 2 diabetes. N Engl J Med. 2016;375(4):323–34.
38. Nicholas SB. Novel anti-inflammatory and anti-fibrotic agents for diabetic kidney disease-from bench to bedside. Adv Chronic Kidney Dis. 2021;28(4):378–90.
39. Inker LA, Schmid CH, Tighiouart H, et al. Estimating glomerular filtration rate from serum creatinine and cystatin C. N Engl J Med. 2012;367(1):20–9.
40. Takir M, Unal AD, Kostek O, Bayraktar N, Demirag NG. Cystatin-C and TGF-β levels in patients with diabetic nephropathy. Nefrologia. 2016;36(6):653–9.
41. Thipsawat S. Early detection of diabetic nephropathy in patient with type 2 diabetes mellitus: a review of the literature. Diab Vasc Dis Res. 2021;18(6):14791641211058856.
42. Jung CY, Yoo TH. Pathophysiologic mechanisms and potential biomarkers in diabetic kidney disease. Diabetes Metab J. 2022;46(2):181–97.
43. UK Prospective Diabetes Study Group. Tight blood pressure control and risk of macrovascular and microvascular complications in type 2 diabetes: UKPDS 38. UK Prospective Diabetes Study Group. BMJ. 1998;317(7160):703–13.
44. Jacobi J, Tsao PS. Asymmetrical dimethylarginine in renal disease: limits of variation or variation limits? A systematic review. Am J Nephrol. 2008;28(2):224–37.
45. Paoletti E, Bellino D, Amidone M, Rolla D, Cannella G. Relationship between arterial hypertension and renal damage in chronic kidney disease: insights from ABPM. J Nephrol. 2006;19(6):778–82.
46. Agarwal R, Andersen MJ. Prognostic importance of ambulatory blood pressure recordings in patients with chronic kidney disease. Kidney Int. 2006;69(7):1175–80.
47. Cruickshank K, Riste L, Anderson SG, Wright JS, Dunn G, Gosling RG. Aortic pulse-wave velocity and its relationship to mortality in diabetes and glucose intolerance: an integrated index of vascular function? Circulation. 2002;106(16):2085–90.
48. Gross ML, Dikow R, Ritz E. Diabetic nephropathy: recent insights into the pathophysiology and the progression of diabetic nephropathy. Kidney Int Suppl. 2005;94:S50–3.
49. KDIGO Blood Pressure Work Group. KDIGO 2021 clinical practice guideline for the management of blood pressure in chronic kidney disease. Kidney Int. 2021;99(3S):S1–S87.
50. Committee ADAPP. 10. Cardiovascular disease and risk management: standards of care in diabetes—2024. Diabetes Care. 2023;47(Suppl_1):S179–218.
51. Pohl MA, Blumenthal S, Cordonnier DJ, et al. Independent and additive impact of blood pressure control and angiotensin II receptor blockade on renal outcomes in the irbesartan diabetic nephropathy trial: clinical implications and limitations. J Am Soc Nephrol. 2005;16(10):3027–37.
52. Bakris GL, Weir MR, Shahinfar S, et al. Effects of blood pressure level on progression of diabetic nephropathy: results from the RENAAL study. Arch Intern Med. 2003;163(13):1555–65.
53. Sanidas EA, Papadopoulos DP, Hatziagelaki E, Grassos C, Velliou M, Barbetseas J. Sodium glucose cotransporter 2 (SGLT2) inhibitors across the spectrum of hypertension. Am J Hypertens. 2020;33(3):207–13.
54. Lv J, Ehteshami P, Sarnak MJ, et al. Effects of intensive blood pressure lowering on the progression of chronic kidney disease: a systematic review and meta-analysis. CMAJ. 2013;185(11):949–57.
55. Sarnak MJ, Greene T, Wang X, et al. The effect of a lower target blood pressure on the progression of kidney disease: long-term follow-up of the modification of diet in renal disease study. Ann Intern Med. 2005;142(5):342–51.
56. ACCORD Study Group, Cushman WC, Evans GW, et al. Effects of intensive blood-pressure control in type 2 diabetes mellitus. N Engl J Med. 2010;362(17):1575–85.

57. Ruggenenti P, Perna A, Gherardi G, et al. Renoprotective properties of ACE-inhibition in non-diabetic nephropathies with non-nephrotic proteinuria. Lancet. 1999;354(9176):359–64.
58. Wright JT Jr, Bakris G, Greene T, et al. Effect of blood pressure lowering and antihypertensive drug class on progression of hypertensive kidney disease: results from the AASK trial. JAMA. 2002;288(19):2421–31.
59. Margolis KL, O'Connor PJ, Morgan TM, et al. Outcomes of combined cardiovascular risk factor management strategies in type 2 diabetes: the ACCORD randomized trial. Diabetes Care. 2014;37(6):1721–8.
60. Emdin CA, Rahimi K, Neal B, Callender T, Perkovic V, Patel A. Blood pressure lowering in type 2 diabetes: a systematic review and meta-analysis. JAMA. 2015;313(6):603–15.
61. Xie X, Atkins E, Lv J, et al. Effects of intensive blood pressure lowering on cardiovascular and renal outcomes: updated systematic review and meta-analysis. Lancet. 2016;387(10017):435–43.
62. Wright JT Jr, Williamson JD, Whelton PK, et al. A randomized trial of intensive versus standard blood-pressure control. N Engl J Med. 2015;373(22):2103–16.
63. de Boer IH, Khunti K, Sadusky T, et al. Diabetes management in chronic kidney disease: a consensus report by the American Diabetes Association (ADA) and Kidney Disease: Improving Global Outcomes (KDIGO). Diabetes Care. 2022;45(12):3075–90.
64. Messerli FH, Mancia G, Conti CR, et al. Dogma disputed: can aggressively lowering blood pressure in hypertensive patients with coronary artery disease be dangerous? Ann Intern Med. 2006;144(12):884–93.
65. Peralta CA, Norris KC, Li S, et al. Blood pressure components and end-stage renal disease in persons with chronic kidney disease: the Kidney Early Evaluation Program (KEEP). Arch Intern Med. 2012;172(1):41–7.
66. Pogue V, Rahman M, Lipkowitz M, et al. Disparate estimates of hypertension control from ambulatory and clinic blood pressure measurements in hypertensive kidney disease. Hypertension. 2009;53(1):20–7.
67. Burrows NR, Li Y, Geiss LS. Incidence of treatment for end-stage renal disease among individuals with diabetes in the U.S. continues to decline. Diabetes Care. 2010;33(1):73–7.
68. Gregg EW, Li Y, Wang J, et al. Changes in diabetes-related complications in the United States, 1990–2010. N Engl J Med. 2014;370(16):1514–23.
69. McMahon EJ, Bauer JD, Hawley CM, et al. A randomized trial of dietary sodium restriction in CKD. J Am Soc Nephrol. 2013;24(12):2096–103.
70. McGuire S. Institute of Medicine. 2013. "Sodium intake in populations: assessment of evidence." Washington, DC: The National Academies Press, 2013. Adv Nutr. 2014;5(1):19–20.
71. American Diabetes Association. 4. Foundations of care: education, nutrition, physical activity, smoking cessation, psychosocial care, and immunization. Diabetes Care. 2015;38 Suppl:S20–30.
72. American Diabetes Association Professional Practice Committee. 2. Classification and diagnosis of diabetes: standards of medical care in diabetes-2022. Diabetes Care. 2022;45(Suppl 1):S17–38.
73. KDIGO Diabetes Work Group. KDIGO 2022 clinical practice guideline for diabetes management in chronic kidney disease. Kidney Int. 2022;102(5S):S1–S127.
74. American Diabetes Association Professional Practice Committee. 7. Diabetes technology: standards of medical care in diabetes-2022. Diabetes Care. 2022;45(Suppl 1):S97–S112.
75. Keane WF, Brenner BM, de Zeeuw D, et al. The risk of developing end-stage renal disease in patients with type 2 diabetes and nephropathy: the RENAAL study. Kidney Int. 2003;63(4):1499–507.
76. Effects of ramipril on cardiovascular and microvascular outcomes in people with diabetes mellitus: results of the HOPE study and MICRO-HOPE substudy. Heart Outcomes Prevention Evaluation Study Investigators. Lancet. 2000;355(9200):253–9.
77. Clase CM, Barzilay J, Gao P, et al. Acute change in glomerular filtration rate with inhibition of the renin-angiotensin system does not predict subsequent renal and cardiovascular outcomes. Kidney Int. 2017;91(3):683–90.

78. Leon SJ, Whitlock R, Rigatto C, et al. Hyperkalemia-related discontinuation of renin-angiotensin-aldosterone system inhibitors and clinical outcomes in CKD: a population-based cohort study. Am J Kidney Dis. 2022;80(2):164–73.e1.
79. Weir MR, Bakris GL, Bushinsky DA, et al. Patiromer in patients with kidney disease and hyperkalemia receiving RAAS inhibitors. N Engl J Med. 2015;372(3):211–21.
80. Spinowitz BS, Fishbane S, Pergola PE, et al. Sodium zirconium cyclosilicate among individuals with hyperkalemia: a 12-month phase 3 study. Clin J Am Soc Nephrol. 2019;14(6):798–809.
81. Fried LF, Emanuele N, Zhang JH, et al. Combined angiotensin inhibition for the treatment of diabetic nephropathy. N Engl J Med. 2013;369(20):1892–903.
82. Pitt B, Filippatos G, Agarwal R, et al. Cardiovascular events with finerenone in kidney disease and type 2 diabetes. N Engl J Med. 2021;385(24):2252–63.
83. Currie G, Taylor AH, Fujita T, et al. Effect of mineralocorticoid receptor antagonists on proteinuria and progression of chronic kidney disease: a systematic review and meta-analysis. BMC Nephrol. 2016;17(1):127.
84. Mancia G, Kreutz R, Brunström M, et al. 2023 ESH Guidelines for the management of arterial hypertension The Task Force for the management of arterial hypertension of the European Society of Hypertension: endorsed by the International Society of Hypertension (ISH) and the European Renal Association (ERA). J Hypertens. 2023;41(12) 1874–2071.
85. Bakris GL, Weir MR, Secic M, Campbell B, Weis-McNulty A. Differential effects of calcium antagonist subclasses on markers of nephropathy progression. Kidney Int. 2004;65(6):1991–2002.
86. James PA, Oparil S, Carter BL, et al. 2014 evidence-based guideline for the management of high blood pressure in adults: report from the panel members appointed to the Eighth Joint National Committee (JNC 8). JAMA. 2014;311(5):507–20.
87. Agarwal R, Sinha AD, Pappas MK, Ammous F. Chlorthalidone for poorly controlled hypertension in chronic kidney disease: an interventional pilot study. Am J Nephrol. 2014;39(2):171–82.
88. Botdorf J, Chaudhary K, Whaley-Connell A. Hypertension in cardiovascular and kidney disease. Cardiorenal Med. 2011;1(3):183–92.
89. Neal B, Perkovic V, Mahaffey KW, et al. Canagliflozin and cardiovascular and renal events in type 2 diabetes. N Engl J Med. 2017;377(7):644–57.
90. Zinman B, Wanner C, Lachin JM, et al. Empagliflozin, cardiovascular outcomes, and mortality in type 2 diabetes. N Engl J Med. 2015;373(22):2117–28.
91. Tikkanen I, Narko K, Zeller C, et al. Empagliflozin reduces blood pressure in patients with type 2 diabetes and hypertension. Diabetes Care. 2015;38(3):420–8.
92. Hesp AC, Schaub JA, Prasad PV, et al. The role of renal hypoxia in the pathogenesis of diabetic kidney disease: a promising target for newer renoprotective agents including SGLT2 inhibitors? Kidney Int. 2020;98(3):579–89.
93. Garvey WT, Mechanick JI, Brett EM, et al. American Association of Clinical Endocrinologists and American College of Endocrinology comprehensive clinical practice guidelines for medical care of patients with obesity. Endocr Pract. 2016;22(Suppl 3):1–203.
94. World Health Organization. WHO acceleration plan to stop obesity. 2023. Available from: https://www.who.int/publications/i/item/9789240075634.
95. Hales CM, Carroll MD, Fryar CD, Ogden CL. Prevalence of obesity and severe obesity among adults: United States, 2017-2018. NCHS Data Brief. 2020;360:1–8.
96. Ward ZJ, Bleich SN, Long MW, Gortmaker SL. Association of body mass index with health care expenditures in the United States by age and sex. PLoS One. 2021;16(3):e0247307.
97. Trends in adult body-mass index in 200 countries from 1975 to 2014: a pooled analysis of 1698 population-based measurement studies with 19·2 million participants. Lancet. 2016;387(10026):1377–96.
98. Jensen MD, Ryan DH, Apovian CM, et al. 2013 AHA/ACC/TOS guideline for the management of overweight and obesity in adults: a report of the American College of Cardiology/American Heart Association Task Force on Practice Guidelines and The Obesity Society. Circulation. 2014;129(25 Suppl 2):S102–38.

99. Eisenberg D, Shikora SA, Aarts E, et al. 2022 American Society for Metabolic and Bariatric Surgery (ASMBS) and International Federation for the Surgery of Obesity and Metabolic Disorders (IFSO): indications for metabolic and bariatric surgery. Surg Obes Relat Dis. 2022;18(12):1345–56.
100. Grunvald E, Shah R, Hernaez R, et al. AGA clinical practice guideline on pharmacological interventions for adults with obesity. Gastroenterology. 2022;163(5):1198–225.
101. ElSayed NA, Aleppo G, Aroda VR, et al. 8. Obesity and weight management for the prevention and treatment of type 2 diabetes: standards of care in diabetes-2023. Diabetes Care. 2023;46(Suppl 1):S128–39.
102. Lakkis JI, Weir MR. Obesity and kidney disease. Prog Cardiovasc Dis. 2018;61(2):157–67.
103. Heymsfield SB, Wadden TA. Mechanisms, pathophysiology, and management of obesity. N Engl J Med. 2017;376(3):254–66.
104. Loos RJF, Yeo GSH. The genetics of obesity: from discovery to biology. Nat Rev Genet. 2022;23(2):120–33.
105. Kessler C. Pathophysiology of obesity. Nurs Clin North Am. 2021;56(4):465–78.
106. Oussaada SM, van Galen KA, Cooiman MI, et al. The pathogenesis of obesity. Metabolism. 2019;92:26–36.
107. Akingbemi BT. Adiponectin receptors in energy homeostasis and obesity pathogenesis. Prog Mol Biol Transl Sci. 2013;114:317–42.
108. Cypess AM, Lehman S, Williams G, et al. Identification and importance of brown adipose tissue in adult humans. N Engl J Med. 2009;360(15):1509–17.
109. Hajer GR, van Haeften TW, Visseren FL. Adipose tissue dysfunction in obesity, diabetes, and vascular diseases. Eur Heart J. 2008;29(24):2959–71.
110. Rayner DV, Trayhurn P. Regulation of leptin production: sympathetic nervous system interactions. J Mol Med (Berl). 2001;79(1):8–20.
111. Yamauchi T, Kamon J, Minokoshi Y, et al. Adiponectin stimulates glucose utilization and fatty-acid oxidation by activating AMP-activated protein kinase. Nat Med. 2002;8(11):1288–95.
112. Yoon MJ, Lee GY, Chung JJ, Ahn YH, Hong SH, Kim JB. Adiponectin increases fatty acid oxidation in skeletal muscle cells by sequential activation of AMP-activated protein kinase, p38 mitogen-activated protein kinase, and peroxisome proliferator-activated receptor alpha. Diabetes. 2006;55(9):2562–70.
113. Manigrasso MR, Ferroni P, Santilli F, et al. Association between circulating adiponectin and interleukin-10 levels in android obesity: effects of weight loss. J Clin Endocrinol Metab. 2005;90(10):5876–9.
114. Putz DM, Goldner WS, Bar RS, Haynes WG, Sivitz WI. Adiponectin and C-reactive protein in obesity, type 2 diabetes, and monodrug therapy. Metabolism. 2004;53(11):1454–61.
115. Ouchi N, Kihara S, Arita Y, et al. Adiponectin, an adipocyte-derived plasma protein, inhibits endothelial NF-kappaB signaling through a cAMP-dependent pathway. Circulation. 2000;102(11):1296–301.
116. Peng Y, Yu S, Li H, Xiang H, Peng J, Jiang S. MicroRNAs: emerging roles in adipogenesis and obesity. Cell Signal. 2014;26(9):1888–96.
117. Arner P, Kulyté A. MicroRNA regulatory networks in human adipose tissue and obesity. Nat Rev Endocrinol. 2015;11(5):276–88.
118. Festa A, D'Agostino R Jr, Williams K, et al. The relation of body fat mass and distribution to markers of chronic inflammation. Int J Obes Relat Metab Disord. 2001;25(10):1407–15.
119. Trayhurn P, Wood IS. Adipokines: inflammation and the pleiotropic role of white adipose tissue. Br J Nutr. 2004;92(3):347–55.
120. Hotamisligil GS. Inflammatory pathways and insulin action. Int J Obes Relat Metab Disord. 2003;27(Suppl 3):S53–5.
121. Sharma K. The link between obesity and albuminuria: adiponectin and podocyte dysfunction. Kidney Int. 2009;76(2):145–8.
122. Kwakernaak AJ, Zelle DM, Bakker SJ, Navis G. Central body fat distribution associates with unfavorable renal hemodynamics independent of body mass index. J Am Soc Nephrol. 2013;24(6):987–94.

123. Chen HM, Liu ZH, Zeng CH, Li SJ, Wang QW, Li LS. Podocyte lesions in patients with obesity-related glomerulopathy. Am J Kidney Dis. 2006;48(5):772–9.
124. Gaynor JJ, Ciancio G, Guerra G, et al. Multivariable risk of developing new onset diabetes after transplant-results from a single-center study of 481 adult primary kidney transplant recipients. Clin Transpl. 2015;29(4):301–10.
125. Obesity: preventing and managing the global epidemic. Report of a WHO consultation. World Health Organ Tech Rep Ser. 2000;894:i–xii, 1–253.
126. Wharton S, Lau DCW, Vallis M, et al. Obesity in adults: a clinical practice guideline. CMAJ. 2020;192(31):E875–E91.
127. Avery A, Langley-Evans SC, Harrington M, Swift JA. Setting targets leads to greater long-term weight losses and 'unrealistic' targets increase the effect in a large community-based commercial weight management group. J Hum Nutr Diet. 2016;29(6):687–96.
128. Ryan DH, Yockey SR. Weight loss and improvement in comorbidity: differences at 5%, 10%, 15%, and over. Curr Obes Rep. 2017;6(2):187–94.
129. Rubino D, Abrahamsson N, Davies M, et al. Effect of continued weekly subcutaneous semaglutide vs placebo on weight loss maintenance in adults with overweight or obesity: the STEP 4 randomized clinical trial. JAMA. 2021;325(14):1414–25.
130. Nolen-Doerr E, Stockman MC, Rizo I. Mechanism of glucagon-like peptide 1 improvements in type 2 diabetes mellitus and obesity. Curr Obes Rep. 2019;8(3):284–91.
131. Wilding JPH, Batterham RL, Calanna S, et al. Once-weekly semaglutide in adults with overweight or obesity. N Engl J Med. 2021;384(11):989–1002.
132. Wadden TA, Bailey TS, Billings LK, et al. Effect of subcutaneous semaglutide vs placebo as an adjunct to intensive behavioral therapy on body weight in adults with overweight or obesity: the STEP 3 randomized clinical trial. JAMA. 2021;325(14):1403–13.
133. Pi-Sunyer X, Astrup A, Fujioka K, et al. A randomized, controlled trial of 3.0 mg of liraglutide in weight management. N Engl J Med. 2015;373(1):11–22.
134. Jastreboff AM, Aronne LJ, Ahmad NN, et al. Tirzepatide once weekly for the treatment of obesity. N Engl J Med. 2022;387(3):205–16.
135. Kosiborod MN, Petrie MC, Borlaug BA, et al. Semaglutide in patients with obesity-related heart failure and type 2 diabetes. N Engl J Med. 2024;390(15):1394–407.
136. Perkovic V, Tuttle KR, Rossing P, et al. Effects of semaglutide on chronic kidney disease in patients with type 2 diabetes. N Engl J Med. 2024;391(2):109–21.
137. Gornik HL, Persu A, Adlam D, et al. First international consensus on the diagnosis and management of fibromuscular dysplasia. Vasc Med. 2019;24(2):164–89.
138. Mezoued M, Habouchi MA, Azzoug S, Mokkedem K, Meskine D. Juxtaglomerular cell cause of secondary hypertension in an adolescent. Acta Endocrinol (Buchar). 2020;16(3):359–61.
139. Conn JW. Primary reninism, a surgically curable form of hypertension. Ergeb Inn Med Kinderheilkd. 1974;34(0):23–44.
140. Wong L, Hsu TH, Perlroth MG, Hofmann LV, Haynes CM, Katznelson L. Reninoma: case report and literature review. J Hypertens. 2008;26(2):368–73.
141. Kim JH, Kim JH, Cho MH, et al. Reninoma: a rare cause of curable hypertension. Korean J Pediatr. 2019;62(4):144–7.

Hypertension in Cystic and Polycystic Kidney Disease

4

Juan Villa, Alvaro Alvarez Lopez, and Nicolás Roberto Robles

4.1 Introduction

Renal cysts are the most common lesion of the kidney and are seen in approximately 40% of patients that undergo imaging studies involving the anatomical region of the kidneys. Renal cysts can be benign or malignant, focal, multifocal, unilateral, or bilateral, and congenital or acquired, though the acquired form is more common (see Table 4.1 for classification). The presence of acquired renal cysts increases with advancing age. Simple renal cysts are the most common cystic renal lesions. Figure 4.1 shows the most common classes of kidney cystic disease.

Autosomal dominant polycystic kidney disease (ADPKD) is generally a late-onset multisystem disorder characterized by bilateral kidney cysts, liver cysts, and an increased risk of intracranial aneurysms. Other manifestations include: cysts in the pancreas, seminal vesicles, and arachnoid membrane; dilatation of the aortic root and dissection of the thoracic aorta; mitral valve prolapse; and abdominal wall hernias. Kidney manifestations include early-onset hypertension, kidney pain, and kidney insufficiency. Approximately, 50% of individuals with ADPKD have end-stage kidney disease (ESKD) by age 60 years. The prevalence of liver cysts increases with age and occasionally results in clinically significant severe polycystic liver disease, most often in females. Overall, the prevalence of intracranial aneurysms is fivefold higher than in the general population and further increased in those with a positive family history of aneurysms or subarachnoid hemorrhage. There is substantial variability in the severity of kidney disease and other extra-kidney manifestations.

J. Villa · A. A. Lopez · N. R. Robles (✉)
Hypertension Unit, Nephrology Department, Badajoz University Hospital, University of Extremadura, Badajoz, Spain
e-mail: nrrobles@unex.es

A. E. Berbari et al. (eds.), *Blood Pressure Disorders in Acute and Chronic Kidney Diseases*, Updates in Hypertension and Cardiovascular Protection
https://doi.org/10.1007/978-3-031-81292-7_4

Table 4.1 Cystic kidney diseases

Renal cyst	An enclosed or communicating segment of nephron or duct that is dilated to a diameter of $200 mmol.
Acquired cystic disease	Spontaneous, idiopathic, bilateral development of multiple cysts in previously noncystic kidneys.
Dialysis-acquired cystic disease	A form of acquired cystic disease found in patients under hemodialysis treatment.
Medullary sponge	Medullary cystic abnormality of sporadic presentation.
Autosomal recessive polycystic kidney disease	A genetically determined cystic (cortical and medullar) lesion of autosomal recessive forms.
Autosomal dominant polycystic kidney disease	A genetically determined cystic lesion (cortical and medullar) of autosomal dominant form.
Multicystic dysplasia	One or both of a baby's kidneys do not develop normally while the baby is still in the uterus. Cysts can replace normal renal tissue. The affected kidney is usually dysfunctional.
Nephronophthisis	Hereditary. Medullary cystic renal disease with renal failure.
Glomerulocystic kidney	Kidney with glomerular cysts but of diverse etiologies.

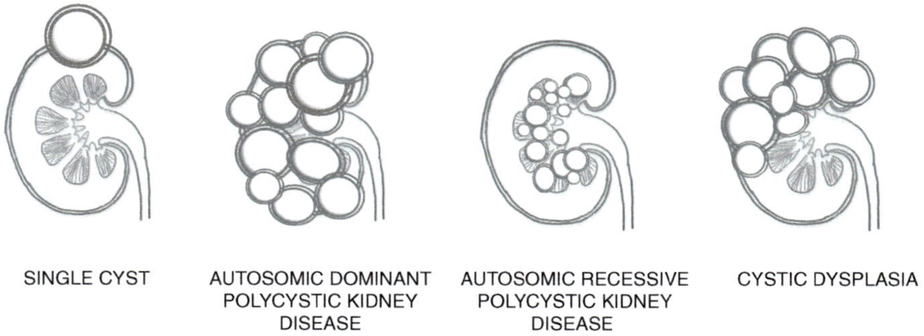

Fig. 4.1 The most common classes of kidney cystic disease

On the other hand, autosomal recessive kidney disease is caused by a mutation in the PKHD1 gene located on chromosome 6 resulting in cyst formation in the collecting ducts. This is an uncommon pediatric disease.

4.2 Adult Polycystic Kidney Disease

Adult polycystic kidney disease is also known as autosomal dominant polycystic kidney disease (ADPKD). This is the most frequent hereditary renal disease and accounts for approximately 6–10% of the patients initiating renal replacement therapies (RRT) worldwide [1]. Although ADPKD is not usually associated with diabetic or hypertensive nephropathy, there is an increase in the rate of CVD in ADPKD patients being the first cause of death [2].

A patient with ADPKD has a normal appearance of the kidneys at birth and begins to develop multiple cysts bilaterally in their 20s to 30s. It is the most common inherited cause of end-stage renal failure with more than 50% of patients requiring dialysis by the age of 60 years. Autosomal dominant kidney disease is caused by a mutation in either the PKD1 gene on chromosome 16 or the PKD2 gene on chromosome 4. There are less common associated genes (ALG5, ALG9, DNAJB11, GANAB, IFT140). Very infrequently, a large deletion which may encompass the genes TSC2 (tuberous sclerosis) and PKD1 causes so-called TSC2/PKD1 contiguous gene syndrome (OMIM #600273) [3].

4.2.1 Diagnostic Criteria of ADPKD

ADPKD should be suspected in individuals with the manifestations shown in Table 4.2 [4]. The diagnosis of ADPKD is established whenever the patient shows any of the following:

- Age-specific ultrasound/MRI criteria and an affected first-degree relative with ADPKD. For patients aged 16–40 years who have an affected first-degree relative, the presence of more than ten cysts in MRI is sufficient for a diagnosis of ADPKD [5]. It has been suggested that MRI criteria may also be more appropriate to use when employing a high-resolution ultrasound scanner that can detect cysts as small as 1–2 mm [6].

The age-specific ultrasound criteria in an individual with an affected first-degree relative are:

- The presence of ≥3 (unilateral or bilateral) kidney cysts in an individual aged 15–39 years
- The presence of ≥2 cysts in each kidney in an individual aged 40–59 years
- Large echogenic kidneys without distinct macroscopic cysts in an infant/child [7]
- Identification of a heterozygous pathogenic variant a PKD1, PKD2, or one of the less common associated genes (ALG5, ALG9, DNAJB11, GANAB, IFT140) identified by molecular genetic testing [6].

Table 4.2 ADPKD suspicion criteria (KDIGO)

• Multiple bilateral kidney cysts and absence of manifestations suggestive of a different cystic kidney disease.
• Cysts in other organs, especially the liver, but also seminal vesicles, pancreas, and arachnoid membrane.
• Enlargement of the kidneys or liver on physical examination.
• Hypertension in an individual younger than age 35 years.
• An intracranial aneurysm.
• Family history consistent with autosomal dominant inheritance (e.g., affected males and females in multiple generations). Absence of a known family history does not preclude the diagnosis.

The sensitivity of ultrasound criteria is lower in subjects with a pathogenic variant in PKD2, families with incompletely penetrant nontruncating PKD1 pathogenic variants, and families with pathogenic variants in less common genes.

4.2.2 Pathogenesis of Hypertension in ADPKD

High blood pressure in ADPKD is salt sensible with normal or increased extracellular fluid volume, plasma volume, and cardiac output. It is characterized by an increased kidney vascular resistance and filtration fraction with normal or high peripheral plasma renin activity. The pressure-natriuresis relationship is reset. An incomplete correction of kidney hemodynamics and sodium handling could be obtained by using converting enzyme inhibitors.

It has been reported that children with ADPKD suffer from increasing prevalence of hypertension during the course of the disease parallel to the increasing number of kidney cysts and size despite normal and stable kidney function and proteinuria [8]. In fact, high blood pressure usually precedes renal function impairing.

High blood pressure is more common and seems to be earlier in patients with PKD1 gene abnormalities [9]. Similarly, the presence of PKD1 gene dysfunction is associated with earlier CKD progression to ESRD compared with patients with PKD2 gene dysfunction (average 58 vs. 79 years in recent series) [9, 10].

The mechanisms involved in the pathogenesis of hypertension and the decline of renal function in ADPKD are not yet fully understood. The most prevalent theory regarding the pathogenesis of hypertension (as well as the initiation and progression of CKD) focuses on the formation and increase of the size of cysts, but this can only incompletely explain the high variability of the disease expression [11]. Results from the CRISP (Consortium for Radiologic Imaging Studies of Polycystic Kidney Disease) study indicated that both the total kidney volume, largely due to the size of the cysts, and renal blood flow as a measure of vascular resistance were independent predictors of renal function decline [12]. Therefore, it has been suggested that increased cyst size could decrease intrarenal perfusion and stimulate the RAAS, but it could also produce direct obstructive phenomena on blood vessels, glomeruli, and the tubules [13].

Earlier theories suggest that the growing cysts in ADPKD may induce displacement and narrowing of renal vessels leading to renal hypoperfusion and, therefore, renin-angiotensin-aldosterone system (RAAS) activation [14]. Although a study in humans reported that systemic RAAS activation in hypertensive patients with ADPKD was no different than in individuals with essential hypertension [15], several lines of evidence indicate that intrarenal RAAS activation may be a pathogenetic factor in ADPKD. In renal tissue specimens from ADPKD patients, vascular stiffening of interlobular arteries and afferent arterioles, as well as interstitial inflammation and fibrosis, was common in normotensive ADPKD patients [16]. Moreover, histological studies examining kidney specimens from ADPKD patients have found accumulation of renin granules within the juxtaglomerular apparatus, raised levels of tubular immunoreactive renin, and higher intracystic renin concentrations [17,

18]. Loghman-Adham et al. reported that renal cysts and dilated tubules were shown to independently produce angiotensinogen and, also, cyst fluids contain high angiotensin-II concentration. Based on these observations, they propose a model of an autocrine/paracrine RAS in polycystic kidney disease, whereby overactivity of the intrarenal system results in sustained increases in intratubular ANG II concentrations [19]. In the same way, it has been suggested that this excessive regional RAAS activation may increase intratubular angiotensin-II presence resulting in enhanced renal tubular sodium reabsorption and consequently high blood pressure and progressive kidney disease [20].

Nevertheless, despite the well-established renoprotection of RAAS blockade in proteinuric nephropathies, there is little evidence to suggest additional benefit from RAAS blockers in ADPKD. So far, randomized studies evaluating the effect of RAAS blocker therapy in ADPKD patients have failed to show any significant improvement in reducing the progression of CKD [21, 22]. In this regard, results from a meta-analysis of 30 studies showed no significant benefits in renal outcomes (kidney volume, eGFR, or serum creatinine levels) from the treatment with angiotensin-converting enzyme inhibitors (ACEi) or angiotensin receptor blockers (ARB) compared with placebo or other pharmacological treatment [23].

In addition to stimulating the RAAS, intrarenal ischemia induces sympathetic stimulation [24]. It has been reported that hypertensive ADPKD patients with normal renal function showed higher muscle sympathetic nerve activity compared with normotensive ADPKD patients or controls [25]. In a rat model of polycystic kidney disease, bilateral renal sympathetic denervation reduced the cystic kidney size, cyst volume density, systolic BP, and serum urea levels compared with controls over an 8-week follow-up [26]. In the same way muscle sympathetic nerve activity was also increased in ADPKD patients with preserved eGFR, compared with patients with essential hypertension [27].

Nitric oxide (NO) bioavailability and NO-dependent vasodilation seem to be affected in patients with ADPKD. Using pressure myography, it was observed a marked defect in ACh-stimulated endothelium-dependent vasodilatation in Pkd2 arterioles. In contrast, Pkd2 vessels responded normally to sodium nitroprusside, phenylephrine, KCl, and pressure, indicating unaltered vascular smooth muscle-dependent responses [28]. In the same context, studies in Han: SPRD-Cy/þ rats with PKD showed decreased NO circulating levels and reduced activity of renal endothelial NO synthase (eNOs) [29]. In a case-control study on endothelium-dependent relaxation of the small resistance vessels, ADPKD patients had impaired vasodilation and higher NO-regulated shear stress compared with healthy individuals, even in the absence of high blood pressure or impaired renal function [30]. Moreover, studies in patients with ADPKD and normal renal function showed a disproportionate reduction in endothelium-dependent vasodilation in the brachial artery and increased reflection of the pulse wave from peripheral sites. These findings have been considered as a deficit in NO release in small arteries [31, 32]. Another way to test the effect of endothelial dysfunction in patients with ADPKD are studies evaluating the prognostic significance of different single nucleotide eNOs gene polymorphisms for CKD progression. It has been shown that the Glu298Aspexon polymorphism, which results in decreased NO synthesis, was associated with faster

CKD progression, but only in male ADPKD patients [33, 34]. In the same context, intron 4 b/a polymorphism was also associated with higher risk for ESRD development in ADPKD patients [35, 36].

Another possible factor is directly related to the pathogenesis of ADPKD. The disease is caused by mutations in PKD1 and PKD2 that encode polycystin 1 (PC1) and polycystin 2 (PC2). PC1/2 localize to cilia of renal epithelial cells, and their function is believed to embody an inhibitory activity that suppresses the cilia-dependent cyst activation (CDCA) signal. Consequently, PC deficiency results in the activation of CDCA and stimulates cyst growth [37]. Abnormal polycystin-1 (PC-1) and polycystin-2 (PC-2) expression in blood vessels results in abnormal vascular structure and function, reduced nitric oxide (NO), and abnormal endothelial response [38].

4.2.3 Clinics

In the early stages of disease, many individuals with ADPKD have no symptoms, although most have high blood pressure. As the kidney cysts increase in size, patients may develop abdominal pain or pressure, blood in the urine, kidney infections, and kidney stones. Over time, more than half of people with ADPKD develop kidney failure and need treatment with dialysis or kidney transplant. Onset of kidney failure is usually after age 50 years but may occur earlier.

Onset of high blood pressure before age 35 years is a poor prognostic factor. Hypertension often develops in young adults, and even in childhood, and usually before any decline in GFR. A reduction in kidney blood flow can be detected in young individuals (when systolic and diastolic blood pressures are still normal) and precedes the development of hypertension [39]. Hypertension is a common early manifestation in ADPKD and occurs in about 60% of patients before renal function impairment [40]. Hypertension occurs earlier and more frequently in PKD1 than in PKD2 and in those ADPKD patients whose affected or unaffected parents also have hypertension [41]. Most importantly, there is an association between hypertension and the decrease in kidney function. A number of studies have shown that high blood pressure is an independent prognostic factor for CKD progression [42].

High blood pressure could be diagnosed much later than when it first occurs in individuals with ADPKD; 24-h monitoring of ambulatory blood pressure (ABPM) of children or young adults may reveal elevated blood pressure, attenuated decrease in nocturnal blood pressure, and exaggerated blood pressure response during exercise. It can also be accompanied by left ventricular hypertrophy and diastolic dysfunction [43]. It has repeatedly shown that children with hypertension and ADPKD have larger kidneys, as well as higher left ventricular mass index, and experience faster progression in kidney dysfunction, especially if glomerular hyperfiltration is present [44–47].

An important issue is the prevalence of hypertension in younger patients. Several single-center cohort analyses have reported frequencies ranging from 6% to 35% [6, 7, 48–50]. Masella et al. [51], using 24 h ambulatory blood pressure monitoring

(ABPM), found that the prevalence of 24 h high blood pressure was 22%, although nighttime hypertension one was 30% and there was a 52% of non-dippers.

Early detection and treatment of hypertension in ADPKD is important because cardiovascular disease is the main cause of death. Uncontrolled high blood pressure also increases the risk for other disease symptoms such as proteinuria, hematuria, and a faster kidney dysfunction progression. It could also produce higher morbidity and mortality from valvular heart disease and aneurysms. In the same way, fetal and maternal complications during pregnancy would be more frequent. Therefore, monitoring blood pressure in children at risk for ADPKD is recommended [52].

Much debate exists as to whether it is appropriate to screen children at risk of ADPKD. Theoretically, these treatments could be more efficient if started during childhood, in particular in patients who are at risk of being fast progressors, if side effects are acceptable [53]. In this regard, the negative psychologic consequences of a diagnosis during childhood could be outweighed by benefits derived from early changes in lifestyle and BP control. Nonetheless, it should be noted that treating hypertension in adults with ADPKD improves cardiac hypertrophy, but benefits on kidney function are less pronounced compared with other chronic kidney diseases [21, 54]. Most importantly, the effect of very early blood pressure treatment in patients with ADPKD, although it is well known to be at high risk of cardiovascular events later in life, is not well established. Therefore, the only possible conclusion is that ABPM helps to identify children who are likely to progress faster and may be candidates for newer treatments [51].

History of CVD is the strongest predictor of mortality among patients with ADPKD [55]. Hypertensive ADPKD patients also have a greater incidence of target organ damage compared with other age-matched hypertensive patients. Nearly 50% of hypertensive ADPKD patients exhibit left ventricular hypertrophy on echocardiography [56].

4.2.4 Treatment of Hypertension in ADPKD

Control of hypertension and other cardiovascular risk factors is a key aspect of early ADPKD management. Cardiovascular disease is the leading cause of premature death in people with ADPKD; therefore, risk management need to be extremely careful.

Current KDIGO Guidelines for Blood Pressure Management [57] suggest an SBP target of <120 mmHg without signaling DBP targets or limits for reduction, and this recommendation could be in line with the results of the HALT study [21]. Contrariwise, no other Guideline on hypertension recommends such a straight target [58–61] (but the Canadian Hypertension Society, only for high-risk patients) [62]. In the HALT-PKD study, intensive BP control (95–110/60–75 mmHg) was associated with 14.2% lower increase in total kidney volume and 3.77% lower urinary albumin excretion, but there was no difference in estimated glomerular filtration rate compared with standard treatment (120–130/70–80 mmHg). In the same way, a greater decline in the left ventricular mass index was observed [21]. A post hoc analysis in patients with ADPKD with rapid chronic kidney disease progression indicated that tight BP control is associated with both slower annual total kidney volume increase (6.4% vs. 7.8%; $p = 0.03$) and estimated glomerular filtration rate slope (−3.57 vs −4.37 mL/min/1.73 m^2 per year; $p = 0.05$) [63]. Nevertheless, this is a small difference. In general, and as in the rest of the population with kidney disease, a goal of BP <140/90 mmHg is recommended (ideally, and in case of good tolerance to treatment, aiming for a goal around 130/80 mmHg). They recommended to lower SBP to a range of 130–139 mmHg, but never below 130 mmHg [60], since the risk for a J curve increase of mortality has been found in CKD patients [64]. However, it has been suggested in young patients (<50 years) with normal renal function that it seems reasonable to seek this stricter BP target, taking into account individual tolerance [65].

ACEIs or ARBs are usually recommended as the first-line antihypertensives in ADPKD since the main etiological mechanism in the genesis of hypertension seems to be the activation of the RAAS [66]. Nonetheless, this recommendation is not based on any randomized clinical trial. In a secondary analysis of the HALT-PKD study [67], patients were categorized into high- and low-dose groups based on the median daily equivalent dose of RAA-blocking drugs used after the initial dose titration period. Subjects in the high-dose group ($n = 252$) did not experience a slower increase in total kidney volume than those in the low-dose ($n = 225$) group, after adjustment for age, sex, genotype, and BP arm. The chronic slope of eGFR decline was similar in both groups.

The combined use of ACE inhibitors and ARBs was tested in the HALT study and did not show additional benefits over the use of one of them, neither in ADPKD progression nor in the cardiovascular risk, so their joint use is not recommended [21]. Calcium channel blockers (due to their theoretical deleterious effect in worsening the disease) and diuretics (because they activate the RAAS) should be reserved for cases of resistant HTN and for those patients with renal failure and fluid overload and beta-blockers would probably be second-line antihypertensive drugs. In spite of these theoretical considerations about diuretics, in the PKD-HALT trials, the second line of treatment after RAAS blockade was a diuretic and the third, metoprolol. Again, there is no available information coming from well-designed clinical trial to answer these questions. Therefore, current recommendations about high blood pressure in CKD should be used [60]. In this regard, the safety of hydrochorotiazide use seems warranted [68].

A Cochrane review included 30 studies (2039 participants) that investigated 11 pharmacological interventions for ADPKD (ACEi, ARBs, calcium channel blockers, beta-blockers, vasopressin receptor 2 antagonists, mammalian target of rapamycin inhibitors, somatostatin analogues, antiplatelet agents, eicosapentaenoic acids, statins, and vitamin D compounds) [23]. ACEi significantly reduced diastolic blood pressure, but had uncertain effects on kidney volumes, GFR, and serum creatinine, in data largely restricted to children. ACEi did not show different effects on GFR and albuminuria when compared with beta-blockers. When compared with ARBs no differences in these parameters were found. Data for calcium channel blockers were inconclusive.

4.2.5 Effects of Tolvaptan on Blood Pressure

The V2 receptor antagonist tolvaptan is prescribed to patients with ADPKD disease to slow CKD progression. Tolvaptan could theoretically induce changes on BP. In the short term, via increased V1a receptor activation, it can produce an increase in vascular resistance and thus, high blood pressure [69, 70]. However, V1a receptor activation may have other effects. It also increases natriuresis, thereby potentially decreasing BP. Moreover, preventing vasopressin binding to the V2 receptor could result in a reduction of BP because of loss of V2 receptor-mediated ENaC channel activation, and therefore, sodium reabsorption, and loss of circulating volume due to aquaresis [71]. In addition, loss of renin-angiotensin-aldosterone system (RAAS) activation due to a decrease in V2 receptor-dependent renin production could also get BP down [72].

The results of a post hoc study of the TEMPO 3:4 trial, which included 1445 patients with autosomal dominant polycystic kidney disease randomized 2:1 to tolvaptan or placebo for 3 years, have been reported [73]. The conclusion was that treatment with tolvaptan in patients with ADPKD does not have a clinically significant short-term effect on BP. During long-term use, however, gradually BP becomes lower in patients on tolvaptan compared with patients on placebo. When after 3 years of treatment tolvaptan was stopped, it was detected an increase in BP in tolvaptan-treated patients up to a level that was again similar to that of the placebo-treated subjects. This increase may produce some concerns since tolvaptan is withdrawn when the patient reaches end-stage renal failure, but there is no clinical data on this issue.

A small study ($n = 13$) has investigated the short-term effects of the addition of hydrochlorothiazide to tolvaptan. During hydrochlorothiazide treatment, there was a statistically significant decrease in GFR (about 4 mL/min per 1.73 m). No serious adverse events were recorded during the study. Plasma potassium was lower during hydrochlorothiazide treatment compared with placebo. Osmolar excretion did not change during hydrochlorothiazide (an important parameter to evaluate the effectivity of tolvaptan treatment). During hydrochlorothiazide treatment, there were decreases in body weight, *N*-terminal pro-brain natriuretic peptide (NTproBNP), systolic BP, and measured GFR, consistent with a decrease in extracellular volume. Urinary aquaporin-2 excretion did not change during any treatment period. Seven (54%) participants experienced better quality of life during hydrochlorothiazide treatment as compared with baseline. Therefore, it seems that the use of hydrochlorothiazide is safe in patients treated with tolvaptan [74].

4.3 Recessive Polycystic Kidney Disease

Autosomal recessive polycystic kidney disease (ARPKD) is an inherited disease characterized by a malformation complex which includes cystically dilated tubules in the kidneys and ductal plate malformation in the liver. It is a cause of significant renal and liver-related morbidity and mortality in children. The majority of individuals with ARPKD present in the neonatal period with enlarged echogenic kidneys. Renal disease is characterized by nephromegaly, hypertension, and varying degrees of renal dysfunction. More than 50% of affected individuals with ARPKD progress to end-stage renal disease within the first decade of life.

All typical forms of ARPKD are caused by mutations in a single gene, PKHD1 (polycystic kidney and hepatic disease 1). This gene encodes polyductin production. This is a 4074-amino acid protein expressed in the cytoplasm, plasma membrane, and primary apical cilia, a structure that has been implicated in the pathogenesis of different polycystic kidney diseases. In fact, cholangiocytes isolated from an ARPKD rat model develop shorter and dysmorphic cilia, suggesting polyductin to be important for normal ciliary morphology. Polyductin seems also to participate in tubule morphogenesis and cell mitotic orientation along the tubular axis [75].

ARPKD has an estimated incidence of 1 in 20,000 live births [76]. The most severely affected cases are identified in utero and characterized by the development of enlarged and echogenic kidneys in diseased fetuses. The decreased fetal urine output, in turn, leads to oligohydramnios and, possibly, to pulmonary hypoplasia. The ARPKD kidney image is typically characterized by bilateral massively enlarged reniform kidneys with poor corticomedullary differentiation on ultrasound. Traditionally, a high death rate (up to 30%) shortly after birth from respiratory insufficiency was found, but a more recent calculation for the United States revealed a survival rate of 79% for the period between 2010 and 2014. Furthermore, the 10-year survival of those patients being managed in the first month of life was found to be very high [77].

The underlying pathophysiology resulting in the high blood pressure in ARPKD is not completely understood, but dysregulation of renal sodium and volume handling with impaired urinary dilution and an activation of the renin-angiotensin system have been suggested [78]. In a rat model of ARPKD, the relationship of intrarenal and systemic RAS activation, hypertension, and renal function at different stages of cystic kidney disease was assessed. The authors reported that increased intrarenal expression of the RAS components, renin, ACE, and angiotensin II is a feature of cystic kidney disease in the polycystic rat. Surprisingly, systemic levels of Ang I and Ang II were not elevated. Therefore, intrarenal renin and ACE gene upregulation were proposed as a novel mechanism for hypertension development or exacerbation in ARPKD [79].

A common and severe problem of ARPKD in the first few months of life is arterial hypertension that may be very severe and may require treatment with multiple drug classes. An ABPM study revealed ambulatory hypertension in 94% of children [80]. RAAS blockers are recommended to be the treatment of choice due to experimental observations, but there is no information from well-designed randomized clinical trials. Antihypertensives should be directed toward optimizing blood pressure control, while minimizing further reduction in GFR in the context of CKD general management. In this regard, the "Effect of Strict Blood Pressure Control and ACE Inhibition on the Progression of CRF in Pediatric Patients" (ESCAPE) trial in children with CKD stages 2–4 indicated that straight blood pressure control (target 24-h mean arterial blood pressure below the 50th percentile for age, height, and sex) might decrease progression to end-stage renal disease [81]. Nonetheless, no specific target for ARPKD has been established.

Hypertension may be aggravated by substitution of sodium chloride given for hyponatremia that is frequently observed as a transient finding in ARPKD mainly in the first year of life. For treatment of hyponatremia in ARPKD, general principles apply. In euvolemic or hypervolemic patients, fluid intake with nutrition should be minimized, e.g., by concentrating feeds [82].

4.4 Renal Cyst

They are thought to be present in up to 5% of the general population. This prevalence increases to more than 25% in people older than 50 years of age. In the elderly population, renal cysts can account for up to 65–70% of the renal masses. The prevalence of renal cysts is higher in patients with hypertension and smoking history [83]. There is no evidence that simple renal cyst can cause hypertension, although it could be possible to find high blood pressure associated with renal neoplasm [84] that could have cystic image at radiology. The Bosniak classification (Table 4.3) [85] is widely used by radiologists and urologists for addressing the clinical problem assessing renal cysts to differentiate from neoplasms. Patients with incidentally found Bosniak type I or II cysts should be assured there is a minimal chance of malignancy and no scheduled follow-up is required [86].

Table 4.3 2019 Bosniak classification for renal cysts

Bosniak I	Well-defined, thin (≤2 mm) smooth wall; homogeneous simple fluid (−9 to 20 HU); no septa or calcifications; the wall may enhance
Bosniak II	
Type 1	Cystic masses with thin (≤2 mm) and few (1–3) septa; septa and wall may enhance; may have calcification of any type
Type 2	Homogeneous hyperattenuating (≥70 HU) masses at non-contrast CT
Type 3	Homogeneous non-enhancing masses >20 HU at renal mass protocol CT. May have calcification of any type
Type 4	Homogeneous masses −9 to 20 HU at non-contrast CT
Type 5	Homogeneous masses 21 to 30 HU at portal venous phase CT
Type 6	Homogeneous low-attenuation masses that are too small to characterize
Bosniak IIF	
Type 1	Cystic masses with a smooth minimally thickened (3 mm) enhancing wall, or smooth minimal thickening (3 mm) of one or more enhancing septa
Type 2	Cystic masses with many (≥4) smooth thin (≤2 mm) enhancing septa
Bosniak III	One or more enhancing thick (≥4 mm width) or enhancing irregular (displaying ≤3 mm obtusely margined convex protrusion[s]) walls or septa
Bosniak IV	One or more enhancing nodules (≥4 mm convex protrusion with obtuse margins, or a convex protrusion of any size that has acute margins)

Torres et al. [87] reported that, at least in some patients, renal cyst formation may be a result of severe hypokalemia rather than a simple association. The study compared patients with aldosteronism and hypokalemia with controls with essential hypertension. Renal cyst formation was significantly more common in patients with hypokalemia and aldosteronism, and the extent of cyst development correlated with lower potassium levels. The cysts were more frequent in patients with adrenal tumors than in those with idiopathic adrenal hyperplasia. Furthermore, removal of the adrenal adenomas resulted in regression of the cysts which also corresponded to the normalization of serum potassium levels. Novello et al. have reported very similar results [88], so that the association of renal cyst and hypokalemia should raise the suspicion of hyperaldosteronism in hypertensive patients.

4.5 Conclusions

ADPKD is frequently associated with arterial hypertension. Uncontrolled high blood pressure seems to be involved in the faster decline of renal function. Therefore, measurement of blood pressure in these patients, even when they are still asymptomatic children, is needed. Adequate, and not delayed, treatment of high blood pressure should be performed, and renin-angiotensin-axis blockers are usually recommended as the main component of antihypertensive therapy.

Recessive polycystic kidney disease is a very less common pathology but has a faster progression to chronic renal dysfunction (usually in the first decade of life). A common problem in the first few months of life is arterial hypertension that may be very severe and may require treatment with multiple drug classes.

Although single kidney cysts are very common ultrasound findings, they are usually not related to high blood pressure. Nevertheless, they could be associated with hypokalemia due to hyperaldosteronism.

References

1. Spithosven EM, Kramer A, Meijer E, et al. Renal replacement therapy for autosomal dominant polycystic kidney disease (ADPKD) in Europe: prevalence and survival - an analysis of data from the ERA-EDTA registry. Nephrol Dial Transplant. 2014;29(Suppl 4):iv15–25.
2. Kuo IY, Chapman AB. Polycystins, ADPKD, and cardiovascular disease. Kidney Int Rep. 2019;5:396–406.
3. Brook-Carter PT, Peral B, Ward CJ, et al. Deletion of the TSC2 and PKD1 genes associated with severe infantile polycystic kidney disease—a contiguous gene syndrome. Nat Genet. 1994;8:328–32.
4. Chapman AB, Devuyst O, Eckardt KU, et al. Autosomal-dominant polycystic kidney disease (ADPKD): executive summary from a Kidney Disease: Improving Global Outcomes (KDIGO) Controversies Conference. Kidney Int. 2015;88:17–27.
5. Pei Y, Hwang YH, Conklin J, et al. Imaging-based diagnosis of autosomal dominant polycystic kidney disease. J Am Soc Nephrol. 2015;26:746–53.
6. Harris PC, Torres VE. Polycystic kidney disease, autosomal dominant. In: Adam MP, Mirzaa GM, Pagon RA, et al., editors. GeneReviews® [Internet]. Seattle (WA): University of Washington, Seattle; 1993–2023. 2002 Jan 10 [updated 2022 Sep 29].

7. Pei Y, Obaji J, Dupuis A, et al. Unified criteria for ultrasonographic diagnosis of ADPKD. J Am Soc Nephrol. 2009;20:205–12.
8. Seeman T, Jansky P, Filip F, Bláhová K, Jaroš A. Increasing prevalence of hypertension during long-term follow-up in children with autosomal dominant polycystic kidney disease. Pediatr Nephrol. 2021;36:3717–23.
9. Dicks E, Ravani P, Langman D, Davidson WS, Pei Y, Parfrey PS. Incident renal events and risk factors in autosomal dominant polycystic kidney disease: a population and family-based cohort followed for 22 years. Clin J Am Soc Nephrol. 2006;1:710–7.
10. Cornec-Le Gall E, Audrézet MP, Chen JM, et al. Type of PKD1 mutation influences renal outcome in ADPKD. J Am Soc Nephrol. 2013;24:1006–13.
11. Grantham JJ. Clinical practice: autosomal dominant polycystic kidney disease. N Engl J Med. 2008;359:1477–85.
12. Grantham JJ, Chapman AB, Torres VE. Volume progression in autosomal dominant polycystic kidney disease: the major factor determining clinical outcomes. Clin J Am Soc Nephrol. 2005;1:148–57.
13. Torres VA, Harris PC. Autosomal dominant polycystic kidney disease. In: Floege J, Johnson RJ, Feehally J, editors. Comprehensive clinical nephrology. St Louis, MO: Elsevier; 2010. p. 529–42.
14. Chapman AB, Johnson A, Gabow PA, Schrier RW. The renin-angiotensinaldosterone system and autosomal dominant polycystic kidney disease. N Engl J Med. 1990;323:1091–6.
15. Doulton TW, Saggar-Malik AK, He FJ, et al. The effect of sodium and angiotensin-converting enzyme inhibition on the classic circulating renin-angiotensin system in autosomal-dominant polycystic kidney disease patients. J Hypertens. 2006;24:939–45.
16. Zeier M, Fehrenbach P, Geberth S, Möhring K, Waldherr R, Ritz E. Renal histology in polycystic kidney disease with incipient and advanced renal failure. Kidney Int. 1992;42:1259–65.
17. Graham PC, Lindop GB. The anatomy of the renin-secreting cell in adult polycystic kidney disease. Kidney Int. 1988;33:1084–90.
18. Torres VE, Donovan KA, Scicli G, et al. Synthesis of renin by tubulocystic epithelium in autosomal-dominant polycystic kidney disease. Kidney Int. 1992;42:364–73.
19. Loghman-Adham M, Soto CE, Inagami T, Cassis L. The intrarenal reninangiotensin system in autosomal dominant polycystic kidney disease. Am J Physiol Renal Physiol. 2004;287:F775–88.
20. Lawson CR, Doulton TW, MacGregor GA. Autosomal dominant polycystic kidney disease: role of the renin-angiotensin system in raised blood pressure in progression of renal and cardiovascular disease. J Renin-Angiotensin-Aldosterone Syst. 2006;7:139–45.
21. Schrier RW, Abebe KZ, Perrone RD, et al. Blood pressure in early autosomal dominant polycystic kidney disease. N Engl J Med. 2014;371:2255–66.
22. van Dijk MA, Breuning MH, Duiser R, van Es LA, Westendorp RG. No effect of enalapril on progression in autosomal dominant polycystic kidney disease. Nephrol Dial Transplant. 2003;18:2314–20.
23. Bolignano D, Palmer SC, Ruospo M, Zoccali C, Craig JC, Strippoli GF. Interventions for preventing the progression of autosomal dominant polycystic kidney disease. Cochrane Database Syst Rev. 2015;2015(7):CD010294.
24. Riccio E, Esposito G, Franzone A, Imbriaco M, Santangelo M, Pisani A. Renal sympathetic-nerve ablation for uncontrolled hypertension in a patient with single-kidney autosomal dominant polycystic kidney disease. J Clin Hypertens. 2014;16:385–6.
25. Klein IHHT, Ligtenberg G, Oey PL, Koomans HA, Blankestijn PJ. Sympathetic activity is increased in polycystic kidney disease and is associated with hypertension. J Am Soc Nephrol. 2001;12:2427–33.
26. Gattone VH 2nd, Siqueira TM Jr, Powell CR, Trambaugh CM, Lingeman JE, Shalhav AL. Contribution of renal innervation to hypertension in rat autosomal dominant polycystic kidney disease. Exp Biol Med (Maywood). 2008;233:952–7.
27. Cerasola G, Vecchi M, Mulè G, et al. Sympathetic activity and blood pressure pattern in autosomal dominant polycystic kidney disease hypertensives. Am J Nephrol. 1998;18:391–8.

28. Brookes ZL, Ruff L, Upadhyay VS, et al. Pkd2 mesenteric vessels exhibit a primary defect in endothelium-dependent vasodilatation restored by rosiglitazone. Am J Physiol Heart Circ Physiol. 2013;304:H33–41.
29. Wang D, Braendstrup O, Larsen S, Horn T, Strandgaard S. The expression and activity of renal nitric oxide synthase and circulating nitric oxide in polycystic kidney disease rats. APMIS. 2004;112:358–68.
30. Wang D, Braendstrup O, Larsen S, Horn T, Strandgaard S. Endothelial dysfunction and reduced nitric oxide in resistance arteries in autosomal-dominant polycystic kidney disease. Kidney Int. 2003;64:1381–8.
31. Heffernan KS, Kuvin JT, Sarnak MJ, et al. Peripheral augmentation index and vascular inflammation in autosomal dominant polycystic kidney disease. Nephrol Dial Transplant. 2011;26:2515–21.
32. Blankestijn PJ. Sympathetic hyperactivity in chronic kidney disease. Nephrol Dial Transplant. 2004;19:1354–7.
33. Stefanakis N, Ziroyiannis P, Trygonis S, Lamnissou K. Modifier effect of the Glu298Asp polymorphism of endothelial nitric oxide synthase gene in autosomal-dominant polycystic kidney disease. Nephron Clin Pract. 2008;110:c101–6.
34. Devuyst O, Persu A, Vo-Cong MT. Autosomal dominant polycystic kidney disease: modifier genes and endothelial dysfunction. Nephrol Dial Transplant. 2003;18:2211–5.
35. Elumalai R, Periasamy S, Ramanathan G, Lakkakula BV. Role of endothelial nitric oxide synthase VNTR (intron 4 a/b) polymorphism on the progression of renal disease in autosomal dominant polycystic kidney disease. J Renal Inj Prev. 2014;3:69–73.
36. Xue C, Zhou CC, Sun LJ, et al. Effects of endothelial nitric oxide synthase gene on end stage renal disease progression in autosomal dominant polycystic kidney disease. Nephrology (Carlton). 2014;19:630–7.
37. Luo L, Roy S, Li L, Ma M. Polycystic kidney disease: novel insights into polycystin function. Trends Mol Med. 2023;29:268–81.
38. Chapman AB, Stepniakowski K, Rahbari-Oskoui F. Hypertension in autosomal dominant polycystic kidney disease. Adv Chronic Kidney Dis. 2010;17:153–63.
39. Torres VE, King BF, Chapman AB, et al. Magnetic resonance measurements of renal blood flow and disease progression in autosomal dominant polycystic kidney disease. Clin J Am Soc Nephrol. 2007;2:112–20.
40. Ecder T, Schrier RW. Cardiovascular abnormalities in autosomaldominant polycystic kidney disease. Nat Rev Nephrol. 2009;5:221–8.
41. Schrier RW, Johnson AM, McFann K, Chapman AB. The role of parental hypertension in the frequency and age of diagnosis of hypertension in offspring with autosomal-dominant polycystic kidney disease. Kidney Int. 2003;64:1792–9.
42. Gabow PA, Johnson AM, Kaehny WD, et al. Factors affecting the progression of renal disease in autosomal-dominant polycystic kidney disease. Kidney Int. 1992;41:1311–9.
43. Seeman T, Dusek J, Vondrichová H, et al. Ambulatory blood pressure correlates with renal volume and number of renal cysts in children with autosomal dominant polycystic kidney disease. Blood Press Monit. 2003;8:107–10.
44. Cadnapaphornchai MA, McFann K, Strain JD, Masoumi A, Schrier RW. Prospective change in renal volume and function in children with ADPKD. Clin J Am Soc Nephrol. 2009;4:820–9.
45. Helal I, Reed B, McFann K, et al. Glomerular hyperfiltration and renal progression in children with autosomal dominant polycystic kidney disease. Clin J Am Soc Nephrol. 2011;6:2439–43.
46. Cadnapaphornchai MA, McFann K, Strain JD, Masoumi A, Schrier RW. Increased left ventricular mass in children with autosomal dominant polycystic kidney disease and borderline hypertension. Kidney Int. 2008;74:1192–6.
47. Cadnapaphornchai MA, Masoumi A, Strain JD, McFann K, Schrier RW. Magnetic resonance imaging of kidney and cyst volume in children with ADPKD. Clin J Am Soc Nephrol. 2011;6:369–76.

48. Selistre L, de Souza V, Ranchin B, Hadj-Aissa A, Cochat P, Dubourg L. Early renal abnormalities in children with postnatally diagnosed autosomal dominant polycystic kidney disease Pediatr Nephrol. 2012;27:1589–93.
49. Mekahli D, Woolf AS, Bockenhauer D. Similar renal outcomes in children with ADPKD diagnosed by screening or presenting with symptoms. Pediatr Nephrol. 2010;25:2275–82.
50. Martínez V, Furlano M, Sans L, et al. Participants in the REPQRAD. Autosomal dominant polycystic kidney disease in young adults. Clin Kidney J. 2022;16:985–95.
51. Massella L, Mekahli D, Paripović D, et al. Prevalence of hypertension in children with early-stage ADPKD. Clin J Am Soc Nephrol. 2018;13:874–83.
52. Gimpel C, Bergmann C, Bockenhauer D, et al. International consensus statement on thediagnosis and management of autosomal dominant polycystic kidney disease in children and young people. Nat Rev Nephrol. 2019;15:713–26.
53. Grantham JJ. Rationale for early treatment of polycystic kidney disease. Pediatr Nephrol. 2015;30:1053–62.
54. Torres VE, Abebe KZ, Chapman AB, et al. HALT-PKD Trial Investigators. Angiotensin blockade in late autosomal dominant polycystic kidney disease. N Engl J Med. 2014;371:2267–76.
55. Abou Heidar N, Chehab O, Morsi RZ, et al. Association of autosomal dominant polycystic kidney disease with cardiovascular disease: a US-National Inpatient Perspective. Clin Exp Nephrol. 2022;26:659–68.
56. Chapman AB, Johnson AM, Rainguet S, Hossack K, Gabow P Schrier RW. Left ventricular hypertrophy in autosomal dominant polycystic kidney disease. J Am Soc Nephrol. 1997;8:1292–7.
57. Kidney Disease: Improving Global Outcomes (KDIGO) Blood Pressure Work Group. KDIGO 2021 clinical practice guideline for the management of blood pressure in chronic kidney disease. Kidney Int. 2021;99(3S):S1–S87.
58. Mancia G, Kreutz R, Brunström M, et al. Authors/Task Force Members. 2023 ESH Guidelines for the management of arterial hypertension The Task Force for the management of arterial hypertension of the European Society of Hypertension Endorsed by the European Renal Association (ERA) and the International Society of Hypertension (ISH). J Hypertens. 2023;41:1874–2071. https://doi.org/10.1097/HJH.0000000000003480.
59. Hypertension in adults: diagnosis and management NICE guideline. 2019 Aug 28 [cited 2023 Jan 21]. Available from: www.nice.org.uk/guidance/ng
60. Unger T, Borghi C, Charchar F, et al. 2020 International Society of Hypertension global hypertension practice guidelines. Hypertension. 2020;75:1334–57.
61. Whelton PK, Carey RM, Aronow WS, et al. 2017 ACC/AHA/AAPA/ABC/ACPM/AGS/APhA/ASH/ASPC/NMA/PCNA Guideline for the prevention, detection, evaluation, and management of high blood pressure in adults: executive summary: a report of the American College of Cardiology/American Heart Association Task Force on clinical practice guidelines. Hypertension. 2018;71:1269–324.
62. Rabi DM, McBrien KA, Sapir-Pichhadze R, et al. Hypertension Canada's 2020 comprehensive guidelines for the prevention, diagnosis, risk assessment, and treatment of hypertension in adults and children. Can J Cardiol. 2020;36:596–624.
63. Irazabal MV, Abebe KZ, Bae KT, et al. Prognostic enrichment design in clinical trials for autosomal dominant polycystic kidney disease: the HALT-PKD clinical trial. Nephrol Dial Transplant. 2017;32:1857–65.
64. Robles NR, Villa J, Fici F. KDIGO guidelines for the management of blood pressure in chronic kidney disease: a sprint to the curve. Eur J Intern Med. 2021;93:21–3.
65. Ars E, Bernis C, Fraga G, et al. Consensus document on autosomal dominant polycystic kidney disease from the Spanish Working Group on inherited kindey diseases. Review 2020. Nefrologia (Engl Ed). 2022;42:367–89.
66. EAF co-chairs, Harris T, Sandford R, EAF members, Roundtable participants. European ADPKD Forum multidisciplinary position statement on autosomal dominant polycystic kidney disease care: European ADPKD Forum and Multispecialist Roundtable participants. Nephrol Dial Transplant. 2018;33 563–73.

67. Brosnahan GM, Abebe KZ, Moore CG, et al. The Halt Pkd Investigators. Determinants of progression in early autosomal dominant polycystic kidney disease: is it blood pressure or renin-angiotensin-aldosterone-system blockade? Curr Hypertens Rev. 2018;14:39–47.
68. Kramers BJ, Koorevaar IW, De Boer R, et al. DIPAK Consortium. Thiazide diuretics and the rate of disease progression in autosomal dominant polycystic kidney disease: an observational study. Nephrol Dial Transplant. 2021;36:1828–36.
69. Miyazaki T, Fujiki H, Yamamura Y, Nakamura S, Mori T. Tolvaptan, an orally active vasopressin V(2)-receptor antagonist - pharmacology and clinical trials. Cardiovasc Drug Rev. 2007;25:1–13.
70. Feng JJ, Arendshorst WJ. Enhanced renal vasoconstriction induced by vasopressin in SHR is mediated by V1 receptors. Am J Phys. 1996;271:F304–13.
71. Bankir L, Bichet DG, Bouby N. Vasopressin V2 receptors, ENaC, and sodium reabsorption: a risk factor for hypertension? Am J Physiol Renal Physiol. 2010;299:F917–28.
72. Gonzalez AA, Cifuentes-Araneda F, Ibaceta-Gonzalez C, et al. Vasopressin/V2 receptor stimulates renin synthesis in the collecting duct. Am J Physiol Renal Physiol. 2016;310:F284–93.
73. Heida JE, Gansevoort RT, Torres VE, et al. The effect of tolvaptan on BP in polycystic kidney disease: a post hoc analysis of the TEMPO 3:4 trial. J Am Soc Nephrol. 2021;32:1801–12.
74. Kramers BJ, Koorevaar IW, van Gastel MDA, et al. Effects of hydrochlorothiazide and metformin on aquaresis and nephroprotection by a vasopressin V2 receptor antagonist in ADPKD: a randomized crossover trial. Clin J Am Soc Nephrol. 2022;17:507–17.
75. Menezes LF, Cai Y, Nagasawa Y, et al. Polyductin, the PKHD1 gene product, comprises isoforms expressed in plasma membrane, primary cilium, and cytoplasm. Kidney Int. 2004;66:1345–55.
76. Guay-Woodford LM, Desmond RA. Autosomal recessive polycystic kidney disease: the clinical experience in North America. Pediatrics. 2003;111:1072–80.
77. Alzarka B, Morizono H, Bollman JW, Kim D, Guay-Woodford LM. Design and implementation of the Hepatorenal Fibrocystic Disease Core Center clinical database: a centralized resource for characterizing autosomal recessive polycystic kidney disease and other hepatorenal fibrocystic diseases. Front Pediatr. 2017;5:80. https://doi.org/10.3389/fped.2017.00080.
78. Loghman-Adham M, Soto CE, Inagami T, Sotelo-Avila C. Expression of components of the reninangiotensin system in autosomal recessive polycystic kidney disease. J Histochem Cytochem. 2005;53:979–88.
79. Goto M, Hoxha N, Osman R, Dell KM. The renin-angiotensin system and hypertension in autosomal recessive polycystic kidney disease. Pediatr Nephrol. 2010;25:2449–57.
80. Seeman T, Blažík R, Fencl F, et al. Ambulatory blood pressure and hypertension control in children with autosomal recessive polycystic kidney disease: clinical experience from two central European tertiary centres. J Hypertens. 2022;40:425–31.
81. ESCAPE Trial Group, Wuhl E, Trivelli A, et al. Strict blood-pressure control and progression of renal failure in children. N Engl J Med. 2009;361:1639–50.
82. Guay-Woodford LM, Bissler JJ, Braun MC, et al. Consensus expert recommendations for the diagnosis and management of autosomal recessive polycystic kidney disease: report of an international conference. J Pediatr. 2014;165:611–7.
83. Mensel B, Kühn JP, Kracht F, et al. Prevalence of renal cysts and association with risk factors in a general population: an MRI-based study. Abdom Radiol (NY). 2018;43:3068–74.
84. Handler J. Renal cell carcinoma and hypertension. J Clin Hypertens (Greenwich). 2005;7:249–51.
85. Schieda N, Davenport MS, Krishna S, et al. Bosniak classification of cystic renal masses, version 2019: a pictorial guide to clinical use. Radiographics. 2021;41:814–28.
86. Warren KS, Mcfarlane J. The Bosniak classification of renal cystic masses. BJU Int. 2005;95:939–42.
87. Torres VE, Young WF Jr, Offord KP, Hattery RR. Association of hypokalemia, aldosteronism, and renal cysts. N Engl J Med. 1990;322:345–51.
88. Novello M, Catena C, Nadalini E, et al. Renal cysts and hypokalemia in primary aldosteronism: results of long-term follow-up after treatment. J Hypertens. 2007;25:1443–50.

Chemically Induced Hypertension: Antineoplastic Agents Associated with High Blood Pressure

5

Emily Moss and Anushree C. Shirali

5.1 Introduction

Cancer and cardiovascular disease (CVD) are leading causes of morbidity and mortality for individuals in the United States and across the globe [1, 2]. As of 2023, the estimated incidence of cancer increased to 1.9 million cases in the United States with over 600,000 cancer-related deaths [3]. Worldwide, the incidence of cancer cases has exceeded 19 million and is estimated to reach >28 million by 2040 [4]. Despite the rising incidence of cancer and its impact on population mortality, cancer death rates have actually decreased in the past few decades. From 1991 to 2020, studies estimate a 33% reduction in the cancer death rate amounting to roughly 3.8 million deaths averted [3]. With a growing population of survivors of cancer, more attention is focused on studying the long-term consequences of anticancer agents.

Hypertension is one of the major risk factors associated with the development of CVD and its prevalence is notably higher in cancer patients or survivors of cancer [5]. One study found that the cumulative prevalence of hypertension increased by age in survivors of childhood cancer, surpassing 70% by age 50 [6]. In comparison, the general prevalence of hypertension in the United States is roughly 45% [7]. Hypertension may develop due to lifestyle choices (e.g., smoking, physical inactivity, poor diet) or the presence of certain comorbid conditions (e.g., obesity, diabetes, chronic kidney disease). However, in patients with cancer, hypertension is also linked to several antineoplastic agents, with increased risk in patients receiving combination anticancer therapy [8].

E. Moss
Department of Internal Medicine, Yale University School of Medicine, New Haven, CT, USA

A. C. Shirali (✉)
Section of Nephrology, Yale University School of Medicine, New Haven, CT, USA
e-mail: anushree.shirali@yale.edu

A. E. Berbari et al. (eds.), *Blood Pressure Disorders in Acute and Chronic Kidney Diseases*, Updates in Hypertension and Cardiovascular Protection,
https://doi.org/10.1007/978-3-031-81292-7_5

Long-standing hypertension increases risks of coronary artery disease, heart failure, valvular disease, arrhythmias, and cardiac death [5]. Given the potential for substantial harm, it is important to recognize the various anticancer agents that increase the risk of high blood pressure so that patients can be appropriately screened and treated. This chapter will focus on the prevalence and mechanism of hypertension with various antineoplastic agents. A summary of the reviewed drug classes and mechanisms of hypertension is included in Table 5.1. The chapter will also briefly touch on recommended screening and management strategies for patients receiving these treatments.

Table 5.1 List of antineoplastic drugs with hypertensive effects and potential mechanisms

Drug class	Drug name(s)	Proposed mechanism(s) for HTN
VEGF antagonists (VEGFi, VEGF-Ri, VEGF-TRAP, and VEGF-TKI)	Bevacizumab, Ramucirumab, Levatinib, Cabozantinib, Pazopanib, Sorafenib, Sunitinib, Vandetanib, Ziv-alibercept. Ponatinib, Axitinib	Inhibition of NO, microvascular rarefaction, decreased GFR/ sodium + water retention, etc. (see Fig. 5.1b)
Bruton TKI	Ibrutinib, Acalabrutinib, Zanubrutinib, Pirtobrutinib	Decreased NO production, inhibition of PI3K
Platinum agents	Cisplatin, carboplatin, oxaliplatin	Endothelial reactivity
Proteosome inhibitors	Bortezomib, Carfilzomib, Ixazomib	Increased oxidative stress, decreased NO production
Alkylating agents	Busulfan, Ifosfamide	Endothelial reactivity
BRAF/MEK inhibitors	Dabrafenib, Vemurafenib, Encorafenib, Trametinib, Binimetinib, Cobimetinib	Decreased NO production
Glucocorticoids	Prednisone, Prednisolone, Methylprednisolone, Dexamethasone	Decreased NO production, sodium + water retention
Calcineurin inhibitors	Tacrolimus, Cyclosporine	Inhibition of NO, sodium retention
Mammalian target of rapamycin inhibitors	Sirolimus, Everolimus	Decreased VEGF leading to decreased NO
RET TKIs	Pralsetinib, Selparcatinib, Vandetanib	Decreased CD47 leading to reduced NO, endothelial reactivity
Antiandrogen drugs	Abiraterone, Enzalutamide	Abiraterone: Inhibition of androgen and cortisol synthesis preferentially leading to increased mineralocorticoid production
PARP inhibitors	Niraparib	Off-target binding to norepinephrine and dopamine receptors

Abbreviations: *BRAF* fibrosarcoma B-type, CD47 cluster of differentiation 47, *GFR* glomerular filtration rate, *PI3K* phosphoinositide 3-kinase, *MEK* mitogen activated protein kinase kinase, *NO* nitric oxide, *PARP* poly ADP ribose polymerase, *R* receptor, *RET* rearranged during transfection, *TKIs* tyrosine kinase inhibitors, *VEGF* vascular endothelial growth factor, *GFR* glomerular filtration rate

5.1.1 Vascular Endothelial Growth Factor Signaling Pathway Inhibitors

Vascular endothelial growth factor (VEGF) signaling pathway inhibitors are the most widely recognized anticancer agents associated with hypertension [9]. Anti-VEGF agents oppose cancer growth by inhibiting angiogenesis, the formation of new blood vessels necessary for tumors to derive oxygen and nutrients for growth [10]. These pathway inhibitors, typically used to treat renal, hepatocellular, thyroid and gastrointestinal stromal cancers among others, include monoclonal antibodies against VEGF, monoclonal antibodies against VEGF-receptor, and tyrosine kinase inhibitors (TKIs). Examples of these medications include bevacizumab, sorafenib, sunitinib, dasatinib, and nilotinib. Less commonly used in cancer patients yet approved for clinical use in oncology is the VEGF-TRAP aflibercept, a fusion protein combining portions of the extracellular domains of VEGFR-1 and VEGFR-2 and the Fc portion of immunoglobulin G.

Incidence of hypertension in patients treated with anti-VEGF agents varies, ranging from 20% to 90% in some studies [9]. Certain factors such as age >60 and BMI higher than 25 appear to be associated with increased risk of anti-VEGF-related hypertension [11]. In patients with preexisting hypertension, use of these therapies increases the risk for significant blood pressure elevation during treatment [11]. Interestingly, the development of hypertension has been associated with increased survival with some suggesting that hypertension is a clinical biomarker to the efficacy of anti-VEGF treatment [12, 13].

VEGF is highly specific to the endothelium and its effects are mediated via its receptors (VEGFR-1, VEGFR-2, and VEGFR-3) [10] (Fig. 5.1). When VEGF binds to its receptors (principally the VEGFR-2 located on endothelial cells), it activates intrinsic tyrosine kinases which jumpstart downstream signaling cascades [14]. This ultimately results in phosphorylation of endothelial nitric oxide synthase (eNOS) and increased nitric oxide (NO) production. As NO migrates to vascular smooth muscle cells, vasodilation occurs. Along with vasodilatory effects, VEGF acts on the endothelial cells to migrate and invade the basement membrane, form fenestrations, and proliferate, thereby explaining its role in angiogenesis [15].

There are several proposed mechanisms for anti-VEGF-associated hypertension (Fig. 5.2). One potential mechanism is reduced NO production which synergizes with increased endothelin production to increase peripheral vasoconstriction. Other studies report increases in reactive oxygen species causing vascular oxidative stress as well as reduced microvascular density, termed rarefaction, leading to increase in peripheral vascular resistance [16]. The nephrotoxicity of VEGF inhibitors may result in reduced glomerular filtration rate and proteinuria, both of which may lead to salt and water retention, further increasing the risk of hypertension.

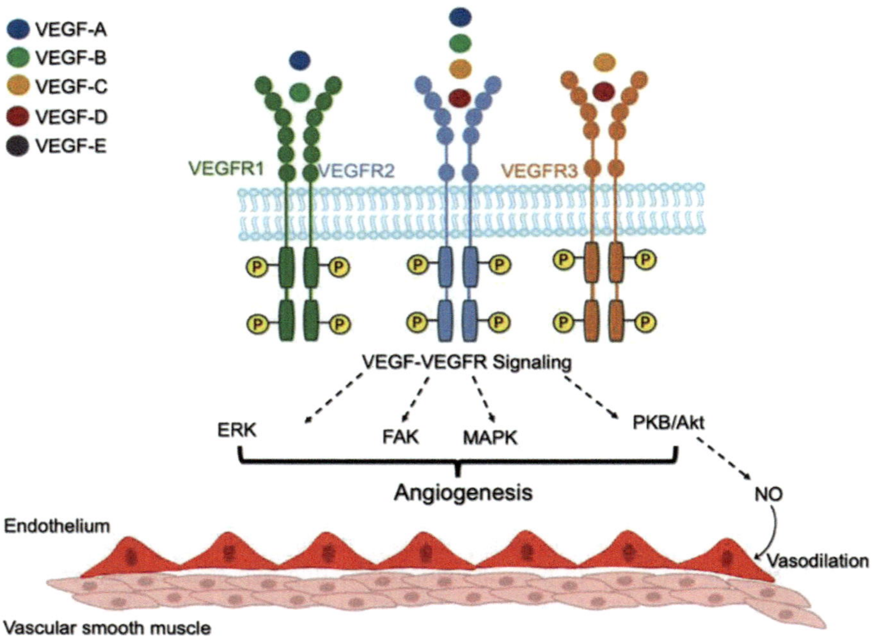

Fig. 5.1 Vascular endothelial growth factor (VEGF) binds to receptors (VEGFR) which initiates tyrosine kinase signaling in blood vascular endothelial (VEGFR-1, VEGFR-2) and lymphatic endothelial (VEGFR-3) cells. This engages a variety of different transcription factors that play a key role in angiogenesis via multiple mechanisms including nitric oxide (NO) production. Abbreviations: *Akt* Ak strain transforming, *ERK* extracellular signal regulating kinases, *FAK* focal adhesion kinase, *MAPK* mitogen activated protein kinase, *PKB* protein kinase B

5.1.2 Bruton Tyrosine Kinase Inhibitors

Bruton tyrosine kinase inhibitors (TKIs) such as ibrutinib, acalabrutinib, or pirtobrutinib are used primarily for the treatment of chronic lymphocytic leukemia and mantle cell leukemia. These small molecules act on Bruton tyrosine kinase to inhibit aberrant signaling of the B-cell production pathway [17]. The prevalence of hypertension related to Bruton TKIs varies with some studies citing rates close to 2–23% and others citing rates as high as 71% when focusing on ibrutinib specifically [18, 19]. In a meta-analysis involving over 2500 patients, this amounted to a 2.8 relative risk of hypertension with use of ibrutinib [19]. It is important to note that patients with chronic lymphocytic leukemia and mantle cell lymphoma may be treated for many years, thus increasing the lifetime risk of hypertension. The exact mechanisms underlying Bruton TKI-related hypertension remain unclear; however, some preliminary data suggest roles of decreased NO production as well as inhibition of the phosphoinositide 3-kinase (PI3K)/Akt pathway which indirectly downregulates PI3k-p110α [20, 21]. Inhibition of PI3k-p110α has been linked to histologic vascular tissue fibrosis [21].

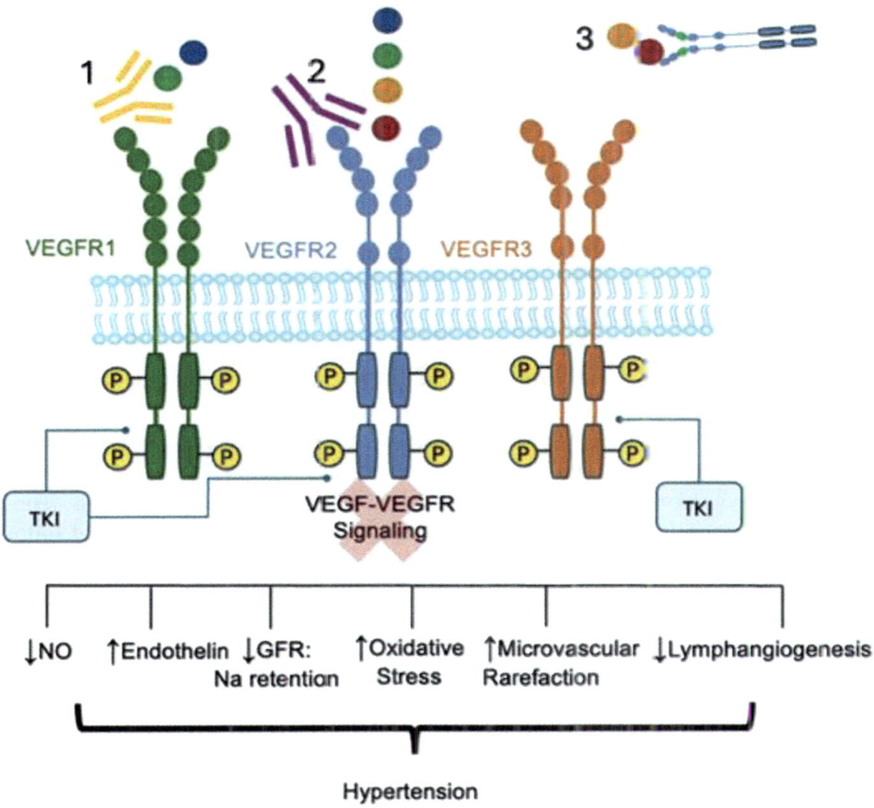

Fig. 5.2 Antagonism of VEGF signaling may occur via: 1. Anti-VEGF antibodies; 2. Anti-VEGFR antibodies; 3. Soluble VEGF decoy receptors (VEGF-Trap); and 4. Tyrosine kinase inhibitors (TKIs). Disruption of VEGF-VEGFR signaling results in hypertension via several mechanisms including changes in nitric oxide (NO) and endothelin levels, reduced glomerular filtration (GFR), increased oxidative stress, increased microvascular rarefaction, and decreased angiogenesis (blood and lymphatic vessels)

5.1.3 Platinum-Based Compounds

Platinum-based compounds, most commonly cisplatin, carboplatin, and oxaliplatin, are indicated in the treatment of bladder, breast, colorectal, ovarian, lung and testicular cancers, among others. Platinum-based chemotherapies assert their anticancer effect when platinum incorporation into DNA results in irreversible apoptotic damage in rapidly dividing cells. It is now recognized that the toxicity of platinum-based compounds extends well beyond the treatment period. Some studies cite detectable platinum levels in the blood up to 20 years after treatment and circulating platinum levels appear to correlate with side effects such as hypertension and renal dysfunction [22, 23]. In a cohort of testicular cancer survivors treated with cisplatin, hypertension was prevalent in 50–53% of the study population which was significantly higher than age- and testosterone-adjusted controls treated with surgery or radiation alone [24]. It is unclear if this effect was related to platinum-related nephrotoxicity as renal function of the participants was not reported. In another study of over 400 childhood cancer survivors, the prevalence of hypertension was more modest at 7–14% [25]. The mechanism of hypertension in these patients is thought to be related to the toxic effects of platinum on blood vessels resulting in endothelial activation and accelerated atherosclerosis [23].

5.1.4 Proteosome Inhibitors

Proteosome inhibitors mainly treat multiple myeloma and include agents such as bortezomib, carfilzomib, and ixazomib. Proteosomes degrade intracellular proteins and contribute to protein homeostasis. Proteosome inhibitors therefore prohibit the breakdown of proteins (including misfolded proteins) which accumulate to produce significant proteotoxic and oxidative stress, eventually triggering apoptosis. These agents preferentially target myeloma cells due to their excessive amount of immunoglobulin production [26, 27]. While effective for myeloma treatment, proteosome inhibition can adversely affect endothelial cells leading to intracellular oxidative stress, reduced NO availability, and accelerated vascular aging [28]. When treated with the proteosome inhibitors bortezomib and carfilzomib, hypertension was seen in 10% and 32% of multiple myeloma patients, respectively [29].

5.1.5 Alkylating Agents

Alkylating agents (busulfan, ifosfamide, and cyclophosphamide) inhibit transcription and replication of DNA, making them useful in the treatment of several hematologic and solid organ malignancies. Hypertension was seen in 25–36% of adults treated with busulfan and 58% of children [9]. In children previously treated with ifosfamide, hypertension was noted in 10% [25]. Data suggest that hypertension may be related to endothelial injury [9]. Ifosfamide specifically is known to cause nephrotoxicity via proximal tubulopathy which may later contribute to hypertension by facilitating development of chronic kidney disease. The role of cyclophosphamide in hypertension is unclear. Some studies do not show an association while others demonstrate decreased VEGF concentrations and endothelial dysfunction which are linked to hypertension [9, 30]. Of note, alkylating agents are often used in combination with other agents, especially glucocorticoids, which may make it more difficult to attribute specific adverse events to these agents.

5.1.6 Glucocorticoids

Glucocorticoids are most often administered in combination with other antineoplastic agents. Dosage of corticosteroids differs, and patients may be exposed to high doses or relatively low doses over longer periods of time. Hypertension is thought to be related to excess sodium and water reabsorption mediated by the mineralocorticoid receptor and decreased NO causing increased peripheral vascular resistance [31, 32]. Understanding of the likelihood or prevalence of high blood pressure with glucocorticoid treatment is mostly derived from studies in patients with chronic inflammatory diseases. In this setting, >30% of patients treated with chronic corticosteroids developed hypertension, especially when treated with doses of at least 7.5 mg prednisone equivalents [33, 34].

5.1.7 Calcineurin Inhibitors

In cancer treatment, calcineurin inhibitors (tacrolimus and cyclophosphamide) are typically used as adjunctive therapies to prevent rejection after bone marrow and solid organ transplantation. They work by decreasing interleukin-2 and interleukin-2 receptor expression, thereby reducing T-cell activation. Given their immunosuppressive effects, calcineurin inhibitors also prove efficacious in managing complications of stem cell transplantation such as graft versus host disease. Cyclosporine was the first calcineurin inhibitor released and its mechanism of hypertension is believed to be secondary to impaired NO-mediated vasodilation and renal sodium retention [35]. The prevalence of hypertension has now grown to 30–60% with more widespread use of cyclosporine [35, 36]. A recent study has shown that tacrolimus may affect blood pressure by inducing sodium retention and increasing angiotensin-II specific vasoconstriction [37].

5.1.8 Fibrosarcoma B-Type and Mitogen-Activated Protein Kinase Kinase Inhibitors

Fibrosarcoma B-type (BRAF) and mitogen-activated protein kinase kinase (MEK) inhibitors are employed to treat melanoma and BRAF-mutated colorectal cancers. These drugs both target aspects of the mitogen-activated protein kinase (MAPK) pathway which transduces signals from the cell surface to the nucleus to promote aspects of cell function, differentiation, and proliferation. By inhibiting mutated proteins involved in the MAPK pathway, BRAF and MEK inhibitors can block uncontrolled cell proliferation and halt tumor growth [38]. Examples of BRAF inhibitors include dabrafenib, vemurafenib, and encorafenib, and examples of MEK inhibitors include trametinib, binimetinib, and cobimetinib. These two drug classes are often coadministered to cause more complete blockage of the MAPK pathway.

In a meta-analysis involving over 2300 patients, the rate of hypertension in patients treated with BRAF inhibitors was 14%. This rose to 19.5% in patients treated with a combination of BRAF and MEK inihibitors [39]. BRAF and MEK inhibition is thought to disrupt the renin-angiotensin-aldosterone-system and decrease NO availability by impairing MAPK-associated VEGF signaling [39]. In melanoma cells in vitro, BRAF and MEK inhibition also upregulates expression of CD47 which blocks NO/cyclic guanosine monophosphate, thus reducing NO availability and leading to hypertension [38].

5.1.9 Mammalian Target of Rapamycin Inhibitors

Everolimus and sirolimus are mammalian target of rapamycin (mTOR) inhibitors typically administered as anticancer agents to patients with renal cell cancer, breast cancer, and pancreatic neuroendocrine tumors. mTOR plays a critical role in cell growth, metabolism, and proliferation, and hyperactivation of mTOR has been implicated in tumor growth. In patients with renal cell cancer treated with mTOR inhibitors, 10% developed high blood pressure [20]. When used in combination with VEGF inhibitors to treat renal cell cancer, hypertension was seen in 41% of patients [40]. In signaling pathways, mTOR also contributes to expression of VEGF. mTOR inhibitors may then lead to mechanisms of hypertension similar to VEGF inhibitors via decreased NO availability [20].

5.1.10 Rearranged During Transfection Receptor Kinase Inhibitors

Rearranged during transfection (RET) tyrosine kinase inhibitors such as selpercatinib and pralsetinib are used to treat non-small-cell lung cancer and thyroid cancers. RET is a tyrosine kinase receptor that, when activated, stimulates signaling pathways necessary for cell survival and proliferation. According to two major drug trials, hypertension is not uncommon in patients treated with RET kinase inhibitors. In fact, 35% of patients treated with selpercatinib and 40% of patients treated with pralsetinib developed hypertension [41]. RET kinase inhibitors may lead to hypertension by upregulating CD47 which eventually reduces NO availability in the endothelium [41].

5.1.11 Antiandrogen Therapies

In patients with metastatic prostate cancer, androgen deprivation therapy (ADT) is the cornerstone of treatment and works by targeting various aspects of the hypothalamic-pituitary-gonadal axis. Leuprolide, a gonadotropin-releasing hormone agonist, results in decreased androgen production by inhibiting luteinizing hormone and follicle stimulating hormone. Abiraterone is a direct inhibitor of androgen synthesis and enzalutamide is an androgen receptor antagonist. Abiraterone and enzalutamide, rather than leuprolide, are most often associated with hypertension. In one meta-analysis, the incidence of all grade hypertension with enzalutamide was 10.5% compared to 26.2% in abiraterone [42]. Abiraterone causes hypertension by inhibiting the 17α-hydroxylase and 17,20-lyase activity of the cytochrome p450 enzyme CYP17. While this prevents the conversion of pregnenolone to androgen hormones as well as cortisol, adrenocorticotropic hormone (ACTH) production increases without negative inhibition of cortisol. As a result of ongoing enzymatic inhibition, abiraterone-induced ACTH production is skewed toward increased mineralocorticoid production leading to hypertension and hypokalemia [43]. Patients treated with abiraterone are typically co-treated with low-dose prednisone to keep ACTH levels suppressed. The mechanism of enzalutamide is less clear.

5.1.12 Poly ADP Ribose Polymerase Inhibitors

Poly ADP ribose polymerase inhibitors (PARPi) induce cellular death by inhibiting enzymes necessary for DNA repair and possess anti-tumor activity in breast, ovarian, and pancreatic cancers. They do not lead to hypertension as class effect; rather, the hypertensive effect appears to be restricted to a particular PARPi niraparib, though others have also reported hypertension with high-dose olaparib monotherapy or standard-dose olaparib combined with cediranib [20, 44]. In the case of niraparib, hypertension may occur as an off-target effect of the drug binding to dopamine and norepinephrine receptors [45].

5.2 Diagnosis and Management of Antineoplastic-Induced Hypertension

To date, optimal blood pressure targets in patients with cancer are not clearly defined and remain based on the 2017 American College of Cardiology/American Heart Association Clinical Practice Guidelines [46]. In these guidelines, normal blood pressure is defined as <120/80 mmHg, elevated blood pressure as 120–129/<80 mmHg, stage 1 hypertension as 130–139/80–89 mmHg, and stage 2 hypertension as ≥140/≥90 mmHg. Accordingly, antihypertensive therapy should aim to lower blood pressure to goal <130/<80. Blood pressure targets may be less stringent in patients pursuing anticancer treatment for palliative intent.

When possible, all patients should be screened for hypertension prior to anticancer treatment initiation either through home blood pressure monitoring or in-office monitoring. In patients with preexisting hypertension, antihypertensive therapy should be optimized, especially if the treatment plan includes known pro-hypertensive agents. While this chapter focuses on hypertension specifically, many anticancer agents have other cardiovascular implications, and patients should also be screened for diabetes mellitus, kidney disease, obesity, hyperlipidemia, and heart failure in certain circumstances.

After initiation of treatment, close monitoring for the development of hypertension is advised. While there are no consensus recommendations, some experts recommend twice weekly home blood pressure monitoring during the first 4–8 weeks of treatment as certain agents can lead to an acute rise in blood pressure [20]. After the first cycle or treatment period, blood pressure monitoring can occur every 1–2 weeks. Blood pressure monitoring should be intensified again around the time of treatment "off-periods" or discontinuation when patients may experience rebound hypotension. Risk of rebound hypotension may be higher in patients for whom antihypertensive therapy was necessary, although data in this area is lacking. As stated previously, antineoplastic-induced hypertension may develop years after initial use of these agents, and ongoing partnership between patients, internists, and oncologists is necessary to discover and treat high blood pressure when it develops.

Choice of antihypertensive agent reflects current hypertension practice guidelines [46]. Clinicians should utilize first-line agents such as angiotensin converting enzyme (ACE) inhibitors or angiotensin receptor blockers (ARBs), dihydropyridine calcium channel blockers, or thiazide diuretics. Selection of individual antihypertensive agents is largely based on patient comorbidities, drug pharmacokinetics and pharmacodynamics, and potential side effects. For example, patients with diabetic nephropathy, proteinuria, or left ventricular systolic failure may benefit from use of an ACE inhibitor or ARB, while patients at high risk of volume depletion should avoid thiazide diuretics. Despite limited implication of the renal-angiotensin-aldosterone system in the underlying mechanisms of hypertension with anticancer agents, ACE inhibitors and ARBs are often utilized for the treatment of VEGF inhibitor–related hypertension [20]. Studies also show success with use of the dihydropyridine calcium channel blocker amlodipine [47]. Combination of ACE inhibitors/ARBs and dihydropyridine calcium channel blockers are often used for uncontrolled blood pressure. Mineralocorticoid receptor antagonists are increasingly used for resistant hypertension, although they carry risk of hyperkalemia. Patients receiving treatment with VEGF inhibitors should avoid non-dihydropyridine calcium channel blockers (verapamil, diltiazem) as these agents may inhibit cytochrome P450 leading to increased drug levels of VEGF inhibitors [20]. While many of the anti-cancer therapies discussed in this chapter appear to mediate their hypertensive effects via NO inhibition, there is a paucity of data to support nitrates as treatment of drug-induced hypertension in patients with cancer. Similarly, while use of endothelin receptor antagonists may seem logical given the proposed mechanisms of VEGF-associated hypertension, their use has not been studied in this setting. Indeed, use of specific drugs in these patients is an area that is ripe for further research.

5.3 Conclusion

Certain antineoplastic drugs contribute to the development of hypertension, which may occur simultaneously with treatment or years after initial drug exposure. The most common mechanism for hypertension appears to involve inhibition of NO activity in the endothelium. In those with preexisting hypertension, use of these agents may exacerbate hypertension or make it difficult to control. For all patients planning to receive anticancer treatment, it is important to perform initial screening for high blood pressure and continue close monitoring during initiation, titration, or discontinuation of agents known to affect blood pressure. Treatment for antineoplastic-induced hypertension is consistent with current standard guideline recommendations for essential hypertension with particular attention to patient comorbidities and drug-drug interactions to further inform choice of anti-hypertensive agents.

References

1. Vos T, Lim SS, Abbafati C, et al. Global burden of 369 diseases and injuries in 204 countries and territories, 1990–2019: a systematic analysis for the Global Burden of Disease Study 2019. Lancet. 2020;396:1204–22. https://doi.org/10.1016/S0140-6736(20)30925-9.
2. Shiels MS, Haque AT, Berrington de González A, Freedman ND. Leading causes of death in the US during the COVID-19 pandemic, March 2020 to October 2021. JAMA Intern Med. 2022;182:883–6. https://doi.org/10.1001/jamainternmed.2022.2476.
3. Siegel RL, Miller KD, Wagle NS, Jemal A. Cancer statistics, 2023. CA Cancer J Clin. 2023;73:17–48. https://doi.org/10.3322/caac.21763.
4. Sung H, Ferlay J, Siegel RL, et al. Global cancer statistics 2020: GLOBOCAN estimates of incidence and mortality worldwide for 36 cancers in 185 countries. CA Cancer J Clin. 2021;71:209–49. https://doi.org/10.3322/caac.21660.
5. Armstrong GT, Oeffinger KC, Chen Y, et al. Modifiable risk factors and major cardiac events among adult survivors of childhood cancer. J Clin Oncol. 2013;31:3673–80. https://doi.org/10.1200/JCO.2013.49.3205.
6. Gibson TM, Li Z, Green DM, et al. Blood pressure status in adult survivors of childhood cancer: a report from the St. Jude lifetime cohort study. Cancer Epidemiol Biomarkers Prev. 2017;26:1705–13. https://doi.org/10.1158/1055-9965.EPI-17-0510.
7. Jaeger BC, Chen L, Foti K, et al. Hypertension statistics for US adults: an open-source web application for analysis and visualization of national health and nutrition examination survey data. Hypertension. 2023;80:1311–20. https://doi.org/10.1161/HYPERTENSIONAHA.123.20900.
8. Guo X, Qian X, Jin Y, et al. Hypertension induced by combination therapy of cancer: a systematic review and meta-analysis of global clinical trials. Front Pharmacol. 2021;12:712995. https://doi.org/10.3389/fphar.2021.712995.
9. Cohen JB, Geara AS, Hogan JJ, Townsend RR. Hypertension in cancer patients and survivors: epidemiology, diagnosis, and management. JACC CardioOncol. 2019;1:238–51. https://doi.org/10.1016/j.jaccao.2019.11.009.
10. Klagsbrun M, Moses MA. Molecular angiogenesis. Chem Biol. 1999;6:R217–24. https://doi.org/10.1016/S1074-5521(99)80081-7.
11. Hamnvik OR, Choueiri TK, Turchin A, et al. Clinical risk factors for the development of hypertension in patients treated with inhibitors of the VEGF signaling pathway. Cancer. 2015;121:311–9. https://doi.org/10.1002/cncr.28972.

12. Scartozzi M, Galizia E, Chiorrini S, et al. Arterial hypertension correlates with clinical outcome in colorectal cancer patients treated with first-line bevacizumab. Ann Oncol. 2009;20:227–30. https://doi.org/10.1093/annonc/mdn637.
13. Osumi H, Shinozaki E, Ooki A, et al. Early hypertension and neutropenia are predictors of treatment efficacy in metastatic colorectal cancer patients administered FOLFIRI and vascular endothelial growth factor inhibitors as second-line chemotherapy. Cancer Med. 2021;10:615–25. https://doi.org/10.1002/cam4.3638.
14. Kruzliak P, Novák J, Novák M. Vascular endothelial growth factor inhibitor-induced hypertension: from pathophysiology to prevention and treatment based on long-acting nitric oxide donors. Am J Hypertens. 2014;27:3–13. https://doi.org/10.1093/ajh/hpt201.
15. Risau W. Development and differentiation of endothelium. Kidney Int Suppl. 1998;54:S3–6. https://doi.org/10.1046/j.1523-1755.1998.06701.x.
16. Mäki-Petäjä KM, McGeoch A, Yang LL, et al. Mechanisms underlying vascular endothelial growth factor receptor inhibition–induced hypertension. Hypertension. 2021;77:1591–9. https://doi.org/10.1161/HYPERTENSIONAHA.120.16454.
17. Aalipour A, Advani RH. Bruton's tyrosine kinase inhibitors and their clinical potential in the treatment of B-cell malignancies: focus on ibrutinib. Ther Adv Hematol. 2014;5:121–33. https://doi.org/10.1177/2040620714539906.
18. Ng J, Ismail H, Rhodes J, Copeland-Halperin RS. Cardiovascular adverse effects of novel bruton tyrosine kinase inhibitors: what all cardiologists should know. American College of Cardiology; 2023.
19. Caldeira D, Alves D, Costa J, Ferreira JJ, Pinto FJ. Ibrutinib increases the risk of hypertension and atrial fibrillation: systematic review and meta-analysis. PLoS One. 2019;14:e0211228. https://doi.org/10.1371/journal.pone.0211228.
20. van Dorst DCH, Dobbin SJH, Neves KB, et al. Hypertension and prohypertensive antineoplastic therapies in cancer patients. Circ Res. 2021;128:1040–61. https://doi.org/10.1161/CIRCRESAHA.121.318051.
21. Dickerson T, Wiczer T, Waller A, et al. Hypertension and incident cardiovascular events following ibrutinib initiation. Blood. 2019;134:1919–28. https://doi.org/10.1182/blood.2019000840.
22. Gietema J, Meinardi M, Messerschmidt J, et al. Circulating plasma platinum more than 10 years after cisplatin treatment for testicular cancer. Lancet. 2000;355:1075–6. https://doi.org/10.1016/S0140-6736(00)02044-4.
23. Boer H, Proost JH, Nuver J, et al. Long-term exposure to circulating platinum is associated with late effects of treatment in testicular cancer survivors. Ann Oncol. 2015;26:2305–10. https://doi.org/10.1093/annonc/mdv369.
24. Sagstuen H, Aass N, Fosså SD, et al. Blood pressure and body mass index in long-term survivors of testicular cancer. J Clin Oncol. 2005;23:4980–90. https://doi.org/10.1200/JCO.2005.06.882.
25. Knijnenburg SL, Jaspers MW, van der Pal HJ, et al. Renal dysfunction and elevated blood pressure in long-term childhood cancer survivors. Clin J Am Soc Nephrol. 2012;7:1416–27. https://doi.org/10.2215/CJN.09620911.
26. Hideshima T, Richardson PG, Anderson KC. Mechanism of action of proteasome inhibitors and deacetylase inhibitors and the biological basis of synergy in multiple myeloma. Mol Cancer Ther. 2011;10:2034–42. https://doi.org/10.1158/1535-7163.MCT-11-0433.
27. Georgiopoulos G, Makris N, Laina A, et al. Cardiovascular toxicity of proteasome inhibitors: underlying mechanisms and management strategies. JACC CardioOncol. 2023;5:1–21. https://doi.org/10.1016/j.jaccao.2022.12.005.
28. Bruno G, Bringhen S, Maffei I, et al. Cardiovascular organ damage and blood pressure levels predict adverse events in multiple myeloma patients undergoing carfilzomib therapy. Cancers (Basel). 2019;11:622. https://doi.org/10.3390/cancers11050622.
29. Dimopoulos MA, Goldschmidt H, Niesvizky R, et al. Carfilzomib or bortezomib in relapsed or refractory multiple myeloma (ENDEAVOR): an interim overall survival analysis of an open-label, randomised, phase 3 trial. Lancet Oncol. 2017;18:1327–37. https://doi.org/10.1016/S1470-2045(17)30578-8.

30. Cohen JB, Brown NJ, Brown SA, et al. Cancer therapy–related hypertension: a scientific statement from the American Heart Association. Hypertension. 2023;80:e46–57. https://doi.org/10.1161/HYP.0000000000000224.
31. Baum M, Moe OW. Glucocorticoid-mediated hypertension. J Am Soc Nephrol. 2008;19(7):1251–3. https://doi.org/10.1681/ASN.2008040410.
32. Goodwin JE, Geller DS. Glucocorticoid-induced hypertension. Pediatr Nephrol. 2012;27:1059–66. https://doi.org/10.1007/s00467-011-1928-4.
33. Costello RE, Yimer BB, Roads P, Jani M, Dixon WG. Glucocorticoid use is associated with an increased risk of hypertension. Rheumatology. 2021;60:132–9. https://doi.org/10.1093/rheumatology/keaa209.
34. Mebrahtu TF, Morgan AW, West RM, Stewart PM, Pujades-Rodriguez M. Oral glucocorticoids and incidence of hypertension in people with chronic inflammatory diseases: a population-based cohort study. CMAJ. 2020;192:E295–301. https://doi.org/10.1503/cmaj.191012.
35. Hoorn EJ, Walsh SB, McCormick JA, Zietse R, Unwin RJ, Ellison DH. Pathogenesis of calcineurin inhibitor-induced hypertension. J Nephrol. 2012;25:269–75. https://doi.org/10.5301/jn.5000174.
36. Textor SC, Canzanello VJ, Taler SJ, et al. Cyclosporine-induced hypertension after transplantation. Mayo Clin Proc. 1994;69:1182–93. https://doi.org/10.1016/S0025-6196(12)65772-3.
37. Wang X, Jiang S, Fei L, et al. Tacrolimus causes hypertension by increasing vascular contractility via RhoA (Ras Homolog Family Member A)/ROCK (Rho-Associated Protein Kinase) pathway in mice. Hypertension. 2022;79:2228–38. https://doi.org/10.1161/HYPERTENSIONAHA.122.19189.
38. Glen C, Tan YY, Waterston A, et al. Mechanistic and clinical overview cardiovascular toxicity of BRAF and MEK inhibitors. JACC CardioOncol. 2022;4:1–18. https://doi.org/10.1016/j.jaccao.2022.01.096.
39. Mincu RI, Mahabadi AA, Michel L, et al. Cardiovascular adverse events associated with BRAF and MEK inhibitors. JAMA Netw Open. 2019;2:e198890. https://doi.org/10.1001/jamanetworkopen.2019.8890.
40. Motzer RJ, Hutson TE, Glen H, et al. Lenvatinib, everolimus, and the combination in patients with metastatic renal cell carcinoma: a randomised, phase 2, open-label, multicentre trial. Lancet Oncol. 2015;16:1473–82. https://doi.org/10.1016/S1470-2045(15)00290-9.
41. Højer Wang L, Wehland M, Wise PM, Infanger M, Grimm D, Kreissl MC. Cabozantinib, vandetanib, pralsetinib and selpercatinib as treatment for progressed medullary thyroid cancer with a main focus on hypertension as adverse effect. Int J Mol Sci. 2023;24:2312. https://doi.org/10.3390/ijms24032312.
42. Iacovelli R, Ciccarese C, Bria E, et al. The cardiovascular toxicity of abiraterone and enzalutamide in prostate cancer. Clin Genitourin Cancer. 2018;16:e645–53. https://doi.org/10.1016/j.clgc.2017.12.007.
43. Zhu X, Wu S. Risks and management of hypertension in cancer patients undergoing targeted therapy: a review. Clin Hypertens. 2022;28:14. https://doi.org/10.1186/s40885-022-00197-3.
44. Chen X, Wen Q, Kou L, Xie X, Li J, Li Y. Incidence and risk of hypertension associated with PARP inhibitors in cancer patients: a systematic review and meta-analysis. BMC Cancer. 2023;23:107. https://doi.org/10.1186/s12885-023-10571-5.
45. Ison G, Howie LJ, Amiri-Kordestani L, et al. FDA approval summary: niraparib for the maintenance treatment of patients with recurrent ovarian cancer in response to platinum-based chemotherapy. Clin Cancer Res. 2018;24:4066–71. https://doi.org/10.1158/1078-0432.CCR-18-0042.
46. Whelton PK, Carey RM, Aronow WS, et al. 2017 ACC/AHA/AAPA/ABC/ACPM/AGS/APhA/ASH/ASPC/NMA/PCNA guideline for the prevention, detection, evaluation, and management of high blood pressure in adults: executive summary: a report of the American College of Cardiology/American Heart Association Task Force on clinical practice guidelines. Circulation. 2018;138(17):e426–83. https://doi.org/10.1161/CIR.0000000000000597.
47. Mir O, Coriat R, Ropert S, et al. Treatment of bevacizumab-induced hypertension by amlodipine. Investig New Drugs. 2012;30:702–7. https://doi.org/10.1007/s10637-010-9549-5.

Post-Kidney Transplantation Hypertension

6

Stefanos Roumeliotis, Francesca Mallamaci, and Carmine Zoccali

6.1 Introduction

In end-stage kidney disease (ESKD), kidney transplantation (KT) is the treatment of choice and is associated with improved outcomes, quality of life, and decreased mortality compared to dialysis treatments. This survival benefit with KT is mainly attributed to improved glomerular filtration rate (GFR) and subsequent delay in cardiovascular disease (CVD) progression [1]. However, the residual risk for CVD morbidity and mortality still remains significantly increased in KT recipients, compared to age-gender-matched controls from the general population, and CVD remains the leading cause of death in these patients [2]. This heavy CVD burden is largely attributed to hypertension (HT), which is common in most KT patients and might be difficult to diagnose and control. Post-kidney transplant HT might be triggered by pre-KT factors associated with the KT procedure per se and by factors

S. Roumeliotis (✉)
Second Department of Nephrology, AHEPA Hospital, Aristotle University of Thessaloniki, Thessaloniki, Greece

F. Mallamaci
CNR-IFC, Clinical Epidemiology of Renal Diseases and Hypertension Unit, Centre of Clinical Physiology, National Research Council of Italy, Reggio Cal., c/o Ospedali Riuniti, Reggio Calabria, Italy

Renal Research Institute, New York, NY, USA

C. Zoccali
Renal Research Institute, New York, NY, USA

Institute of Molecular Biology and Genetics (Biogem), Ariano Irpino, Italy

Associazione Ipertensione Nefrologia Trapianto Renale (IPNET), c/o Nefrologia, Grande Ospedale Metropolitano, Reggio Calabria, Italy
e-mail: carmine.zoccali@tin.its

A. E. Berbari et al. (eds.), *Blood Pressure Disorders in Acute and Chronic Kidney Diseases*, Updates in Hypertension and Cardiovascular Protection,
https://doi.org/10.1007/978-3-031-81292-7_6

occurring after KT and is associated with dysfunction and decreased survival of the graft, loss of kidney function, CV outcomes, and increased mortality [3]. KT recipients present a significant prevalence of masked, white-coat, resistant HT and abnormal diurnal blood pressure (BP) changes [4] and, thus, traditional recommendations for office BP assessment should be reconsidered to include systemic methodologies.

6.2 Epidemiology

BP rises immediately after the KT procedure, mainly due to the interaction of normal saline with high-dose immunosuppressive treatment, but then declines. However, in the long term, the prevalence of post-KT HP is very high, ranging from 70% to 90% in early reports, but it exceeds 95% in more recent studies [5]. This broad variability is attributed to the heterogeneity among studies regarding definitions for HT diagnosis and methods of BP measurement. Misclassification and misdiagnosis of HT by office BP are usual in KT patients, whereas the optimal method of BP measurement, the 24-hour ambulatory blood pressure monitoring (24-h ABPM), is more sensitive in detecting uncontrolled HT and should be preferred [6]. Masked HT has been reported in 33–39% of this population [7, 8], whereas optimal control of BP is observed only in approximately 50% [9]. Epidemiological data from the large RETENAL study from 30 centers and 868 KT patients showed that uncontrolled management of BP was detected in 64% of this population using the more sensitive 24-h ABPM [10], whereas refractory, uncontrolled HT was found only in 6.8% using the office BP measurements and the 140/90 mmHg criterion [11]. In another cohort of hypertensive KT patients aged <70 years and with functional graft for at least 12 months, ABPM detected true resistant HT in 18.9% of all cases. Notably, these patients had accumulating CV risk factors and were mostly receiving glucocorticoids, and thus could benefit from optimal BP control [12]. Therefore, one unresolved issue in the diagnosis and management of post-KT HT still remains the method of BP measurement. Another overlooked issue is the adherence to anti-hypertensive treatment. Remarkably, although the adherence to anti-rejection immunosuppression drugs has been investigated [13–15], whether KT patients receive their anti-hypertensive medications as prescribed has not been studied so far.

Interestingly, despite the fact that our understanding regarding the pathophysiology of HT has been improved and new drug agents have been discovered, BP control in KT recipients has been suboptimal from the 1970s until today [3, 16]. This might be largely attributed to using calcineurin inhibitors (CNI) as initial immunosuppressive treatment. The launch of CNI was accompanied by a significant 10–30% rise in the prevalence of HT, 3–5 years following KT [17, 18].

It has been coherently shown by large epidemiological studies that among recipients' characteristics, male gender, obesity, the presence of native kidneys (due to renin secretion), diabetes, African-American ethnicity, pre-transplant HP and acute rejection, delayed and/or chronic graft dysfunction, recurrence of primary kidney disease in the allograft, immunosuppressive agents (including glucocorticoids and CNI), and post-transplant albuminuria or proteinuria are strong, independent risk factors for post-transplant HT [3, 16]. Chronic pre-transplantation HT might accelerate vascular calcification/stiffness of the media and the intima layer of the aorta, which might not be fully regressed after KT [19].

6.3 Post-KT HT and Target Organ Damage

6.3.1 Kidney Graft and Patient Survival

Post-KT HP is associated with target organ injury and adverse clinical outcomes, including deterioration of kidney function and both allograft and patient survival [3, 16, 20–22] independently of acute rejection and creatinine clearance. It has been shown that every 10 mmHg of systolic BP confers increased 17–18%, increased risks for death-censored allograft failure, and death [16]. In agreement with these findings, data from the large, multicenter Collaborative Transplant Study, which enrolled 24,404 first cadaver KT recipients followed for more than a decade, showed that poor management of systolic BP at 1 and 3 years following KT increased the risk for allograft failure (relative risk (RR) 1.61; 95% confidence interval (CI) 1.50–1.72) and death (RR 1.35; CI 1.23–1.48) [3]. Conversely, increased systolic BP during the first post-transplant year that was later on successfully managed (<140 mmHg) for the following 2 years was associated with improved 10-year allograft survival and death-censored functional survival, thus suggesting that optimal management of BP even after the first post-KT-year benefits the allograft outcome [3]. In this study, the authors did not examine whether lower values of SBP could be more clinically relevant, even though an analysis of this Collaborative Transplant Study dated 7 years before indicated that SBP below 120 mmHg was more beneficial in terms of allograft survival [23]. Although the association between post-KT HP and kidney graft survival has been repeatedly documented in both adults [3, 16, 20–22] and children [24], one study reported no association between HT at 3 and 12 months following KT and graft survival [17] probably due to the increased prevalence of HT in this study (>80%) and the fact that the effect of serum creatinine on the outcome of graft survival was so pronounced that, inevitably, other risk factors including HT were excluded from the risk models.

6.3.2 CV Outcomes

Moreover, hypertension following KT increases the risk of premature CV death and CV morbidity. Similar results to the Kasiske et al. and Collaborative Transplant Study were reported by a post hoc analysis of the Folic Acid for Vascular Outcome Reduction in Transplantation (FAVORIT) trial [25]. In a cohort of 3474 prevalent KT recipients, every 20 mmHg increase in SBP over baseline was correlated with a 32% increase in CVD and a 13% increase in mortality, independently of traditional

CVD risk factors. Interestingly, this study also reported that every 10 mmHg decrease in diastolic BP level below 70 mmHg was related to a 31% increase in CVD and mortality, whereas higher DBP levels were not [25]. A French national retrospective study included 17,526 KT recipients and 3,288,857 non-transplanted, non-dialysis patients and found that during a 5-year follow-up, there was a 3% higher incidence of myocardial infarction (MI) in the KT compared to the control group (5.8% vs, 2.8%, HR 1.45, CI 95% 1.35–1.55). This finding might be partially explained by the fact that patients in the KT group who experienced a novel MI episode were more likely to be hypertensive compared to their non-transplanted counterparts (76.0% vs. 48.1%, $p < 0.0001$) [26]. Similarly, a Norwegian national study showed that each 10 mmHg rise in SBP above baseline increased the 5-year risk for death from ischemic heart disease by 20% [27]. In disagreement with these, one study reported no association between HT at 3 and 12 months following KT and CV mortality [17], probably due to the increased prevalence of HT in this study (>80%) and the fact that the effect of serum creatinine on the outcome of CV survival was so pronounced that, inevitably, other risk factors including HT were excluded from the risk models. The clinical superiority of 24-h methods compared to office BP regarding the detection of CV risk profiles was highlighted in a study including 868 hypertensive KT patients aged <70 years with functional graft for at least 12 months, where ABPM detected true resistant HT in 18.9% of all cases. Notably, these patients had a pronounced CV risk profile (advanced age, male gender) and were mostly receiving glucocorticoids and thus could benefit from optimal BP control [12].

6.3.3 Kidney Function

Besides CVD, death, and graft dysfunction, post-KT HT has also been associated with target organ damage, including kidney function (GFR and albuminuria) and early surrogate markers of CVD and atherosclerosis. However, the association between kidney function and BP is less robust using the traditional office measurements; night-time SBP is the strongest predictor of GFR decrease and allograft function over time [28, 29]. To investigate the possible association between BP measurements by different methodologies and target organ damage, Pisano et al. [30] performed a meta-analysis of 22 studies and 2078 participants. The 24-h ABPM outperformed traditional office BP assessment regarding the prediction of GFR/creatinine clearance decline, and serum creatinine rises in 10 out of 12 studies with available data. These findings agree with other studies reporting that abnormal dipping patterns (reverse dippers and non-dippers) occurring in the first year post-KT are strong, independent predictors of subsequent decline in GFR [29, 31]. Albuminuria (including micro- and macro-albuminuria) is also associated with HT in the KT population and is a strong, independent predictor of ESKD, graft loss, and death. Interestingly, in non-proteinuric KT recipients, microalbuminuria still predicts kidney graft loss and, thus, albuminuria and proteinuria are both markers of organ damage in this population [32]. The Spanish Chronic Allograft Nephropathy

Study included 3365 KT patients and found that de novo proteinuria developed in the first 12 months after KT was detected in 15.3% of all patients. There was a progressive increase in the risk of kidney graft loss and patient death as the degree of proteinuria increased [for graft loss—0.5–1 g/day: HR 2.33 (1.79–3.01); >1 g/day HR: 3.46 (2.73–4.39); for mortality—0.5–1 g/day: HR 2.05 (1.39–3.01); >1 g/day HR 2.3 (1.55–3.39)]. The tight association between proteinuria and HT in this population was highlighted by the fact that across the categories of proteinuria, both SBP and DBP were gradually increased (<0.5 g/day: SBP 139 ± 18 mmHg, DBP 82 ± 10 mmHg; 0.5–1 g/day: SBP 145 ± 20 mmHg, DBP 83 ± 12 mmHg; >1 g/day: SBP 148 ± 20 mmHg, DBP 86 ± 12 mmHg) [33]. Similarly, a retrospective study in 321 patients with functional graft 1-year post-transplant reported that proteinuria was correlated with post-KT HT (RR 1.84, 95% CI 1.06–3.18) [34]. Compared to normoalbuminuric, KT patients with microalbuminuria present significantly impaired SBP levels; this association becomes more pronounced in macroalbuminuric subjects [35].

6.3.4 Atherosclerosis and Cardiac Function

Several researchers found a tight association between post-KT HT, cardiovascular damage markers, and atherosclerotic complications. A large inclusive survey of 170 KT patients showed that 24-h systolic ABPM was strongly correlated with carotid intima-media thickness (CIMT), whereas office BP failed to show the same association [36]. The authors used the night-day SBP ratio, which, compared to the nocturnal BP decrease, depends less on the BP value and found that 36% of this population were non-dippers. The association between CIMT and BP was even more pronounced using the night-day SBP ratio, compared to the 24-h average SBP [36]. Moreover, MHT and sustained HT, quite common among KT patients, are strong, independent predictors of LVH [7]. These findings highlight the need to detect non-dipping status and night-time HT and suggest that optimal management of nocturnal HT and MHT might ameliorate the heavy CV burden of KT recipients. The meta-analysis by Pisano et al. showed that compared to office BP, the 24-h ABPM was reported to be a stronger predictor of CV surrogate markers, including left ventricular mass index (LVMI), CIMT, diffuse thickening, and endothelial dysfunction [30]. In agreement with these findings, increased BP in KT patients has been reported to be associated with endothelial dysfunction and arterial stiffness, assessed by pulse-wave velocity (PWV) [37]. Furthermore, an altered circadian BP pattern (dipping status) identified a subgroup of KT recipients at high risk for adverse CVD and kidney outcomes. The effect of KT on LVMI remains controversial. There are reports that not only HT is associated with left ventricular hypertrophy in KT, but also, during the first 2 or 3 years post-KT, there is a progressive regression of this hypertrophy, which might be blunted if BP is poorly controlled or by excessive dietary sodium intake and hyperuricemia, regardless the BP control [38–40]. This regression of LVMI in the first 2 years following KT is approximately -15 g/m^2 [38] and is also consistent in children after KT [41]. However, Patel et al. reported that KT failed to improve LVMI as assessed by cardiac magnetic resonance [42], and a meta-analysis by Pickup et al. included data from six studies and 26 patients and indicated no difference in LVMI between groups following transplantation (standardized mean difference −0.07, 95% CI −0.41 to 0.26) and no difference in left ventricular ejection fraction or left ventricular end-diastolic volume [43]. This failure to improve LVH was associated with high pulse pressure and persistent HT [38].

6.4 Pathophysiology

The pathogenesis of HT following KT is multifactorial and involves risk factors present before KT, risk factors associated with the KT procedure per se, and parameters present after KT.

6.4.1 Kidney Graft Dysfunction

Acute, delayed, and chronic kidney graft injury might trigger post-transplant HT. Acute rejection might cause HT by increased renin-angiotensin-aldosterone system (RAAS), sodium retention, kidney graft dysfunction, and high-dose glucocorticoid treatment. BP control requires the reversal or management of graft rejection. In the setting of delayed graft function, the transplant does not work right away and, therefore, patients need dialysis treatment during the first 7 days after KT. This might cause volume overload accompanied by an acute rise in BP almost immediately after the procedure, where patients are typically administered normal saline intravenously. In this scenario, diuretics and/or ultrafiltration dialysis to remove fluid overload is usually effective in controlling hypertension. Chronic allograft injury due to previous, recurrent glomerulopathy, thrombotic microangiopathy, tubulointerstitial fibrosis and necrosis and immunological chronic rejection episodes are frequently associated with HT, progressive GFR decline, and proteinuria. The pathophysiological mechanisms underlying this association are practically the same as those responsible for the pathogenesis of hypertensive nephrosclerosis.

6.4.2 Immunosuppressive Agents

Corticoids and CNI are the main immunosuppressive drug agents responsible for the anti-rejection therapy-mediated HT. In the early post-KT period, corticosteroids are usually administered at high doses and contribute to HT. However, later on, due to the timely dose tapering, this immunosuppressive drug class is not regarded as a strong determinant of chronic HT in KT patients. Data from the Astellas Corticosteroid Withdrawal Study Group randomized controlled trial showed that compared to chronic low-dose corticosteroid therapy, early discontinuation of corticosteroids in KT patients receiving CNIs was associated with a significantly reduced weight gain (median change: 7.7 vs. 5.1 kg, $p = 0.05$), but failed to reduce BP during the first 5 years following transplantation [44].

Conversely, CNIs are major risk factors for the development of post-transplant HT. Notably, after this anti-rejection drug class was implemented in clinical practice, the prevalence of post-transplant HT increased by 10–50%, and almost all KT patients receiving CNIs present HT, which in some cases might be overt [45]. Cyclosporine increases peripheral vascular resistance locally (affecting the afferent arteriole) and systemically. Although the exact pathophysiological mechanisms have not yet been fully elucidated, the kidney vascular effects, along with stimulation of vasoconstrictors like endothelin and suppression of prostaglandins, cause renal hypoperfusion and a subsequent GFR decline. Additionally, cyclosporine upregulates the function of sodium transporter of the loop of Henle (NKCC2), causing impaired sodium excretion [46], which in turn gives rise to BP [47].

6.4.3 Renal Artery Stenosis

Transplant renal artery stenosis (TRAS) is a common and potentially reversible vascular complication of KT causing post-transplant HT, graft dysfunction, and eventually loss of the graft and premature death. The incidence rate is approximately 8.3 cases per 1000 patient-years [48], whereas the prevalence of this complication ranges from 1% to 23% [49] due to the large heterogeneity among studies regarding the diagnostic criteria and other surgical factors. TRAS commonly occurs 3–24 months after KT, with a mean diagnosis time of 9.9 ± 9.7 months, but might also present earlier or later in this timeframe [48, 50]. It frequently presents near the anastomosis between the donor and the recipient renal arteries and rarely at the feeding native artery and the donor renal artery. Risk factors associated with TRAS are delayed graft function, laborious organ procurement, suboptimal surgical techniques, ischemic heart disease, and atherosclerosis [48, 49, 51, 52], while there are contraindicatory reports regarding cytomegalovirus status [48, 52]. The clinical manifestation of TRAS is quite similar to that of renovascular disease in non-transplanted subjects, including worsening or refractory HT, recurrent episodes of flash pulmonary edema, hypokalemia, graft dysfunction without rejection, ureteric infection or obstruction, and worsening kidney function after treatment with RAAS inhibitors. The pathophysiology of this common vascular complication is multifractional. Kidney hypoperfusion activates the RAAS system, leading to a salt-avid state and fluid retention. Recurrent bouts of flash pulmonary edema occur in critical, bilateral renal artery stenosis or unilateral stenosis in a solitary kidney. These bouts might occur and resolve quite rapidly, whereas between the episodes, patients might experience only HT as a clinical sign. Early, timely diagnosis of TRAS might prevent allograft loss and bouts and control BP. KT recipients with resistant, worsening, or new-onset HT and other relevant clinical characteristics should be screened for TRAS, whereas others suggest routine evaluation after KT. The initial diagnostic screening should be done by Doppler ultrasonography, which is easy, cheap, quick, and reliable (sensitivity 58–100%, specificity 87–100%) but highly dependent on the operator's experience [53, 54]. The Doppler findings consistent with TRAS diagnosis include the presence of ultrasound spectral waveform with tardus parvus pattern (a Doppler pattern resulting from arterial stenosis), peak systolic velocity above 200 cm/sec in the renal artery, ratio of the peak systolic velocity to external iliac arteries >1.8, and acceleration time of 0.1 s or higher in the transplant renal and intrarenal arteries [55]. If Doppler raises the suspicion of TRAS, the next step in the diagnosis algorithm is usually computed tomography (CTA) or magnetic resonance angiography (MRA). The advantage of CTA over Doppler is that it depends less on operator experience and uses lower intravenous radiocontrast volume compared to classic, interventional arteriography. Reported specificities of MRA for the diagnosis of renal stenosis >50% range from 75% to 98%, and sensitivity reaches 100% [56, 57]. However, the administration of gadolinium might cause nephrogenic systemic fibrosis in moderate and severe CKD and thus should be avoided in the acute kidney injury setting, in dialysis, and in patients with CKD stage 4. Angiography of the renal artery is the optimal test to confirm the diagnosis of TRAS and provides the option for angioplasty with stent placement. It is an invasive test with the use of a radiocontrast agent and, therefore, should not be a first-line examination but should be reserved for inconclusive cases or those who need angioplasty. An interesting approach before renal angiography is the kidney allograft biopsy to exclude chronic rejection and kidney parenchymal disease forms [58].

6.4.4 Donor Characteristics

It has been repeatedly demonstrated that advanced donor age is a strong, independent risk factor for adverse clinical outcomes and development of HT after KT [34]. Moreover, marked mismatch between somatometric parameters of donors/recipients like female to male pairs, pediatric to adult pairs, low BMI to high BMI pairs also lead to adverse clinical outcomes, due to inadequate graft nephron mass to cover the recipient's metabolic needs, thus leading to glomerular hypertrophy and hyperfiltration and intraglomerular hypertension [59, 60].

The genetic background of the transplanted kidney might also predispose to pro- or anti-hypertensive states. Genetic variants affecting the function of apolipoprotein L1, P-glycoprotein, cytochrome P450, and multidrug resistance protein in the donor genome might trigger the development of post-transplant HT [61, 62]. Transplantation studies in genetic hypertensive animal models have coherently shown that this inherited message for HT might mainly reside within the kidney [63]. In human clinical studies, it is not that easy to replicate this finding on a large scale. However, an interesting study published in 1983 reported the clinical course of six patients with essential HT-derived nephrosclerosis who developed ESKD and underwent dialysis. Although these patients presented resistant HT during dialysis, KT from normotensive donors with no familial predispose to HT was accompanied by amelioration of the primary, essential HT. This study suggests that the genetic background and characteristics of the kidney play a major role in the pathogenesis of essential HT [64]. The hypothesis that, along with the graft, the risk for HT might also be "transplanted" and passed on to the KT recipient was suggested by a landmark prospective study enrolling 85 KT patients [65]. Neither the patients nor the physicians treating them have access to the family history data of donors or recipients. During the 8 years following KT, recipients with negative familial history for HT who received a kidney from a family with HT were more likely to develop HT and start antihypertensive treatment, compared to those receiving a kidney from a "normotensive" family (odds ratio 5.0, 95% CI 1.4–17.8). Conversely, in recipients coming from a "hypertensive" family themselves, the effect of the origin of the kidney graft was blunted [65]. After these interesting results the authors expanded their analysis in an extension study showing that recipients from a "normotensive" family receiving a "hypertensive" kidney presented a higher hypertensive response and much worse acute kidney injury during episodes of acute rejections compared to all other recipient-donor combinations. This finding implies that the transplanted kidney might transmit susceptibility to HT and risk for steeper BP rises and more critical kidney injury during acute rejections [66]. Similarly, APOL1 risk variants in donors but not recipients are associated with poor graft survival [67]. These natural clinical experiments suggest that the kidney is the main factor underlying genetic predisposition for HT. To further elucidate the clinical impact of genetic predisposal in KT, the NIH APOL1 Long-Term Kidney Transplantation Outcomes Network (APOLLO) study is currently assessing the effects of *APOL1* polymorphism on KT outcomes (including GFR decline, increase in proteinuria, and graft survival) in a large cohort of over 3000 kidney donors and 260 transplant programs [68]. The results of the APOLLO study might provide novel insights in the risk assessment of KT donors and recipients; current risk calculators such as the Kidney Donor Risk Index might be revised to include these genomic data, whereas low-risk *APOL1* genotype donors might be reconsidered as safe options. As these years are considered the era of precision medicine, this initiative might enhance our understanding, improve KT clinical outcomes, and expand the KT programs.

6.4.5 Post-Transplant Obesity

In maintenance dialysis, the obesity paradox establishes high BMI as a protective factor regarding mortality. However, this reverse epidemiology does not apply after dialysis patients receive a kidney transplant. A systematic review and meta-analysis of 11 studies and 305,392 KT recipients showed that abnormal values of BMI increased all-cause mortality. HRs for mortality were 1.09 for underweight (95% CI 1.02–1.20), 1.07 for overweight (95% CI 1.04–1.12), and 1.20 for underweight (95% CI 1.14–1.23) in adults, whereas in children (only one study) obesity was related with death [69]. BMI under 30 post-KT favors acute graft rejection (RR = 1.17), delayed graft function (RR = 1.52), both graft (RR = 0.97) and patient survival (RR = 0.99) during the first 3 years after KT, and HT (RR = 1.35) [70]. The favorable effect of low BMI on various outcomes might imply that dialysis patients with BMI >30 might consider losing weight before KT.

KT recipients gain approximately 2.2 kg during the first 3 months and 6.6 kg of body weight in the first year after a successful KT, mainly attributed to the accumulation of adipose tissue in the central body [71]. Conversely, there is no change in muscle mass and fluid status. These findings suggest that post-transplant weight gain should not be falsely regarded as a positive outcome reflecting recovery from kidney failure because, in that case, all body compartments would grow proportionally. Longitudinal data showed that BMI was progressively increased during follow-up visits in KT patients, leading to worsening quality of sleep, a well-known factor for post-transplant HT [72]. Moreover, every kilogram added post-KT increases proportionally the risk for insulin resistance, HT, and CV disease [71, 73].

6.4.6 Sleep Apnea

KT is considered the optimal treatment choice for ESKD patients owing to its beneficial outcomes in survival, cardiovascular health, and quality of life. However, sleep disorders, mainly sleep apnea, are still highly common and might not always improve after KT and increase the susceptibility for HT and other adverse clinical outcomes [74]. It has been reported that the prevalence of sleep apnea might reach even 28% in patients following KT and is quite similar to patients undergoing maintenance hemodialysis (HD) on the waiting list for a kidney transplant [75, 76]. However, broader terms of sleep disorders have been reported to be 37.5% prevalent in dialysis patients before transplant, which is reduced to 20% in the first 6 months post-transplantation [77]. An Indian polysomnographic study showed that among 18 patients (14 men, 4 women) with a median age of 28 years, the prevalence (44.4% pre-transplantation vs 5.6% post-transplantation) and severity of sleep-disordered breathing (5.8 events/h in pre-transplantation vs 0 events/h in post-transplantation) significantly improved shortly after KT [78]. In KT patients, sleep apnea is associated with traditional CV risk factors, including obesity and age, and resistant and/or uncontrolled HT. Restored kidney function following KT suppresses volume overload and uremia, but after 5 years, approximately 33% of KT recipients present with fluid overload and post-transplant obesity [69]. In the long term, sleep apnea is progressively worsened in KT patients, which is directly associated with a parallel increase in the BMI, thus highlighting obesity and sleep apnea as interrelated, strong, and modifiable factors underlying the pathophysiology of post-transplant HT [72]. An extended analysis of this study showed that sleep disorders were associated with a significant rise in SBP (daytime, nighttime, and 24-h) independently of GFR, BMI, and traditional CV risk factors, thus suggesting a causal relationship between these two entities [79]. The cross-sectional SLeep disorders Evaluation in Patients after kidney Transplantation [SLEPT] Study showed that the proportion of KT recipients receiving three or more antihypertensive medications was significantly increased (56% vs. 31%) in those with sleep apnea. A large study of 823 KT patients showed that 28% were at increased risk of sleep apnea at baseline. This high-risk group presented advanced age, increased prevalence of diabetes and obesity, and lower GFR. However, only in women KT recipients, this high risk for sleep apnea, independently of HT, age, BMI, GFR, duration of CKD, and other transplant-related parameters, conferred a threefold risk for loss of graft function [75]. The sleep apnea risk assessment was based on the Berlin questionnaire, a rather subjective and unreliable surrogate marker of sleep apnea. Similar results were published by a retrospective study merging two databases; sleep apnea was associated with a 2.61 increased risk for graft loss or CV death with functional graft in patients transplanted between 2009 and 2017. Of note, in patients that were transplanted a decade before this era, sleep apnea reduced by 37% the risk for graft failure [80]. These contradictory results might be attributed to the misdiagnosis of sleep apnea in the first decade. In disagreement with these, other studies failed to show an association between sleep apnea and all-cause mortality and/or deterioration of kidney function [81, 82], which might be due to denervation of the kidney graft. To investigate this area, a meta-analysis included four observational studies, 5259 KT patients followed for 14 years, and found no association between sleep apnea and graft loss or failure and mortality [83].

Sleep disturbances are associated with post-transplant HT and poor quality of life. It remains unknown whether sleep apnea affects the allograft function and increases the CV risk of KT recipients.

6.5 Clinical Aspects

6.5.1 Methods of BP Measurement

Standard office BP measurement often provides unreliable readings, resulting in misclassification and misdiagnosis of HT in the KT population. On the other hand, 24-h ABPM is the optimal method to characterize BP. To investigate the clinical utility of the later method, Pisano et al. performed a meta-analysis including 27 studies and 3481 KT patients and found that the prevalence of uncontrolled HT detected by office BP measurement was 47% (95% CI 36–58%) and by 24-h ABPM was 56% (95% CI 46–65%) [6]. Moreover, the mean concordance ratio between these two methods regarding the classification of controlled/uncontrolled HT was 66%. Only a few studies reported home BP measurements, whereas 24-h ABPM also provided insight into the HT phenotypes among the KT population; masked HP (MHT) was detected in 26% of all cases and white-coat HT (WCHT) in 10%. Data analyzed from 28 studies showed that non-dippers' prevalence was 54% (95% CI 45–63%), which could be attributed to the disturbance of circadian rhythm post-KT. These results highlight the clinical superiority of 24-h methods of BP over office measurements to detect uncontrolled HT, MHT, and WCHT [6]. Moreover, in a cohort of 170 KT patients, when the night-time (>120/70 mm Hg) criterion for the diagnosis of HT replaced the daytime criterion, there were 43% more diagnoses for HT. In this cohort, 36% were clear-cut nondippers [36] and MHT was diagnosed in 33–39% [7, 8]. The broader use of ABPM helped identify non-dipper phenotype in 36–95% [36, 84, 85] and nocturnal HT in 69% to 77% [36, 72]. It should be noted that there was a poor agreement in a cohort of 260 KT patients where 785 paired measurements of office and 24-h ABPM were obtained during a follow-up of 3.9 years (37% disagreement in visits) [72]. Applying the cutoffs for office values ≥140/90 and ≥130/80 mmHg for ABPM, another study reported WCHT at 12% and MHT at 20% [12]. In contrast, using the 130/80 for office and 125/75 mmHg for ABPM thresholds, a retrospective study estimated the prevalence of WCHT at 3% and MHT at 56% [86]. Moreover, in this population, resistant HT is found in 17.5–23.5% of patients despite treatment with 1–3 antihypertensive regimens [12, 87].

Despite this accumulating evidence, the optimal BP goal and the method of BP assessment are yet unclear in KT recipients. There are limited efforts to shift BP assessment from casual office measurements to 24-h ABPM or home BP readings in KT recipients. On the contrary, various guidelines promote using 24-h methods for diagnosis and stratification of HT in high-risk patients (such as CKD 1–4 and dialysis). The American College of Cardiology/American Heart Association (ACC/AHA) 2017 guidelines suggested a threshold of 130/80 for office and 125/75 mmHg for 24-h ABPM (after exclusion of MHT and WCHT), based on the 10-year risk for CVD [88]. One year later, the Task Force for the Management of Arterial Hypertension of the European Society of Cardiology and the European Society of Hypertension (ESC/ESH) defined HT as office values ≥140/90 and ≥130/80 mmHg for ABPM [89], whereas similarly to ACC/AHA, the Kidney Disease: Improving Global Outcomes (KDIGO) Blood Pressure Work Group 2021 Clinical Practice Guidelines recommended the cutoff values of 130/80 for office and 125/75 mmHg for ABPM [90].

The optimal BP target in KT recipients has not yet been clearly defined, mainly because there is no high-quality evidence from RCTs examining the clinical benefits of different BP targets in hard outcomes. Therefore, traditionally and rather arbitrary, BP optimal goals in this population have been adopted from high-risk populations, including pre-dialysis CKD, diabetics, and patients with CVD. Large RCTs, such as the Systolic Blood Pressure Intervention Trial (SPRINT), graded differences in CVD and death in more intensive BP management and had KT among the exclusion criteria. Moreover, there is an excessive risk of AKI and loss of GFR with lower BP targets because graft denervation and use of CNIs might hinder the graft's autoregulation ability and raise its susceptibility to AKI and subsequent GFR decrease when SBP is <120 mmHg. However, this hypothesis has not been supported by research data. A secondary analysis of the Systolic Blood Pressure Intervention trial showed that when targeting even lower, below 120 mmHg for SBP in CKD patients, there was an improvement in all-cause mortality [91]. However, in this study, BP recordings were performed unattended, and these results were perceived with skepticism. Similarly, a secondary analysis of the Folic Acid for Vascular Outcome Reduction in Transplantation (FAVORIT) trial showed that among 3598 KT patients, followed for a mean period of 4 years, there were no cutoffs identified at which lower BP values increased the risk for GFR decline or graft failure [92].

Post-KT, the routine follow-up at each visit should include office BP measurements at the beginning and, if elevated, a second measurement at the end of the visit, seated at rest. Supine and standing BP measurements might reveal orthostatic hypotension, especially in diabetics or in those treated with alpha-blockers. However, all KT recipients should be advised to self-monitor their BP at home, especially in the first 90 days following KT. Although 24-h ABPM has not yet been implemented in everyday, routine clinical practice for KT recipients, it might be helpful to identify WCHT or resistant HT. In a consensus statement, the "hypertension and the kidney" working group of the European Society of Hypertension (ESH) nicely framed this discrepancy and pointed out that there are currently no specific target goals for HT in KT recipients. The ESH suggests a reduction of BP to 140/90 and further to 130/80 mmHg in CKD patients, but there is no separate recommendation for KT recipients. According to ACC/AHA 2017 and KDIGO guidelines, the office BP goal should be below 130/80 mmHg [93].

6.5.2 Therapeutic Management

In the KT population, the management of HT is a complex and multifactorial problem. Post-transplantation development of de novo HT or worsening of preexisting HT indicates potential reversible causes. Therefore, in these cases, all patients should be evaluated for volume overload, which might be present in the early post-KT period but also occur later due to sodium retention or graft dysfunction. Since acute and chronic graft dysfunction might cause post-transplant HT, assessing graft function includes estimating GFR and albuminuria. Following in this stepwise approach is the evaluation of immunosuppressive regimens (including CNIs and corticosteroids), and if TRAS is suspected, patients should also be monitored with Doppler ultrasonography. Notably, in the early post-KT period, anxiety, pain, and poor sleeping habits might also raise BP.

The first-line management of post-KT HT includes lifestyle changes that might exert clinical benefits irrespectively of BP control, such as a low-salt diet (<2 g/24 h), physical activity of moderate intensity (>3 h/week), balanced diet with fiber, fruits, and vegetables, and calories to maintain a healthy BMI, smoking cessation, and limited alcohol consumption, as described in the 2021 KDIGO HT guidelines [90]. The second step in this multifactorial approach is the management of immunosuppressive therapy. Generally, CNIs and low-dose corticosteroids should not be discontinued to manage HT in KT recipients. However, when the patients are treated with high doses of corticosteroids for a long time to prevent rejection, and post-KT HT occurs, timely tapering of prednisone might also help control HT. Finally, the optimal choice of antihypertensive medications is the cornerstone of post-transplant HT. In hypertensive CKD patients, the antihypertensive treatment of choice includes RAASi, diuretics (loops or thiazide, depending on eGFR), and calcium channel blockers (CCBs). However, the use of RAASi in the early post-KT period is an area for debate; it is not uncommon in everyday clinical practice for nephrologists to discontinue RAASi because of the risk of acute rejection, AKI, and hyperkalemia. ACC/AHA guidelines suggest calcium channel blockers (CCBs) as first-line treatment for post-KT HT, due to their beneficial effects on graft survival, improved kidney function, and neutralizing the vasoconstriction caused by CNIs [94]. In contrast, RAASi should be used only when heart failure or albuminuria is present [88]. Conversely, KDIGO BP Working Group guidelines recommend the use of CCBs (dihydropyridine) or ARBs as a first-line therapy for KT patients with 1C level of evidence [95]. A meta-analysis of 71 RCTs showed that compared to CCBs, ACEi were associated with hyperkalemia and decreased kidney function. RAASi improved graft survival, whereas the data on other clinical hard endpoints including mortality, rejection, and graft loss were extremely limited [96]. However, after the early post-KT period, the choice of optimal antihypertensive treatment should be individualized according to comorbidities, kidney function, and pre-KT medication management.

6.6 Conclusions

Hypertension after kidney transplantation is quite common and might be triggered by preexisting factors, factors associated with the KT procedure per se, and by factors occurring after KT. Since post-kidney transplant HT is associated with increased mortality and morbidity, including dysfunction and decreased survival of the graft, loss of kidney function, and cardiovascular disease, accurate diagnosis and optimal control of post-kidney transplant HT are mandatory, which still remain challenging, mainly due to the lack of RCTs and controversial guidelines. In order to elucidate this topic, future, large, well-designed RCTs are needed.

References

1. Rangaswami J, Mathew RO, Parasuraman R, et al. Cardiovascular disease in the kidney transplant recipient: epidemiology, diagnosis and management strategies. Nephrol Dial Transplant. 2019;34:760–73.
2. Collins AJ, Foley RN, Chavers B, et al. US renal data system 2011 annual data report. Am J Kidney Dis. 2012;59:A7.
3. Opelz G, Dohler B, Collaborative Transplant Study. Improved long-term outcomes after renal transplantation associated with blood pressure control. Am J Transplant. 2005;5:2725–31.
4. Wadei HM, Amer H, Taler SJ, et al. Diurnal blood pressure changes one year after kidney transplantation: relationship to allograft function, histology, and resistive index. J Am Soc Nephrol. 2007;18:1607–15.
5. Korogiannou M, Sarafidis P, Theodorakopoulou MP, et al. Diagnostic performance of office versus ambulatory blood pressure in kidney transplant recipients. Am J Nephrol. 2021;52:548–58.
6. Pisano A, Mallamaci F, D'arrigo G, et al. Assessment of hypertension in kidney transplantation by ambulatory blood pressure monitoring: a systematic review and meta-analysis. Clin Kidney J. 2022;15:31–42.
7. Hamdani G, Nehus EJ, Hanevold CD, et al. Ambulatory blood pressure, left ventricular hypertrophy, and allograft function in children and young adults after kidney transplantation. Transplantation. 2017;101:150–6.
8. Kayrak M, Gul EE, Kaya C, et al. Masked hypertension in renal transplant recipients. Blood Press. 2014;23:47–53.

9. Forconi C, Gatault P, Miquelestorena-Standley E, et al. Polymorphism in programmed cell death 1 gene is strongly associated with lung and kidney allograft survival in recipients from CMV-positive donors. J Heart Lung Transplant. 2017;36:315–24.
10. Fresnedo GF, Esteve AF, Huertas EG, et al. Ambulatory blood pressure monitoring in kidney transplant patients: RETENAL study. Transplant Proc. 2012;44:2601–2.
11. Fraile MG, Fresnedo GF, Gómez-Alamillo C, de Castro SS, Arias M. Clinical and epidemiological characteristics of refractory hypertension in renal transplant patients. Transplant Proc. 2009;41:2132–3.
12. Arias-Rodríguez M, Fernández-Fresnedo G, Campistol JM, et al. Prevalence and clinical characteristics of renal transplant patients with true resistant hypertension. J Hypertens. 2015;33:1074–81.
13. Joost R, Dörje F, Schwitulla J, Eckardt K-U, Hugo C. Intensified pharmaceutical care is improving immunosuppressive medication adherence in kidney transplant recipients during the first post-transplant year: a quasi-experimental study. Nephrol Dial Transplant. 2014;29:1597–607.
14. Low JK, Williams A, Manias E, Crawford K. Interventions to improve medication adherence in adult kidney transplant recipients: a systematic review. Nephrol Dial Transplant. 2015;30:752–61.
15. Nevins TE, Nickerson PW, Dew MA. Understanding medication nonadherence after kidney transplant. J Am Soc Nephrol. 2017;28:2290–301.
16. Kasiske BL, Anjum S, Shah R, et al. Hypertension after kidney transplantation. Am J Kidney Dis. 2004;43:1071–81.
17. Campistol JM, Romero R, Paul J, Gutierrez-Dalmau A. Epidemiology of arterial hypertension in renal transplant patients: changes over the last decade. Nephrol Dial Transplant. 2004;19(Suppl 3):iii62–6.
18. Zhang R, Leslie B, Reisin E, Boudreaux JP, Frey D. Hypertension after kidney transplantation: impact, pathogenesis and therapy. Am J Med Sci. 2003;325:202–8.
19. Korogiannou M, Xagas E, Marinaki S, Sarafidis P, Boletis JN. Arterial stiffness in patients with renal transplantation; associations with co-morbid conditions, evolution, and prognostic importance for cardiovascular and renal outcomes. Front Cardiovasc Med. 2019;6:67.
20. Ponticelli C, Montagnino G, Aroldi A, Angelini C, Braga M, Tarantino A. Hypertension after renal transplantation. Am J Kidney Dis. 1993;21(5 Suppl 2):73–8
21. Mange KC, Cizman B, Joffe M, Feldman HI. Arterial hypertension and renal allograft survival. JAMA. 2000;283:633–8.
22. Mange KC, Feldman HI, Joffe MM, Fa K, Bloom RD. Blood pressure and the survival of renal allografts from living donors. J Am Soc Nephrol. 2004;15:187–93.
23. Opelz G, Wujciak T, Ritz E. Association of chronic kidney graft failure with recipient blood pressure. Kidney Int. 1998;53:217–22.
24. Seeman T. Hypertension after renal transplantation. Pediatr Nephrol. 2009;24:959–72.
25. Carpenter MA, John A, Weir MR, et al. BP, cardiovascular disease, and death in the folic acid for vascular outcome reduction in transplantation trial. J Am Soc Nephrol. 2014;25:1554–62.
26. Didier R, Yao H, Legendre M, et al. Myocardial infarction after kidney transplantation: a risk and specific profile analysis from a nationwide French medical information database. J Clin Med. 2020;9:3356. https://doi.org/10.3390/jcm9103356.
27. Aakhus S, Dahl K, Wideroe TE. Cardiovascular disease in stable renal transplant patients in Norway: morbidity and mortality during a 5-yr follow-up. Clin Transpl. 2004;18:596–604.
28. Mallamaci F, D'arrigo G, Tripepi R, et al. Office, standardized and 24-h ambulatory blood pressure and renal function loss in renal transplant patients. J Hypertens. 2018;36:119–25.
29. Wadei HM, Amer H, Griffin MD, Taler SJ, Stegall MD, Textor SC. Abnormal circadian blood pressure pattern 1-year after kidney transplantation is associated with subsequent lower glomerular filtration rate in recipients without rejection. J Am Soc Hypertens. 2011;5:39–47.
30. Pisano A, Mallamaci F, D'Arrigo G, et al. Blood pressure monitoring in kidney transplantation: a systematic review on hypertension and target organ damage. Nephrol Dial Transplant. 2021;36:1326–46.

31. Ibernon M, Moreso F, Sarrias X, et al. Reverse dipper pattern of blood pressure at 3 months is associated with inflammation and outcome after renal transplantation. Nephrol Dial Transplant. 2012;27:2089–95. https://doi.org/10.1093/ndt/gfr587.
32. Halimi JM, Buchler M, Al-Najjar A, et al. Urinary albumin excretion and the risk of graft loss and death in proteinuric and non-proteinuric renal transplant recipients. Am J Transplant. 2007;7:618–25. https://doi.org/10.1111/j.1600-6143.2007.01665.x.
33. Fernandez-Fresnedo G, Plaza JJ, Sanchez-Plumed J, Sanz-Guajardo A, Palomar-Fontanet R, Arias M. Proteinuria: a new marker of long-term graft and patient survival in kidney transplantation. Nephrol Dial Transplant. 2004;19(Suppl 3):iii47–51. https://doi.org/10.1093/ndt/gfh1015.
34. Ducloux D, Motte G, Kribs M, et al. Hypertension in renal transplantation: donor and recipient risk factors. Clin Nephrol. 2002;57:409–13.
35. Halimi JM. Albuminuria, proteinuria, and graft survival in kidney transplantation. Am J Kidney Dis. 2011;58:1037; author reply 1037–8. https://doi.org/10.1053/j.ajkd.2011.09.003.
36. Mallamaci F, Tripepi R, Leonardis D, et al. Nocturnal hypertension and altered night-day BP profile and atherosclerosis in renal transplant patients. Transplantation. 2016;100:2211–8. https://doi.org/10.1097/TP.0000000000001023.
37. Ozkayar N, Altun B, Yildirim T, et al. Blood pressure measurements, blood pressure variability and endothelial function in renal transplant recipients. Clin Exp Hypertens. 2014;36:392–7.
38. Rigatto C, Foley RN, Kent GM, Guttmann R, Parfrey PS. Long-term changes in left ventricular hypertrophy after renal transplantation. Transplantation. 2000;70:570–5. https://doi.org/10.1097/00007890-200008270-00006.
39. du Cailar G, Oudot C, Fesler P, et al. Left ventricular mass changes after renal transplantation: influence of dietary sodium and change in serum uric acid. Transplantation. 2014;98:202–7. https://doi.org/10.1097/TP.0000000000000043.
40. Montanaro D, Gropuzzo M, Tulissi P, et al. Effects of successful renal transplantation on left ventricular mass. Transplant Proc. 2005;37:2485–7.
41. Becker-Cohen R, Nir A, Ben-Shalom E, et al. Improved left ventricular mass index in children after renal transplantation. Pediatr Nephrol. 2008;23:1545–50.
42. Patel RK, Mark PB, Johnston N, McGregor E, Dargie HJ, Jardine AG. Renal transplantation is not associated with regression of left ventricular hypertrophy: a magnetic resonance study. Clin J Am Soc Nephrol. 2008;3:1807–11.
43. Pickup LC, Law JP, Radhakrishnan A, et al. Changes in left ventricular structure and function associated with renal transplantation: a systematic review and meta-analysis. ESC Heart Fail. 2021;8:2045–57.
44. Woodle ES, First MR, Pirsch J, et al. A prospective, randomized, double-blind, placebo-controlled multicenter trial comparing early (7 day) corticosteroid cessation versus long-term, low-dose corticosteroid therapy. Ann Surg. 2008;248:564–77. https://doi.org/10.1097/SLA.0b013e318187d1da.
45. Textor SC, Canzanello VJ, Taler SJ, et al. Cyclosporine-induced hypertension after transplantation. Mayo Clin Proc. 1994;69:1182–93. https://doi.org/10.1016/s0025-6196(12)65772-3.
46. Esteva-Font C, Ars E, Guillen-Gomez E, et al. Ciclosporin-induced hypertension is associated with increased sodium transporter of the loop of Henle (NKCC2). Nephrol Dial Transplant. 2007;22:2810–6. https://doi.org/10.1093/ndt/gfm390.
47. Perico N, Ruggenenti P, Gaspari F, et al. Daily renal hypoperfusion induced by cyclosporine in patients with renal transplantation. Transplantation. 1992;54:56–60. https://doi.org/10.1097/00007890-199207000-00009.
48. Hurst FP, Abbott KC, Neff RT, et al. Incidence, predictors and outcomes of transplant renal artery stenosis after kidney transplantation: analysis of USRDS. Am J Nephrol. 2009;30:459–67.
49. Audard V, Matignon M, Hemery F, et al. Risk factors and long-term outcome of transplant renal artery stenosis in adult recipients after treatment by percutaneous transluminal angioplasty. Am J Transplant. 2006;6:95–9. https://doi.org/10.1111/j.1600-6143.2005.01136.x.
50. Chen W, Kayler LK, Zand MS, Muttana R, Chernyak V, DeBoccardo GO. Transplant renal artery stenosis: clinical manifestations, diagnosis and therapy. Clin Kidney J. 2015;8:71–8.

51. Humar A, Matas AJ. Surgical complications after kidney transplantation. Semin Dial. 2005;18:505–10. https://doi.org/10.1111/j.1525-139X.2005.00097.x.
52. Pouria S, State OI, Wong W, Hendry BM. CMV infection is associated with transplant renal artery stenosis. QJM. 1998;91:185–9. https://doi.org/10.1093/qjmed/91.3.185.
53. Loubeyre P, Abidi H, Cahen R, Tran Minh VA. Transplanted renal artery: detection of stenosis with color Doppler US. Radiology. 1997;203:661–5. https://doi.org/10.1148/radiology.203.3.9169685.
54. Baxter GM, Ireland H, Moss JG, et al. Colour Doppler ultrasound in renal transplant artery stenosis: which Doppler index? Clin Radiol. 1995;50:618–22. https://doi.org/10.1016/s0009-9260(05)83291-x.
55. de Morais RH, Muglia VF, Mamere AE, et al. Duplex Doppler sonography of transplant renal artery stenosis. J Clin Ultrasound. 2003;31:135–41. https://doi.org/10.1002/jcu.10147.
56. Huber A, Heuck A, Scheidler J, et al. Contrast-enhanced MR angiography in patients after kidney transplantation. Eur Radiol. 2001;11:2488–95. https://doi.org/10.1007/s003300100992.
57. Luk SH, Chan JH, Kwan TH, Tsui WC, Cheung YK, Yuen MK. Breath-hold 3D gadolinium-enhanced subtraction MRA in the detection of transplant renal artery stenosis. Clin Radiol. 1999;54:651–4. https://doi.org/10.1016/s0009-9260(99)91085-1.
58. Sankari BR, Geisinger M, Zelch M, Brouhard B, Cunningham R, Novick AC. Post-transplant renal artery stenosis: impact of therapy on long-term kidney function and blood pressure control. J Urol. 1996;155:1860–4. https://doi.org/10.1016/s0022-5347(01)66030-0.
59. Brenner BM, Milford EL. Nephron underdosing: a programmed cause of chronic renal allograft failure. Am J Kidney Dis. 1993;21(5 Suppl 2):66–72. https://doi.org/10.1016/0272-6386(93)70097-i.
60. el-Agroudy AE, Hassan NA, Bakr MA, Foda MA, Shokeir AA, Shehab el-Dein AB. Effect of donor/recipient body weight mismatch on patient and graft outcome in living-donor kidney transplantation. Am J Nephrol. 2003;23:294–9. https://doi.org/10.1159/000072819.
61. Hauser IA, Kruck S, Gauer S, et al. Human pregnane X receptor genotype of the donor but not of the recipient is a risk factor for delayed graft function after renal transplantation. Clin Pharmacol Ther. 2012;91:905–16. https://doi.org/10.1038/clpt.2011.346.
62. Joy MS, Hogan SL, Thompson BD, Finn WF, Nickeleit V. Cytochrome P450 3A5 expression in the kidneys of patients with calcineurin inhibitor nephrotoxicity. Nephrol Dial Transplant. 2007;22:1963–8. https://doi.org/10.1093/ndt/gfm133.
63. Cowley AW Jr, Roman RJ. The role of the kidney in hypertension. JAMA. 1996;275:1581–9.
64. Curtis JJ, Luke RG, Dustan HP, et al. Remission of essential hypertension after renal transplantation. N Engl J Med. 1983;309:1009–15. https://doi.org/10.1056/NEJM198310273091702.
65. Guidi E, Menghetti D, Milani S, Montagnino G, Palazzi P, Bianchi G. Hypertension may be transplanted with the kidney in humans: a long-term historical prospective follow-up of recipients grafted with kidneys coming from donors with or without hypertension in their families. J Am Soc Nephrol. 1996;7:1131–8. https://doi.org/10.1681/ASN.V781131.
66. Guidi E, Cozzi MG, Minetti E, Bianchi G. Donor and recipient family histories of hypertension influence renal impairment and blood pressure during acute rejections. J Am Soc Nephrol. 1998;9:2102–7. https://doi.org/10.1681/ASN.V9112102.
67. Freedman BI, Pastan SO, Israni AK, et al. APOL1 genotype and kidney transplantation outcomes from deceased African American donors. Transplantation. 2016;100:194–202.
68. Freedman BI, Moxey-Mims MM, Alexander AA, et al. APOL1 long-term kidney transplantation outcomes network (APOLLO): design and rationale. Kidney Int Rep. 2020;5:278–88.
69. Ahmadi S-F, Zahmatkesh G, Streja E, et al. Body mass index and mortality in kidney transplant recipients: a systematic review and meta-analysis. Am J Nephrol. 2014;40:315–24.
70. Lafranca JA, IJermans JN, Betjes MG, Dor FJ. Body mass index and outcome in renal transplant recipients: a systematic review and meta-analysis. BMC Med. 2015;13:111.
71. Workeneh B, Moore LW, Fong JVN, Shypailo R, Gaber AO, Mitch WE. Successful kidney transplantation is associated with weight gain from truncal obesity and insulin resistance. J Ren Nutr. 2019;29:548–55.

72. Mallamaci F, Tripepi R, D'Arrigo G, et al. Long-term changes in sleep disordered breathing in renal transplant patients: relevance of the BMI. J Clin Med. 2020;9:1739.
73. El-Agroudy AE, Wafa EW, Gheith OE, El-Dein ABS, Ghoneim MA. Weight gain after renal transplantation is a risk factor for patient and graft outcome. Transplantation. 2004;77:1381–5.
74. Zoccali C, Roumeliotis S, Mallamaci F. Sleep apnea as a cardiorenal risk factor in CKD and renal transplant patients. Blood Purif. 2021;50:642–8.
75. Szentkiralyi A, Czira ME, Molnar MZ, et al. High risk of obstructive sleep apnea is a risk factor of death censored graft loss in kidney transplant recipients: an observational cohort study. Sleep Med. 2011;12:267–73.
76. Molnar MZ, Lazar AS, Lindner A, et al. Sleep apnea is associated with cardiovascular risk factors among kidney transplant patients. Clin J Am Soc Nephrol. 2010;5:125–32.
77. Ekici M, Aksoy N. Sleep disorders in kidney transplant recipients. Exp Clin Transplant. 2024;22(Suppl 1):192–4.
78. Mahajan S, Gupta K, Sinha S, Malhotra A, Mahajan S. Effect of kidney transplantation on sleep-disordered breathing in patients with end stage renal disease: a polysomnographic study. Sleep Med. 2018;45:140–5.
79. Mallamaci F, Tripepi R, D'Arrigo G, et al. Sleep-disordered breathing and 24-hour ambulatory blood pressure monitoring in renal transplant patients: longitudinal study. J Am Heart Assoc. 2020;9:e016237.
80. Lubas MM, Ware JC, Szklo-Coxe M. Sleep apnea and kidney transplant outcomes: findings from a 20-year (1997–2017) historical cohort study. Sleep Med. 2019;63:151–8.
81. Fornadi K, Ronai KZ, Turanyi CZ, et al. Sleep apnea is not associated with worse outcomes in kidney transplant recipients. Sci Rep. 2014;4:6987.
82. Tiwari R, Lyu B, Alagusundaramoorthy S, Astor BC, Mandelbrot DA, Parajuli S. Association of diagnosed obstructive sleep apnea with kidney transplant outcomes. Clin Transpl. 2019;33:e13747. https://doi.org/10.1111/ctr.13747.
83. Hansrivijit P, Kanderi T, Puthenpura MM, Ghahramani N, Thongprayoon C, Cheungpasitporn W. The clinical impacts of sleep apnea on mortality and allograft function in kidney transplant patients: a meta-analysis. Clin Nephrol. 2021;95:195–200.
84. Kooman JP, Christiaans MH, Boots JM, van der Sande FM, Leunissen KM, van Hooff JP. A comparison between office and ambulatory blood pressure measurements in renal transplant patients with chronic transplant nephropathy. Am J Kidney Dis. 2001;37:1170–6.
85. Wen KC, Gourishankar S. Evaluating the utility of ambulatory blood pressure monitoring in kidney transplant recipients. Clin Transpl. 2012;26:E465–70.
86. Ahmed J, Ozorio V, Farrant M, Van Der Merwe W. Ambulatory vs office blood pressure monitoring in renal transplant recipients. J Clin Hypertens (Greenwich). 2015;17:46–50.
87. Fernando V, Vincent P, Ilan S, et al. Prevalence and risk factors of noncontrolled and resistant arterial hypertension in renal transplant recipients. Transplantation. 2015;99:1016–22.
88. Whelton PK, Carey RM, Aronow WS, et al. 2017 ACC/AHA/AAPA/ABC/ACPM/AGS/APhA/ASH/ASPC/NMA/PCNA guideline for the prevention, detection, evaluation, and management of high blood pressure in adults: a report of the American College of Cardiology/American Heart Association Task Force on clinical practice guidelines. JACC. 2018;71:e127–248.
89. Williams B, Mancia G, Spiering W, et al. 2018 ESC/ESH guidelines for the management of arterial hypertension: the Task Force for the management of arterial hypertension of the European Society of Cardiology (ESC) and the European Society of Hypertension (ESH). Eur Heart J. 2018;39:3021–104.
90. Cheung A, Chang T, Cushman W, et al. Kidney Disease: Improving Global Outcomes (KDIGO) Blood Pressure Work Group KDIGO 2021 clinical practice guideline for the management of blood pressure in chronic kidney disease. Kidney Int. 2021;99(3S):S1–87.
91. Cheung A, Chertow G, Greene T, et al. Benefits and risks of intensive blood-pressure lowering in advanced chronic kidney disease. J Intern Med. 2018;284:106–7.
92. Malhotra R, Katz R, Weiner DE, et al. Blood pressure, chronic kidney disease progression, and kidney allograft failure in kidney transplant recipients: a secondary analysis of the FAVORIT Trial. Am J Hypertens. 2019;32:816–23.

93. Halimi J-M, Ortiz A, Sarafidis PA, et al. Hypertension in kidney transplantation: a consensus statement of the 'hypertension and the kidney' working group of the European Society of Hypertension. J Hypertens. 2021;39:1513–21.
94. Cross NB, Webster AC, Masson P, O'Connell PJ, Craig JC. Antihypertensive treatment for kidney transplant recipients. Cochrane Database Syst Rev. 2009;2009(3):CD003598.
95. Becker GJ, Wheeler DC, De Zeeuw D, et al. Kidney disease: improving global outcomes (KDIGO) blood pressure work group. KDIGO clinical practice guideline for the management of blood pressure in chronic kidney disease. Kidney Int Suppl. 2012;2:337–414.
96. Pisano A, Bolignano D, Mallamaci F, et al. Comparative effectiveness of different antihypertensive agents in kidney transplantation: a systematic review and meta-analysis. Nephrol Dial Transplant. 2020;35:878–87.

Part III

Renovascular Disorders

Renovascular Disease

7

Constantina Chrysochou, Tom Robberechts, Maria Simona Stoenoiu, and Alexandre Persu

7.1 Introduction

Renal artery stenosis (RAS) is one of the leading causes of secondary hypertension. With an ageing population, increased awareness and wider use of imaging modalities, it is increasingly encountered in daily clinical practice.

With about 90% of cases, atherosclerotic renovascular disease (ARVD) accounts for the vast majority of patients. Non-atherosclerotic disease is found in about 10% of cases, with fibromuscular dysplasia (FMD) being the leading aetiology. Since

C. Chrysochou
Renal Department, Salford Royal Hospital, Northern Care Alliance, Salford, UK

Cardiovascular Sciences, School of Medical Sciences, University of Manchester, Manchester, UK

T. Robberechts
Department of Nephrology and Hypertension, Universitair Ziekenhuis Brussel, Vrije Universiteit Brussel (VUB), Brussels, Belgium

Department of Cardiology, Cliniques Universitaires Saint-Luc, Université Catholique de Louvain, Brussels, Belgium

M. S. Stoenoiu
Department of Internal Medicine, Rheumatology, Cliniques Universitaires Saint-Luc, Institut de Recherche Expérimentale et Clinique, Université Catholique de Louvain, Brussels, Belgium

A. Persu (✉)
Department of Cardiology, Cliniques Universitaires Saint-Luc, Université Catholique de Louvain, Brussels, Belgium

Pole of Cardiovascular Research, Institut de Recherche Expérimentale et Clinique, Université Catholique de Louvain, Brussels, Belgium
e-mail: alexandre.persu@saintluc.uclouvain.be

A. E. Berbari et al. (eds.), *Blood Pressure Disorders in Acute and Chronic Kidney Diseases*, Updates in Hypertension and Cardiovascular Protection
https://doi.org/10.1007/978-3-031-81292-7_7

global cardiovascular risk profile, concomitant atherosclerotic burden and disease management largely differ between both groups, it is important to make the distinction. Differences in patient characteristics, clinical presentation and disease associations will be covered in this chapter.

Although the interplay between renal artery stenosis, arterial hypertension and chronic kidney disease (CKD) has been described for decades, the optimal management of RAS remains under debate. In ARVD, negative outcomes of major randomised controlled trials in the last two decades raised controversy regarding the role of revascularisation in management of the disease. Taking this controversy into account, a consensus regarding selection of patients likely to benefit from revascularisation is presented below. In patients with FMD, controversy is mainly fuelled by the lack of randomised studies assessing the role of revascularisation on blood pressure and kidney outcomes. Although FMD guidelines are partly extrapolated from studies on ARVD, some important differences in treatment will be highlighted, particularly concerning the role of stenting (usually contra-indicated in FMD). Besides revascularisation, the role of medical treatment in both diseases will be discussed as well.

7.2 Atheromatous Renovascular Disease (ARVD)

- **What is ARVD?**

  Any degree of RAS due to atheroma deposition is referred to as ARVD. ARVD tends to affect the proximal third and ostium of the renal arteries, in some cases being the extension of an aortic plaque. ARVD is associated with ageing and other traditional macrovascular atheromatous diseases. The reduction in blood flow and perfusion pressure to the kidney initiates a series of pathophysiological changes and compensatory mechanisms, ultimately resulting in parenchymal injury. These changes include downstream disruption of renal function, blood pressure dysregulation, fluid and salt retention and renal endocrine dysfunction, increased sympathetic activity, arterial remodelling and vasoconstriction, activation of inflammatory and oxidative stress pathways.
- **What is the prevalence of ARVD?**

  There has been a steady increase in the number of patients diagnosed with ARVD in the last few decades [1]. ARVD occurs in 14.1% of all patients with hypertension and in 20% of patients with hypertension and diabetes [2]. Given this strong association, international consensus guidelines [3, 4] recommend screening for ARVD in patients with hypertension with a more severe phenotype such as resistant hypertension, accelerated hypertension, or coexisting heart failure [5].
- **Why is ARVD regarded as a marker of cardiovascular burden?**

  ARVD is frequently identified concurrent with other vascular manifestations and has significant impact on the progression and outcomes of co-existent cardiac disease. The prevalence of ARVD is strongly associated with ageing [6], hypertension (91%), heart failure (up to 68% [5], aorto-iliac and more distal peripheral vascular disease (12–56% [1, 7], coronary artery disease (5–67% [8]), abdominal aortic aneurysms (33% [2], carotid artery stenosis and cerebrovascular disease (5.2–22% [9]) and diabetes mellitus with coexistent hypertension (20% [2]). Around half of patients with ARVD are current or ex-smokers [10]. ARVD is, as such, regarded as a marker of more significant atheromatous burden.

Abnormal cardiac structure and/or function is present in 95 % of ARVD patients [11] with left ventricular hypertrophy (LVH) and diastolic dysfunction being the predominant abnormalities.

- **Why is ARVD regarded as a marker of CKD burden?**

  In middle-aged patients with advanced CKD, ARVD is prevalent in 5–24% of cases, with twice as high prevalence rates in dialysis patients [12]. Nearly 10 3% of patients with acute kidney injury (AKI) have underlying ARVD [1].

  Pre-dialysis patients with ARVD have 1.5 times, and those on dialysis, 3.3 times higher mortality risk than patients with other causes of CKD [13].

7.2.1 What Is the Pathophysiology of Ischaemic Nephropathy?

Lumen stenoses >70% are regarded as sufficient to reduce blood flow and hypoperfuse the juxtaglomerular apparatus [8, 14].

This in turn activates the renin-angiotensin-aldosterone system (RAAS) pathway via renin secretion from renal baroreceptors that sense decreased perfusion to the kidney, low sodium chloride levels detected by the macula densa, beta-adrenergic stimulation and an increase in the number of renin-expressing cells due to prolonged ischaemia. Renin cleaves angiotensinogen to angiotensin I, which is then converted to angiotensin II. Angiotensin II raises blood pressure by multiple mechanisms such as vasoconstriction, sympathetic nervous stimulation causing a presynaptic release of norepinephrine, aldosterone secretion by the adrenal cortex causing sodium and water retention, increased collagen type I and III synthesis in fibroblasts leading to thickening of the vascular wall and myocardium, and fibrosis [4, 8, 14]. These processes result in rarefaction of microvessels, cortical hypoxia, stimulation of inflammatory cytokines and recruitment of progenitor and inflammatory cells, which have been implicated in the development of glomerulosclerosis and tubulointerstitial fibrosis.

Lesser degrees of stenosis may still have haemodynamic effects. Bearing in mind the heavy burden of concomitant atherosclerotic disease, ageing and diabetes in ARVD, renal autoregulation may be compromised [14, 15] with secondary impact on renal flow. At some point in the natural history of ARVD, the systemic inflammatory response triggered by chronic subclinical ischaemia may become the predominant driver of kidney impairment, rather than the reduced blood flow itself [16].

In unilateral RAS, the contralateral healthy kidney may compensate for the above-mentioned adverse effects of renin-dependent hypertension through pressure natriuresis. However, this compensation is lost in bilateral RAS, causing sodium/volume retention and leading to a volume-dependent hypertension phenotype and higher risk of 'flash' pulmonary oedema.

In addition to the endocrine consequences of mechanical flow reduction, glomerular hypoperfusion and deoxygenation result in vascular rarefaction, oxidative stress injury and an inflammatory cytokine release that ultimately produces mitochondrial and microvascular dysfunction, leading to kidney fibrosis [14]. Consequently, in case of longstanding RAS, mechanical intervention to restore renal arterial flow may not reverse ischaemic nephropathy. However, the optimal window of opportunity for revascularisation is still unclear.

7.2.2 How Does ARVD Present?

Patients with ARVD may present in a variety of ways (Table 7.1). While some remain asymptomatic, others may present severe renal and/or cardiac manifestations.

7.2.3 How to Diagnose ARVD?

Angiography, either invasive or non-invasive, remains the cornerstone of diagnosis. In daily practice, Doppler ultrasound is generally used as screening tool for RAS, due to its low cost and easy availability. However, it is operator-dependant and thus subject to inter- and intra-observer variability. Computed tomography angiography (CTA) and magnetic resonance angiography (MRA) are less subjective and more reliable for diagnosis and assessment of severity. Due to improvement of sensitivity of CTA and MRA, captopril renography is largely abandoned. Catheter-based angiography remains the gold standard, in particular when renal revascularisation is considered.

7.2.3.1 Doppler Ultrasound

Diagnostic criteria: a peak systolic velocity (PSV) >200 cm/s or a renal/aorta PSV ratio ≥3.5.

Advantages: Sensitive (in experienced hands), non-invasive, easily available investigative tool. Doppler waveforms can provide resistive index (RI), a surrogate marker of viability of the renal parenchyma (if RI <0.8).

Table 7.1 When to suspect ARVD

Incidentally, e.g., detected whilst undergoing vascular imaging for another purpose
Difficult-to-control or resistant hypertension
Chronic kidney disease (CKD)
Acute kidney injury (>30% increase in serum creatinine level) ≤1 week after initiating ACE-inhibitors or angiotensin receptor blockers
Renal asymmetry (size difference >1.5 cm)
Acute 'flash' pulmonary oedema
Decompensated heart failure, particularly in patients with CKD Grade 3–5 and hypertension

Disadvantages: Time consuming, views difficult to obtain in obese patients or those with a distended small or large bowel. Operator and centre-dependent, subject to wide intra- and inter-observer variations.

7.2.3.2 Magnetic Resonance Angiography (MRA)

Advantages: Non-invasive, accurate, renal artery ostium visibility better than in DSA (Fig. 7.1).

Disadvantages: Contra-indicated with non-compatible metallic implants such as pacemakers, false positive artefacts from respiration, noisy, difficult to tolerate for patients with claustrophobia. Older gadolinium agents were implicated in nephrogenic systemic fibrosis in patients with severe renal impairment, but this risk is marginal (<0.07%) in CKD Grade 4–5 [17] with newer agents.

7.2.3.3 Computed Tomography Angiography (CTA)

Advantages: Non-invasive, readily available in most hospitals, fast, similar sensitivity/specificity to MRA for detection of RAS, allows detection of renal arterial calcification (Fig. 7.2).

Disadvantages: Use of iodinated contrast may result in contrast-induced nephropathy, exposure to ionising radiation.

7.2.3.4 Catheter-Based or Digital Subtraction Angiography (DSA)

Advantages: Accurate assessment of degree of RAS, regarded as a gold standard assessment, concomitant diagnosis and treatment during renal revascularisation procedure.

Disadvantages: Invasive procedure, bleeding risk due to arterial puncture, costly, provides only 2D images and poses a risk of contrast nephropathy.

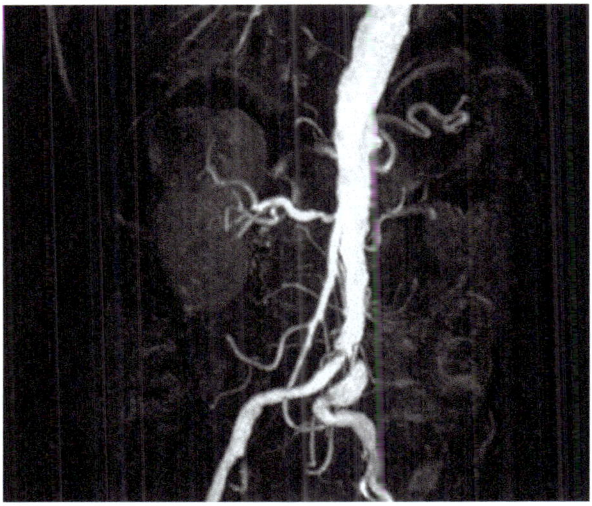

Fig. 7.1 Magnetic resonance angiogram showing atheromatous and irregular aorto-iliac and renovascular disease

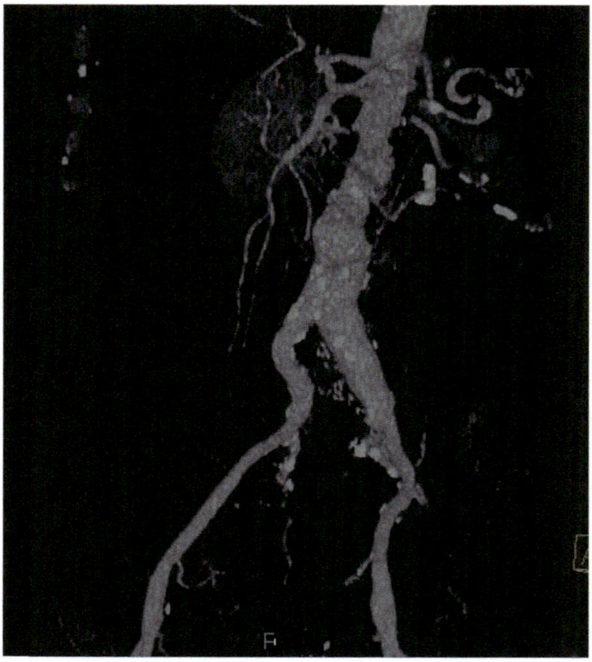

Fig. 7.2 Computed tomography angiography showing ARVD and areas of calcification in aorta

7.2.3.5 Intravascular Ultrasound

Advantages: Assessment of distal vascular disease using intra-renal blood flow velocity measurements.

Disadvantages: Invasive, not generally applicable in clinical practice.

7.2.3.6 Captopril Renography

Advantages: Non-invasive, good sensitivity and specificity.

Disadvantages: Offers no anatomical information on renal artery or degree of stenosis, has limited reliability in case of associated CKD or bilateral RAS. Inferior to CTA and MRA.

7.2.4 What Is the Management of ARVD and Why Is It Controversial?

The diagnosis and management of atherosclerotic renovascular disease (ARVD) remain controversial. Whilst there is agreement on optimal medical management, endovascular treatment requires individual consideration [18].

7.2.4.1 How to Medically Optimise a Patient with ARVD?

Medical management of ARVD should aim to reduce cardiovascular risk and protect renal function. KDIGO and European Renal Best Practice guidelines [4, 8]

underscore the importance of medical therapy, including a statin [19] and antihypertensive medications, just as in generalised atheromatous disease. Supportive adjuncts such as smoking cessation, weight loss, regular physical exercise and reduced sodium consumption remain cornerstones in the general management of vascular diseases.

Targets for blood pressure control in ARVD follow the general BP management guidelines [3, 4]. Since reduced renal perfusion triggers RAAS activation, pharmacological targeting of this overactivity can improve blood pressure control. The use of renin-angiotensin-aldosterone system blockers (RAB) is now considered the first-line choice to treat hypertension in the setting of ARVD [20]. RAB are well tolerated even in bilateral ARVD and have been shown to reduce mortality [21]. However, there remains reservation using RAB in significant, bilateral ARVD or in a single kidney affected by ARVD due to concerns with renal functional decline. After initiation of RAB, kidney function should be carefully monitored. In case of significant kidney function decline, renal artery revascularisation should be considered. As several antihypertensive agents are often needed to achieve blood pressure targets, selection of specific treatment should follow general guidelines.

The role of antiplatelet therapy is established in patients with atherosclerotic coronary or peripheral artery disease, and observational studies suggest that the use of low-dose aspirin is also associated with reduced mortality risk in patients with ARVD [22].

Potential therapies in development are aimed at regenerating the ischaemic parenchyma in addition to revascularisation, thereby remedying renal function and blood pressure more effectively. Pathophysiological mechanisms include oxidative stress, microvascular disease, inflammation, mitochondrial injury and cellular senescence and may, for example, be targeted by vascular endothelial growth factor, endothelin antagonists or stem cells [23–25].

7.2.4.2 Is There an Added Value of Percutaneous Renal Artery Revascularisation?

Opinions regarding gains from renal artery intervention have shifted considerably in the last few decades. The 1990s saw observational evidence supporting the efficacy and safety of percutaneous transluminal renal artery angioplasty (PTRA) with or without stenting for the treatment of ARVD. Increasing awareness of the association between coronary artery disease (CAD) and ARVD, and the adverse prognosis engendered in CAD patients by significant RAS, fuelled enthusiasm of interventionalists to 'shoot the renal arteries' by 'drive by angioplasty' during coronary investigation [26]. This resulted in an increase in PTRA [27].

This trend lost popularity after multiple randomised controlled trials (RCTs) in the 2000s showed no significant benefit of revascularisation compared to medical treatment alone, either on renal function or on blood pressure (Table 7.2). It is widely acknowledged that these trials had individual design weaknesses, lack of pre-specified sub-groups and recruitment difficulties [18, 35]. Nonetheless, the results were consistent in the message that routinely restoring vessel patency alone

Table 7.2 Randomised controlled trials comparing renal revascularisation to medical therapy alone

Author	Patients (*n*)	Follow-up (months)	Randomisation	Difference in BP outcome between treatment arms	Difference in renal functional outcome	Other key clinical outcomes
Weibull et al, 1993 [28]	58	24	29—PTRA 29—surgery	No	No	More complications in surgical arm. 96% primary patency rate at 24 months for surgery vs 75% for PTRA
Plouin et al. (EMMA study), 1998 [10]	49	6	23—PTRA 26—Medical treatment	No. Reduced anti-hypertensive use in PTRA group		26% complications in PTRA group
Webster et al, 1998. [29]	55	3–54	25—PTRA 30—Medical treatment	Statistically significant BP drop only in patients with bilateral disease randomised to PTRA	No	No significant difference in survival
Van de Ven et al, 1999 [30]	85	6	42—PTRA 43—PTRAS	No	No	PTRAS technically more successful. 12 patients who failed PTRA required secondary PTRAS
Van Jaarsveld et al, 2000 [31]	106	12	56—PTRA 50—Medical treatment	No	No	
Bax et al, 2009. [32] (STAR)	140	24	76—Medical treatment 64—Medical treatment + PTRAS		22% medical vs 16% PTRAS had >20% decrease in CrCl from baseline	Significant number of PTRAS-related complications

Wheatley et al, 2009. [33] (ASTRAL)	806	33.6 (median)	403—Medical treatment 403—Medical treatment + PTRAS (95%) or PTRA	No. Diastolic BP lower in medically treated group	No statistically significant difference in rates of renal decline or end-stage kidney disease	No statistically significant difference in rates of CVE or death. PTRAS associated with 6.7% serious adverse events
Marcantoni et al, 2012. [34] (RAS-CAD)	84	12	41—Medical therapy 43—Medical therapy + PTRAS	No		No statistically significant difference in CVE, left ventricular mass index or mortality
Cooper et al, 2014. [35] (CORAL)	947	43 (median)	480—Medical treatment 467—Medical treatment + PTRAS (95%) or PTRA	Non-significant BP improvement in PTRA group	No	No benefit of PTRA(S) over optimal medical treatment in terms of clinical outcomes

BP blood pressure, *CrCl* creatinine clearance, *CVE* cardiovascular events, *PTRA* percutaneous transluminal renal angioplasty, *PTRAS* percutaneous transluminal renal artery stenting was insufficient to recover kidney function for most patients and did not add clinical benefit beyond that achievable with best medical therapy.

Viability of renal parenchyma is an important predictor of successful revascularisation. Certain radiological features may support a potential for renal recovery, e.g. preserved cortical thickness >0.5 cm, renal resistive index <0.8 or renal diameter >8 cm [8]. In contrast, a urine albumin-creatinine ratio (UACR) >300 mg/g (30 mg/mmol) could be seen as a relative contra-indication for revascularisation, since it potentially marks underlying parenchymal atrophy or secondary glomerular damage [37]. Newer imaging techniques such as blood oxygen level–dependent (BOLD) MRI allow evaluation of tissue oxygenation, with the possibility of detecting so-called 'hibernating parenchyma' [38]: parenchyma with attenuated activity due to reduced blood flow but without irreversible hypoxic damage. However, these techniques are still in the research realm.

7.2.4.3 What Are the Risks of Revascularisation?

Due to its invasive nature, revascularisation is not devoid of risk, with major complications occurring in 9% [33] of patients. Most complications are minor and linked to the arterial access site, including bruising, groin haematoma or pseudoaneurysm formation. Major vascular complications such as renal artery dissection, rupture or thrombosis occur rarely (1–2% of procedures [39]). Decline in kidney function in some cases leading to end-stage renal disease is possible, either due to contrast-induced AKI or due to cholesterol embolisation. The presence of extensive aortic atherosclerosis, significant cardiovascular disease and advanced CKD increases the risk of complications. As most patients are elderly and have extra-renal atherosclerotic disease, this risk is not to be underappreciated.

Optimal renal stent deployment and sizing is important. Technical developments, such as drug eluting or low-profile stents that allow better stent deployment in smaller vessels, and distal protection devices may increase the safety and effectiveness of revascularisation [40].

7.2.5 Which Clinical Scenarios Benefit from Intervention? A Practical Guide

Despite the negative results of randomised controlled studies, well-conducted observational studies have shown that particular clinical phenotypes may derive substantial benefit from revascularisation [41, 42]. Their identification is thus cornerstone to decision-making [8, 18]. In so-called 'high-risk clinical presentations', revascularisation is associated with preservation of kidney function, blood pressure improvement, decreased risk of both acute and chronic cardiovascular events, improved cardiac remodelling [43, 44] and/or lower mortality [41, 42, 45].

A decision aid is proposed below and summarised in Fig. 7.3 [8]:

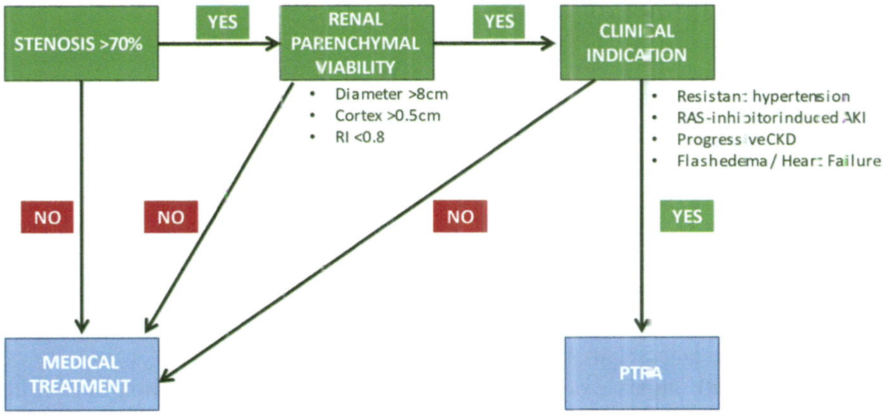

Fig. 7.3 Decision aid to guide which patients to refer for renal artery angioplasty. *CKD* chronic kidney disease, *PTRA* percutaneous transluminal renal angioplasty, *RAS* renin angiotensin system

1. Is there a high-grade RAS lesion (>70%) or radiologic evidence suggesting compromised blood flow?
2. Is there remaining viable renal parenchyma?
   (a) Renal diameter >8 cm
   (b) Preserved cortical thickness (>0.5 cm)
   (c) Renal resistive index <0.8
3. Are we in presence of a high-risk clinical syndrome likely to benefit from intervention [8]?

   As per consensus guidelines [8], these syndromes, in the presence of high-grade RAS, are:

   (a) Definite indications:
   - Resistant hypertension
   - ACE-i or ARB-induced AKI
   - Acute pulmonary oedema or acute decompensation of heart failure
   - Progressive CKD in high-grade RAS (bilateral stenosis or solitary kidney)
   - AKI due to acute renal artery occlusion or high-grade RAS with anuria
   - Kidney transplant with RAS (symptomatic or asymptomatic)

   (b) Possible indications:
   - Chronic heart failure
   - Coexistence of progressive CKD and uncontrolled hypertension
   - Asymptomatic high-grade RAS (either bilateral or solitary kidney) with viable renal parenchyma
   - New (<3 months) dialysis patient with non-functioning but possibly viable kidney

7.2.6 What Is the Prognosis?

The natural history of ARVD involves progression of RAS lesions, cardiovascular disease, hypertension and renal damage if left untreated [13]. The strong link between ARVD and other co-morbid cardiovascular diseases is reflected in the high incidence of cardiovascular events and death in patients with ARVD [46, 47]. In ARVD, the risk of death is nearly six times greater than the risk of evolving towards renal replacement therapy (RRT), with respective incidence rates of 166.3 vs. 28.8 cases per 1000 patient years [1, 12]. Patients who present with flash pulmonary oedema and do not undergo revascularisation have a twofold increased risk of death and threefold increase in cardiovascular events. Patients who do require RRT have a poor life expectancy, with a 4-year mortality rate of 35% [1, 12].

However, with improvements in medical management and selection of patients suitable for revascularisation, outcomes are more favourable [8, 44, 48, 49]. The use of more effective antihypertensive, statins and renal protective medical therapies in RCTs resulted in slower renal function deterioration, improved blood pressure control and mortality [20, 33, 49].

Beyond medical treatment, revascularisation in selected cohorts with the above-mentioned 'high risk features' results in cardiac benefits with improved symptom relief, improved left ventricular diastolic function [43], reduced hospital admissions for heart failure/flash pulmonary oedema, and reduced cardiovascular events and mortality [42, 45]. In patients with resistant hypertension, it may contribute to improved blood pressure control. In a retrospective single-centre study, a mean reduction in daytime ambulatory blood pressure of 14 mmHg was described after angioplasty, with use of less anti-hypertensives [50]. Concerning renal benefits, data are heterogeneous. Some studies report no benefit on renal function [50] while others do report improvement of eGFR in selected populations [51].

7.2.7 Which Studies Are Needed to Cover Current Knowledge Gaps? (Adapted from [4, 8])

- RCTs enrolling patients with haemodynamically significant ARVD and high-risk clinical presentations
- RCTs aiming to discern true renovascular hypertension rather than patients with primary hypertension and incidental RAS through systematic use of, e.g., trans-lesional pressure gradient
- Studies testing the impact of functional non-invasive imaging, e.g., blood oxygenation level–dependent (BOLD) imaging, arterial spin labelling (ASL) or markers of hibernating parenchyma, to identify patients more likely to benefit from revascularisation
- Studies examining the efficacy of revascularisation at all levels of CKD
- Studies establishing the optimal timeline of revascularisation
- Studies evaluating the efficacy of revascularisation in combination with novel therapeutic strategies (e.g. targeting inflammation-related pathways, mesenchymal stem cells or angiogenic/growth factors)

7.3 Fibromuscular Dysplasia (FMD)

- **What is FMD?**

  FMD is a non-atherosclerotic, non-inflammatory arterial disease which involves medium-sized muscular arteries throughout the body. The causes of FMD remain poorly understood. It is likely that a variety of genetic, mechanical, hormonal and environmental factors play a role in its pathogenesis.

  FMD phenotype shows high variability, with arterial stenosis, dissection, aneurysm and tortuosity being part of the disease spectrum. Arterial stenosis is classified as either focal or multifocal. Multifocal FMD is characterised by a 'string-of-beads' pattern, an arterial lesion with alternating dilatations and stenoses. It represents ~70% of cases and usually occurs in the mid and distal portions of the artery. Focal FMD may occur in any part of the artery. Multifocal and focal FMD roughly correspond to the medial and intimal histological forms of FMD, although the histological classification is no longer used.

- **What is the prevalence of FMD?**

  FMD may occur in subjects of any age, including children and elderly patients, but is most commonly seen in young and middle adulthood, with a mean age of diagnosis of 43–53 years [52, 53]. The majority of patients with FMD are women (82–95%). However, compared to women, men with FMD have higher rates of focal FMD and arterial dissection [54, 55].

  Smoking seems to be a relevant risk factor in FMD, with higher prevalence of current smoking in FMD compared to matched controls with essential hypertension. Current smoking may be associated with a more severe disease presentation and a higher prevalence of aneurysms [56]. However, not all publications confirm these associations [57].

- **How does FMD present?**

  While FMD most commonly involves the renal (66–91%), cerebrovascular (25–80%), and less often mesenteric (14–21%) and lower extremity (10–45%) arteries, involvement of most arteries throughout the body has been reported [52, 58–60] (Fig. 7.4a–c). Independent predictors of multivessel FMD include higher age at diagnosis, stroke, multifocal subtype, presence of aneurysm or dissection, and family history of FMD [53].

  Much has been learnt from dedicated international FMD registries [52, 53, 58, 60]. Symptoms of FMD are mostly related to arterial stenosis, with clinical presentation depending on the localisation of the lesion. Aneurysms, dissections and tortuosity are commonly detected at presentation, while progression of lesions is rare. Dissections are most often found in cerebrovascular arteries, with prevalence rates of 9–39.5% in (inter)national registries [52, 61–63]. Carotid artery dissections are two to four times more frequent than vertebral artery dissections, in agreement with the higher prevalence of carotid vs. vertebral FMD. Independent factors associated with arterial dissections include male gender, older age at FMD diagnosis, stroke/neurovascular presentation and multivessel FMD [53]. In contrast, arterial hypertension/renovascular presentation is negatively correlated with dissections.

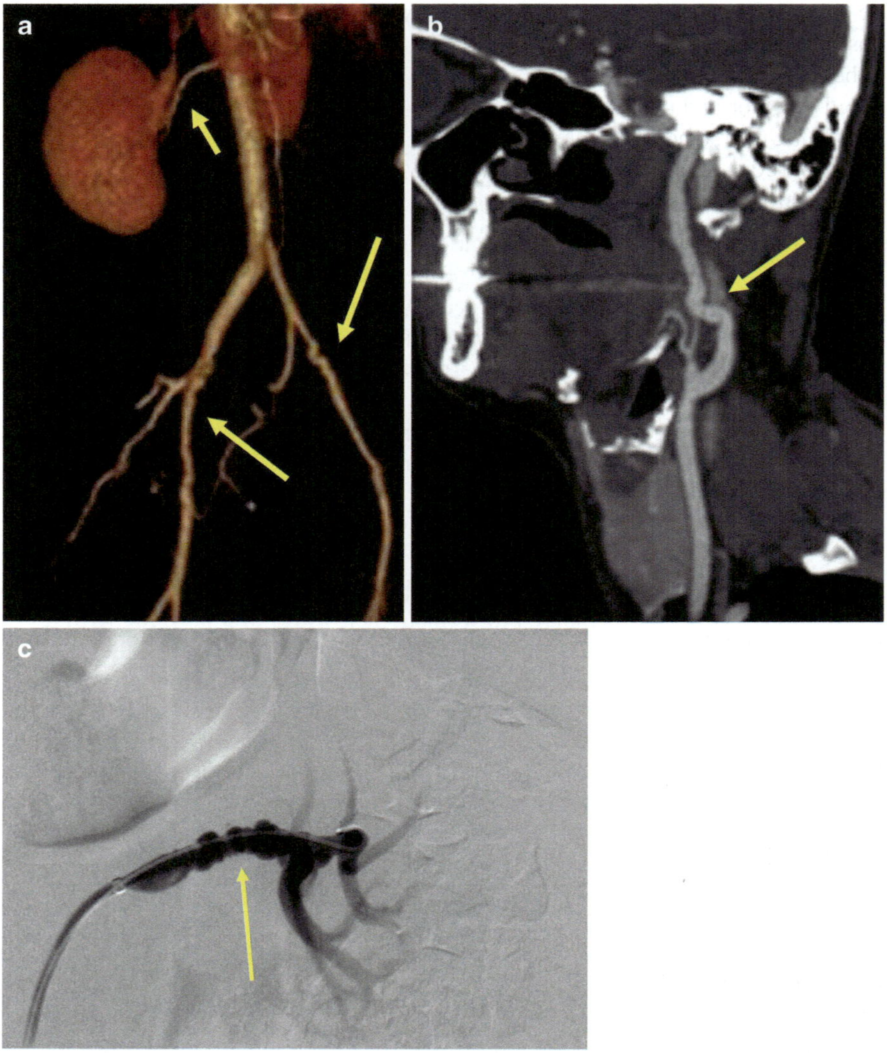

Fig. 7.4 3D volume rendered CTA of aorta highlighting renal and external iliac artery FMD involvement (**a**) and left internal carotid artery FMD (**b**) in same patient. (**c**) Left renal artery string-of-beads detected during intra-arterial angiography

Clinical manifestations of renal FMD include:

- Hypertension in patients <50 years of age, especially women
- Accelerated, malignant or grade 3 (>180/110 mmHg) hypertension
- Drug-resistant hypertension (blood pressure target not achieved despite three drug therapies at optimal doses including a diuretic)
- Unilateral small kidney without a causative urological abnormality

- Abdominal bruit in the absence of atherosclerotic disease or risk factors for atherosclerosis
- Suspected renal artery dissection/infarction

Clinical manifestations of cerebrovascular FMD include:

- Stroke, transient ischaemic attack or amaurosis fugax
- Cerebrovascular aneurysms and/or dissections (associated with male gender)
- Severe and/or chronic migraine headaches, especially in the presence of other suggestive symptoms or signs
- Pulsatile tinnitus
- Cervical bruit
- Unilateral head/neck pain or focal neurologic findings (e.g. partial Horner's syndrome with ipsilateral ptosis and miosis) suggestive of a cervical artery dissection
- A 'carotid web' or 'carotid bulb diaphragm' is possibly an atypical presentation of FMD and described predominantly in black/Afro-Caribbean patients [64]. It is associated with a high risk of ischaemic stroke, likely via an embolic mechanism, which may justify carotid stenting or endarterectomy in the setting of recurrent ischaemic events despite appropriate medical management

In contrast to ARVD, FMD lesions do not impact cardiac or renal parenchymal integrity [65, 66] unless an acute ischaemic event has occurred [67] or long-standing hypertension impacts parenchymal integrity.

- **What is the relation between FMD and Spontaneous Coronary Artery Dissection (SCAD)?**

Spontaneous coronary artery dissection (SCAD) is increasingly recognised as an important cause of acute coronary syndrome, myocardial infarction and sudden death, particularly among young women <60 years of age and individuals with few conventional atherosclerotic risk [52, 68, 69]. In initial reports studying overlap with FMD, FMD prevalence rates of up to 86% were reported in cohorts with confirmed SCAD [69, 70]. However, true prevalence is probably lower, as shown in more recent publications, including a blinded analysis case series by Persu et al., showing an FMD prevalence rate of 31.8% [71].

SCAD and FMD appear to be overlapping entities which share common features such as female sex predominance, mean age at diagnosis, pregnancy, physical and emotional stress triggers phenotype and association with the *PHACTR1* variant [68, 72]. However, both diseases show some important differences in clinical presentation, type and distribution of arterial lesions, and genetic background [62, 71, 73, 74]. Therefore, despite the similarities at certain points (see Table 7.3), SCAD and FMD should probably be considered as distinct entities.

7.3.1 What Is the Pathophysiology of FMD Lesions?

Extensive studies have correlated the arterial lesions of FMD to histopathological findings of arterial fibrosis, cellular hyperplasia and distortion of the abnormal architecture of the arterial wall. The vascular phenotype of lesions associated with

Table 7.3 Similarities and differences between FMD and SCAD

	Similarities	Differences
Age, gender	Majority occur in women. Similar age range (young–middle aged) at diagnosis	Strong association of dissections with male gender in patients with FMD, whereas female gender in SCAD
Clinical presentation	Both FMD and SCAD are associated with extra-coronary dissections and aneurysms As such, full-body CT/MR-angiography recommended	Less frequent extra-coronary multivessel involvement, aneurysms and dissections in SCAD vs. FMD FMD but not SCAD associated with extra-coronary arterial tortuosity
Histology and imaging	Non-inflammatory Non atherosclerotic Spontaneous formation of intramural haematoma within tunica media of artery compressing the true lumen during dissections	Continuous, alternating, irregular distribution of FMD within arteries. FMD lesions predominantly medial (medial fibroplasia, perimedial fibroplasia or medial hyperplasia), less commonly intimal or adventitial. No similar lesions documented in SCAD
Genetics	Some shared common genetic determinants including *PHACTR1* variant	A polygenic risk score for SCAD allows prediction of an increased risk of SCAD also in patients with FMD, suggesting distinct genetic determinants
Treatment	Anti-platelets on an individual risk–benefit analysis	Renal FMD presenting with hypertension likely to benefit from angioplasty. SCAD best treated conservatively in most cases.

FMD has been expanded to include arterial aneurysms, dissections, and tortuosity. However, in the absence of a string-of-beads or focal stenosis, the presence of these lesions alone is deemed not sufficient to establish the diagnosis.

New evidence suggests that FMD is a systemic arterial disease. Subclinical alterations can be found in even non-affected arterial segments, such as the 'triple signal' pattern in the brachial and common carotid artery [75, 76]. This 'triple signal', an ultrasonic finding characterised by a supernumerary acoustic interface located between the blood-intima and the media-adventitia interfaces of the arterial wall, might correspond to focal zones of fibrosis in the outer media. Preliminary data on 'triple signal' in FMD suggest an association with increased stiffness of the vascular wall and impaired endothelial function but its specificity as a hallmark of FMD has been questioned.

Mechanical factors, e.g., repeated stretching of an artery, may contribute to the formation of FMD in certain arterial locations such as right renal artery, mid to distal internal carotid and external iliac arteries, but specific mechanisms are currently unknown.

7.3.2 Is There a Genetic Cause?

There are currently no genetic tests specific to FMD, but genetic susceptibility studies are a rapidly evolving field. At the present, time there is no justification for genetic testing of asymptomatic relatives. Familial cases are reported only in a minority of cases (<5%), some with potential autosomal dominant inheritance with incomplete penetrance. The impact of potential environmental modifiers (e.g., female hormones, lifetime mechanical stress and tobacco smoking) is not yet clear.

Using a genome-wide association study approach, a single nucleotide polymorphism (SNP) rs9349379-A, in the phosphatase and actin regulator 1 (*PHACTR1*) gene, has been consistently associated with FMD. The protein encoded by this gene is involved in regulating reorganisation of the actin cytoskeleton, tubule formation and endothelial cell survival. The associated SNP confers an odds ratio of ~1.4 for FMD and ~ 1.8 SCAD [72, 77]. The *PHACTR1* variant is also associated with an increased odds ratio for carotid artery dissection, hypertension and migraine headache, as well as interestingly an inverse association with coronary atherosclerotic arterial disease and related myocardial infarction [78]. In view of its mild effect, there is no clinical indication to test for this variant in clinical practice.

Gene variants in *collagen type V alpha 1 chain (COL5A1)* and prostaglandin I2 receptor (PTGIR) have been labelled the first clinically actionable genetic test [73]. In particular, the phenotype associated with the recurrent *COL5A1* variant is a more severe multifocal FMD with arterial dissections, aneurysms and tortuosity [52]. Genetic forms are rare; their identification may allow forward planning of surveillance angiographic imaging, blood pressure monitoring and control, consideration of pregnancy risk, avoidance of contact sports and surgical precautions. Variants reported, but not meeting a statistical criteria, have been also described in genes *COL3A1*, *LOX*, *FLNA*, *LOX SMAD2*, *TGFB2*, *TGFB3*, *TGFBR1*, *TGFBR2* and *YY1AP1* [73].

7.3.3 How to Diagnose FMD?

The First International FMD Consensus guidelines specify the presence of a stenotic lesion to validate the diagnosis and differentiate FMD from FMD mimics [52]. To confirm a FMD diagnosis, ≥1 multifocal or focal arterial stenotic lesion must be present. Aneurysm, dissection or tortuosity without multifocal/focal lesion(s) is not sufficient to diagnose FMD. Many patients present arterial lesions in two or more arterial beds, which correspond to so-called multivessel FMD. Once the diagnosis of FMD is confirmed based on ≥1 stenotic lesion, all other lesions (including aneurysm, dissection and tortuosity) can be considered as part of the FMD-spectrum.

CTA is regarded as the first-line investigation for renal FMD, especially if the level of suspicion is high, with MRA as alternative in case of contraindication for CTA. Benefits and shortcomings of imaging techniques are discussed higher in the section on ARVD and are roughly similar in FMD [52]. CTA has better spatial resolution and visualises small calcifications, thereby providing a more accurate discrimination of FMD from ARVD.

Strong data are lacking to recommend one imaging modality over another for assessment of suspected cerebrovascular FMD. At most centres, CTA or MRA is the initial diagnostic modality of choice, as determined by local resources and experience. In high-volume centres with extensive expertise in duplex ultrasound for FMD, this modality may be used for initial assessment of suspected carotid artery FMD, though not adequate to assess the distal internal carotid, vertebral or intracranial arteries.

The consensus guidelines advocate a CTA or MRA brain to pelvis imaging at diagnosis, in light of the high proportion of patients with multi-vessel FMD [52]. Systematic screening of all potentially affected vascular beds helps to assess the global vascular burden in individual patients and to identify hitherto asymptomatic lesions (e.g. aneurysms) that might require follow-up or treatment.

7.3.4 How to Manage FMD?

7.3.4.1 What Is the Optimal Medical Treatment in FMD?

In the absence of RCTs, antiplatelet agents such as aspirin are reasonable to prescribe, as FMD patients may be at risk for thrombotic and thromboembolic events due to flow disturbances linked to string-of-beads and marked arterial tortuosity. This should be weighted on an individual risk–benefit analysis in both symptomatic and asymptomatic FMD and seen as part of a global prevention strategy [52], e.g., patients >60 years of age and with carotid cerebrovascular FMD may benefit more from antiplatelet treatment.

As the ideal blood pressure target in patients with FMD is unknown, generic guideline recommendations are applied [3, 79]. No specific anti-hypertensive is recommended but certain medications may benefit individual scenarios, e.g., beta blockers may have protective effect on SCAD; beta-blockers, calcium channel blockers, angiotensin receptor blockers (ARBs) may prevent migraines; and angiotensin converting enzyme (ACE) inhibitors or ARBs are more commonly used in FMD [52, 68].

Migraines may occur in patients with FMD even in the absence of cerebrovascular involvement. Usual migraine management (lifestyle modification to avoid triggering factors, preventive and treatment therapies) can be considered. Caution is however advised in prescribing tryptans, ergots and other vasoconstrictive agents, especially in patients with a prior history of cervical artery dissection or SCAD. Sound or cognitive behavioural therapy and multi-disciplinary input may be needed for pulsatile tinnitus [52, 80].

The safety of fluoroquinolones warrants further study due to the increased risk of aortic rupture and dissection with their use [52].

7.3.4.2 What Is the Role of Angioplasty?

In contrast to ARVD, renal FMD lesions, especially focal, are more likely to benefit from renovascular intervention. In a meta-analysis, the rate of hypertension cure (defined as blood pressure <140/90 mmHg without treatment) after angioplasty or surgery was estimated to be 46% and 58% [81]. The probability of being cured was negatively associated with patient age. The latter may partially be explained by the

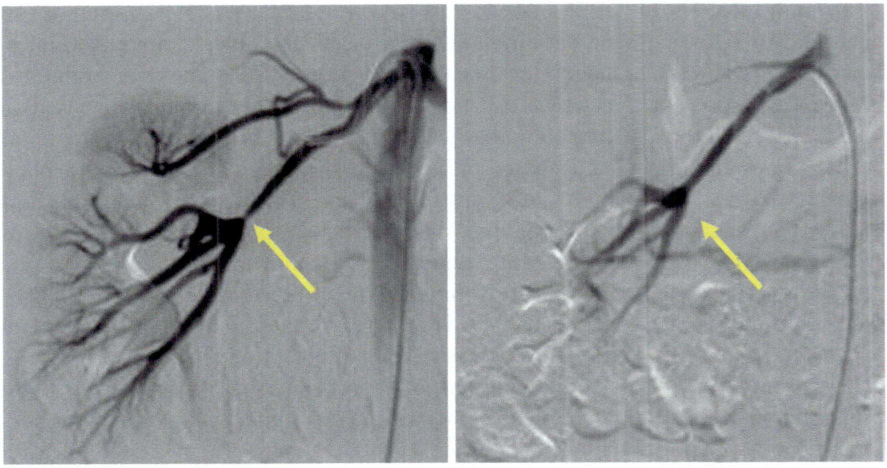

Fig. 7.5 Pre- and post-catheter angiography of the right renal artery with resolution of focal non-ostial stenosis (yellow arrow)

higher prevalence of essential hypertension in the ageing population, thereby diluting the potential benefits of revascularisation on blood pressure profile.

In patients with renal FMD requiring revascularisation, angioplasty without stent placement is recommended (Fig. 7.5) [52]. Stent placement in FMD is indeed associated with a higher risk of stent-related complications including stent kinking and fracture. Recent observational data report in-stent restenosis and/or stent occlusion in up to 58% of cases of patients with FMD treated by renal artery stenting [32]. In addition, in cases of subsequent surgical revascularisation, previous stenting may hinder this procedure. Stenting in renal artery FMD is only used as a bail out strategy if the gradient cannot be obliterated with angioplasty alone, or as treatment of a dissection or aneurysm. The combined risks of periprocedural complications are 12% and 17% after angioplasty and surgery, respectively, with fewer major complications after angioplasty compared to surgery (6% versus 15%).

An agreed protocol for catheter-based angiography and angioplasty in patients with renal artery FMD is published in the International Consensus guidelines [52].

7.3.5 How to Assess the Haemodynamic Significance of a Renal Lesion?

Haemodynamic impact of FMD-related stenosis on renal perfusion is not well studied.

In focal FMD, the aspect of stenosis is anatomically quite similar to stenosis in ARVD, making the evaluation of its haemodynamic severity quite straightforward. This may partly explain the higher success rate of balloon angioplasty in improving hypertension in patients with focal compared to multifocal FMD [52].

In multifocal FMD, string-of-beads are characterised by a high variability in anatomical phenotype, with varying number of beads and diverse degrees of inter-bead stenosis. Assessing haemodynamic impact of successive stenosis and dilations is complex, which explains why estimation of haemodynamic significance based on visual aspects of the lesion is particularly challenging and often erroneous.

Initial evaluation is usually based on non-invasive imaging. Duplex ultrasound gives some idea of haemodynamic impact, but has significant limitations. It is operator-dependent and is only advised as a diagnostic tool in specialised centres with extensive experience [52]. More importantly, diagnostic criteria for haemodynamic significance are extrapolated from atherosclerotic stenosis and are not validated in (multifocal) FMD. CTA or MRA offer further insights in anatomical aspects of lesions but do not allow assessing haemodynamic impact.

According to the international consensus [52], catheter-based angiography with translesional pressure gradient measurement is the recommended approach for haemodynamic evaluation of multifocal FMD. Typically, invasively measured pressure gradients can be used to decide whether to perform balloon angioplasty, with a gradient threshold of 10% (i.e. Pd/Pa <0.90) [52, 81]. Notably however, this cut-off is extrapolated from studies in ARVD and has not been validated in patients with FMD. Furthermore, this approach implies potentially unnecessary exposure to an invasive, costly and time-consuming procedure. Finally, the expertise to perform renal translesional pressure gradient measurements is lacking in a majority of centres.

Based on centre expertise, other techniques such as fractional flow reserve, intravascular ultrasound imaging or optical coherence tomography (OCT) may provide thresholds to perform balloon angioplasty. Again, validated data are lacking in FMD, with thresholds generally extrapolated from ARVD populations.

Tools to non-invasively evaluate renal artery haemodynamics in patients with FMD and help selecting cases most likely to benefit from renal artery revascularisation are currently under study, but not yet ready for application in daily clinical practice.

7.3.6 Are There Any Data on Safety During Pregnancy and Exogenous Hormone Use?

Whilst the prevalence of pregnancy-related complications such as gestational hypertension and preterm birth and, to a lesser extent, pre-eclampsia, is higher in patients with FMD (likely related to renal FMD severity), the risk of arterial complications (aneurysm rupture, dissection) seems fortunately low [83]. It is important to consider screening hypertensive women of childbearing age for FMD and to perform renal angioplasty prior to pregnancy if indicated. Pregnancy is not to be discouraged in FMD, but warrants closer monitoring and follow-up [83, 84].

Despite theoretical concerns due to female predominance of FMD, there is no data to support the safety or harm associated with exogenous female hormones in FMD.

7.3.7 Can You Donate a Kidney with FMD?

International guidelines advise against donating a kidney in which FMD has been found incidentally on pre-surgery screening tests or peri-operatively. Some long-term studies, however, have shown comparable hypertension and renal and cardiovascular outcomes in donors with FMD compared to controls. While long-term data is awaited for recipients, as a practical guide it has been advocated to only consider kidney donation in the event of no other suitable living kidney donor, mild or non-multi-vessel FMD, no or mild hypertension or cardiovascular disease, no systemic dissections or aneurysms, no pregnancy considered after donation and written informed consent [85].

7.3.8 What Is the Prognosis?

There are very few prospective analyses formally assessing progression rate in FMD. However, current understanding of the natural history of FMD is that substantial progression is rare. For example, one pilot study showed no progression in arterial lesions after 2–3 years of CT angiographic follow-up [86]. Additionally, in patients with known FMD, development of new arterial complications is rare.

In a study on patients with cerebrovascular FMD and a mean follow-up time of 35 months, de novo carotid dissection was identified in only 3/146 (2%) of patients [55].

However, in patients with arterial dissection, underlying FMD may be associated with an increased—though still low risk of recurrence. In particular, in a national Italian cohort of patients with cervical artery dissection, 3.3% of subjects experienced recurrent cervical dissection after a median follow-up of 34 months (mostly asymptomatic presentation occurring within 6 months after the index event) [61]. In multivariable analysis, the presence of FMD was associated with a higher risk (hazard ratio: 3.4) of dissection recurrence.

Longer term studies are needed to look into this further and understand risk factors of progression of FMD and its complications.

Current guidelines recommend follow-up at least annually by a health care provider with experience in the field of FMD. In patients with renal FMD, follow-up should include blood pressure control, assessment of renal function and imaging. The timing of follow-up imaging should be customised to each patient's pattern and severity of disease, including the need for monitoring of aneurysms or dissections or following revascularisation, as well as local imaging resources and experience.

7.3.9 What Are the Knowledge Gaps Future Research Might Want to Target? (Adapted from [52, 78])

- Identification of causative and regulatory genes associated with FMD
- Study of familial patterns of FMD, including intermediate phenotypes, and feasibility/utility of different modalities of screening

- Dissection of the main molecular/pathologic processes underlying FMD, e.g. molecular and genetic characteristics of fibroblasts from individuals with FMD
- Unravelling of both shared and distinct biologic mechanisms of FMD, SCAD and cervical artery dissection
- Establishment of a tissue bank of pathology specimens to allow for study of the arterial wall properties associated with FMD
- Risk stratification: what are the factors that determine major adverse cardiovascular events in patients with known FMD? Distinguishing 'benign' from 'severe' phenotypes, including those with increased risk of dissection/aneurysm
- Identification of factors associated with disease progression
- Understanding the cause and impact of arterial tortuosity in patients with FMD
- Determination of the prevalence of FMD in at-risk patient populations (e.g. young and middle-aged patients with stroke and transient ischaemic attack without apparent cardiovascular risk factors, women with severe migraine headaches)
- Studies to explore the efficacy of antiplatelet therapy
- Studies to demonstrate the effectiveness of haemodynamic-guided angioplasty (i.e. pressure gradient measurement) for renal FMD in terms of clinical outcomes, including cure or control of hypertension.

Further research on a blood signature, proteomics and blood test to diagnosis FMD [87, 88] (Table 7.4).

- Proteomic tests which provide a blood 'signature' and ultimately blood test to diagnose FMD [87, 88].

Table 7.4 Comparative differences and similarities between ARVD and FMD

	ARVD	FMD
Age	Disease of ageing	Young to middle-aged
Gender	M > F Males more likely to have significant RAS	F > M (80–90% female) Males more likely to have a more severe phenotype, dissections
Ethnicity	Similar in Caucasian and African-American population	Predominantly (95%) Caucasian ethnicity
Location of lesions	90% *ostial,* i.e. occur within 1 cm (proximal third) of the origin of the renal artery	Often mid to distal third of renal artery (multifocal FMD)
Nature of lesions	Atherosclerotic Stenotic	Non-atherosclerotic, non-inflammatory Stenotic, aneurysmal or dissection
Lesions in other vascular beds	Strong association with multi-vessel atheromatous vascular disease	Up to two-thirds have multi-vessel FMD
Renal blood flow	Reduced	May be preserved [89]
Renal parenchymal involvement	Impaired	Preserved (at early stage)

(continued)

Table 7.4 (continued)

	ARVD	FMD
Cardiac involvement	Frequent association with coronary atherosclerosis/ ischaemic heart disease	No differences in left ventricular morphology and function between FMD patients and matched controls. This holds true regardless of FMD extent, type, hypertension or serious vascular complications [66]
Activation of renin–angiotensin system	Increased renin and angiotensin II release and disturbed regulation in majority of patients	Normal renin release and intact response to renin modulation in majority of patients [89]
Correlation between renin release and blood pressure	Positive correlation	No correlation [89]
Revascularisation	Angioplasty and stenting only in selected populations manifesting a clinical syndrome	Angioplasty cures hypertension in a high proportion of patients, especially when diagnosed at a young age
Anti-platelets, renin–angiotensin blockade	Generally recommended	To be considered based on individual characteristics
Statins	Recommended	No documented benefit

7.4 Rare Causes of Renovascular Hypertension

Rare causes of renovascular hypertension are increasingly identified due to extensive use of non-invasive imaging techniques (Fig. 7.6). Clinical management of the underlying condition should be individualised because of marked differences in aetiologies.

Examples include inflammatory arteritides, Takayasu's arteritis and giant cell arteritis, all requiring multi-disciplinary involvement and consideration of immunosuppression. Other less common aetiologies of RAS include aortic or renal artery dissection, non-specific aortic arteritis, aortic arch syndrome, thrombotic or cholesterol embolisation, collagen vascular disease, neurofibromatosis, mechanical trauma, post-transplantation stenosis, Williams syndrome, Alagille syndrome, Loeys-Dietz syndrome, post-inflammatory remodelling and post-radiation fibrosis [90].

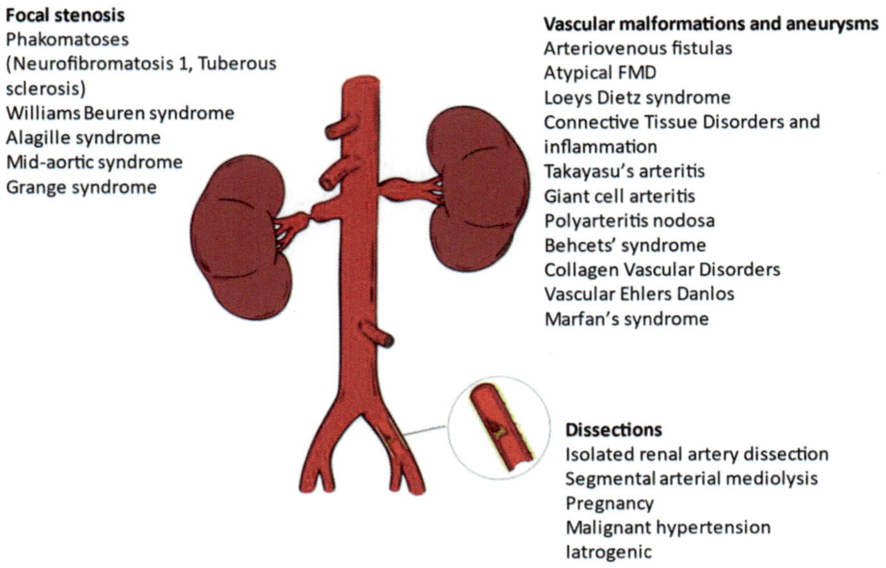

Fig. 7.6 Rare causes of renovascular hypertension

7.5 Conclusion

Renal artery stenosis remains an important contributor to hypertensive and cardiovascular disease burden. In ARVD, it must be seen as a manifestation of a usually diffuse atherosclerotic disease. Therefore, optimal medical treatment of cardiovascular risk factors remains the cornerstone of management, in order to improve patients' cardiovascular prognosis. Major clinical trials have failed to establish the role of revascularisation as a universal first-line treatment in ARVD. However, due to study design shortcomings and selection bias, these trials have been largely criticized. In selected patients with significant renal artery stenosis, viable renal parenchyma and specific clinical presentation, revascularisation remains a valid treatment option.

In FMD, international consensus guidelines recommend revascularisation as first-line treatment in young/middle-aged patients with haemodynamically significant renal artery stenosis. The role of pharmacological cardiovascular prevention in FMD remains unclear, the use of low-dose aspirin is usually advised.

Like ARVD, FMD should be seen as a systemic disease. Indeed, the majority of patients with FMD present lesions in two or more vascular beds. Therefore, a systematic screening of arterial beds by CT- or MR angiography is recommended.

While the landscape and management of RAS has evolved in the last few decades, numerous relevant clinical and scientific questions remain unanswered. Awaiting future knowledge, optimal treatment should be tailored on individual level, taking patient-specific characteristics into account.

References

1. Kalra PA, Guo H, Kausz AT, et al. Atherosclerotic renovascular disease in United States patients aged 67 years or older: risk factors, revascularization, and prognosis. Kidney Int. 2005;68:293–301.
2. de Mast Q, Beutler JJ. The prevalence of atherosclerotic renal artery stenosis in risk groups: a systematic literature review. J Hypertens. 2009;27:1333–40.
3. Mancia G, Kreutz R, Brunström M, et al. 2023 ESH Guidelines for the management of arterial hypertension The Task Force for the management of arterial hypertension of the European Society of Hypertension. J Hypertens. 2023;41:1874–2071.
4. Sarafidis PA, Theodorakopoulou M, Ortiz A, et al. Atherosclerotic renovascular disease: a clinical practice document by the European Renal Best Practice (ERBP) board of the European Renal Association (ERA) and the Working Group Hypertension and the Kidney of the European Society of Hypertension (ESH). Nephrol Dial Transplant. 2023;38:2835–50.
5. de Silva R, Loh H, Rigby AS, et al. Epidemiology, associated factors, and prognostic outcomes of renal artery stenosis in chronic heart failure assessed by magnetic resonance angiography. Am J Cardiol. 2007;100:273–9.
6. Hansen KJ, Edwards MS, Craven TE, et al. Prevalence of renovascular disease in the elderly: a population-based study. J Vasc Surg. 2002;36:443–51.
7. Missouris CG, Buckenham T, Cappuccio FP, MacGregor GA. Renal artery stenosis: a common and important problem in patients with peripheral vascular disease. Am J Med. 1994;96:10–4.
8. Hicks CW, Clark TWI, Cooper CJ, et al. Atherosclerotic renovascular disease: a KDIGO (Kidney Disease: Improving Global Outcomes) controversies conference. Am J Kidney Dis. 2022;79:289–301.
9. Kawarada O, Yokoi Y, Morioka N, Takemoto K. Renal artery stenosis in cardio-and cerebrovascular disease renal duplex ultrasonography as an initial screening examination. Circ J. 2007;71:1942–7.
10. Plouin PF, Chatellier G, Darné B, Raynaud A. Blood pressure outcome of angioplasty in atherosclerotic renal artery stenosis. Hypertension. 1998;31:823–9.
11. Wright JR, Shurrab AE, Cooper A, Kalra PR, Foley RN, Kalra PA. Left ventricular morphology and function in patients with atherosclerotic renovascular disease. J Am Soc Nephrol. 2005;16:2746–53.
12. Guo H, Kalra PA, Gilbertson DT, et al. Atherosclerotic renovascular disease in older US patients starting dialysis, 1996 to 2001. Circulation. 2007;115:50–8.
13. Ritchie J, Green D, Alderson HV, Chiu D, Sinha S, Kalra PA. Risks for mortality and renal replacement therapy in atherosclerotic renovascular disease compared with other causes of chronic kidney disease. Nephrology. 2015;20:688–96.
14. Textor SC, Lerman LO. Paradigm shifts in atherosclerotic renovascular disease. J Am Soc Nephrol. 2015;26:2074–80.
15. Hill GS, Heudes D, Bariéty J. Morphometric study of arterioles and glomeruli in the aging kidney suggests focal loss of autoregulation. Kidney Int. 2003;63:1027–36.
16. Wright JR, Duggal A, Thomas R, Reeve R, Roberts ISD, Kalra PA. Clinicopathological correlation in biopsy-proven atherosclerotic nephropathy: implications for renal functional outcome in atherosclerotic renovascular disease. Nephrol Dial Transplant. 2001;16:765–70.
17. Woolen SA, Shankar PR, Gagnier JJ, MacEachern MP, Singer L, Davenport MS. Risk of nephrogenic systemic fibrosis in patients with stage 4 or 5 chronic kidney disease receiving a group II gadolinium-based contrast agent. JAMA Intern Med. 2020;180:223–30.
18. Bhalla V, Textor SC, Beckman JA, et al. Revascularization for renovascular disease: a scientific statement from the American Heart Association. Hypertension. 2022;79:e128–43.
19. Sun D, Chen Z, Eirin A, et al. Hypercholesterolemia impairs nonstenotic kidney outcomes after reversal of experimental renovascular hypertension. Am J Hypertens. 2016;29:853–9.
20. Vassallo D, Kalra PA. Progress in the treatment of atherosclerotic renovascular disease: the conceptual journey and the unanswered questions. Nephrol Dial Transplant. 2016;31:1595–605.

21. Chrysochou C, Foley RN, Young JF, Khavandi K, Cheung CM, Kalra PA. Dispelling the myth: the use of renin-angiotensin blockade in atheromatous renovascular disease. Nephrol Dial Transplant. 2012;27:1403–9.
22. Ritchie J, Green D, Alderson HV, et al. Associations of antiplatelet therapy and beta blockade with patient outcomes in atherosclerotic renovascular disease. J Am Soc Hypertens. 2016;10:149–58.e3.
23. Chade AR, Bidwell GL. Novel drug delivery technologies and targets for renal disease. Hypertension. 2022;79:1937–48.
24. Harvey TW, Engel JE, Chade AR. Vascular endothelial growth factor and podocyte protection in chronic hypoxia: effects of endothelin-a receptor antagonism. Am J Nephrol. 2016;43:74–84.
25. Engel JE, Williams ML, Williams E, et al. Recovery of renal function following kidney-specific VEGF therapy in experimental renovascular disease. Am J Nephrol. 2020;51:891–902.
26. White CJ, Jaff MR, Haskal ZJ, et al. Indications for renal arteriography at the time of coronary arteriography. Circulation. 2006;114:1892–5.
27. Murphy TP, Soares G, Kim M. Increase in utilization of percutaneous renal artery interventions by medicare beneficiaries, 1996–2000. Am J Roentgenol. 2004;183:561–8.
28. Weibull H, Bergqvist D, Bergentz SE, Jonsson K, Hulthén L, Manhem P. Percutaneous transluminal renal angioplasty versus surgical reconstruction of atherosclerotic renal artery stenosis: a prospective randomized study. J Vasc Surg. 1993;18:841–52.
29. Webster J, Marshall F, Abdalla M, et al. Randomised comparison of percutaneous angioplasty vs continued medical therapy for hypertensive patients with atheromatous renal artery stenosis. J Hum Hypertens. 1998;12:329–35.
30. van de Ven PJ, Kaatee R, Beutler JJ, et al. Arterial stenting and balloon angioplasty in ostial atherosclerotic renovascular disease: a randomised trial. Lancet. 1999;353:282–6.
31. van Jaarsveld BC, Krijnen P, Pieterman H, et al. The effect of balloon angioplasty on hypertension in atherosclerotic renal-artery stenosis. New Engl J Med. 2000;342:1007–14.
32. Bax L. Stent placement in patients with atherosclerotic renal artery stenosis and impaired renal function. Ann Intern Med. 2009;150:840–8.
33. ASTRAL Investigators, Wheatley K, Ives N, et al. Revascularization versus medical therapy for renal-artery stenosis. N Engl J Med. 2009;361:1953–62.
34. Marcantoni C, Zanoli L, Rastelli S, et al. Effect of renal artery stenting on left ventricular mass: a randomized clinical trial. Am J Kidney Dis. 2012;60:39–46.
35. Cooper CJ, Murphy TP, Cutlip DE, et al. Stenting and medical therapy for atherosclerotic renal-artery stenosis. New Engl J Med. 2014;370:13–22.
36. Pappaccogli M, Robberechts T, Lengelé JP, et al. Endovascular versus medical management of atherosclerotic renovascular disease: update and emerging concepts. Hypertension. 2023;80:1150–61.
37. Thadhani R, Pascual M, Tolkoff-Rubin N, Nickeleit V, Colvin R. Preliminary description of focal segmental glomerulosclerosis in patients with renovascular disease. Lancet. 1996;347:231–3.
38. Chrysochou C, Green D, Ritchie J, Buckley DL, Kalra PA. Kidney volume to GFR ratio predicts functional improvement after revascularization in atheromatous renal artery stenosis. PLoS One. 2017;12:e0177178.
39. Ivanovic V, McKusick MA, Johnson CM, et al. Renal artery stent placement: complications at a single tertiary care center. J Vascr Interv Radiol. 2003;14:217–25.
40. Holden A, Hill A. Renal angioplasty and stenting with distal protection of the main renal artery in ischemic nephropathy: early experience. J Vasc Surg. 2003;38:962–8.
41. Vassallo D, Ritchie J, Green D, Chrysochou C, Kalra PA. The effect of revascularization in patients with anatomically significant atherosclerotic renovascular disease presenting with high-risk clinical features. Nephrol Dial Transplant. 2018;33:497–506.
42. Ritchie J, Green D, Chrysochou C, Chalmers N, Foley RN, Kalra PA. High-risk clinical presentations in atherosclerotic renovascular disease: prognosis and response to renal artery revascularization. Am J Kidney Dis. 2014;63:186–97.

43. Kawarada O, Yokoi Y, Morioka N, Shiotani S, Higashimori A. Cardiac benefits of renal artery stenting. EuroIntervention. 2010;6:485–91.
44. Chrysochou C, Sharma R, Kalra PA, Kalra PR. Improved left ventricular filling following bilateral renal artery stenting. Int J Cardiol. 2011;150:e40–1.
45. Reinhard M, Schousboe K, Andersen UB, et al. Renal artery stenting in consecutive high-risk patients with atherosclerotic renovascular disease: a prospective 2-centercCohort study. J Am Heart Assoc. 2022;11:e024421.
46. Wright JR, Shurrab AE, Cheung C, et al. A prospective study of the determinants of renal functional outcome and mortality in atherosclerotic renovascular disease. Am J Kidney Dis 2002;39:1153–61.
47. Edwards MS, Craven TE, Burke GL, Dean RH, Hansen KJ. Renovascular disease and the risk of adverse coronary events in the elderly: a prospective, population-based study. Arch Intern Med. 2005;165:207–13.
48. de Bhailis Á, Al-Chalabi S, Hagemann R, et al. Managing acute presentations of atheromatous renal artery stenosis. BMC Nephrol. 2022;23:210.
49. Chrysochou C, Kalra PA. Current management of atherosclerotic renovascular disease - what have we learned from astral? Nephron Clin Pract. 2010;115:c73–81.
50. Courand PY, Dinic M, Lorthioir A, et al. Resistant hypertension and atherosclerotic renal artery stenosis. Hypertension. 2019;74:1516–23.
51. Ramos F, Kotliar C, Alvarez D, et al. Renal function and outcome of PTRA and stenting for atherosclerotic renal artery stenosis. Kidney Int. 2003;63:276–82.
52. Gornik HL, Persu A, Adlam D, et al. First international consensus on the diagnosis and management of fibromuscular dysplasia. Vasc Med. 2019;24:164–89.
53. Pappaccogli M, Di Monaco S, Warchoł-Celińska E, et al. The European/International Fibromuscular Dysplasia Registry and Initiative (FEIRI)—clinical phenotypes and their predictors based on a cohort of 1000 patients. Cardiovasc Res. 2021;117:950–9.
54. Arnaud C, Boulanger M, Lorthioir A, et al. Male sex is associated with cervical artery dissection in patients with fibromuscular dysplasia. J Am Heart Assoc. 2021;10:e018311.
55. Kadian-Dodov D, Goldfinger JZ, Gustavson S, Olin JW. Natural history of cervical artery fibromuscular dysplasia and associated neurovascular events. Cerebrovasc Dis. 2018;45:33–9.
56. Lather HD, Gornik HL, Olin JW, et al. Prevalence of intracranial aneurysm in women with fibromuscular dysplasia. JAMA Neurol. 2017;74:1081–7.
57. Dobrowolski P, Januszewicz M, Witowicz H, et al. Prevalence of smoking and clinical characteristics in fibromuscular dysplasia. The ARCADIA-POL study. Blood Press. 2019;28 49–56.
58. Olin JW, Froehlich J, Gu X, et al. The United States registry for fibromuscular dysplasia. Circulation. 2012;125:3182–90.
59. Wuerzner G, Krieger C, Bouchardy J, et al. Fibromuscular dysplasia and hypertension: beyond renal arteries. Rev Med Suisse. 2017;13:1580–3.
60. Plouin PF, Baguet JP, Thony F, et al. High prevalence of multiple arterial bed lesions in patients with fibromuscular dysplasia: the ARCADIA Registry (assessment of renal and cervical artery dysplasia). Hypertension. 2017;70:652–8.
61. Bonacina S, Grassi M, Zedde M, et al. Clinical features of patients with cervical artery dissection and fibromuscular dysplasia. Stroke. 2021;52:821–9.
62. Huart J, Stoenoiu MS, Zedde M, Pascarella R, Adlam D, Persu A. From fibromuscular dysplasia to arterial dissection and back. Am J Hypertens. 2023;36:573–85.
63. Kadian-Dodov D, Gornik HL, Gu X, et al. Dissection and aneurysm in patients with fibromuscular dysplasia: findings from the U.S. Registry for FMD. J Am Coll Cardiol. 2016;68:176–85.
64. Haussen DC, Grossberg JA, Bouslama M, et al. Carotid web (intimal fibromuscular dysplasia) has high stroke recurrence risk and is amenable to stenting. Stroke. 2017;48:3134–7.
65. Januszewicz M, Januszewicz A, Michałowska I, et al. Intra-renal blood flow parameters assessed by doppler sonography in hypertensive patients with fibromuscular dysplasia – relationship to renal function and target organ damage. The ARCADIA-POL study. Pol Arch Intern Med. 2019;129:234–41.

66. Dobrowolski P, Januszewicz M, Klisiewicz A, et al. Echocardiographic assessment of left ventricular morphology and function in patients with fibromuscular dysplasia. J Hypertens. 2018;36:1318–25.
67. Al-Hussaini A, Abdelaty AMSEK, Gulsin GS, et al. Chronic infarct size after spontaneous coronary artery dissection: implications for pathophysiology and clinical management. Eur Heart J. 2020;41:2197–205.
68. Adlam D, Alfonso F, Maas A, et al. European Society of Cardiology, acute cardiovascular care association, SCAD study group: a position paper on spontaneous coronary artery dissection. Eur Heart J. 2018;39:3353–68.
69. Hayes SN, Kim ESH, Saw J, et al. Spontaneous coronary artery dissection: current state of the science: a scientific statement from the American Heart Association. Circulation. 2018;137:e523–57.
70. Saw J, Ricci D, Starovoytov A, Fox R, Buller CE. Spontaneous coronary artery dissection: prevalence of predisposing conditions including fibromuscular dysplasia in a tertiary center cohort. JACC Cardiovasc Interv. 2013;6:44–52.
71. Persu A, Lopez-Sublet M, Al-Hussaini A, et al. Prevalence and disease spectrum of extra-coronary arterial abnormalities in spontaneous coronary artery dissection. JAMA Cardiol. 2022;7:159–66.
72. Adlam D, Olson TM, Combaret N, et al. Association of the PHACTR1/EDN1 genetic locus with spontaneous coronary artery dissection. J Am Coll Cardiol. 2019;73:58–66.
73. Kim ESH, Saw J, Kadian-Dodov D, Wood M, Ganesh SK. FMD and SCAD: sex-biased arterial diseases with clinical and genetic pleiotropy. Circ Res. 2021;128:1958–72.
74. Adlam D, Berrandou TE, Georges A, et al. Genome-wide association meta-analysis of spontaneous coronary artery dissection identifies risk variants and genes related to artery integrity and tissue-mediated coagulation. Nat Genet. 2023;55:964–72.
75. Bruno RM, Marais L, Khettab H, et al. Deep vascular phenotyping in patients with renal multifocal fibromuscular dysplasia. Hypertension. 2019;73:371–8.
76. Boutouyrie P, Gimenez-Roqueplo AP, Fine E, et al. Evidence for carotid and radial artery wall subclinical lesions in renal fibromuscular dysplasia. J Hypertens. 2003;21:2287–95.
77. Kiando SR, Tucker NR, Castro-Vega LJ, et al. PHACTR1 is a genetic susceptibility locus for fibromuscular dysplasia supporting its complex genetic pattern of inheritance. PLoS Genet. 2016;12:e1006367.
78. Persu A, Dobrowolski P, Gornik HL, et al. Current progress in clinical, molecular, and genetic aspects of adult fibromuscular dysplasia. Cardiovasc Res. 2022;118:65–83.
79. Whelton PK, Carey RM, Aronow WS, et al. 2017 ACC/AHA/AAPA/ABC/ACPM/AGS/APhA/ASH/ASPC/NMA/PCNA Guideline for the prevention, detection, evaluation, and management of high blood pressure in adults: executive summary: a report of the American College of Cardiology/American Heart Association Task Force on clinical practice guidelines. Hypertension. 2018;71:1269–324.
80. Dicks AB, Gornik HL, Gu X, et al. Association of fibromuscular dysplasia and pulsatile tinnitus: a report of the US Registry for Fibromuscular Dysplasia. J Am Heart Assoc. 2021;10:e021962.
81. Trinquart L, Mounier-Vehier C, Sapoval M, Gagnon N, Plouin PF. Efficacy of revascularization for renal artery stenosis caused by fibromuscular dysplasia. Hypertension. 2010;56:525–32.
82. Kądziela J, Jóźwik-Plebanek K, Pappaccogli M, et al. Risks and benefits of renal artery stenting in fibromuscular dysplasia: lessons from the ARCADIA-POL study. Vasc Med. 2024;29:50–7.
83. Pappaccogli M, Prejbisz A, Ciurică S, et al. Pregnancy-related complications in patients with fibromuscular dysplasia: a report from the European/International Fibromuscular Dysplasia Registry. Hypertension. 2020;76:545–53.
84. Berra E, Dominiczak AF, Touyz RM, et al. Management of a pregnant woman with fibromuscular dysplasia. Hypertension. 2018;71:540–7.
85. Chrysochou C, Devresse A, Kanaan N, Persu A. Kidney donors with fibromuscular dysplasia, is it time to open the doors? Nephrol Dial Transplant. 2021;36:1365–8.

86. de Leeuw PW, Zelis P, Kleijnen B, Schutten M, Kroon A. Follow-up of vascular lesions in fibromuscular dysplasia. No evidence for progression yet. J Hypertens. 2023;41(Suppl 3):e48.
87. Latosinska A, Bruno RM, Pappaccogli M, et al. Increased collagen turnover is a feature of fibromuscular dysplasia and associated with hypertrophic radial remodeling: a pilot, urine proteomic study. Hypertension. 2022;79:93–103.
88. Olin JW, Di Narzo AF, d'Escamard V, et al. A plasma proteogenomic signature for fibromuscular dysplasia. Cardiovasc Res. 2020;116:63–77.
89. van Twist DJL, Houben AJHM, de Haan MW, de Leeuw PW, Kroon AA. Renal hemodynamics and renin–angiotensin system activity in humans with multifocal renal artery fibromuscular dysplasia. J Hypertens. 2016;34:1160–9.
90. Persu A, Canning C, Prejbisz A, et al. Beyond atherosclerosis and fibromuscular dysplasia: rare causes of renovascular hypertension. Hypertension. 2021;78:898–911.

Part IV

Hypertension in Chronic Kidney Disease in Pediatrics and Adolescents

CKD as a Cause of Hypertension in Children and Adolescents

8

Empar Lurbe

8.1 Introduction

Hypertension (HTN) is one of the most important cardiovascular (CV) and renal disease factors increasing the risk of mortality worldwide. Although the majority of cases of HTN are primary, i.e., in the absence of a disease leading to elevated blood pressure (BP) levels, secondary HTN is the norm in children. In contrast to adults, where chronic kidney disease (CKD) is considered to be hypertension-mediated organ damage (HMOD) as a consequence of primary HTN, in children and adolescents, HTN is secondary to renal lesions in at least 85% of cases. In this case, the prevalence ranges from 20% to 60% and is directly related to the degree of renal dysfunction, even starting in children with stage 2 CKD when the eGFR is between 60 and 90 mL/min/1.73 m^2 [1]. Although HTN may not be the primary cause of kidney disease, BP affects the rate of progression to kidney failure.

Chronic kidney disease in children has some unique features and challenges. These include the variable spectrum of clinical presentation, from completely silent disease to severe renal dysfunction with a significant impact on life expectancy and quality of life, the challenge of measuring renal function and defining CKD, and the role of therapeutic options. To date, our knowledge of antihypertensive pharmacological treatment in children and adolescents is limited by the paucity of randomized clinical trials, which hampers well-supported management.

This chapter reviews information on the prevalence and causes of CKD in children, the contribution of HTN to disease progression, and the therapeutic approach.

E. Lurbe (✉)
Pediatric Department, University of Valencia, Valencia, Spain

CIBERObn, ISCIII, Madrid, Spain
e-mail: empar.lurbe@uv.es

A. E. Berbari et al. (eds.), *Blood Pressure Disorders in Acute and Chronic Kidney Diseases*, Updates in Hypertension and Cardiovascular Protection,
https://doi.org/10.1007/978-3-031-81292-7_8

8.2 CKD and HTN Definitions in Children

The most important step in making accurate clinical decisions is to consider the specific characteristics of the children at that time to identify both CKD and HTN.

The definition of CKD is based on the assessment of glomerular filtration rate (GFR) and urinary excretion of albuminuria/proteinuria. The eGFR classification of CKD included arbitrary cut-off values and applies only to children over 2 years of age.

Glomerular filtration rate is calculated by assessing blood levels of substances that are filtrated and excreted without being reabsorbed by the kidney, but it varies according to age, sex, race, ethnicity, and size. The most commonly used is creatinine, with the addition of cystatin C in recent years. The 2009 Schwartz formula [2] estimates GFR from serum creatinine, patient height, and a constant (k) for all children, 0.413. The adult equation, MDRD and CKD-EPI define CKD by GFR <60 mL/min/1.73 m^2 but have some limitations and lack accuracy in defining CKD in children with eGFR >75 mL/min/1.73 m^2 and hyperfiltration [3]. A new formula was developed and validated in the Chronic Kidney Disease in Children cohort (CKiDU25), which enrolled patients up to 25 years of age [4]. The formula used serum creatinine, cystatin C, patient age, and sex and appears to be more reliable in adolescents and young adults.

KDIGO stratification [5] based on GFR and urinary albumin excretion is considered relevant for risk assessment when the majority of children with CKD have non-glomerular disease. Despite the new developments in the definition, clinical information should be included for better risk assessment. These include low birth weight, prematurity, previous episodes of acute kidney injury, exposure to nephrotoxic drugs, reduced kidney size, and low nephron endowment. Consequently, the classic KDIGO scheme for CKD classification should be considered in the context of clinical information that may shift the risk between the boxes, increasing the risk according to the individual circumstances of each child [6] (Fig. 8.1).

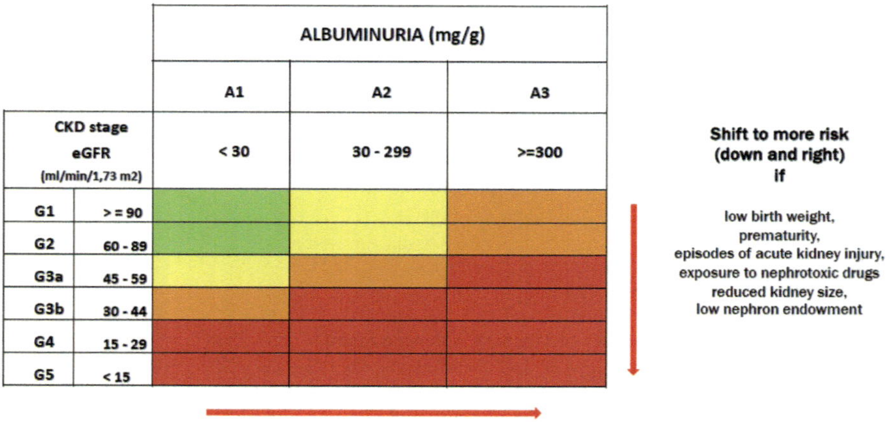

Fig. 8.1 KDIGO 2012 stratification of risk in CKD. Factors to consider for risk assessment in children based on factors associated

The definition of HTN in children varies from guideline to guideline. Between 2016 and 2020, three guidelines were published with different criteria to define HTN. In 2016, the European Society of Hypertension (ESH) [7] recommended the 95th percentile for age, sex, and height for children up to 16 years and the ESH/ESC adult criteria ≥140/90 mmHg for those 16 years and older. One year later, the American Academy of Pediatrics [8] recommended the use of percentiles for children up to 13 years of age and ≥130/80 mmHg for those 13 years and older, following the AHA adult definition. In 2020, the Canadian guidelines [9] established different criteria from the previous ones; in this case, percentiles were used up to 6 years, between 6 and 11 years ≥120/80 mmHg, 12–17 years ≥130/85 mmHg, and ≥18 years ≥140/90 mmHg. For reference tables of percentiles, all guidelines use the Fourth Report of the National High Blood Pressure Education Program Working Group on High Blood Pressure in Children and Adolescents, but the ESH guidelines did not exclude overweight/obese children (BMI ≥85th percentile) at the time the percentiles were calculated [10]. A table showing the different criteria has recently been published [11].

8.3 Etiology and Prevalence of CKD

The etiology of CKD includes a large number of conditions with different clinical characteristics, prognosis, and prevalence, making it difficult to estimate incidence and prevalence. The most common underlying condition in pediatric CKD and renal failure is congenital anomalies of the kidney and urinary tract (CAKUT), which are about 40% across studies. The others are podocytopathies 10%, cystic diseases 13%, hemolytic uremic syndrome 5%, tubulopathies 3%, and a miscellany 29%, which includes glomerulopathies, glomerulonephritis, and focal segmental glomerulosclerosis, although these account for a relatively small proportion of CKD in children [6]. Diseases that primarily affect the tubular-interstit al compartment tend to progress slowly, whereas those that originate in the glomerular structures affect older children and progress rapidly.

The prevalence of CKD in children, unlike that in adults, is not well estimated because the figures have been obtained from different sources that underestimate the prevalence for different reasons [12, 13]. Information from European registries estimated 30–100 per million age-related populations of CKD stages 2–5, but published hospital-based studies underestimated the real figs [14]. In contrast, population-based studies in the pediatric population suggested a prevalence of around 0.1–1%, 100 times higher than hospital-based data, and the National Health and Nutrition Examination Surveys expected a 0.9% prevalence [15, 16].

8.4 Prevalence and Characteristics of HTN

The prevalence of HTN in CKD is high, although the figures vary between reports due to differences in the criteria used to define HTN, the method of BP measurement, and the etiology of the underlying disease causing CKD. Several reports have estimated the prevalence to be as low as 22% [17], 26% [18], 28–41% in the NAPRTCS [19], and as high as 50%, 52% [20], and 54% [21]. What is relevant is the confirmation that the prevalence is high, that the presence of masked HTN even reduces the prevalence, and that the control rate among those treated is relatively low [22]. Data coming from the Chronic Kidney Disease in Children (CKiD) study regarding the lack of improvement after years when the problem had been assessed by office and ambulatory BP monitoring (ABPM) seem to be more relevant [23, 24].

In CKD patients, the presence of masked HTN is not uncommon, and blunted circadian variability is often present, with less BP fall at night. The non-dipping pattern is present in a large proportion of patients with CKD and increases with decreasing GFR. Both conditions support the recommendation to use 24-h ABPM to obtain more accurate BP values and targets to improve outcomes during follow-up [25].

8.5 Mechanisms of HTN in CKD

HTN in children develops in parallel with, or as a consequence of, the pathophysiology of the underlying kidney disease. While children with CAKUT have a gradual progression, those with acquired forms of CKD develop HTN in parallel with the progression of the primary lesion. In children, the main mechanisms of BP elevation are impaired sodium handling, overactivity of the renin-angiotensin-aldosterone system (RAAS) and the sympathetic nervous system, and disturbances in autoregulatory elements. In addition, other elements contribute to the increase in BP [26].

In children with CKD, a decrease in GFR is followed by a state of sodium retention with an increase in blood and extravascular volume, even in the absence of edema [27, 28]. The contribution of sodium retention depends on the underlying disease, as tubular diseases with polyuria are sodium depleting.

The RAAS is activated by the secretion of renin when the GFR is reduced in poorly perfused and scarred areas [29]. Renin increases levels of angiotensin II, which causes vasoconstriction, sodium retention, and aldosterone secretion, with activation of the mineralocorticoid receptor pathway with multiple systemic effects, including increased sodium reabsorption in the distal tubule [30].

Overactivity of the SNS is another relevant mechanism [31] with bidirectional cross-talk with the RAAS. In addition, secretion of renalase, an amine oxidase that metabolizes catecholamines secreted by the glomerulus and renal tubule, is reduced with consequent increase in sympathetic activity. Blood levels of renalase are inversely proportional to GFR, contributing to the increase in sympathetic activity [26].

Autoregulatory mechanisms in the endothelium and at the vascular level also contribute to BP elevation in children with CKD. Nitric oxide (NO) and endothelin-1 (ET-1) levels and vascular stiffness increase peripheral resistance [32]. Nitric oxide, a potent vasodilator, is reduced by low levels of L-arginine, which is required for its production, and by increases in ADMA, an inhibitor of NO synthase. Elevated levels of ET-1 increase peripheral resistance by acting on the vascular endothelium.

Chronic inflammation and calcification of the arterial wall increase vascular stiffness and contribute to blood pressure elevation.

Other factors to consider include:

- Pharmacological treatments for underlying diseases, such as glucocorticoids (volume retention and RAAS activation), calcineurin inhibitors (SNS hyperactivity, endothelin increase and NO reduction), and erythropoietin-stimulating agents (reduction of NO activity and increased vasoconstriction) [33].
- Mineral bone disease with reduced levels of 1–25(OH)$_2$ vitamin D increases renin synthesis [34] and fibroblast growth factor 23 (FGF-23) increase associated with RAAS activation and endothelial dysfunction and/or Klotho deficiency associated with endothelial dysfunction and vascular calcifications [35].
- Hyperuricemia—although uric acid increases in CKD and has been associated with HTN, its relationship and impact have not been established.
- Obesity has also been associated with increased BP and an increased risk of developing HTN-related organ damage [36].

8.6 HTN and Progression of Renal Damage

Hypertension is the most important modifiable factor influencing the progression of kidney disease. This has been supported by studies over the last 30 years. The first evidence came from a study examining the effect of a low-protein diet on the progression of renal function. A surrogate endpoint of the study found that SBP >120 mmHg predicted faster decline in renal function [37]. The CKD data from the North American Pediatric Renal Transplant Cooperative Study (NAPRTCS) found that SBP in the 95th percentile increased the risk of progression [38]. This evidence was also confirmed in the CKiD study, mainly in subjects with glomerular disease [39].

Although these observations point to the need for treatment and control of HTN, additional studies have provided relevant information. First, the importance of time in varying SBP, which is more relevant than baseline values for disease progression. This study also demonstrated the prognostic value of DBP >90th percentile [40]. Second, monitoring patients with 24-h ABPM describes that mean arterial pressure (MAP) >90th percentile increases the risk of progression with an uneven time effect, faster in glomerular disease and slower in non-glomerular [41]. Third is the level of circadian variation in BP. While no association is observed between non-dipping pattern and disease progression, nocturnal HTN induces faster disease progression in addition to diurnal HTN [42].

Regarding the impact of HTN on the progression of renal disease, a landmark trial provided relevant confirmatory evidence of the need for intensified BP control to protect renal function in children with CKD. The ESCAPE (Effect of Strict Blood Pressure Control and ACE Inhibition on Progression of Chronic Renal Failure in Pediatric Patients) trial [43] provided evidence that strict BP control, aimed at a 24-h BP target below the 50th percentile, leads to improved long-term renal survival

[44]. On average, 1.9 antihypertensive medications (including the fixed-dose ACE inhibitor ramipril) were required to achieve the lower BP target. A post-hoc analysis suggests that similar renal outcomes occurred with any 24-h BP below the 75th percentile, whereas 5-year renal survival progressively worsened as achieved BP remained above this cut-off. The renoprotective effect was independent of RAAS inhibition, as all subjects followed in ESCAPE received a fixed daily dose of ramipril (6 mg/m^2). Children with glomerular disease had the greatest benefit from tight BP control. The presence of proteinuria exerts an additive effect on GFR decline and is a modifier of the renoprotective effect of tighter BP control. The renal survival benefit of BP control appears to be limited to children with even mild proteinuria. Intensive BP lowering is recommended in proteinuric children.

8.7 HMOD in CKD Children

In addition to the effects of HTN on the kidney, other hypertension-mediated organ damage (HMOD) increases the risk of cardiovascular events, which usually develop after childhood. In this regard, systematic studies have been reported in the CKiD study. Left ventricular hypertrophy (LVH) was associated with poor BP control. One-third of the cohort with persistent ambulatory HTN had LVH [45]. Similarly, clinic BP was not inferior to ambulatory BP in the risk of developing LVH [46]. Similarly, in a cross-sectional study, median carotid intima-media thickness (cIMT) was thicker in children with CKD compared with healthy controls. However, the severity of renal dysfunction was not relevant to cIMT levels. A surrogate marker of arterial stiffness, pulse wave velocity (PWV), has been reported to be elevated in small cross-sectional studies, although no increase in GFR was observed [18]. Finally, in a cross-sectional study using neurocognitive assessments, children with elevated BP had lower performance IQ scores [47]. Similarly, in a longitudinal study, visit-to-visit variability in SBP was associated with poorer performance on a test of cognitive efficiency and processing speed [48].

8.8 Treatment

8.8.1 Goals of Therapy

Recommendations for BP targets in patients with CKD are inconsistent in published guidelines due to the small number of studies and the different designs and methods used. The most recognized are:

- ESH (7): Target <75th percentile or <130/80 at 16 years. Proteinuria: <50th percentile or <125/75 at 16 years. The same BP percentile targets have been suggested for office and home BP measurement.
- American Academy of Pediatrics clinical practice guideline [8]: Target BP <90th percentile or 130/80 for those >13 years of age, whichever is lower.

- Canada´s Hypertension Guidelines [9]: Target <90th percentile or age 6–11 years <120/80, age 12–17 years <130/85.
- KDIGO [49]: Target <50th percentile MAP on ABPM or <90th percentile cBP. Practice points recommend monitoring BP once a year with ABPM and monitoring every 3–6 months with standardized auscultatory office BP in children with CKD. In children with high BP and CKD, when ABPM is not available, manual auscultatory office BP obtained in a protocol-driven standardized setting aiming to achieve SBP <90th percentile for age, sex, and height of normal children is a reasonable approach.

Evidence for BP reduction in patients with CKD comes from the only clinical trial in which the risk of progression to ESRD was the primary outcome, the ESCAPE trial, published in 2009. The trial enrolled children with CKD secondary to glomerular and non-glomerular diseases who were randomized to two different BP targets assessed by 24-h ABPM (24-h MBP between 50–90 percentile vs <50 percentile) and treatment with ramipril, an ACEi. Additional medication was allowed to achieve the BP target. The study concluded that children with the most challenging BP targets had a reduced rate of progression compared to standard treatment. A greater reduction in proteinuria was also observed [43]. More recently, the CKiD study confirmed that BP reduction protects against CKD progression during follow-up using 24-h ABPM sleep or wake MAP and clinical BP [41, 50].

8.8.2 Non-pharmacologic Treatment

Lifestyle interventions, including dietary modification, physical activity, and weight loss, are recommended as adjuncts to medication, with or without effects on BP, although the application of specific interventions depends on the physiopathology of the entity causal to CKD. While the beneficial effects of some of these interventions appear to be small or irrelevant, others require careful consideration in specific clinical conditions, as is the case with dietary salt.

The Dietary Approaches to Stop Hypertension (DASH) diet, with a reduction in protein and whole grains and a high intake of fruit and vegetables, has been recommended together with a reduction in salt consumption. Despite the traditional view on the impact of salt intake in HTN, it is not clear that salt is a relevant factor for HTN in children with CKD. However, if salt restriction is implemented, it should be monitored by a dietician to avoid growth retardation. In addition, it is not recommended in children with CKD who may not be able to concentrate urine and may have salt-wasting nephropathy [33].

8.8.3 Pharmacologic Treatment

CKD children require antihypertensive drugs to reduce BP levels and to protect against progression of renal dysfunction and cardiovascular risk. These drugs have demonstrated to be safe like in children with primary HTN [51], but comparative prospective trials tested superiority of one class of drugs over others when they are not available.

Overall, clinical trials of antihypertensive drugs in the pediatric population are scarce. Three publications in recent years have attempted to draw conclusions from the identified clinical trials (CTs). A Cochrane review [52] included 21 randomized CTs and concluded that among the classes of drugs tested, ACEi, ARB, and CCB did not show a consistent dose-response relationship. Furthermore, a meta-analysis [53] with 13 CTs of better quality than the previous ones increased the available experience with drugs that block the renin-angiotensin system (i.e., ACEIs and ARBs), the greater proportion of treatment in the patients recruited. In a narrative study [54], 51 CTs were collected, of which 30 included children with both primary and secondary HTN, mainly renal disease. Significant reductions in both systolic and diastolic BP were observed by ACEIs, ARBs, or diuretics treatment. Only four trials assessed the effect on the reduction of albuminuria or proteinuria [55–58].

Clinical guidelines recommend the use of monotherapy with dose intensification and the addition of a second drug if goals are not achieved with monotherapy [7, 8]. RAAS blockers, angiotensin converting enzyme inhibitors (ACEi), and angiotensin II receptor blockers (ARBs) are the first to be recommended based on the impact of the RAAS on the progression of renal damage, with superiority over other drug classes demonstrated in the CKiD trial [59]. Similarly, Abraham and coworkers demonstrated the superiority of ACEi/ARB in reducing progression to renal replacement therapy [60]. Finally, RAAS blockers demonstrated superiority over other classes of drugs in reducing proteinuria, a relevant player in the progression to ESRD [61].

If monotherapy with RAAS blockers does not achieve the desired goal despite dose optimization, the addition of a second or third antihypertensive drug is required. The addition of another RAAS blocker, combining ACEi plus ARB, is not recommended due to the risk of side effects, despite the potential effect on BP and reduction of proteinuria. The choice of second-line drug should first be based on other changes present in the affected children. This is the case with volume overload or hyperkaliemia, which requires diuretic therapy with a thiazide-like drug such as chlorthalidone [62] or a loop diuretic. The most commonly used second-line agents are the dihydropyridine calcium channel blockers (CCBs), which have shown additional BP reduction with good tolerability and are recommended to be prescribed as single-pill combination therapy to improve adherence. In the presence of intolerance or contraindication to RAAS blockers, dihydropyridine CCB monotherapy is recommended over the use of beta-blockers.

KDIGO 2021 [50] states in practice point 5.3 the "Use ACEi or ARB as first-line therapy for high BP in children with CKD". These drugs reduce proteinuria and are usually well tolerated, but they carry a risk of hyperkalemia and have adverse fetal risks in pregnant women. Figure 8.2 summarizes how to face pharmacologic treatment.

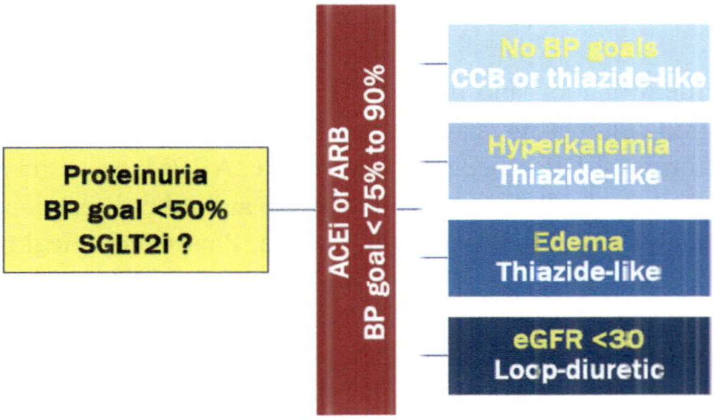

Fig. 8.2 Recommendations for BP lowering in CKD children

8.8.4 New Developments

Two new classes of drugs with demonstrated renal protection in adults are on the horizon for pediatric CKD: the sodium-glucose cotransporter-2 inhibitors (SGLT2i) and the non-steroidal mineralocorticoid receptor blocker finerenone.

The SGLT2i, a new class of drugs introduced for the treatment of type 2 diabetes, has been shown to have beneficial effects on diabetic and non-diabetic CKD and heart failure, although these benefits are not directly related to the primary effect of sodium-glucose co-transporter blockade. Modulation of tubular-glomerular feedback appears to be a key element in the renal protection observed. Results from CTs in adults have demonstrated the effect in reducing proteinuria and preserving GFR, so a similar beneficial effect is expected in children with proteinuria due to primary or secondary glomerular damage, as a potential adjuvant therapy to RAAS blockers [63]. Clinical trials in children need to demonstrate efficacy and safety in children with proteinuria.

The mineralocorticoid receptor (MRA) is a key player in the mechanisms leading to the development and progression of renal and cardiovascular damage. A non-steroidal potent MRAs blocker, finerenone, inhibits the recruitment of transcriptional cofactors that bind less hypertrophic, proinflammatory, and profibrotic gene expression and induces a dose-dependent moderate increase in K+ retention. Finerenone has been shown in clinical trials to reduce albuminuria and protect against the development of renal failure, but the reduction in BP is small (1–2 mmHg) [64]. Ongoing studies in children will determine whether this class of drugs can be safely used and their potential beneficial effect on renal protection.

The potential use of new drugs in children, based on targeting endothelin blockers, inhibition of aldosterone synthase, and even blockade of angiotensinogen mRNA or activation of the natriuretic receptor gene, may open new horizons.

8.9 Conclusions

Identification and treatment of HTN in children with CKD are essential to reduce and delay progression of renal damage to ESRD. The best approach requires monitoring of BP, office and, if available, ABPM, assessment of HMOD and planning of therapy, including appropriate diet and other lifestyle aspects, based on the physiopathology of the underlying cause. Pharmacological treatment with ACEi or ARB as first-line therapy is now the recommended first step, with the addition of a second antihypertensive class, CCB, or diuretics, depending on the need or not to reduce volume overload. The BP targets to be achieved must be more stringent in the presence of proteinuria, which has an additive effect on GFR decline and is a modifier of renoprotective efficacy. New drugs may offer additional benefits that have been clearly demonstrated in adults but need to be tested for safety and efficacy in children.

References

1. Van Sickle JS, Warady BA. Chronic kidney disease in children. Pediatr Clin N Am. 2022;69:1239–54. https://doi.org/10.1016/j.pcl.2022.07.010.
2. Schwartz GJ, Muñoz A, Schneider MF, et al. New equations to estimate GFR in children with CKD. J Am Soc Nephrol. 2009;20:629–37. https://doi.org/10.1681/ASN.2008030287.
3. Gao A, Cachat F, Faouzi M, et al. Comparison of the glomerular filtration rate in children by the new revised Schwartz formula and a new generalized formula. Kidney Int. 2013;83:524–30. https://doi.org/10.1038/ki.2012.388.
4. Pierce CB, Muñoz A, Ng DK, Warady BA, Furth SL, Schwartz GJ. Age- and sex-dependent clinical equations to estimate glomerular filtration rates in children and young adults with chronic kidney disease. Kidney Int. 2021;99:948–56. https://doi.org/10.1016/j.kint.2020.10.047.
5. KDIGO Blood Pressure Work Group. KDIGO clinical practice guideline for the management of blood pressure in chronic kidney disease. Kidney Int Suppl. 2012;2:337–414.
6. Cirillo L, De Chiara L, Innocenti S, Errichiello C, Romagnani P, Becherucci F. Chronic kidney disease in children: an update. Clin Kidney J. 2023;16:1600–11. https://doi.org/10.1093/ckj/sfad097.
7. Lurbe E, Agabiti-Rosei E, Cruickshank JK, et al. 2016 European Society of Hypertension guidelines for the management of high blood pressure in children and adolescents. J Hypertens. 2016;34:1887–920. https://doi.org/10.1097/HJH.0000000000001039.
8. Flynn JT, Kaelber DC, Baker-Smith CM, et al. Subcommittee on Screening and Management of High Blood Pressure in Children. Clinical practice guideline for screening and management of high blood pressure in children and adolescents. Pediatrics. 2017;140:e20171904. https://doi.org/10.1542/peds.2017-1904.
9. Rabi DM, McBrien KA, Sapir-Pichhadze R, et al. Hypertension Canada's 2020 comprehensive guidelines for the prevention, diagnosis, risk assessment, and treatment of hypertension in adults and children. Can J Cardiol. 2020;36:596–624. https://doi.org/10.1016/j.cjca.2020.02.086.
10. National High Blood Pressure Education Program Working Group on High Blood Pressure in Children and Adolescents. The fourth report on the diagnosis, evaluation, and treatment of high blood pressure in children and adolescents. Pediatrics. 2004;114(2 Suppl 4th Report):555–76.
11. Lurbe E, Redon J. The changing epidemiology of hypertension in children and adolescents. Hypertens News. 2022;Opus 69:14–8. https://doi.org/10.30824/2204-1.

12. Annual reports ESPN/ERA Registry [Internet]. Available from: https://espn-reg.org/index.jsp?p=pua
13. Annual data report US Department of Health and Human Services, USRDS 2022 annual data report [Internet]. Available from: https://adr.usrds.org/
14. Harada R, Hamasaki Y, Okuda Y, Hamada R, Ishikura K. Epidemiology of pediatric chronic kidney disease/kidney failure learning from registries and cohort studies. Pediatr Nephrol. 2022;37:1215–29. https://doi.org/10.1007/s00467-021-05145-1.
15. Harambat J, Madden I. What is the true burden of chronic kidney disease in children worldwide? Pediatr Nephrol. 2023;38:1389–93. https://doi.org/10.1007/s00467-022-05816-7.
16. Geylis M, Coreanu T, Novack V, Landau D. Risk factors for childhood chronic kidney disease: a population-based study. Pediatr Nephrol. 2023;38:1569–76. https://doi.org/10.1007/s00467-022-05714-y.
17. Ashoor IF, Mansfield SA, O'Shaughnessy MM, et al. CureGN Consortium. Prevalence of cardiovascular disease risk factors in childhood glomerular diseases. JAMA. 2019;8:e012143.
18. Schaefer F, Doyon A, Azukaitis K, et al. 4C Study Consortium. Cardiovascular phenotypes in children with CKD: the 4C study. Clin J Am Soc Nephrol. 2017;12:19–28.
19. Mitsnefes M, Stablein D. Hypertension in pediatric patients on long-term dialysis: a report of the North American Pediatric Renal Transplant Cooperative Study (NAPRTCS). Am J Kidney Dis. 2015;45:309–15.
20. Thompson M. Gaps in the evidence for screening children for hypertension to prevent adult cardiovascular disease-response to the editorial by Samuels and colleagues. J Clin Hypertens. 2014;16:80–1.
21. Flynn JT, Mitsnefes M, Pierce C, et al. Blood pressure in children with chronic kidney disease a report from the Chronic Kidney Disease in Children Study. Hypertension. 2008;52 631–7.
22. Primack W, Kleeman S, Boineau F, Jernigan S. Are my pediatric patients at increased risk of developing chronic kidney disease? Clin Pediatr (Phila). 2020;59:801–8. https://doi.org/10.1177/0009922820920015.
23. Wilson AC, Flynn JT. Blood pressure in children with chronic kidney disease: lessons learned from the Chronic Kidney Disease in Children Cohort Study. Pediatr Nephrol. 2020;35:1203–9. https://doi.org/10.1007/s00467-019-04288-6.
24. Barletta GM, Pierce C, Mitsnefes M, et al. Is blood pressure improving in children with chronic kidney disease? A period analysis. Hypertension. 2018;71:444–50. https://doi.org/10.1161/HYPERTENSIONAHA.117.09649.
25. Samuels J, Ng D, Flynn JT, et al. Chronic Kidney Disease in Children Study Group. Ambulatory blood pressure patterns in children with chronic kidney disease. Hypertension. 2012;60:43–50. https://doi.org/10.1161/HYPERTENSIONAHA.111.189266.
26. Ameer OZ. Hypertension in chronic kidney disease: what lies behind the scene. Front Pharmacol. 2022;13:949260. https://doi.org/10.3389/fphar.2022.949260.
27. Hall JE. Renal dysfunction, rather than non-renal vascular dysfunction, mediates salt-induced hypertension. Circulation. 2016;133:894–906. https://doi.org/10.1161/CIRCULATIONAHA.115.018526.
28. Bovée DM, Cuevas CA, Zietse R, et al. Salt-sensitive hypertension in chronic kidney disease: distal tubular mechanisms. Am J Physiol Renal Physiol. 2020;319:F729–45. https://doi.org/10.1152/ajprenal.00407.2020.
29. Gupta A, Nagaraju SP, Bhojaraja MV, Swaminathan SM, Mohan PB. Hypertension in chronic kidney disease: an update on diagnosis and management. South Med J. 2023;116:237–44. https://doi.org/10.14423/SMJ.0000000000001516.
30. Liang L, Shimosawa T. Molecular mechanisms of Na-Cl cotransporter in relation to hypertension in chronic kidney disease. Int J Mol Sci. 2022;24:286. https://doi.org/10.3390/ijms24010286.
31. Tanaka S, Okusa MD. Crosstalk between the nervous system and the kidney. Kidney Int 2020;97(3):466–76. https://doi.org/10.1016/j.kint.2019.10.032

32. Frąk W, Kućmierz J, Szlagor M, Młynarska E, Rysz J, Franczyk B. New insights into molecular mechanisms of chronic kidney disease. Biomedicines. 2022;10:2846. https://doi.org/10.3390/biomedicines10112846.
33. Halbach SM. Hypertension in chronic kidney disease. In: Flynn JT, Ingelinger JR, Brady TM, editors. Pediatric hypertension. 5th ed. Springer; 2023. p. 477–98.
34. Aguilar A, Gifre L, Ureña-Torres P, et al. Pathophysiology of bone disease in chronic kidney disease: from basics to renal osteodystrophy and osteoporosis. Front Physiol. 2023;14:1177829. https://doi.org/10.3389/fphys.2023.1177829.
35. Freundlich M, Gamba G, Rodriguez-Iturbe B. Fibroblast growth factor 23-Klotho and hypertension: experimental and clinical mechanisms. Pediatr Nephrol. 2021;36:3007–22. https://doi.org/10.1007/s00467-020-04843-6.
36. Brady TM, Roem J, Cox C, et al. Adiposity, sex, and cardiovascular disease risk in children with CKD: a longitudinal study of youth enrolled in the Chronic Kidney Disease in Children (CKiD) Study. Am J Kidney Dis. 2020;76:166–73. https://doi.org/10.1053/j.ajkd.2020.01.011.
37. Wingen AM, Fabian-Bach C, Schaefer F, Mehls O. Randomised multicentre study of a low-protein diet on the progression of chronic renal failure in children. European Study Group of Nutritional Treatment of Chronic Renal Failure in Childhood. Lancet. 1997;349:1117–23.
38. Mitsnefes M, Ho PL, McEnery PT. Hypertension and progression of chronic renal insufficiency in children: a report of the North American Pediatric Renal Transplant Cooperative Study (NAPRTCS). J Am Soc Nephrol. 2003;14:2618–22.
39. Warady BA, Abraham AG, Schwartz GJ, et al. Predictors of rapid progression of glomerular and nonglomerular kidney disease in children and adolescents: the chronic kidney disease in children (CKiD) cohort. Am J Kidney Dis. 2015;65:878–88.
40. Reynolds BC, Roem JL, Ng DKS, et al. Association of time-varying blood pressure with chronic kidney disease progression in children. JAMA Netw Open. 2020;3:e1921213.
41. Dionne JM, Jiang S, Ng DK, et al. Group CKs. Mean arterial pressure and chronic kidney disease progression in the CKiD cohort. Hypertension. 2021;78:65–73.
42. Guzman-Limon ML, Jiang S, Ng D, et al. Nocturnal hypertension in children with chronic kidney disease is common and associated with progression to kidney replacement therapy. Hypertension. 2022;79:2288–97.
43. Wühl E, Trivelli A, Picca S, et al. Strict blood-pressure control and progression of renal failure in children. N Engl J Med. 2009;361:1639–50.
44. Schaefer B, Wühl E. Educational paper: progression in chronic kidney disease and prevention strategies. Eur J Pediatr. 2012;171:1579–88. https://doi.org/10.1007/s00431-012-1814-5.
45. Mitsnefes M, Flynn J, Cohn S, et al. CKiD Study Group. Masked hypertension associates with left ventricular hypertrophy in children with CKD. J Am Soc Nephrol. 2010;21:137–44. https://doi.org/10.1681/ASN.2009060609.
46. Ku E, McCulloch CE, Warady BA, Furth SL, Grimes BA, Mitsnefes MM. Twenty-four-hour ambulatory blood pressure versus clinic blood pressure measurements and risk of adverse outcomes in children with CKD. Clin J Am Soc Nephrol. 2018;13:422–8. https://doi.org/10.2215/CJN.09630917.
47. Lande MB, Gerson AC, Hooper SR, et al. Casual blood pressure and neurocognitive function in children with chronic kidney disease: a report of the children with chronic kidney disease cohort study. Clin J Am Soc Nephrol. 2011;6:1831–7. https://doi.org/10.2215/CJN.00810111.
48. Lande MB, Mendley SR, Matheson MB, et al. Association of blood pressure variability and neurocognition in children with chronic kidney disease. Pediatr Nephrol. 2016;31:2137–44. https://doi.org/10.1007/s00467-016-3425-2.
49. Kidney Disease: Improving Global Outcomes (KDIGO) Glomerular Diseases Work Group. KDIGO 2021 clinical practice guideline for the management of glomerular diseases. Kidney Int. 2021;100(4S):S1–S276. https://doi.org/10.1016/j.kint.2021.05.021.
50. Flynn JT, Carroll MK, Ng DK, Furth SL, Warady BA. Achieved clinic blood pressure level and chronic kidney disease progression in children: a report from the Chronic Kidney Disease in Children cohort. Pediatr Nephrol. 2021;36:1551–9. https://doi.org/10.1007/s00467-020-04833-8.

51. Watt KM, Avant D, Sherwin J, et al. Effect of renal function on antihypertensive drug safety and efficacy in children. Pediatr Nephrol. 2018;33:139–46. https://doi.org/10.1007/s00467-017-3763-8.
52. Chaturvedi S, Lipszyc DH, Licht C, Craig JC, Parekh RS. Cochrane in context: pharmacological interventions for hypertension in children. Evid Based Child Health. 2014;9:581–3. https://doi.org/10.1002/ebch.1975.
53. Burrello J, Erhardt EM, Saint-Hilary G, et al. Pharmacological treatment of arterial hypertension in children and adolescents: a network meta-analysis. Hypertension. 2018;72:306–13. https://doi.org/10.1161/HYPERTENSIONAHA.118.10862.
54. Redon J, Seeman T, Pall D, et al. Narrative update of clinical trials with antihypertensive drugs in children and adolescents. Front Cardiovasc Med. 2022;9:1042190. https://doi.org/10.3389/fcvm.2022.1042190.
55. Soergel M, Verho M, Wühl E, Gellermann J, Teichert L, Schärer K. Effect of ramipril on ambulatory blood pressure and albuminuria in renal hypertension. Pediatr Nephrol. 2000;15:113–8. https://doi.org/10.1007/s004670000422.
56. Seeman T, Dusek J, Vondrák K, Flögelová H, Geier P, Janda J. Ramipril in the treatment of hypertension and proteinuria in children with chronic kidney diseases. Am J Hypertens. 2004;17:415–20. https://doi.org/10.1016/j.amjhyper.2004.01.008.
57. Webb NJ, Wells TG, Shahinfar S, et al. A randomized, open-label, dose-response study of losartan in hypertensive children. Clin J Am Soc Nephrol. 2014;9:1441–8. https://doi.org/10.2215/CJN.11111113.
58. Lou-Meda R, Stiller B, Antonio ZL, et al. Long-term safety and tolerability of valsartan in children aged 6 to 17 years with hypertension. Pediatr Nephrol. 2019;34:495–506. https://doi.org/10.1007/s00467-018-4114-0.
59. Ferguson MA, Flynn JT. Rational use of antihypertensive medications in children. Pediatr Nephrol. 2014;29:979–88. https://doi.org/10.1007/s00467-013-2510-z.
60. Abraham AG, Betoko A, Fadrowski JJ, et al. Renin-angiotensin II-aldosterone system blockers and time to renal replacement therapy in children with CKD. Pediatr Nephrol. 2017;32:643–9. https://doi.org/10.1007/s00467-016-3512-4.
61. Fathallah-Shaykh SA, Flynn JT, Pierce CB, et al. Progression of pediatric CKD of nonglomerular origin in the CKiD cohort. Clin J Am Soc Nephrol. 2015;10:571–7. https://doi.org/10.2215/CJN.07480714.
62. Agarwal R, Sinha AD, Cramer AE, et al. Chlorthalidone for hypertension in advanced chronic kidney disease. N Engl J Med. 2021;385:2507–19. https://doi.org/10.1056/NEJMoa2110730.
63. Cirillo L, Ravaglia F, Errichiello C, Anders HJ, Romagnani P, Becherucci F. Expectations in children with glomerular diseases from SGLT2 inhibitors. Pediatr Nephrol. 2022;37:2997–3008. https://doi.org/10.1007/s00467-022-05504-6.
64. Redon J. New insights of cardiovascular and renal protection in diabetic chronic kidney disease with finerenone. Cardiovasc Res. 2022;118:e36–7. https://doi.org/10.1093/cvr/cvac024.

Part V

Pathophysiologic Mechanisms

Pivotal Role of the Kidneys in Blood Pressure Regulation and Hypertension

9

Joey P. Granger, Ana C. Palei, and Frank T. Spradley

9.1 Introduction

Regulation of blood pressure involves the integration of numerous factors including neural, hormonal, physical, and autacoid factors [1–8]. Short-term blood pressure regulation is achieved through rapid alterations in cardiac output and/or total peripheral resistance. In contrast, long-term control of blood pressure is intimately linked to the regulation of sodium excretion and ultimately extracellular fluid volume. A central factor in the regulation of sodium balance is the relationship between arterial pressure and sodium excretion or the so-called pressure natriuresis relationship [5–7]. Thus, hypertension develops only when factors impair the sodium and fluid excretory ability of the kidney and shifts the relation between sodium excretion and arterial pressure toward higher levels [1, 5, 6]. While there is strong theoretical and experimental evidence that the kidney is a major determinant of the long-term

J. P. Granger (✉)
Department of Physiology and Biophysics, University of Mississippi Medical Center, Jackson, MS, USA
e-mail: jgranger@umc.edu

A. C. Palei
Department of Surgery, University of Mississippi Medical Center, Jackson, MS, USA
e-mail: apalei@umc.edu

F. T. Spradley
Department of Physiology and Biophysics, University of Mississippi Medical Center, Jackson, MS, USA

Department of Surgery, University of Mississippi Medical Center, Jackson, MS, USA

Department of Pharmacology and Toxicology, University of Mississippi Medical Center, Jackson, MS, USA
e-mail: fspradley@umc.edu

A. E. Berbari et al. (eds.), *Blood Pressure Disorders in Acute and Chronic Kidney Diseases*, Updates in Hypertension and Cardiovascular Protection,
https://doi.org/10.1007/978-3-031-81292-7_9

control of arterial pressure, the initial cause of abnormal pressure natriuresis and hypertension need not be intrinsic to the kidney [1–3]. The focus of this chapter is to review the importance of the kidneys in the long-term regulation of extracellular volume and blood pressure and briefly summarize the various intra- and extra-renal factors that contribute to abnormal pressure natriuresis in hypertension. In addition, we will discuss how the two new classes of glucose-lowering drugs, sodium-glucose cotransporter 2 (SGLT-2) inhibitors and glucagon-like peptide 1 (GLP-1) receptor agonists, lower blood pressure through their renal actions [9–13].

9.2 Long-Term Regulation of Extracellular Volume and Blood Pressure

Extracellular fluid volume is determined by the balance between intake and excretion of salt and water by the kidneys. The renal-body fluid system concept predicts that a higher intake than output would lead to an increase in extracellular volume and arterial pressure (Fig. 9.1). If the excretory ability of the kidney is not impaired, the increase in arterial pressure raises sodium excretion and extracellular fluid

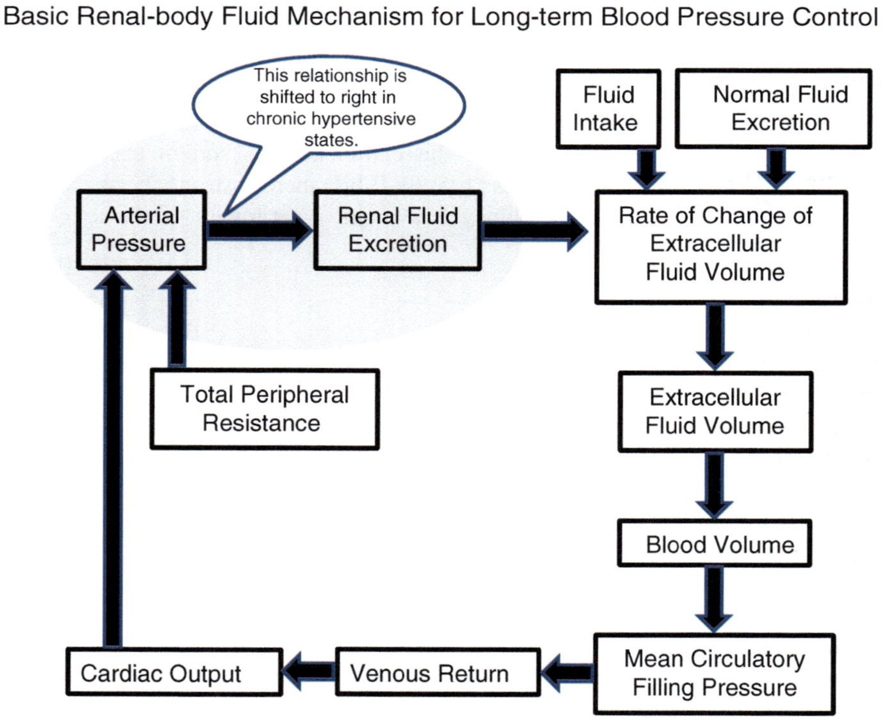

Fig. 9.1 Basic renal-body fluid feedback mechanism for long-term regulation of blood pressure and body fluid volumes

volume would then decrease, thereby reducing venous return and cardiac output until blood pressure returns to normal and fluid intake and output are reestablished. Conversely, when sodium output exceeds intake, extracellular fluid volume, blood volume, venous return, and cardiac output fall ultimately leading to a decrease in blood pressure below normal. This decrease in arterial pressure causes the kidneys to retain sodium and water until arterial pressure is restored to the normal set point. Thus, according to renal-body fluid feedback mechanism concept, the set point for long-term blood pressure control is the arterial pressure at which sodium and water intake and output are at equilibrium [1, 5, 6].

A key component of this mechanism for regulating salt and water balance is pressure natriuresis/diuresis which is the effect of increased arterial pressure to raise sodium and water excretion. An important feature of pressure natriuresis is that various hormonal and neural control systems can amplify or blunt the pressure natriuresis mechanism [5, 6, 8]. For example, in most individuals, chronic increases in sodium intake are associated with only small changes in arterial pressure. The lack of significant increases in arterial pressure in response to elevations in sodium intake is due to a number of very effective volume control systems that are activated by extracellular volume expansion. For example, in response to increases in sodium intake, decreased formation of antinatriuretic hormones and/or increased formation of natriuretic factors enhance the effectiveness of pressure natriuresis and allow sodium balance to be maintained with little or no increase in arterial pressure [5, 6, 8]. On the other hand, excessive activation of antinatriuretic systems or abnormalities in natriuretic systems can reduce the effectiveness of pressure natriuresis, thereby necessitating greater increases in arterial pressure to maintain sodium and water balance. Thus, excessive activation of antinatriuretic systems or abnormalities in natriuretic systems impair the excretory ability of the kidney and shift the relation between sodium excretion and arterial pressure toward higher levels and reset the set point for long-term blood pressure control (Fig. 9.2). In contrast, antihypertensives that act to improve renal excretory function shift the renal pressure natriuresis relationship to the left (red arrows).

While total peripheral resistance and cardiac output are determinants of arterial pressure, one prediction of the renal-body fluid feedback mechanism is that if the pressure natriuresis mechanism is not impaired, a primary increase in total peripheral resistance without changes in renal resistance would not result in long-term alterations in arterial pressure [14]. For instance, an increase in total peripheral resistance would result in an immediate elevation in arterial pressure (Fig. 9.3). The increase in arterial pressure would immediately increase sodium and water excretion, via pressure natriuresis. As long as fluid excretion exceeds fluid intake, extracellular fluid volume will continue to decrease, reducing venous return and cardiac output, until blood pressure returns to normal and fluid balance is reestablished (Fig. 9.3, panel B). Thus, primary increases in total peripheral resistance without changes in renal function do not result in long-term alterations in arterial pressure. A sustained elevation in blood pressure can only be achieved when physiological and/or pathophysiological factors impair the excretory ability of the kidney and shift the relation between sodium excretion and arterial pressure toward higher levels [14].

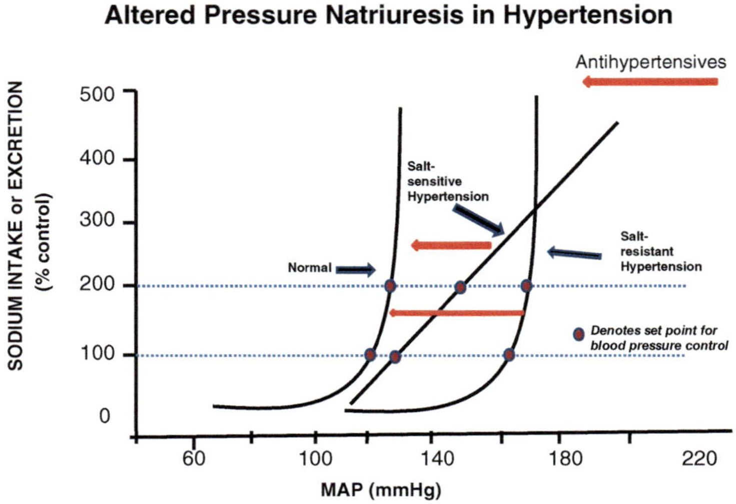

Fig. 9.2 Steady-state relationships between arterial pressure and urinary sodium excretion and sodium intake for control subjects with normal kidneys and for subjects with a rightward hypertensive shift in the pressure-natriuresis relationship. A shift in the pressure-natriuresis relationship can occur as a result of *intrarenal* abnormalities such as enhanced formation of angiotensin II (Ang II), reactive oxygen species (ROS), inflammatory cytokines and endothelin-1 (ET-1 via ET_A receptor activation) or decreased synthesis of natriuretic substances like nitric oxide (NO), eicosanoids (20-HETE), and prostaglandins (PG) or inherent genetic defects in renal Na^+ handling. In other instances, the altered kidney function is caused by *extrarenal* disturbances, such as increased renal sympathetic nervous system activity (RNSA) or excessive formation of anti-natriuretic hormones such as aldosterone or decreased atrial natriuretic peptide (ANP)

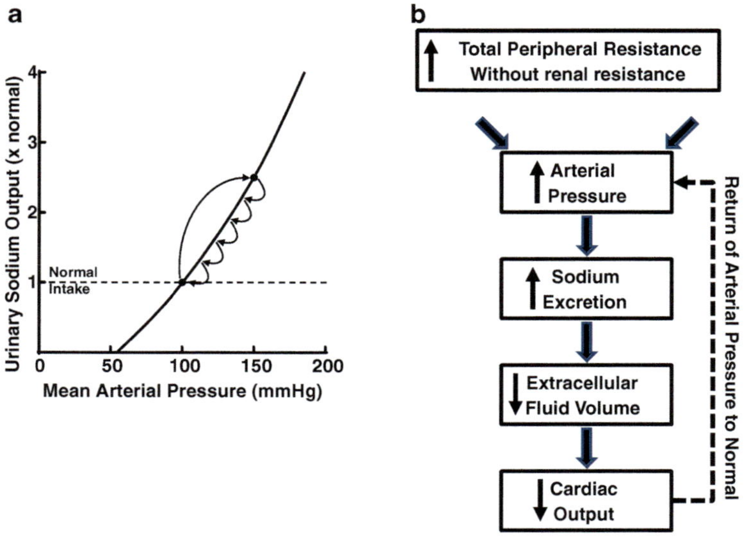

Fig. 9.3 Effect of increasing total peripheral resistance without changes in renal resistance on arterial pressure

9.3 Pressure Natriuresis: A Key Factor in Maintaining Sodium Balance in Hypertension

Another important prediction of the renal body fluid feedback control system concept is that an increase in blood pressure in hypertensive states is an essential compensatory mechanism that allows sodium balance to be maintained in the face of an underlying sodium retaining defect [4, 15]. To determine the importance of the pressure-natriuresis mechanism in achieving sodium balance caused by aldosterone excess, Hall and colleagues examined the long-term effects of aldosterone on sodium excretion and arterial pressure in normal dogs and in dogs in which renal artery pressure was prevented from increasing with an electronically servo-controlled aortic occlude [15]. In dogs in which renal artery pressure was permitted to increase during chronic aldosterone infusion, sodium excretion decreased markedly on the first day and then returned to control levels on days 2–3 of aldosterone infusion as arterial pressure increased. In contrast, in dogs in which renal artery pressure was prevented from increasing, sodium excretion decreased on the first day and remained below sodium intake for the 7 days of aldosterone infusion. The sustained sodium retention resulted in dramatic increases in cumulative sodium balance and systemic arterial pressure. The results from this study clearly demonstrated that an increase in renal arterial pressure is essential in allowing the kidneys to override the chronic sodium-retaining actions of aldosterone and to achieve normal sodium balance. Similar findings were reported from the same group during chronic administration of other sodium-retaining hormones, such as angiotensin II and norepinephrine [4].

9.4 Impaired Renal-Pressure Natriuresis in Hypertension Caused by Intra- and Extrarenal Factors

An important observation that points toward abnormal kidney function as a key factor in causing hypertension is that almost all forms of experimental hypertension are caused by perturbations to the kidneys that alter renal hemodynamics or tubular reabsorption and reduce the kidney's ability to excrete sodium and water [4–6, 15]. For example, constriction of the renal arteries or compression of the kidneys, or administration of sodium-retaining hormones such as angiotensin II or aldosterone are all associated with either decreases in renal blood flow and glomerular filtration rate and/or increases in renal tubular reabsorption prior to development of hypertension [5, 6]. Further evidence supporting the important role of the kidneys in the development and maintenance of hypertension is that in all known monogenic forms of human hypertension, the common pathway to hypertension appears to be increased renal tubular reabsorption caused by mutations that directly increase renal electrolyte transport (e.g., Liddle's or Gordon's syndromes) or the synthesis and/or activity of antinatriuretic hormones (e.g., glucocorticoid remediable aldosteronism) [6, 8].

Table 9.1 Partial list of factors affecting renal pressure natriuresis in hypertension

Prohypertensive—Antinatriuretic Factors
• Angiotensin II (Ang II)
• Aldosterone
• Renal sympathetic nervous activity (RSNA)
• Endothelin (via ET_A receptor activation)
• Vascular 20 hydroxyeicosatetraenoic acid (20-HETE)
• Immune factors and inflammatory cytokines
• Reactive oxygen species (ROS)
• Renal vascular stenosis
• Glomerular disease
• Genetic defects in renal sodium transporters
Antihypertensive Natriuretic Factors
• Nitric oxide (NO)
• Prostaglandins (PGs)
• Renal tubular 20-HETE
• Epoxyeicosatrienoic acids (EETs)
• Atrial natriuretic peptide (ANP)
• Endothelin (via ET_B receptor activation)
• Sodium glucose cotransporter-2 (SGLT-2) inhibitors
• Glucagon-like peptide-1 (GLP-1) receptor agonists

A shift in the pressure natriuresis relationship can occur as a result of *intrarenal* abnormalities such as excess formation of angiotensin II, reactive oxygen species, inflammatory cytokines, and endothelin (via ET_A receptor activation), or decreased synthesis of nitric oxide and natriuretic prostanoids and decreased renal medullary production of endothelin (and decreased ET_B receptor activation), or even genetic defects that enhance renal sodium transport systems (Table 9.1). In other instances, the altered kidney function is caused by *extrarenal* disturbances, such as increased renal sympathetic nervous activity (RSNA) or excessive formation of antinatriuretic hormones such as aldosterone (Table 9.1). The remaining portion of this chapter will discuss how these and other intra- and extrarenal factors impair renal pressure natriuresis and lead to chronic hypertension.

9.4.1 Excess Levels of Angiotensin II (Ang II) Cause Chronic Hypertension by Enhancing Renal Tubular Sodium Reabsorption

The renin-angiotensin system (RAS) plays a critical role in the long-term regulation extracellular fluid volume and blood pressure [7, 16–23]. The classical arm of the RAS consists of the enzymes, renin and angiotensin-converting enzyme, generating Ang II from angiotensinogen, which activates its Ang II type 1 (AT1) receptor, thereby causing retention of salt and water and ultimately hypertension [16, 19, 22, 23]. Under normal conditions, the RAS, via AT1 receptor, plays an important role in maintaining sodium balance and a relatively normal pressure as sodium intake is altered from low to high levels [21]. Excess activation of the RAS has also been implicated in the pathogenesis of various forms of hypertension including renovascular hypertension and human essential hypertension [8, 19, 22, 24].

The effect of Ang II to reduce renal pressure natriuresis and increase blood pressure is the result of its effects to directly or indirectly stimulate sodium transport [7]. While AT1 receptors are prominently expressed in the kidney, they are also expressed in the heart, blood vessels, adrenal glands, and the brain [7, 22]. Because AT1 receptors are ubiquitously expressed, dissecting the quantitative importance of each individual organ system, including the kidney, in the long-term regulation of blood pressure has been difficult. Utilizing a combined gene targeting with renal cross-transplantation approach, Coffman and colleagues examined the role of AT1 receptors in the kidney and their contribution to the development of Ang II-induced hypertension [1, 2, 17]. They found that Ang II causes hypertension primarily through effects on AT1 receptors in the kidney associated with reduced urinary sodium excretion, independent of actions of the sympathetic nervous system or aldosterone. When AT1 receptors are eliminated from the kidney, the extrarenal AT1 receptors are not sufficient to induce hypertension. Coffman and colleagues also reported that deletion of AT1 receptors in the proximal tubule alone reduces proximal fluid reabsorption, alters expression of key sodium transporters, improves pressure natriuresis, and significantly attenuates Ang II hypertension (Fig. 9.4).

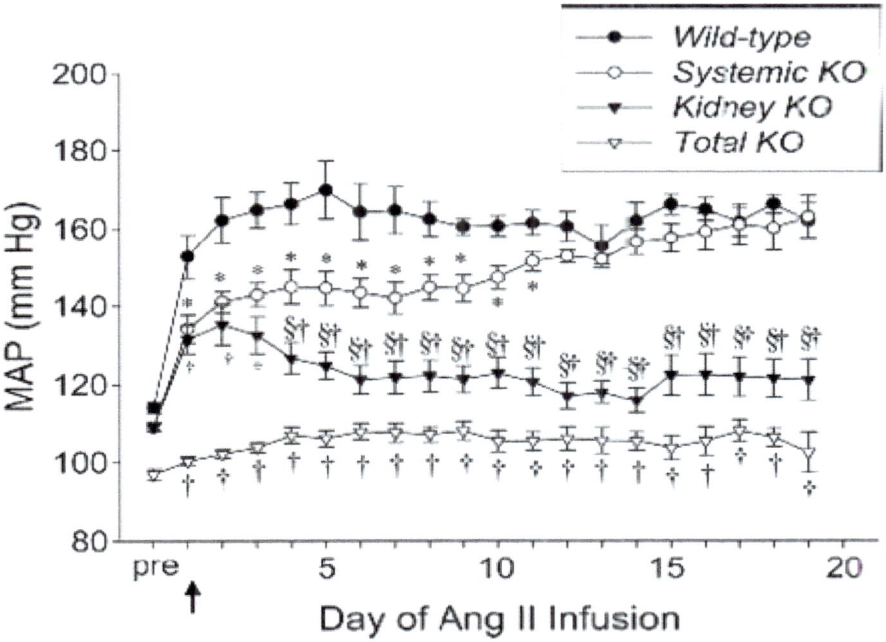

Fig. 9.4 A dominant role for renal AT_{1A} receptors in blood pressure control was demonstrated using four groups of cross-kidney transplanted mice, namely whole-body AT_{1A} expressing (Wild-type); AT_{1A} expressing systemically but not in the kidney (Systemic KO); AT_{1A} expressing only in the kidney (Kidney KO); and no AT_{1A} in either location (Total KO). Mice then received 21 days of Ang II infusion. Blood pressure response to Ang II in the systemic KO recapitulated that of the wild-type group by day 12 of Ang II infusion. Absence of renal AT_{1A} receptors in the kidney KO animals ameliorated Ang II-induced hypertension. Total KO blood pressure shows minimal response to Ang II infusion [1, 17] https://www.ahajournals.org/doi/10.1161/HYPERTENSIONAHA.105.063636

Collectively, these findings highlight the critical role of the kidney in the pathogenesis of Ang II-dependent hypertension. In addition, they suggest that the major mechanism of action of RAS blockade in hypertension is attenuation of Ang II effects in the kidney.

In addition to activation of the AT1 receptor, Ang II can also activate a second receptor, the AT2 receptor [19, 23, 24]. Moreover, the removal of the C-terminal phenylalanine from Ang II by angiotensin-converting enzyme 2 (ACE2) yields angiotensin-(1–7), and this peptide interacts with its receptor Mas. When the aminoterminal Asp of angiotensin-(1–7) is decarboxylated, alamandine is generated, which activates the Mas-related G-protein-coupled receptor D (MrgD) [19, 23, 24]. The Mas, MrgD, and the AT2 receptor have opposing effects to the classical AT1 receptor. While results from animal studies suggest a potential physiological role for these opposing receptors, the importance of these pathways in regulating renal function and arterial pressure in humans remains unclear.

9.4.2 Aldosterone Acts on the Distal Tubules and Cortical Collecting Ducts to Enhance Sodium Transport and Leads to Increases in Extracellular Fluid Volume and Hypertension

In addition to primary hyperaldosteronism, excess activation of mineralocorticoid receptor (MR) by aldosterone has also been implicated in several forms of human hypertension including renovascular hypertension, patients with resistant hypertension, and obesity-related hypertension [7, 11, 25–28]. Aldosterone plays an important role in the chronic regulation of blood pressure via its sodium-retaining actions on the kidney [7, 11]. Aldosterone alters the renal pressure natriuresis relationship by enhancing sodium transport in the distal tubules and cortical collecting ducts. The sodium-retaining effect of aldosterone is due to binding of aldosterone to intracellular MR and activation of transcription by target genes. These target genes, in turn, stimulate synthesis or activation of the sodium-potassium ATPase pump on the basolateral epithelial membrane and activation of amiloride-sensitive sodium channels on the luminal side of the epithelial membrane [7, 26].

As sodium intake is increased to high levels, aldosterone levels are suppressed allowing sodium excretion to increase to match sodium intake. Conversely, when sodium intake is restricted, aldosterone levels increase and sodium excretion is reduced to match the low sodium intake [11]. Thus, a change in aldosterone production in response to changes in sodium intake is another important hormone in the maintenance of sodium balance. An inability to suppress aldosterone production in response to increases in sodium intake therefore is another potential mechanism for salt-sensitive hypertension in humans [11].

MRs also exist in the vasculature, and the advent of technology to specifically knockout the MR from smooth muscle cells (SMCs) in mice has led to a better understanding of the SMC-MR in cardiovascular function and disease [29]. Results of studies using SMC-MR knockout animals suggest that the SMC may contribute to the regulation of vasomotor function and blood pressure and vascular remodeling in response to hypertension and vascular injury [29].

9.4.3 Excess Renal Sympathetic Nervous System Reduces Sodium Excretion by Increasing Tubular Reabsorption or Decreasing the Filtered Load of Sodium Via Alpha Adrenergic Receptor Activation

Another system that can reduce the renal pressure natriuresis relationship and cause chronic hypertension is the renal sympathetic nervous system [7, 30, 31]. The kidneys receive extensive sympathetic innervation, and increases in RSNA reduce sodium excretion by increasing tubular reabsorption or decreasing the filtered load of sodium via alpha-adrenergic receptor activation [30, 31]. Renal nerves can act directly on the tubule to increase sodium reabsorption or indirectly by increasing renal vascular resistance and reducing medullary blood flow and renal interstitial pressure [7, 30, 31]. In addition, increased RSNA can enhance tubule reabsorption by activating the RAS [7, 30, 31].

Excessive activation of the renal sympathetic nervous system has been implicated in the pathogenesis of several experimental and genetic forms of hypertension [30, 31]. Evidence for the role of the renal nerves in hypertension derives from animal studies showing that renal denervation attenuates or delays the development of hypertension in several forms of experimental hypertension [30, 31]. One particular experimental form of hypertension that is mediated via enhanced RSNA is obesity-related hypertension [32]. Obesity is often associated with increased sympathetic activity [30–32]. To determine the role of renal nerves in mediating the sodium retention and hypertension associated with obesity, Kassab and colleagues determined the hemodynamic and renal excretory responses to a high-fat diet in control and bilaterally renal-denervated dogs (Fig. 9.5) [32]. In response to a high-fat diet, body weight increased similarly (about 40%) in the control and bilaterally renal-denervated groups. Arterial pressure increased by 15% in the control group; but in sharp contrast, 5 weeks of a high-fat diet in the bilaterally renal-denervated group did not significantly increase arterial pressure. Furthermore, after 5 weeks of a high-fat diet, cumulative sodium retention was 455 ± 85 mmol in the control group and only 252 ± 47 mmol in the bilaterally renal-denervated group. Similar increases in glomerular filtration rate and renal plasma flow occurred in both groups in response to the high-fat diet, indicating that the sodium retention in response to a high fat diet was due to enhanced sodium reabsorption [32]. The results of this study indicate that the renal nerves play an important role in mediating the sodium retention and hypertension associated with obesity.

While there is growing evidence for the role of the renal sympathetic nervous system in the development of several animal models of hypertension, the importance of renal nerves in the pathogenesis of human hypertension has yet to be fully elucidated [33–35]. Application of the norepinephrine spillover methodology in humans has demonstrated activation of the sympathetic nervous outflow to the

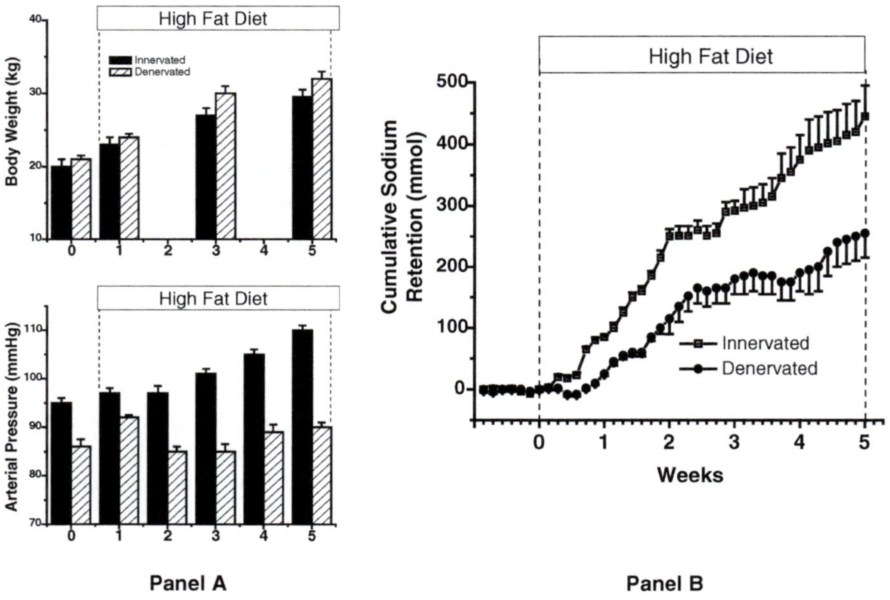

Fig. 9.5 Changes in body weight and arterial pressure (Panel A) and cumulative sodium balance (Panel B) in response to a high-fat diet in dogs with innervated and denervated kidneys. (Redrawn from [32]) https://www.ahajournals.org/doi/full/10.1161/01.hyp.26.3.471

kidneys in humans with essential hypertension [36]. Renal norepinephrine spillover, on average, is elevated two- to threefold in both normal-weight patients with essential hypertension and in obesity-related hypertension [30, 31, 36].

Evidence for a potential role of renal nerves in human hypertension is the findings that ablation of the renal sympathetic nerves with a radiofrequency-emitting catheter inserted percutaneously significantly reduces blood pressure in patients with resistant hypertension [30, 33–36]. Symplicity HTN-1 and HTN-2 studies demonstrated significant reductions of blood pressure within 6 months of the procedure [30, 33–35]. In contrast, the Symplicity HTN-3 trial, which controlled for factors believed to influence the outcome, including the addition of a sham arm, yielded a much lower blood pressure reduction compared with the Symplicity HTN-1 and HTN-2 trials [33–35]. While the initial enthusiasm was sparked by the results of early clinical trials, it was dampened by the findings of the Symplicity HTN-3 study. However, recent advances in catheter technology and more refined patient selection criteria have yielded more promising results. Subsequent studies, such as SPYRAL HTN-OFF MED and RADIANCE II, demonstrated significant reductions in blood pressure, even in patients with mild to moderate hypertension [33–35]. Future research is needed to address many unanswered questions in this field and investigate the impact of blood pressure lowering with renal denervation on clinical outcomes and potential clinical indications beyond hypertension.

9.4.4 Endothelin Can Either Elicit a Prohypertensive, Antinatriuretic Effect by Activating Endothelin Type A (ET_A) Receptors and Causing Renal Vasoconstriction or an Antihypertensive, Natriuretic Effect Via Endothelin Type B (ET_B) Receptor Activation

Endothelin-1 (ET-1) is derived from preproendothelin which is cleaved after translation to form proendothelin [37–42]. Proendothelin is cleaved in the presence of a converting enzyme to produce the 21 amino acid peptide, ET-1. ET-1 receptor binding sites have been identified throughout the body with the greatest numbers of receptors in the kidneys. ET-1 can either elicit a prohypertensive, antinatriuretic effect by activating ET_A receptor and causing renal vasoconstriction or an antihypertensive, natriuretic effect via ET_B receptor activation (Fig. 9.6). Thus, the ability of ET-1 to influence blood pressure regulation and renal pressure-natriuresis is highly dependent on where ET-1 is produced in the kidney and which renal ET receptor type is activated [16, 43].

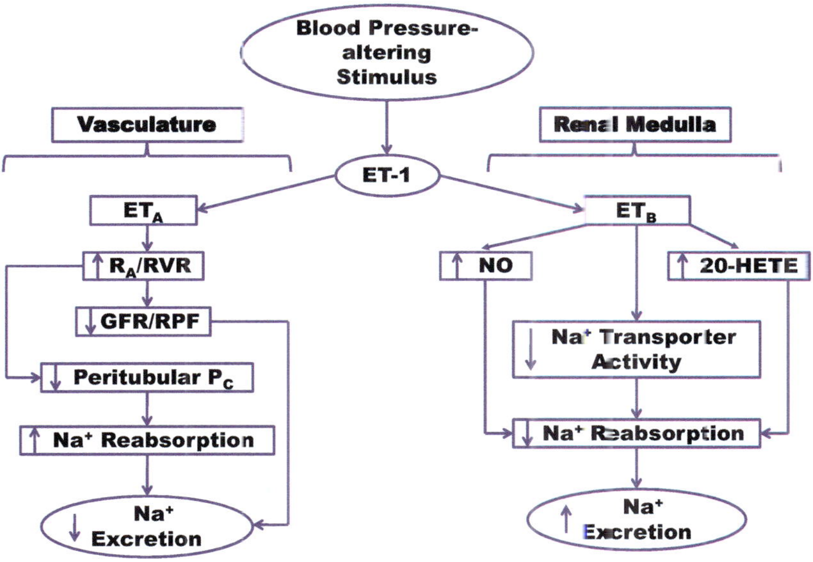

Fig. 9.6 Pro- and antihypertensive actions of endothelin-1 (ET-1). The ability of ET-1 to influence blood pressure regulation and renal pressure-natriuresis is highly dependent on where ET-1 is produced and which renal ET receptor type is activated. ET-1 can elicit a prohypertensive, antinatriuretic effect by activating ET_A receptors in the kidneys. Activation of renal ET_A receptors increases renal vascular resistance (RVR), which decreases renal plasma flow (RPF) and glomerular filtration rate (GFR), and enhances sodium reabsorption by decreasing peritubular capillary hydrostatic pressure (Pc). The net effect of renal ET_A receptor activation would be increased in sodium retention and blood pressure. Conversely, ET-1 can elicit an antihypertensive, natriuretic effect via ET_B receptor activation. Activation of the renal ET_B receptor leads to enhanced synthesis of nitric oxide (NO) and prostaglandin E_2 (PG) and suppression of the RAS. The net effect of renal ET_B receptor activation would be decreased in sodium retention and blood pressure

ET-1, via ET_A receptor activation, exerts a variety of actions within the kidney that, if sustained chronically, could contribute to the development of hypertension and progressive renal injury [37, 41, 42]. ET-1 decreases glomerular filtration rate and renal plasma flow [44, 45]. Long-term effects of ET-1 on the kidney include stimulation of mesangial cell proliferation and extracellular matrix deposition as well as stimulation of vascular smooth muscle hypertrophy in renal resistance vessels [37–39, 46]. Previous studies have indicated that expression of ET-1 is greatly enhanced in animal models of severe hypertension with renal vascular hypertrophy and in models of progressive renal injury [37–42]. In addition, treatment with endothelin receptor antagonists attenuated the hypertension and small artery morphologic changes and improved kidney function in these models [39, 40, 44, 45, 47]. An interesting unanswered question that emerges is whether the beneficial effect of the ET_A blockade in reducing renal injury is mediated through reducing blood pressure or through direct renal mechanisms.

While much attention has been given to the role of ET-1 in the pathophysiology of cardiovascular and renal disease acting via an ET_A receptor, recent studies indicate an important physiological role for ET-1 in the regulation of sodium balance and arterial pressure via ET_B receptor activation [39, 40, 43, 47, 48]. The most compelling evidence that the endothelin system may play a significant role in the regulation of sodium balance and arterial pressure are the reports that transgenic animals deficient in ET_B receptors develop a severe form of salt-sensitive hypertension [16, 43, 47–49]. Additional evidence comes from studies indicating that pharmacological antagonism of ET_B receptors produces significant hypertension in rats [38, 39, 46].

The collecting duct ET_B receptor appears to be an important physiologic regulator of renal sodium excretion and blood pressure. Ge and colleagues reported that disruption of the ET_B receptor in the collecting duct cells of mice was found to produce significant hypertension that was salt-sensitive [47, 48]. Collecting duct ET_B knockout mice on a normal sodium diet were hypertensive [47, 48]. Collecting duct ET_B knockout mice on a high sodium diet had worsened hypertension, reduced urinary sodium excretion, and excessive weight gain [47, 48]. Similar findings were found in mice with combined ET_B and ET_A receptor knockout in the collecting duct cells [47, 48]. These findings provide strong evidence that the collecting duct ET_B receptor is an important physiologic regulator of renal sodium excretion and blood pressure.

An improved understanding of the pathophysiological processes involving endothelin, in conjunction with the development of new antagonists of endothelin receptors, has led to a flourishing of new clinical trials [39–42, 50]. The favorable results of some of them have extended the proven indications for targeting the endothelin system to a variety of clinical conditions, including resistant arterial hypertension and glomerulopathies.

The hypertension with preeclampsia and with inhibitors of vascular endothelial growth factors (VEGFs) used in cancer therapy are associated with increased ET-1 production [51–53]. Thus, it is possible that the resulting hypertension could be prevented by endothelin receptor antagonist. Preclinical studies have confirmed that endothelin receptor blockade can prevent VEGF inhibitor-induced and placental ischemia-induced hypertension; however, there have been no clinical studies to support this as a therapeutic approach [51–53]. These recent preclinical and clinical studies may yet bring new life to the translation of endothelin targeting strategies in clinical practice.

9.4.5 Nitric Oxide (NO) Deficiency Decreases Sodium Excretion and Causes Hypertension

All components of the NO system are located within the kidney and pharmacological or genetic disruption of this system results in sustained hypertension associated with reductions in renal hemodynamics and pressure-natriuresis [7, 28, 54–57]. The magnitude of the increase in blood pressure is also dependent on the dietary sodium intake [7, 55, 56, 58]. These findings have led to the concept that NO is not only important in the long-term regulation of sodium balance and blood pressure but also to the notion that abnormalities in NO production result in altered pressure natriuresis and a salt-sensitive form of hypertension. Several lines of evidence suggest that NO may play an important role in the regulation of sodium balance and in the pathogenesis of salt-sensitive hypertension [7, 28, 55]. An increase in renal NO production or release as evidence by increased urinary excretion of NO metabolites or the NO second messenger, cyclic guanosine monophosphate (cGMP), has been reported to be essential for the maintenance of normotension during a dietary salt challenge. Prevention of this increase in renal NO production results in salt-sensitive hypertension [59].

Reductions in NO synthesis also reduce sodium excretory function either through direct effects on tubular transport or through changes in intrarenal physical factors such as renal interstitial hydrostatic pressure or medullary blood flow [7]. Consistent with this concept are observations that the acute infusion of a NO synthase inhibitor directly into the renal medulla significantly reduces papillary blood flow and renal interstitial hydrostatic pressure and decreases urinary sodium and water excretion without affecting glomerular filtration rate or systemic pressure [7, 59]. Chronic medullary interstitial infusion of NO synthase inhibitors in conscious rats results in sustained reductions in medullary blood flow, sustained sodium and water retention and hypertension which are reversed when the infusion is discontinued [59]. These findings demonstrate that reductions in medullary blood flow may be another important mechanism whereby inhibition of NO in the kidney leads to a hypertensive shift in pressure natriuresis.

NO-sGC-cGMP signaling is impaired human hypertension [56, 57, 60, 61]. A key component of this pathway is soluble guanylate cyclase (sGC). This second messenger consecutively interacts with intracellular proteins, including cGMP-dependent protein kinases, cGMP-regulated ion channels, and phosphodiesterases. These signal cascades mediate several physiological effects, such as inhibition of sodium transport, dilation of blood vessels, antifibrotic and anti-inflammatory effects, and platelet function. There is increasing interest in the development of drugs targeting NO-sGC-cGMP signaling to treat hypertension [57, 60]. For example, a recent study demonstrated that sGC stimulation (BAY 41-2272) significantly lowers blood pressure in a new canine model of resistant hypertension [61]. BAY 41-2272 was highly efficient as a standalone treatment for resistant hypertension but was also effective in addition to standard-of-care treatment. These data strongly suggest that sGC stimulators might provide an effective pharmacologic therapy for patients with resistant hypertension.

9.4.6 Atrial Natriuretic Peptide (ANP) Enhances Sodium Excretion Via Multiple Mechanisms and Reduces Blood Pressure

ANP elicits an antihypertensive, natriuretic effect via its receptor, the natriuretic peptide receptor A (NPR-A). ANP is 28 amino acid peptide synthesized and released from atrial cardiomyocytes in response to stretch [7]. Once ANP is released from the atria, it enhances sodium excretion through extrarenal and intrarenal mechanisms [7]. A deficiency in ANP production or a defect in its receptors may reduce pressure natriuresis and lead to hypertension by enhancing tubular sodium reabsorption either directly by enhancing the active tubular transport of sodium or indirectly via alterations in medullary blood flow, physical factors, and intrarenal hormones [7].

Plasma levels of ANP are elevated in numerous physiological conditions associated with enhanced sodium excretion [7]. Acute saline of blood volume expansion consistently elevates circulating levels of ANP. Some, but not all, investigators have reported that chronic increases in dietary sodium intake raise circulating levels of ANP [7]. Several studies have reported that infusions of exogenous ANP at rates that result in physiologically relevant plasma concentrations, comparable to those observed during volume expansion, have significant renal and cardiovascular effects [7, 62]. Infusion of ANP at a rate that causes a twofold increase in plasma ANP elicits significant natriuresis, especially in the presence of other natriuretic stimuli, such as high renal perfusion pressure [62]. Long-term physiological elevations in plasma ANP also shift the renal-pressure natriuresis relationship and reduce arterial pressure [7, 62].

The development of genetic mouse models that exhibit chronic alterations in the expression of the genes for ANP or its receptors (NPR-A, NPR-C) has also provided compelling evidence for the role of ANP in chronic regulation of renal pressure natriuresis and blood pressure [63]. Transgenic mice overexpressing ANP gene are hypotensive relative to the non-transgenic littermates, whereas mice harboring functional disruptions of the ANP or NPR-A genes are hypertensive [63]. The ANP gene knockout mice develop a salt-sensitive form of hypertension in association with failure to adequately suppress the RAS [64]. These findings suggest that genetic deficiencies in ANP or natriuretic receptor activity could play a role in the pathogenesis of salt-sensitive hypertension.

Recent drug development targeting the natriuretic peptide system has been found promising and effective against cardiovascular diseases, including hypertension [65]. For example, after discovering crosstalk between the natriuretic peptide system and the renin-angiotensin-aldosterone system, various combinations such as neprilysin/AT_1 receptor inhibitors and neprilysin/renin inhibitors have been preclinically and clinically tested in cardiovascular diseases [65]. However, the therapeutic effects of such combinations on the pathophysiology of hypertension are poorly understood and more research in this area is warranted.

9.4.7 Arachidonic Acid Metabolites, Sodium Excretion, and Hypertension

Cyclooxygenase metabolizes arachidonic acid into prostaglandin (PG) G_2 and subsequently to PGH_2, which is then further metabolized by tissue-specific isomerases to PGs and thromboxane [66]. Although the kidney produces many types of PGs with multiple functions, the major renal PG controlling sodium excretion is PGE_2 [66]. However, production of other arachidonic acid metabolites, such as prostacyclin, thromboxane, and 20 hydroxyeicosatetraenoic acid (20-HETE), may also influence renal pressure natriuresis and blood pressure regulation. The largest production of PGE_2 occurs in the medulla with decreasing synthesis in the cortex. PGE_2 is synthesized and rapidly inactivated and, once synthesized, is released and not stored. Once released, PGE_2 influences sodium transport by several intrarenal mechanisms [7, 66].

Inhibition of PG synthesis with nonselective or selective inhibitors of cyclooxygenase 2 (COX-2) activity induces or exacerbates salt-sensitive hypertension, an effect that has been attributed to inhibition of renal COX-2 activity and subsequent increase in renal sodium transport [67]. Zhang et al. recently reported that macrophages isolated from the kidneys of high-salt-treated mice have increased levels of COX-2 and microsomal PGE synthase-1 (mPGES-1). Furthermore, they showed that bone marrow transplantation from either COX-2-deficient or mPGES-1-deficient mice into wild-type mice or macrophage-specific deletion of the PGE2 type 4 (EP4) receptor induced salt-sensitive hypertension and increased phosphorylation of the renal sodium chloride cotransporter (NCC) [67]. These studies suggest that COX-2-derived PGE2 in hematopoietic cells plays an important role in response to chronically increased dietary sodium intake and also indicate that inhibiting COX-2 expression or activity in hematopoietic cells can result in a predisposition to salt-sensitive hypertension.

In addition to renal PGs generated via the COX pathway, other eicosanoids that inhibit tubular sodium transport are produced by cytochrome P450 (CYP) monooxygenase metabolism of arachidonic acid [68]. CYP enzymes metabolize arachidonic acid primarily to 20-HETE and epoxyeicosatrienoic acids (EETs). 20-HETE is a potent constrictor of renal vasculature and 20-HETE and EETs also inhibit sodium reabsorption in the proximal tubule and thick ascending limb of the loop of Henle [68].

The renal production of CYP metabolites of arachidonic acid is altered in genetic and experimental models of hypertension, and this system contributes to the resetting of pressure natriuresis and the development of hypertension [68]. 20-HETE can elicit a pro- or antihypertensive effect depending upon where it is produced in the kidney (Fig. 9.7). Vascular production of 20-HETE increases renal vascular resistance by direct constriction of preglomerular vessels or by enhancing myogenic tone or tubuloglomerular feedback (Fig. 9.7). These effects ultimately lead to chronic hypertension. In the spontaneously hypertensive rat (SHR) model, the renal production of 20-HETE is increased, and inhibitors of the formation of 20-HETE decrease arterial pressure [68]. Blockade of 20-HETE synthesis also reduces blood pressure or improves renal function in deoxycorticosterone acetate (DOCA)-salt, Ang II-infused, and Lyon hypertensive rats [68].

In contrast, 20-HETE formation is reduced in the thick ascending limb of Dahl salt-sensitive rats and this contributes to elevated sodium reabsorption [68]. Enhanced 20-HETE synthesis improves pressure natriuresis and lowers blood pressure in Dahl salt-sensitive rats, whereas inhibitors of 20-HETE production promote the development of hypertension in Lewis rats [68].

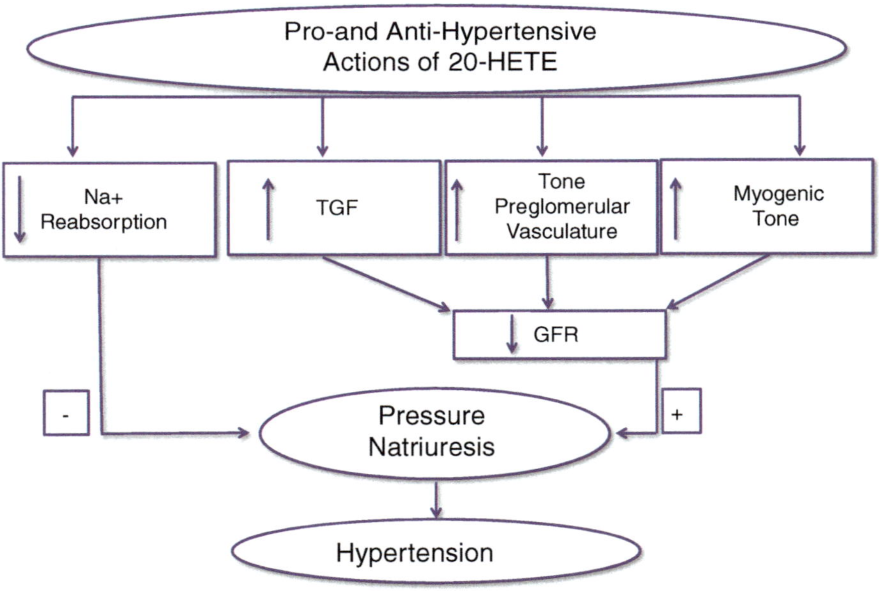

Fig. 9.7 Pro- and antihypertensive actions of 20 hydroxyeicosatetraenoic acid (20-HETE) on the kidney

9.4.8 Oxidative Stress Reduces the Ability of the Kidneys to Excrete Sodium

Recent studies suggest that reactive oxygen species (ROS) may play a role in the initiation and progression of cardiovascular dysfunction associated with diseases such as hyperlipidemia, diabetes mellitus, and hypertension [69, 70]. In many forms of hypertension, the increased ROS are derived from nicotinamide adenine dinucleotide phosphate hydrogen (NADPH) oxidases, which could serve as a triggering mechanism for uncoupling endothelial NO synthase by oxidants [69, 70].

ROS produced by migrating inflammatory cells and/or vascular cells have distinct functional effects on each cell type [69, 70]. These effects include endothelial dysfunction, renal tubule sodium transport, cell growth, migration, inflammatory gene expression, and extracellular matrix regulation. ROS, by renal hemodynamics and renal tubule cell function, can play a role in altering renal pressure natriuresis and blood pressure regulation.

Growing experimental evidence supports the role of ROS in various animal models of sodium-sensitive hypertension [49, 69–71]. The Dahl salt-sensitive rat has increased vascular and renal superoxide production and increased levels of H_2O_2. The renal protein expression of superoxide dismutase (SOD) is decreased in the kidney of Dahl salt-sensitive rats, and long-term administration of Tempol, a superoxide mimetic, significantly decreases arterial pressure and renal damage [67, 69, 70, 72]. Another salt-sensitive model, the stroke-prone spontaneously hypertensive rat (SHRSP), has elevated levels of superoxide and decreased total plasma antioxidant capacity. Superoxide production is also increased in the DOCA-salt hypertensive rat. Treatment of the DOCA-salt rats with apocynin, an NADPH oxidase inhibitor, decreases aortic superoxide production and arterial pressure [69, 70].

The importance of oxidative stress in human hypertension is unclear. An imbalance between total oxidant production and the antioxidant capacity in human hypertension has been reported to occur in some but not all studies [67, 69, 70, 73]. The equivocal findings in human studies are most likely due to the difficulty of assessing oxidative stress in humans. Moreover, most recent human studies have found that vitamin E and C supplementation has little or no effect on blood pressure [67, 69, 70, 73]. However, it should be noted that these are relatively weak antioxidants and further studies are needed to assess the role of ROS in human hypertension.

9.4.9 Inflammatory Cytokines and the Immune System Contribute to the Initiation and Progression of Hypertension

Inflammation has been implicated in the pathogenesis of hypertension [74–76]. Numerous studies have reported a strong association between inflammation and blood pressure [77–79]. Underlying mechanisms whereby inflammation contributes to hypertension include elicitation of oxidative stress, endothelial dysfunction, increased vascular stiffness and constriction, and abnormal extracellular matrix deposition. An important organ involved in inflammation-induced hypertension is the kidney [74–76, 80]. Macrophages and T cells accumulate in the kidneys of hypertensive animals and are thought to contribute to altered renal hemodynamics and tubular function in hypertension [80–84]. Findings that plasma levels of proinflammatory cytokines correlate with increased blood pressure in human hypertension and in some experimental animal models of hypertension also provide additional support for the role of cytokines in hypertension [74–76]. Moreover, several studies have demonstrated that chronic increases in plasma cytokines, comparable to concentrations observed in the hypertension associated with preeclampsia, cause significant and sustained increases in blood pressure [52].

Animal studies utilizing genetic deletion of cytokines or their receptors support the role of cytokines in hypertension. For example, mice with knockout of interleukin 6 (IL-6) have significantly lower blood pressure than wild-type mice during 2 weeks of Ang II infusion [83]. Although these findings demonstrate a significant role for IL-6 in mediating the chronic hypertensive response to Ang II in mice, the importance of inflammatory cytokines in the pathogenesis and progression of the various forms of human hypertension is unclear and is currently an area of active investigation.

Results from several recent studies also suggest that T cells play a role in the progression of hypertension [74, 80–82, 84, 85]. Harrison and colleagues proposed that hypertensive stimuli lead to renal injury, neoantigen formation, and eventual T cell activation within the kidney [86]. T cell-derived signals promote the entry of other inflammatory cells such as macrophages which result in renal vasoconstriction and increased sodium reabsorption, thereby increasing the severity of the hypertension (Fig. 9.8). Supporting this concept are results from studies in recombination-activating gene 1 (RAG-1) mice, which lack T cells and B cells. These mice do not develop the degree of hypertension in response to Ang II infusion as the wild-type mice, an observation that was attributed to lack of T cells [86]. Moreover, chronic Ang II infusion was associated with a greater number of activated T cells as well as increased Rantes, a chemotaxis protein, in the vasculature and perivascular fat. These observations were confirmed by Crowley et al. using a model very similar to the RAG-1 knockout mice [81]. They reported that Ang II hypertension, renal injury, left ventricular hypertrophy, and cardiac fibrosis were prevented in severe combined immunodeficiency (SCID) mice lacking T cells [81].

Although there is growing evidence that the immune system may play a role in the progression of hypertension, the mechanisms by which hypertension stimulates an immune response remain unclear, but might involve the formation of neoantigens that activate adaptive immunity. Moreover, while findings in experimental models of hypertension are intriguing, the importance of the immune system in the pathogenesis of hypertension in humans remains to be determined. However, in a very interesting recent study, Itani and colleagues used a humanized mouse model in which the murine immune system was replaced by the human immune system to determine whether human T cells are activated in hypertension [82]. They reported that a hypertensive stimulus of Ang II promoted the accumulation of human T cells in the kidney, aorta, and lymph nodes of humanized mice. The cells exhibited an

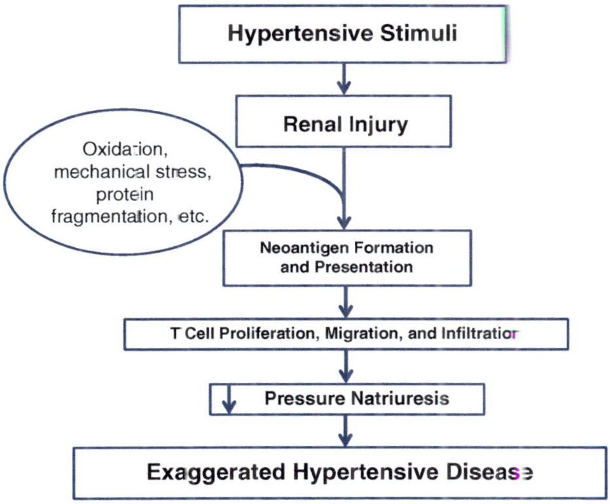

Fig. 9.8 Proposed role of T cells and inflammation in progression of chronic hypertension. Initial hypertensive stimuli lead to renal injury, neoantigen formation, and eventual T cell activation within the kidney. T cell–derived signals promote entry of other inflammatory cells, such as macrophages, which result in renal vasoconstriction and sodium reabsorption, thereby increasing the severity of hypertension and cardiovascular-renal disease

increase in the memory cell marker CD45RO. In addition, $CD3^-$ $CD45^+$ cells were increased in the lymph nodes of Ang II-infused mice. They also demonstrated that circulating T cells of humans with hypertension exhibit evidence of activation, as indicated by an increased percent of memory T cells and an increase in production of IL-17A and interferon γ (IFN-γ) [82]. Thus, human T cells become activated and invade critical end-organ tissues in response to Ang II hypertension in the humanized mouse model.

9.5 Impact of Antihypertensive Drugs on Renal Pressure Natriuresis

In all forms of chronic hypertension studied to date, the renal pressure natriuresis and diuresis mechanisms are abnormal, since increased arterial pressure is required to maintain normal excretion of sodium and water, and therefore fluid balance [3, 4, 14]. Likewise, drugs that are used to treat hypertension improve renal pressure natriuresis by reversing and or counteracting the underlying defect in renal sodium handling. Antihypertensives that act to improve renal excretory function shift the renal pressure natriuresis relationship to the left (red arrows) (Fig. 9.2).

Indeed, the impact of antihypertensive agents on the pressure natriuresis relationship has been extensively examined in animal models as well as in humans [87, 88]. For example, Gross and colleagues examined the impact of drugs that block the RAS in hypertensive transgenic rats harboring an extra mouse renin gene

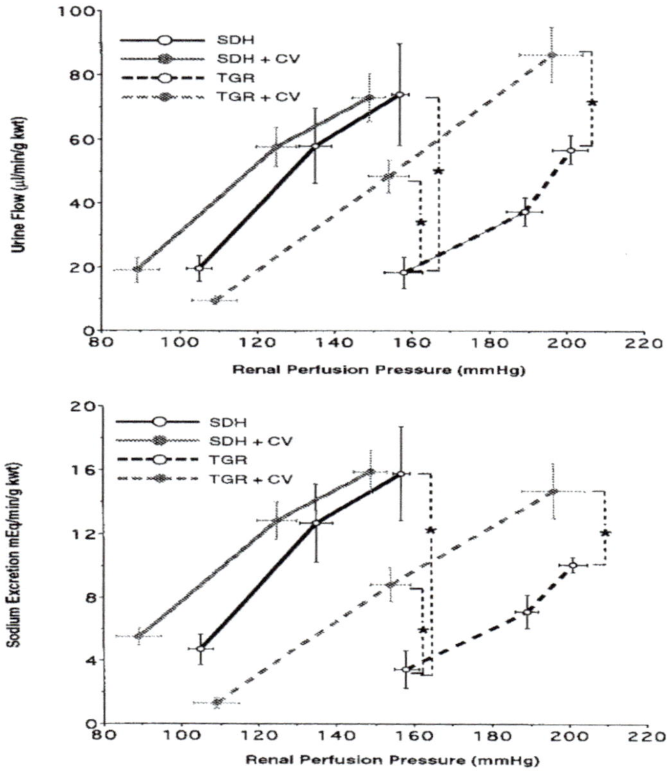

Fig. 9.9 Effect of captopril and angiotensin II receptor blockade on pressure natriuresis in transgenic TGR (mRen-2)27 rats [89]

[TGR(mRen-2)27] and have shifted rightward in the pressure natriuresis relationship [89]. They infused the converting enzyme inhibitor captopril or the Ang II receptor blocker CV11974 into transgenic and normotensive Sprague-Dawley Hannover (SDH) control rats (Fig. 9.9). Their experiments showed that blockade of Ang II generation by captopril or blockade of the AT_1 receptor in TGR is accompanied by a shift of the pressure-natriuresis and -diuresis relationships to a lower operating level of arterial pressure [89]. The results underscore the importance of the RAS for sodium and water balance in TGR at the level of the kidney.

Saito et al. analyzed the hypotensive mechanisms of a thiazide-type diuretic, mefruside, on the basis of the pressure-natriuresis relationship in humans [88]. The hypotensive effect of mefruside during a high sodium diet correlated positively with both the hypotensive effect of sodium restriction and the increase in the slope by mefruside (Fig. 9.10). Thus, mefruside lowers blood pressure especially in patients with high sodium sensitivity mainly by making blood pressure sodium insensitive through its diuretic action. Kimura and colleagues also previously reported the

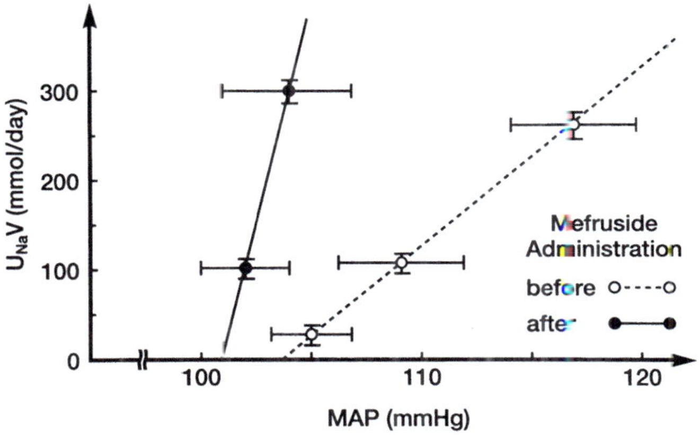

Fig. 9.10 Antihypertensive mechanism of diuretics based on pressure-natriuresis relationship [88]

effect of antihypertensives nicardipine, propranolol, and captopril in the pressure natriuresis relationship in humans [87]. The pressure-natriuresis curve was shifted left, without a change in the slope, by nicardipine and propranolol and also left, but with a decrease in the slope, by captopril [87]. The hypotensive effect of nicardipine and propranolol, being independent of the amount of sodium intake, was based on the leftward shift of the pressure-natriuresis curve that was probably due to the decrease in renal vascular resistance.

9.5.1 Glucose-Lowering Drugs, Sodium-Glucose Cotransporter-2 (SGLT-2) Inhibitors and Glucagon-Like Peptide-1 (GLP-1) Receptor Agonists Increase Sodium Excretion and Reduce Blood Pressure

The coexistence of diabetes and elevated blood pressure is an increased risk for cardiovascular disability and death worldwide. Recently, the management of diabetes has been dramatically changed by two new classes of glucose-lowering drugs, sodium-glucose cotransporter-2 (SGLT-2) inhibitors and glucagon-like peptide-1 (GLP-1) receptor agonists [90–94]. In patients with type 2 diabetes, the reduction in mortality and cardiovascular events were significantly associated with hypotensive effects of SGLT-2 inhibitors and GLP-1 receptor agonists [12, 91]. These findings suggest that the blood pressure-lowering effect could be seen as an additive indicator of cardiovascular protection by SGLT-2 inhibitors and GLP-1 receptor agonists. While the mechanisms underlying this beneficial effect on blood pressure are not well understood, they may be related to the renal natriuretic effects of SGLT-2 inhibitors and GLP-1 receptor agonists (Figs. 9.11 and 9.12).

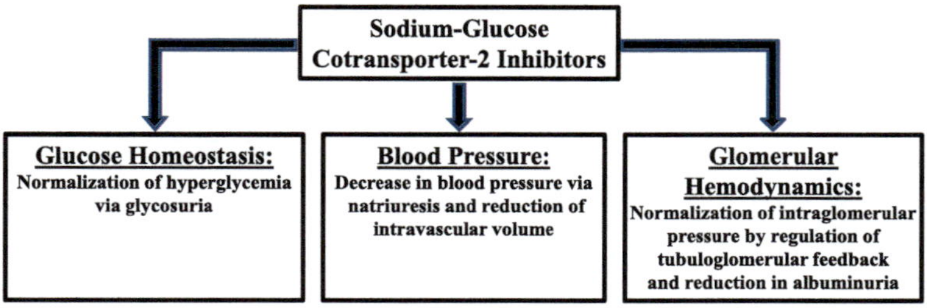

Fig. 9.11 Multiple beneficial actions of sodium-glucose cotransporter-2 inhibitors including reduction in blood pressure

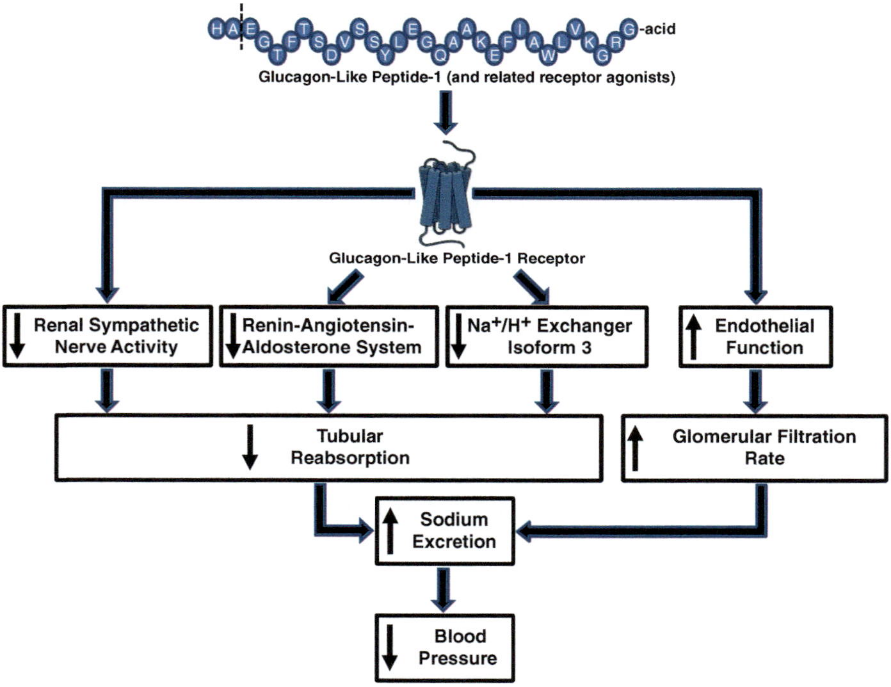

Fig. 9.12 Potential renal mechanisms for blood pressure lowering effects of glucagon-like peptide-1 (and related receptor agonists)

9.5.1.1 Effect of SGLT-2 Inhibitors on Sodium Excretion and Blood Pressure

Under normal conditions, filtered glucose is fully reabsorbed at the proximal tubules, and glucose is not excreted in the urine. SGLT-2 is a low-affinity and high-capacity glucose transporter and is located in the convoluted proximal tubule. SGLT-2 is responsible for reabsorbing around 90% of filtered glucose in the kidney [12, 13]. SGLT-2 inhibitors are a relatively new class of antidiabetic drugs. SGLT-2 inhibitors improve hyperglycemia by inhibiting reabsorption of filtered glucose, thereby increasing glycosuria [12, 13]. SGLT-2 inhibitors are also thought to reduce hyperfiltration and physical glomerular stress via tubuloglomerular feedback and improve or preserve renal function in diabetic patients [12].

The EMPA-REG OUTCOME study and CANVAS program have shown that the selective SGLT-2 inhibitors, empagliflozin and canagliflozin, significantly decrease the risk of cardiovascular death or hospitalized heart failure in type 2 diabetic patients who suffer a high risk of cardiovascular diseases [92–95]. The mechanisms underlying this beneficial outcome are not well understood, although SGLT-2 inhibitors result in reduced blood pressure. Clinical studies have shown that SGLT-2 inhibitors initially cause natriuresis after treatment is initiated [12]. SGLT-2 inhibitors do not have long-term natriuretic effects in type 2 diabetes patients, and the literature on the mechanisms of the transient effects of SGLT-2 inhibitors on sodium and water excretion is limited [12]. While studies in humans have shown SGLT-2 inhibitors increase sodium and water excretion only transiently, as most diuretics, one would expect a return to sodium balance as blood pressure decreases with chronic administration of SGLT-2 inhibitors.

SGLT-2 inhibitors increase sodium and water excretion and presumably play an important role in cardioprotection via reductions in blood pressure. SGLT-2 inhibitors have been reported in animal models as well as in humans [12]. Administration of SGLT-2 inhibitors acutely caused an increase in urinary sodium excretion in non-diabetic rats and in diabetic rats [12]. Likewise, SGLT-2 inhibitors increase urinary sodium excretion in type 2 diabetic patients [12]. Therefore, it is highly likely that the antihypertensive effects of SGLT-2 inhibitors found in the EMPA-REG OUTCOME study and the CANVAS program are probably due to natriuresis. Supporting this concept, there are studies indicating that SGLT-2 inhibitors reduce plasma volume and an increase in hematocrit [12, 13, 95].

9.5.1.2 Effects of GLP-1 Receptor Agonists on Sodium Excretion and Blood Pressure

GLP-1 is a key component of the signaling mechanisms promoting glucose homeostasis [9]. GLP-1 exerts insulinotropic effects via a G protein-coupled receptor, stimulation of adenylyl cyclase, and cyclic adenosine monophosphate (cAMP) generation [9]. There is growing evidence from recent clinical and experimental studies that GLP-1 receptor agonists, including GLP-1 itself, reduce blood pressure and the risk of major cardiovascular events independent of its actions on glucose [9, 93]. Since GLP-1 receptors are present in various regions of the body including the brain, vasculature, and the kidneys, there are a variety of potential mechanisms whereby activation of GLP-1 receptor signaling exerts its blood pressure-lowering effects [9]. However, the long-term effects of GLP-1 receptor agonist on blood pressure are most likely related to the direct and indirect actions on the kidney.

Several studies have reported that GLP-1 increases sodium and water excretion via inhibition of sodium reabsorption [10]. Hormonal systems such as the ANP or the renin-angiotensin-aldosterone system may also be indirectly involved in the signaling of GLP-1-mediated renal actions [94]. There is also evidence to suggest that the diuretic and natriuretic effects of GLP-1 are partly mediated via activation of afferent renal nerves by GLP-1 acting on sensory nerve fibers within the pelvis of the kidney [96, 97].

GLP-1 directly inhibits sodium reabsorption through inhibition of the sodium-hydrogen ion exchanger isoform-3 (NHE-3) in the proximal tubule [94, 98]. Inhibition of NHE-3 activity in the renal proximal tubule by GLP-1 is associated with increased urinary cAMP excretion, renal cortical protein kinase A (PKA) activation, and a significant increase of PKA-mediated NHE-3 phosphorylation [94, 98]. Administration of PKA and adenylate cyclase inhibitors further confirmed the involvement of the cAMP/PKA pathway in mediating the inhibitory effects of GLP-1 on NHE-3 activity and natriuresis [94, 98].

GLP-1 receptor agonists may also increase sodium excretion by enhancing glomerular filtration rate. Jensen and colleagues reported GLP-1 receptor expression on vascular smooth cells of the afferent arterioles and demonstrated that receptor activation causes vasodilation and increases renal blood flow and glomerular filtration rate [99, 100]. Thus, renal GLP-1 receptor activation most likely increases glomerular filtration rate by decreasing preglomerular resistance.

9.6 Conclusion

The kidneys, via the regulation of sodium excretion and body fluid volume, play a central role not only in the long-term control of blood pressure but ultimately in the pathogenesis of hypertension. The renal-pressure natriuresis relationship plays a pivotal part in the renal body fluid feedback control system for long-term volume and pressure regulation. Renal-pressure natriuresis is abnormal (rightward shift to higher blood pressure levels) in all types of experimental and clinical hypertension. Abnormal pressure natriuresis may occur as a result of *intrarenal* abnormalities, and in some instances, the altered kidney function is caused by *extrarenal* disturbances. Drugs used to treat hypertension reduce blood pressure by correcting and/or counteracting the intra- and/or extrarenal abnormalities that alter the pressure natriuresis relationship.

References

1. Coffman TM, Crowley SD. Kidney in hypertension: guyton redux. Hypertension. 2008;51:811–6.
2. Guyton AC, Coleman TG, Cowley AV Jr, Scheel KW, Manning RD Jr, Norman RA Jr. Arterial pressure regulation. Overriding dominance of the kidneys in long-term regulation and in hypertension. Am J Med. 1972;52:584–94.
3. Hall JE, Granger JP, do Carmo JM, et al. Hypertension: physiology and pathophysiology. Compr Physiol. 2012;2:2393–442.
4. Hall JE, Granger JP, Hester RL, Montani JP. Mechanisms of sodium balance in hypertension: role of pressure natriuresis. J Hypertens Suppl. 1986;4:S57–65.

5. Hall JE, Mizelle HL, Hildebrandt DA, Brands MW. Abnormal pressure natriuresis. A cause or a consequence of hypertension? Hypertension. 1990;15:547–59.
6. Hall JE, Granger JP. Regulation of fluid and electrolyte balance in hypertension: role of hormones and peptides. In: Battegay EJ, Lip GYH, Bakris GL, editors. Hypertension: principles and practice. Boca Raton, FL: Taylor & Francis; 2005.
7. Knox FG, Granger JP. Control of sodium excretion: an integrative approach. In: Windhager EE, editor. Handbook of physiology - section 8: renal physiology. New York, NY: Oxford University Press; 1992. p. 927–67.
8. Lifton RP. Molecular genetics of human blood pressure variation. Science. 1996;272:676–80.
9. Boshchenko AA, Maslov LN, Mukhomedzyanov AV, et al. Peptides are cardioprotective drugs of the future: the receptor and signaling mechanisms of the cardioprotective effect of glucagon-like peptide-1 receptor agonists. Int J Mol Sci. 2024;25:4900.
10. Crajoinas RO, Oricchio FT, Pessoa TD, et al. Mechanisms mediating the diuretic and natriuretic actions of the incretin hormone glucagon-like peptide-1. Am J Physiol Renal Physiol. 2011;301:F355–63.
11. Shibata S, Fujita T. The kidneys and aldosterone/mineralocorticoid receptor system in salt-sensitive hypertension. Curr Hypertens Rep. 2011;13:109–15.
12. Vallon V, Verma S. Effects of SGLT2 inhibitors on kidney and cardiovascular function. Annu Rev Physiol. 2021;83:503–28.
13. Wright EM. SGLT2 inhibitors: physiology and pharmacology. Kidney. 2021;360(2):2027–37.
14. Hall JE. Renal dysfunction, rather than nonrenal vascular dysfunction, mediates salt-induced hypertension. Circulation. 2016;133:894–906.
15. Hall JE, Granger JP, Smith MJ Jr, Premen AJ. Role of renal hemodynamics and arterial pressure in aldosterone “escape”. Hypertension. 1984;6:I183–92.
16. Bagnall AJ, Kelland NF, Gulliver-Sloan F, et al. Deletion of endothelial cell endothelin B receptors does not affect blood pressure or sensitivity to salt. Hypertension. 2006;48:286–93.
17. Coffman TM. Under pressure: the search for the essential mechanisms of hypertension. Nat Med. 2011;17:1402–9.
18. Crowley SD, Zhang J, Herrera M, Griffiths R, Ruiz P, Coffman TM. Role of AT(1) receptor-mediated salt retention in angiotensin II-dependent hypertension. Am J Physiol Renal Physiol. 2011;301:F1124–30.
19. Gironacci MM, Bruna-Haupt E. Unraveling the crosstalk between renin-angiotensin system receptors. Acta Physiol (Oxf). 2024;240:e14134.
20. Gurley SB, Riquier-Brison ADM, Schnermann J, et al. AT1A angiotensin receptors in the renal proximal tubule regulate blood pressure. Cell Metab. 2011;13:469–75.
21. Hall JE, Guyton AC, Smith MJ Jr, Coleman TG. Blood pressure and renal function during chronic changes in sodium intake: role of angiotensin. Am J Phys. 1980;239:F271–80.
22. Navar LG, Harrison-Bernard LM, Nishiyama A, Kobori H. Regulation of intrarenal angiotensin II in hypertension. Hypertension. 2002;39:316–22.
23. Te Riet L, van Esch JH, Roks AJ, van den Meiracker AH, Danser AH. Hypertension: renin-angiotensin-aldosterone system alterations. Circ Res. 2015;116:960–75.
24. Bader M, Steckelings UM, Alenina N, Santos RAS, Ferrario CM. Alternative renin-angiotensin system. Hypertension. 2024;81:964–76.
25. Arroyo JP, Lagnaz D, Ronzaud C, et al. Nedd4-2 modulates renal Na+-Cl- cotransporter via the aldosterone-SGK1-Nedd4-2 pathway. J Am Soc Nephrol. 2011;22:1707–19.
26. Calhoun DA, Nishizaka MK, Zaman MA, Thakkar RB, Weissmann P. Hyperaldosteronism among black and white subjects with resistant hypertension. Hypertension. 2002;40:892–6.
27. Epstein M, Calhoun DA. Aldosterone blockers (mineralocorticoid receptor antagonism) and potassium-sparing diuretics. J Clin Hypertens (Greenwich). 2011;13:644–8.
28. Granger J, Novak J, Schnackenberg C, Williams S, Reinhart GA. Role of renal nerves in mediating the hypertensive effects of nitric oxide synthesis inhibition. Hypertension. 1996;27:613–8.

29. Camarda ND, Ibarrola J, Biwer LA, Jaffe IZ. Mineralocorticoid receptors in vascular smooth muscle: blood pressure and beyond. Hypertension. 2024;81:1008–20.
30. DiBona GF. Neural control of the kidney: past, present, and future. Hypertension. 2003;41:621–4.
31. DiBona GF, Esler M. Translational medicine: the antihypertensive effect of renal denervation. Am J Physiol Regul Integr Comp Physiol. 2010;298:R245–53.
32. Kassab S, Kato T, Wilkins FC, Chen R, Hall JE, Granger JP. Renal denervation attenuates the sodium retention and hypertension associated with obesity. Hypertension. 1995;25:893–7.
33. Gomez-Rosero JA, Duque-Gonzalez L, Senior-Sanchez JM. The current state of renal sympathetic denervation in hypertension. Arch Cardiol Mex. 2024;94:366–72.
34. Krum H, Schlaich M, Whitbourn R, et al. Catheter-based renal sympathetic denervation for resistant hypertension: a multicentre safety and proof-of-principle cohort study. Lancet. 2009;373:1275–81.
35. Verdecchi P, Cavallini C, Sclafani R, et al. Catheter-based renal artery denervation: facts and expectations. Eur J Intern Med. 2023;117:66–77.
36. Esler MD, Krum H, Schlaich M, Schmieder RE, Böhm M, Sobotka PA. Symplicity HTN-2 Investigators. Renal sympathetic denervation for treatment of drug-resistant hypertension: one-year results from the Symplicity HTN-2 randomized, controlled trial. Circulation. 2012;126:2976–82.
37. Dhaun N, Goddard J, Kohan DE, Pollock DM, Schiffrin EL, Webb DJ. Role of endothelin-1 in clinical hypertension: 20 years on. Hypertension. 2008;52:452–9.
38. Kohan DE, Rossi NF, Inscho EW, Pollock DM. Regulation of blood pressure and salt homeostasis by endothelin. Physiol Rev. 2011;91:1–77.
39. Pollock DM, Pollock JS. Evidence for endothelin involvement in the response to high salt. Am J Physiol Renal Physiol. 2001;281:F144–50.
40. Prasad VS, Palaniswamy C, Frishman WH. Endothelin as a clinical target in the treatment of systemic hypertension. Cardiol Rev. 2009;17:181–91.
41. Schiffrin EL, Pollock DM. Endothelin system in hypertension and chronic kidney disease. Hypertension. 2024;81:691–701.
42. Schinzari F, Tesauro M, Cardillo C. Is endothelin targeting finally ready for prime time? Clin Sci (Lond). 2024;138:635–44.
43. Gariepy CE, Ohuchi T, Williams SC, Richardson JA, Yanagisawa M. Salt-sensitive hypertension in endothelin-B receptor-deficient rats. J Clin Invest. 2000;105:925–33.
44. Kassab S, Miller MT, Novak J, Reckelhoff J, Clower B, Granger JP. Endothelin-A receptor antagonism attenuates the hypertension and renal injury in Dahl salt-sensitive rats. Hypertension. 1998;31:397–402.
45. Kassab S, Novak J, Miller T, Kirchner K, Granger J. Role of endothelin in mediating the attenuated renal hemodynamics in Dahl salt-sensitive hypertension. Hypertension. 1997;30:682–6.
46. Ohuchi T, Kuwaki T, Ling GY, et al. Elevation of blood pressure by genetic and pharmacological disruption of the ETB receptor in mice. Am J Phys. 1999;276:R1071–7.
47. Ge Y, Bagnall A, Stricklett PK, Webb D, Kotelevtsev Y, Kohan DE. Combined knockout of collecting duct endothelin A and B receptors causes hypertension and sodium retention. Am J Physiol Renal Physiol. 2008;295:F1635–40.
48. Ge Y, Bagnall A, Stricklett PK, et al. Collecting duct-specific knockout of the endothelin B receptor causes hypertension and sodium retention. Am J Physiol Renal Physiol. 2006;291:F1274–80.
49. Garvin JL, Ortiz PA. The role of reactive oxygen species in the regulation of tubular function. Acta Physiol Scand. 2003;179:225–32.
50. Krum H, Viskoper RJ, Lacourciere Y, Budde M, Charlon V. The effect of an endothelin-receptor antagonist, bosentan, on blood pressure in patients with essential hypertension. Bosentan Hypertension Investigators. N Engl J Med. 1998;338:784–90.
51. Alexander BT, Rinewalt AN, Cockrell KL, Massey MB, Bennett WA, Granger JP. Endothelin type a receptor blockade attenuates the hypertension in response to chronic reductions in uterine perfusion pressure. Hypertension. 2001;37:485–9.

52. Granger JP, Alexander BT, Llinas MT, Bennett WA, Khalil RA. Pathophysiology of preeclampsia: linking placental ischemia/hypoxia with microvascular dysfunction. Microcirculation. 2002;9:147–60.
53. Lankhorst S, Kappers MH, van Esch JH, et al. Treatment of hypertension and renal injury induced by the angiogenesis inhibitor sunitinib: preclinical study. Hypertension. 2014;64:1282–9.
54. Granger JP, Alberola AM, Salazar FJ, Nakamura T. Control of renal hemodynamics during intrarenal and systemic blockade of nitric oxide synthesis in conscious dogs. J Cardiovasc Pharmacol. 1992;20(Suppl 12):S160–2.
55. Granger JP, Alexander BT. Abnormal pressure-natriuresis in hypertension: role of nitric oxide. Acta Physiol Scand. 2000;168:161–8.
56. Schnackenberg C, Patel AR, Kirchner KA, Granger JP. Nitric oxide, the kidney and hypertension. Clin Exp Pharmacol Physiol. 1997;24:600–6.
57. Schnackenberg CG, Wilkins FC, Granger JP. Role of nitric oxide in modulating the vasoconstrictor actions of angiotensin II in preglomerular and postglomerular vessels in dogs. Hypertension. 1995;26:1024–9.
58. Mattson DL, Lu S, Nakanishi K, Papanek PE, Cowley AW Jr. Effect of chronic renal medullary nitric oxide inhibition on blood pressure. Am J Phys. 1994;266:H1918–26.
59. Cowley AW Jr, Mori T, Mattson D, Zou A-P. Role of renal NO production in the regulation of medullary blood flow. Am J Physiol Regul Integr Comp Physiol. 2003;284:R1355–69.
60. Vakalopoulos A, Wunder F, Hartung IV, et al. New generation of sGC stimulators: discovery of imidazo[1,2-a]pyridine carboxamide BAY 1165747 (BAY-747), a long-acting soluble guanylate cyclase stimulator for the treatment of resistant hypertension. J Med Chem. 2023;66:7280–303.
61. Vogel J, Boehme P, Homann S, et al. sGC stimulation lowers elevated blood pressure in a new canine model of resistant hypertension. Hypertens Res. 2021;44:1568–77.
62. Granger JP, Opgenorth TJ, Salazar J, Romero JC, Burnett JC Jr. Long-term hypotensive and renal effects of atrial natriuretic peptide. Hypertension. 1986;8:II112–6.
63. Melo LG, Steinhelper ME, Pang SC, Tse Y, Ackermann U. ANP in regulation of arterial pressure and fluid-electrolyte balance: lessons from genetic mouse models. Physiol Genomics. 2000;3:45–58.
64. Melo LG, Veress AT, Chong CK, Pang SC, Flynn TG, Sonnenberg H. Salt-sensitive hypertension in ANP knockout mice: potential role of abnormal plasma renin activity. Am J Phys. 1998;274:R255–61.
65. Shelke V, Dagar N, Puri B, Gaikwad AB. Natriuretic peptide system in hypertension: current understandings of its regulation, targeted therapies and future challenges. Eur J Pharmacol. 2024;976:176664.
66. Chen HF, Harris RC. Cyclooxygenases, the kidney, and hypertension. Hypertension. 2004;43:525–30.
67. Zhang MZ, Yao B, Wang Y, et al. Inhibition of cyclooxygenase-2 in hematopoietic cells results in salt-sensitive hypertension. J Clin Invest. 2015;125:4281–94.
68. Roman RJ. P-450 metabolites of arachidonic acid in the control of cardiovascular function. Physiol Rev. 2002;82:131–85.
69. Taniyama Y, Griendling KK. Reactive oxygen species in the vasculature: molecular and cellular mechanisms. Hypertension. 2003;42:1075–81.
70. Wilcox CS. Reactive oxygen species: roles in blood pressure and kidney function. Curr Hypertens Rep. 2002;4:160–6.
71. Schreck C, O'Connor PM. NAD(P)H oxidase and renal epithelial ion transport. Am J Physiol Regul Integr Comp Physiol. 2011;300:R1023–9.
72. Manning RD Jr, Meng S, Tian N. Renal and vascular oxidative stress and salt-sensitivity of arterial pressure. Acta Physiol Scand. 2003;179:243–50.
73. Zhang T, Huo H, Zhang Y, et al. Th17 cells: a new target in kidney disease research. Int Rev Immunol. 2024;43:263–79.

74. Aboukhater D, Morad B, Nasrallah N, et al. Inflammation and hypertension: underlying mechanisms and emerging understandings. J Cell Physiol. 2023;238:1148–59.
75. Shokoples BG, Paradis P, Schiffrin EL. Immunological insights into hypertension: unraveling triggers and potential therapeutic avenues. Hypertens Res. 2024;47:2115–25.
76. Wenzel U, Turner JE, Krebs C, Kurts C, Harrison DG, Ehmke H. Immune mechanisms in arterial hypertension. J Am Soc Nephrol. 2016;27:677–86.
77. Cai X, Song S, Hu J, et al. Systemic inflammation response index as a predictor of stroke risk in elderly patients with hypertension: a cohort study. J Inflamm Res. 2023;16:4821–32.
78. Caiazzo E, Sharma M, Rezig AOM, et al. Circulating cytokines and risk of developing hypertension: a systematic review and meta-analysis. Pharmacol Res. 2024;200:107050.
79. Chen Y, Li Y, Liu M, Xu W, Tong S, Liu K. Association between systemic immunity-inflammation index and hypertension in US adults from NHANES 1999-2018. Sci Rep. 2024;14:5677.
80. De Miguel C, Das S, Lund H, Mattson DL. T lymphocytes mediate hypertension and kidney damage in Dahl salt-sensitive rats. Am J Physiol Regul Integr Comp Physiol. 2010;298:R1136–42.
81. Crowley SD, Song YS, Lin EE, Griffiths R, Kim HS, Ruiz P. Lymphocyte responses exacerbate angiotensin II-dependent hypertension. Am J Physiol Regul Integr Comp Physiol. 2010;298:R1089–97.
82. Itani HA, McMaster WG Jr, Saleh MA, et al. Activation of human T cells in hypertension: studies of humanized mice and hypertensive humans. Hypertension. 2016;68:123–32.
83. Lee DL, Sturgis LC, Labazi H, et al. Angiotensin II hypertension is attenuated in interleukin-6 knockout mice. Am J Physiol Heart Circ Physiol. 2006;290:H935–40.
84. Mattson DL. Effector memory T lymphocytes in renal disease. Am J Physiol Renal Physiol. 2010;299:F1257.
85. De Miguel C, Guo C, Lund H, Feng D, Mattson DL. Infiltrating T lymphocytes in the kidney increase oxidative stress and participate in the development of hypertension and renal disease. Am J Physiol Renal Physiol. 2011;300:F734–42.
86. Harrison DG, Guzik TJ, Lob HE, et al. Inflammation, immunity, and hypertension. Hypertension. 2011;57:132–40.
87. Kimura G, Deguchi F, Kojima S, et al. Antihypertensive drugs and sodium restriction. Analysis of their interaction based on pressure-natriuresis relationship. Am J Hypertens. 1988;1:372–9.
88. Saito F, Kimura G, Shimozaki Y, et al. Mechanism of hypotensive action of a diuretic, mefruside, based on the pressure-natriuresis relationship. Nihon Jinzo Gakkai Shi. 1987;29:461–7.
89. Gross V, Lippoldt A, Schneider W, Luft FC. Effect of captopril and angiotensin II receptor blockade on pressure natriuresis in transgenic TGR(mRen-2)27 rats. Hypertension. 1995;26:471–9.
90. Benham JL, Booth JE, Sigal RJ, Daskalopoulou SS, Leung AA, Rabi DM. Systematic review and meta-analysis: SGLT2 inhibitors, blood pressure and cardiovascular outcomes. Int J Cardiol Heart Vasc. 2021;33:100725.
91. Diallo A, Carlos-Bolumbu M, Galtier F. Blood pressure-lowering effects of SGLT2 inhibitors and GLP-1 receptor agonists for preventing of cardiovascular events and death in type 2 diabetes: a systematic review and meta-analysis. Acta Diabetol. 2023;60:1651–62.
92. Radholm K, Figtree G, Perkovic V, et al. Canagliflozin and heart failure in type 2 diabetes mellitus: results from the CANVAS program. Circulation. 2018;138:458–68.
93. Rivera FB, Lumbang GNO, Gaid DRM, et al. Glucagon-like peptide-1 receptor agonists modestly reduced blood pressure among patients with and without diabetes mellitus: a meta-analysis and meta-regression. Diabetes Obes Metab. 2024;26:2209–28.
94. Skov J. Effects of GLP-1 in the kidney. Rev Endocr Metab Disord. 2014;15:197–207.
95. Zinman B, Wanner C, Lachin JM, et al. Empagliflozin, cardiovascular outcomes, and mortality in type 2 diabetes. N Engl J Med. 2015;373:2117–28.

96. Katsurada K, Nandi SS, Sharma NM, Zheng H, Liu X, Patel KP. Does glucagon-like peptide-1 induce diuresis and natriuresis by modulating afferent renal nerve activity? Am J Physiol Renal Physiol. 2019;317:F1010–21.
97. Liu X, Patel KP, Zheng H. Role of renal sympathetic nerves in GLP-1 (glucagon-like peptide-1) receptor agonist exendin-4-mediated diuresis and natriuresis in diet-induced obese rats. J Am Heart Assoc. 2021;10:e022542.
98. Farah LX, Valentini V, Pessoa TD, Malnic G, McDonough AA, Girardi AC. The physiological role of glucagon-like peptide-1 in the regulation of renal function. Am J Physiol Renal Physiol. 2016;310:F123–7.
99. Jensen EP, Poulsen SS, Kissow H, et al. Activation of GLP-1 receptors on vascular smooth muscle cells reduces the autoregulatory response in afferent arterioles and increases renal blood flow. Am J Physiol Renal Physiol. 2015;308:F867–77.
100. Kim M, Platt MJ, Shibasaki T, et al. GLP-1 receptor activation and Epac2 link atrial natriuretic peptide secretion to control of blood pressure. Nat Med. 2013;19:567–75.

Miscellaneous Factors

10

Monica Cortinovis, Norberto Perico,
and Giuseppe Remuzzi

10.1 Introduction

Hypertension is a frequent disorder in patients with chronic kidney disease, and contributes to progressive decline in kidney function. The present chapter provides mechanistic insights into some of the multiple and interlinked processes involved in the pathophysiology of hypertension and its attendant damage to organs, such as the kidney and vasculature. To begin with, we focused on endothelial dysfunction secondary to reduced nitric oxide supply or due to a shift in the balance between endothelium-derived relaxing and contracting factors toward the latter. This is followed by a presentation of our current understanding of the roles of inflammation and the immune response in hypertension and its associated kidney damage, dissecting the relative contribution of specific immune cell subsets. Furthermore, we outlined clinical overlap and differences between malignant hypertension-associated thrombotic microangiopathy and atypical hemolytic uremic syndrome, highlighting features that can help to differentiate the two conditions, thereby guiding toward the most appropriate therapy.

M. Cortinovis · N. Perico
Istituto di Ricerche Farmacologiche Mario Negri IRCCS, Clinical Research Center for Rare Diseases "Aldo & Cele Daccò", Bergamo, Italy
e-mail: monica.cortinovis@marionegri.it; norberto.perico@marionegri.it

G. Remuzzi (✉)
Istituto di Ricerche Farmacologiche Mario Negri IRCCS, Centro Anna Maria Astori, Science and Technology Park Kilometro Rosso, Bergamo, Italy
e-mail: giuseppe.remuzzi@marionegri.it

A. E. Berbari et al. (eds.), *Blood Pressure Disorders in Acute and Chronic Kidney Diseases*, Updates in Hypertension and Cardiovascular Protection,
https://doi.org/10.1007/978-3-031-81292-7_10

10.2 Impaired Regulation of Vasoactive Substances

The vascular system plays a key role in regulating blood pressure, mainly by changes in peripheral arterial resistance in order to maintain blood flow to organs and tissues in response to oxygen demands [1]. This is associated with structural and functional adaptations within the three layers of the vessels, which from inside to outside comprise the tunica intima, tunica media, and the tunica adventitia. Nevertheless, under pathological conditions, these adaptive changes do not return to baseline levels, but instead lead to the maladaptive vascular alterations associated with hypertension, including endothelial dysfunction, increased vascular contraction, and arterial remodeling [2, 3]. These processes are triggered by complex interacting systems, such as the sympathetic nervous system, the renin–angiotensin–aldosterone system, the endothelin system, and other vasoactive agents, along with inflammation and immunity [3].

10.2.1 Endothelial Dysfunction

The tunica intima consists of a single layer of endothelial cells which regulate vascular homeostasis through the synthesis and release of a plethora of vasoactive substances [4]. Given its biological features, nitric oxide (NO) is probably one of the most important endothelium-derived mediators [5]. NO is a gaseous molecule continuously synthesized by the endothelial enzyme nitric oxide synthase (NOS) in response to flow-induced shear stress starting from the amino acid L-arginine and oxygen, in the presence of various cofactors, including tetrahydrobiopterin (BH4) [5]. Once released, it freely diffuses into adjacent smooth muscle cells leading to relaxation by activation of guanylate cyclase and generation of cyclic guanosine monophosphate [5]. Endothelial cells also secrete other vasodilators, such as prostacyclin and endothelium-derived hyperpolarizing factors, as well as vasoconstrictors, including endothelin-1 (ET-1), tromboxane A2, and locally produced angiotensin II [6]. In particular, ET-1 promotes potent and prolonged vasoconstriction through stimulation of ET type A (ET_A) and B (ET_B) receptors on vascular smooth muscle cells. On the other hand, it also has counter-regulatory properties, since it can stimulate ET_B receptors on the endothelial cells inducing nitric oxide- and prostacyclin-mediated vasodilation [7, 8]. The balance between endothelial-derived relaxing and contracting factors eventually determines the vascular tone [6]. Endothelial dysfunction, characterized by impaired endothelium-dependent vascular relaxation, especially due to reduced NO release or bioavailability, plays a seminal part in the pathogenesis of hypertension [9]. Defects in NO production can be attributed to several factors, including reduced NOS expression, limited substrate bioavailability, and increased levels of endogenous NOS inhibitors, such as asymmetrical dimethylarginine [10, 11]. Moreover, oxidative stress can cause NOS uncoupling, a dysfunctional state of the enzyme that leads to the generation of superoxide anion instead of NO, and the eventual formation of the potent oxidant peroxynitrite [12]. Oxidative depletion of BH4 as a trigger for NOS uncoupling has been described in the aorta of mice with deoxycorticosterone acetate (DOCA)-salt hypertension [13]. In both this model of hypertension and in spontaneously hypertensive rats, treatment with BH4 prevented NOS uncoupling and blunted blood pressure elevation [13, 14]. Nonetheless, administration of sepiapterin, a BH4 precursor, did not prevent glucocorticoid-induced hypertension in rats, suggesting that NOS uncoupling does not play a critical role in all hypertension models [15].

Besides reduced NO availability, dysregulation of ET-1 expression has also been involved in the development of hypertension and vascular damage [7]. Indeed, various animal models, such as DOCA-salt rats, angiotensin II-infused rats, and stroke-prone spontaneously hypertensive rats, have been associated with increased vascular expression of ET-1, and responded to endothelin receptor antagonists with blood pressure lowering and correction of vascular remodeling [16–19]. Consistent with these observations, constitutive overexpression of human ET-1 restricted to the endothelium of mice resulted in endothelial dysfunction and hypertrophic vascular remodeling [20]. These effects were at least partially attributed to enhanced oxidative stress induced by ET-1. Moreover, mice with inducible endothelial-specific overexpression of human ET-1 showed sustained elevation of blood pressure at 3 weeks [21] and 3 months [22]. At the latter time point, small artery stiffening, kidney injury, and renal infiltration of immune cells were also observed, all of which were normalized or reduced by 2 week treatment with the selective ET_A receptor antagonist atrasentan [22]. The renal effects of ET-1 have also been investigated in rodent models of malignant hypertension. In particular, salt-loaded stroke-prone spontaneously hypertensive rats, which are characterized by severe hypertension and proteinuria, also exhibit enhanced renal expression of ET-1, transforming growth factor-β1 and procollagens [23]. These effects were attenuated by selective ET_A receptor antagonism. Additional evidence comes from the use of double transgenic rats overexpressing both human renin and angiotensinogen genes, which feature malignant hypertension along with severe kidney and cardiac injury [24]. In this model, treatment with the dual ET_A/ET_B receptor antagonist bosentan reduced blood pressure and cardiac hypertrophy, while providing considerable renal protection, as assessed by reduced albuminuria and inhibition of nuclear factor κB (NFκB) activation in the kidney [24]. In the same experimental model, combination therapy with the ET_A receptor antagonist avosentan and the angiotensin receptor blocker valsartan reduced albuminuria, renal histopathological lesions, and mortality rate to a greater extent than each drug given alone [25].

Overactivation of the endothelin system has also emerged as a potential contributor to hypertension and glomerular injury observed during vascular endothelial growth factor (VEGF) inhibition, a key therapeutic strategy for some types of cancers [26, 27]. Indeed, the elevation of blood pressure and albuminuria induced in rats by treatment with sunitinib, which inhibits the tyrosine kinase activity of VEGF receptors, could be prevented by the simultaneous administration of the selective ET_A receptor antagonist sitaxentan [27].

Angiotensin II, a key effector peptide of the renin–angiotensin–aldosterone system (RAAS), plays a critical role in the pathogenesis of hypertension and its associated vascular changes. In particular, angiotensin II-induced hypertension in rats was associated with impaired endothelium-dependent vascular relaxation, an effect mediated in large part by increased oxidative stress [28]. Moreover, angiotensin II can promote proliferation of vascular smooth muscle cells through activation of mitogenic signaling pathways, including mitogen-activated protein kinases and tyrosine kinases [29, 30]. Angiotensin II-induced proliferative effects appear to be mediated also by transactivation of growth factor receptors, such as epidermal growth factor receptor (EGFR). Indeed, mice with vascular smooth muscle cell-specific knockout for EGFR were protected against angiotensin II-induced tunica media hypertrophy of mesenteric arteries, renal arterioles, and the aorta [31]. Consistent with the above experimental findings is that in patients with primary hypertension RAAS blockade with an angiotensin II type 1 receptor antagonist or an angiotensin-converting enzyme inhibitor corrected the altered structure and endothelial dysfunction of resistance arteries, while treatment with a β-blocker led to a similar degree of blood pressure lowering but had no effects on vascular remodeling or endothelial function [32, 33].

10.2.2 Activation of Intrarenal Renin–Angiotensin System

The RAAS plays a critical role in the regulation of blood pressure and fluid homeostasis [34]. Besides the systemic, circulating RAAS, a local RAAS has been identified in a variety of organs, including the kidney. All of the components necessary for angiotensin II generation (angiotensinogen, renin, and angiotensin-converting enzymes) and action (type 1 and type 2 angiotensin II receptors) are present along the nephron, even though there is still debate regarding the possible extrarenal origin of angiotensinogen and other RAAS constituents within the kidney [35]. A growing body of experimental evidence has pointed to an important role for inappropriate activation of the intrarenal RAAS in the pathogenesis of hypertension. Kidney cross-transplantation strategies have shown that angiotensin II mainly mediates hypertension through activation of renal rather than extrarenal type 1 angiotensin II receptors (AT_1R) [36]. Further research has sought to dissect the contribution of angiotensin II signaling in specific nephron segments and/or cellular types in the development and maintenance of hypertension. Mice with conditional deletion of AT_1R from the proximal tubule exhibited reduced baseline blood pressure and attenuated hypertension in response to angiotensin II infusion [37]. This hypotensive phenotype was accompanied by enhanced natriuresis and reduced expression of epithelial sodium transporter proteins, including sodium hydrogen exchanger 3 [37]. Two approaches have been used to delete AT_1R from the distal segments of the nephron. Cell-specific deletion of AT_1R in the principal cells of the collecting duct, which play a major role in sodium and water reabsorption, had negligible effects on baseline blood pressure, but it did attenuate the early phase of angiotensin II-induced hypertension [38]. Instead, deleting AT_1R from the entire collecting duct, both principal and intercalated cells, had no effects on baseline blood pressure, but led to an exaggerated hypertensive response to angiotensin II infusion [39]. This worsened hypertensive phenotype was attributed to a failure to upregulate cyclooxygenase-2 (COX-2) in intercalated cells and the eventual reduced generation of vasodilator prostanoids [39]. Overall, these findings point to the complexity of angiotensin II effects across the nephron.

The importance of intrarenal RAAS has also been suggested by studies showing that genetically modified mice with minimal or no renal angiotensin-converting enzyme (ACE) expression exhibited blunted blood pressure elevation in response to either angiotensin II infusion or NO synthase inhibitor NG-nitro-L-arginine methyl ester (L-NAME) treatment [40, 41]. While angiotensin II infusion and L-NAME administration upregulated renal ACE 1.5- to 2-fold in wild-type mice, thereby increasing local angiotensin II production and the activation of renal sodium transporters, these effects were markedly attenuated in mice lacking renal ACE, with consequent natriuresis [40, 41]. A further investigation showed that mice expressing ACE in the tubular epithelial brush border developed salt-sensitive hypertension following L-NAME exposure, while mice selectively lacking tubular epithelial ACE did not [42]. Therefore, angiotensin II produced by tubular epithelial ACE appears to provide a major contribution to salt-sensitive hypertension.

Evidence from experimental and clinical studies has suggested that urinary angiotensinogen excretion may serve as a specific biomarker of intrarenal RAAS activity in hypertension and kidney disease. In particular, a strong and direct correlation has been reported between renal angiotensin II levels and urinary angiotensinogen excretion rate in a rat model of angiotensin II-induced hypertension [43]. Moreover, in a cohort of 106 adults, urinary angiotensinogen concentrations directly correlated with blood pressure levels, and were higher in hypertensive patients not treated with RAAS blockers than in normotensive individuals [44]. On the other hand, a recent study in a cohort of 2076 patients with chronic kidney disease showed that higher systolic blood pressure was associated with an increased risk of disease progression in participants with low, but not in those with high, urinary angiotensinogen concentrations [45]. These findings highlight the complexity of the relationship between blood pressure and poor kidney outcomes, which may be affected by intrarenal RAAS activity [45].

10.3 Inflammation and Immune System in Hypertension

It has been known for decades that renal infiltration of inflammatory and immune cells is a common characteristic of both experimental and clinical hypertension [46–48]. In more recent years, several studies, mainly in experimental models, have pointed to a critical role of the immune system in the pathogenesis of hypertension. In this context, both innate and adaptive immune cells infiltrate into target organs, including the kidney, where in response to various hypertensive stimuli, such as high salt, angiotensin II, or catecholamines, they release cytokines or directly act on organ cells, thereby promoting blood pressure elevation and/or tissue injury (Fig. 10.1) [49, 50]. There is also some preliminary evidence that the immune system contributes to salt-sensitive hypertension in mouse models of chronic kidney disease, but further investigation is required to determine which immune cell types and mediators are involved and the underlying molecular mechanisms [51, 52].

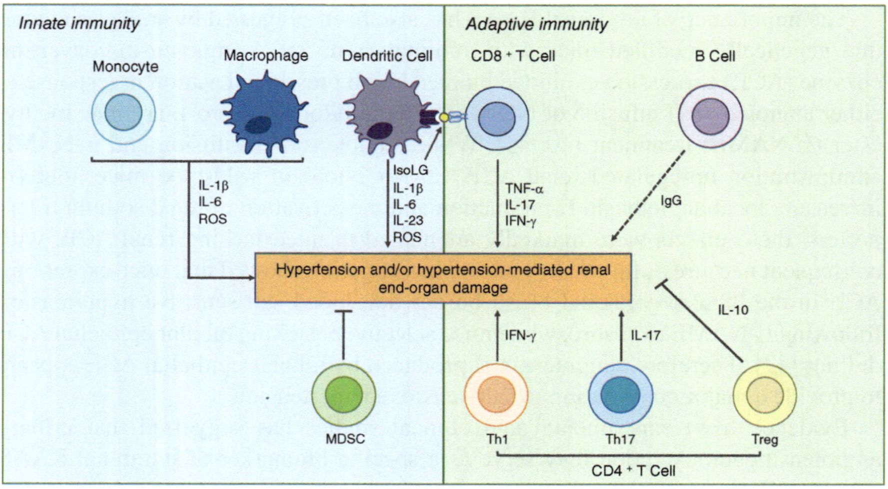

Fig. 10.1 Overview of innate and adaptive immune cells that have been involved in the pathogenesis of hypertension and/or hypertension-mediated renal end-organ damage. Both innate and adaptive immune cells release factors, such as cytokines and reactive oxygen species, which promote or inhibit hypertension and/or hypertension-mediated renal end-organ damage. The role of B cells remains ill-defined. *IFN-γ* interferon γ, *Ig* immunoglobulin, *IL* interleukin, *IsoLG* isolevuglandin, *MDSC* myeloid-derived suppressor cells, *ROS* reactive oxygen species, *TNF-α* tumor necrosis factor α

10.3.1 Experimental Hypertension

10.3.1.1 Innate Immune Cells in Hypertension

Several studies documented the involvement of innate immune cells, especially monocytes, macrophages, and dendritic cells, in the development of hypertension and its attendant target organ damage. In particular, mice with monocyte/macrophage deficiency due to an inactivating mutation in the macrophage colony-stimulating factor gene had blunted blood pressure rise, vascular remodeling, and endothelial dysfunction following either angiotensin II infusion or treatment with the aldosterone precursor DOCA and salt [53, 54]. Moreover, ablation of lysozyme M-positive (LysM$^+$) myelomonocytic cells attenuated angiotensin II-induced blood pressure elevation and vascular dysfunction [55]. Adoptive transfer of wild-type monocytes, but not neutrophils, into mice depleted of LysM$^+$ myelomonocytic cells restored the angiotensin II-mediated disease phenotype [55]. In various animal models of hypertension, macrophages were found to infiltrate into the kidney, where they acquired an M1 pro-inflammatory phenotype [56–58]. Macrophage recruitment in the hypertensive kidney appears to be modulated by complex interactions among chemokines. In the angiotensin II-induced mouse model of hypertension, genetic deletion of C–C motif chemokine 5 (CCL5)—a chemokine known to drive accumulation of inflammatory cells into injured tissues—was found to markedly increase renal infiltration of macrophages with pro-inflammatory signature and kidney damage [59]. These observations may be ascribed to a compensatory local upregulation of other chemokine(s) which could have exacerbated the effects of angiotensin II. In fact, pharmacological inhibition of CCL2 abrogated the augmented renal macrophage infiltration and interstitial fibrosis in CCL5-deficient mice [59]. Macrophages within the kidney may act as mediators of hypertensive kidney injury. In both angiotensin II-infused mice and Dahl salt-sensitive rats, depletion of macrophages by liposome-encapsulated clodronate to reduce their recruitment in the kidney attenuated blood pressure elevation while protecting against glomerular injury and fibrosis, probably by lowering local oxidative stress and inflammation [58]. Macrophages not only release pro-inflammatory cytokines, but can also be targets of them. In this regard, IL-1β from tubular epithelial cells of diabetic mice was recently found to promote the polarization of macrophages toward a pro-inflammatory phenotype characterized by high release of IL-6 which in turn activates the epithelial sodium channel, leading to salt-sensitive hypertension [60, 61].

As highly specialized antigen-presenting cells, dendritic cells also participate to hypertension through T cell activation, especially under the influence of elevated sodium concentrations in the microenvironment [62]. Increased extracellular sodium enters dendritic cells by the epithelial sodium channel, leading to subsequent calcium influx via the sodium-calcium exchanger [63]. In turn, increased intracellular calcium activates nicotinamide adenine dinucleotide phosphate (NADPH) oxidase, resulting in the production of highly reactive γ-ketoaldehydes, also known as isolevuglandins, which rapidly bind to self-proteins to form immunogenic protein adducts [63]. During this process, dendritic cells acquire a pro-inflammatory phenotype and increase surface expression of the co-stimulatory molecules CD80 and CD86 [64]. Such activated dendritic cells can process and present isolevuglandin-protein adducts as neoantigens to T cells, leading to their proliferation and elaboration of the pro-inflammatory cytokines tumor necrosis factor-α (TNF-α), interleukin-17A (IL-17A), and interferon-γ (IFN-γ) [63, 64], all of which contribute to blood pressure elevation [65, 66]. Accordingly, the adoptive transfer of isolevuglandin-activated dendritic cells primed hypertension to a generally subpressor dose of angiotensin II in recipient mice [64]. Moreover, treatment with isolevuglandin scavengers reduced blood pressure, kidney injury, and renal T cell infiltration in mice with angiotensin II-induced hypertension [64].

The kidney appears as a major site of dendritic cell activation in the setting of experimental hypertension, since renal denervation, besides attenuating blood pressure elevation, prevented the formation of isolevuglandin-protein adducts in dendritic cells, while reducing their surface expression of costimulatory molecules and production of pro-inflammatory cytokines [67].

Among dendritic cell subsets, classical dendritic cells, whose differentiation is driven by the growth factor Fms-like tyrosine kinase 3 ligand (FLT3L), are required to maintain the full hypertensive response, since FLT3L-deficient mice had blunted blood pressure elevation during chronic infusion of angiotensin II [68]. Mechanistically, classical dendritic cells were found to sustain blood pressure elevation by promoting oxidative stress and cytokine production by renal T cells [68]. These effects were accompanied by increased expression of multiple tubular sodium channels, with ensuing fluid retention [68]. By contrast, dendritic cells expressing A20, an ubiquitin editor which inhibits NF-κB signaling, appear to mitigate hypertension by limiting T cell activation. Accordingly, mice with heterozygous deletion of A20 in dendritic cells showed an exaggerated hypertensive response to low-dose angiotensin II infusion, along with augmented renal accumulation of IFN-γ- and TNF-α-producing T lymphocytes [69]. Another subset of myeloid cells, myeloid-derived suppressor cells, was found to provide protection against the increase of blood pressure and renal end-organ damage in murine models of hypertension [70]. Depletion of these cells in angiotensin II-treated mice exacerbated hypertension and proteinuria, while increasing renal infiltration of T cells producing IFN-γ and TNF-α [70].

10.3.1.2 Adaptive Immune Cells in Hypertension

The specific role of T cells in the pathogenesis of hypertension was demonstrated in 2007 by Guzik et al. who showed that recombination-activating gene 1 deficient ($Rag1^{-/-}$) mice, which lack T and B cells, were protected against angiotensin II-induced hypertension [71]. Adoptive transfer of T cells, but not B cells, restored the full hypertensive response. These findings were then confirmed and expanded by several other studies using different animal models [49, 72], with evidence that T cells infiltrating the kidney participate in the pathogenesis of hypertension by promoting oxidative stress and renal sodium reabsorption [48, 73]. T cells mediate these effects by releasing pro-inflammatory cytokines, such as TNF-α, IL-7A, and IFN-γ, which regulate the abundance or activity of sodium transporters along the nephron [65, 66], but also engaging in direct interactions with tubular cells [74]. Even though both $CD4^+$ T cells and $CD8^+$ T cells accumulate within the kidney of hypertensive mice, the latter T cell subset appears to provide a major contribution in driving blood pressure elevation [69, 75]. In fact, selective depletion of $CD8^+$ T cells in mice conferred partial protection against angiotensin II-induced hypertension, whereas selective depletion of $CD4^+$ T cells did not [75]. Moreover, the exacerbated hypertensive response to low-dose angiotensin II observed in mice with heterozygous deletion of the ubiquitin-editing protein A20 in dendritic cells was accompanied by increased renal infiltration of IFN-γ- and TNF-α-producing effector memory $CD8^+$ but not $CD4^+$ T lymphocytes [69]. $CD8^+$ T cells can influence blood pressure also by enhancing sodium and water retention. Indeed, wild-type but not CD8 knockout mice showed an impaired capability to excrete an intraperitoneal salt load after angiotensin II infusion [75]. Consistent with these observations, $CD8^+$ T cells were found to infiltrate into the kidney of DOCA-salt-treated mice, where they directly interact with distal convoluted tubule cells, increasing the expression and activity of the sodium chloride co-transporter, leading to sodium retention and the development of salt-sensitive hypertension [74]. Mechanistically, the interaction between activated $CD8^+$ T cells and distal convoluted tubule cells seems mediated by the IFN-γ-programmed cell death ligand 1 (PDL1) pathway [76, 77]. Abrogation of the IFN-γ response limited renal T cell infiltration and blunted blood pressure elevation in two mouse models of hypertension [76, 77].

Several studies have sought to dissect the relative contribution of specific $CD4^+$ T cell subsets in the pathogenesis of hypertension and related target-organ damage. In particular, evidence that mice deficient in the T helper 1 (Th1)-promoting transcription factor T-bet had a preserved hypertensive response to angiotensin II but were protected against glomerular injury, points to a role for Th1 cells in driving hypertensive renal damage without affecting blood pressure [78, 79]. By contrast, Th17 cells have been involved in angiotensin II-dependent blood pressure elevation in mice through the production of IL-17A [80]. Mechanistically, this cytokine acts on proximal and distal tubular cells, where it increases the expression or activity of multiple sodium transporters, including the epithelial sodium channel, sodium chloride co-transporter, and sodium hydrogen exchanger-3, thereby enhancing salt and water reabsorption [81, 82]. Moreover, mice with T cell-specific deletion of serum and glucocorticoid-regulated kinase 1 (*Sgk1*)—a serine/threonine-protein kinase which enhances the generation of Th17 cells in response to salt [83, 84]—exhibited blunted blood pressure elevation along with marked amelioration of kidney injury and endothelial dysfunction following angiotensin II infusion [85]. In another experimental model of hypertension, rats treated with mineralocorticoid-salt exhibited activation of Th17 and downregulation of Treg cells in their heart and kidneys [86]. Besides preventing blood pressure elevation, spironolactone treatment also shifted the balance of $CD4^+$ T cells from Th17 toward Treg cells [86]. A reduction in renal Treg cells has also been reported in spontaneously hypertensive rats and in angiotensin II-treated mice [87, 88]. In keeping with their immunosuppressive functions, adoptive transfer of $CD4^+CD25^+$ splenic Tregs into aldosterone-infused mice reduced cardiac and renal infiltration of T cells and macrophages, while ameliorating hypertension and endothelial dysfunction [89]. The protective effect of Treg cells on microvascular endothelial function in hypertension may be ascribed to their release of the anti-inflammatory cytokine IL-10, which was found to ameliorate endothelium-dependent artery relaxation in hypertensive mice by mitigating vascular oxidative stress [90]. Another approach to promote Treg cell expansion, that is treatment with low-dose IL-2, led to attenuation in hypertension and glomerular injury in a murine model of systemic lupus erythematosus [91]. The modulatory activity of Treg cells in the setting of hypertension appears to be counter-regulated by complement receptors. In this regard, angiotensin II was found to raise the expression of complement component 3a receptor (C3aR) and complement component 5a receptor (C5aR) on Treg cells in vitro and in vivo, while mice with double knockout (DKO) for both complement receptors exhibited blunted blood pressure elevation and renal damage in response to angiotensin II, coupled with an increase of Treg cells in the kidney [92]. Depletion of Treg cells by anti-CD25 antibody abrogated these protective effects in DKO mice [92]. By contrast, adoptive transfer of Treg cells from DKO mice into wild-type recipients markedly reduced angiotensin II-induced hypertension and kidney injury. These elegant experiments suggest that blocking C3aR and C5aR specifically on Treg cells could protect against hypertension and its attendant end-organ damage, even though the exact mechanism(s) behind this protection remains to be investigated.

Experimental studies have shown an inconsistent role of B cells and immunoglobulins in the pathogenesis of hypertension and renal end-organ damage. In a mouse model of systemic lupus erythematosus, treatment with an anti-CD20 monoclonal antibody prevented the onset of hypertension and renal injury, as assessed by urinary protein excretion, glomerulosclerosis, and tubulointerstitial fibrosis [93]. Anti-CD20 antibody therapy also attenuated the hypertensive response to angiotensin II in mice, as did genetic deficiency in B cell-activating factor receptor (BAFF-$R^{-/-}$), which is required for B cell maturation and survival [94]. However, neither mice with global B cell deficiency caused by deletion of IgM heavy chain ($\mu MT^{-/-}$) nor those unable to produce high-affinity class-switched immunoglobulins due to deletion of activation-induced deaminase ($Aicda^{-/-}$) were protected from angiotensin II-induced hypertension and kidney damage [95]. Such discrepancies were attributed to differences in the B cell subtypes targeted in the experimental models used. While $\mu MT^{-/-}$ and $Aicda^{-/-}$ mice are characterized by the lack of both B1 cells (i.e., innate-like cells mainly found in the peritoneal and pleural cavities) and B2 cells (i.e., conventional B cells) [95], BAFF-$R^{-/-}$ mice and those given anti-CD20 antibody have a preferential decline in B2 cells, with some extent of B1 cell sparing [96, 97]. Whether these B1 cells serve a protective function in hypertension which might be masked by whole B cell depletion is an intriguing hypothesis that needs to be tested.

10.3.2 Human Hypertension

Although data in humans are still scant, various lines of evidence suggest that inflammation and immunity may participate in the development of hypertension and its associated kidney damage also in the clinical setting. Histological examination of kidney autopsy samples showed that, compared to normotensive individuals, patients with hypertension had a greater degree of glomerulosclerosis and fibrosis, as well as an increased density of $CD68^+$ macrophages, primarily localized to areas of glomerular damage [47]. Moreover, kidney biopsy specimens from patients with hypertensive nephrosclerosis showed increased infiltration of $CD4^+$ and $CD8^+$ T cells compared to those from normotensive controls, coupled with augmented tubular expression of interferon-inducible T cell α chemoattractant, a tissue-homing chemokine for T cells [98].

These observations have been corroborated by studies showing that immunomodulatory therapies ameliorated hypertension when prescribed for the management of other diseases. In particular, treatment with mycophenolate mofetil, besides reducing renal T lymphocyte infiltration and blood pressure in animal models of hypertension [99, 100], led to blood pressure lowering also in patients with psoriasis or rheumatoid arthritis [101]. More recently, 4-week treatment with the IL-1 receptor inhibitor anakinra in obese patients was found to reduce systolic blood pressure and peripheral vascular resistance while increasing the plasma levels of the vasodilatory peptide angiotensin-(1–7) [102]. Instead, the results of the CANTOS (Canakinumab Anti-inflammatory Thrombosis Outcomes Study) trial showed that treatment with the anti-IL-1β monoclonal antibody canakinumab reduced major cardiovascular events in patients with established atherosclerotic disease, but did not lower the incidence of hypertension or blood pressure values [103, 104]. Nevertheless, several patients were receiving evidence-based blood pressure-lowering therapies at baseline, which may have masked any anti-hypertensive effect of canakinumab [104, 105].

Data from genome-wide association studies also point to an involvement of inflammation and immunity in hypertension [106, 107], which is further supported by integrative network analysis [84] and Mendelian randomization strategies [108, 109]. In particular, the gene SH2B adaptor protein 3 (*SH2B3*, also known as lymphocyte adaptor protein), which encodes for a modulator of T cell activation, has been identified as a key driver of human hypertension in a systems biology-based network analysis [110]. A missense single-nucleotide polymorphism (SNP) in *SH2B3* (rs3184504), which results in the conversion of an arginine to a tryptophan, has been associated with hypertension in multiple genome-wide association studies in humans [106, 107, 110]. Recently, the CRISPR-Cas9 technology has been employed to create mice that were homozygous for either the tryptophan (Trp/Trp) or the arginine allele (Arg/Arg) in this *SH2B3* polymorphism [111]. Trp/Trp mice exhibited greater blood pressure elevation and kidney damage in response to angiotensin II infusion compared to control Arg/Arg mice, suggesting a causal role for the rs3184504 SNP in *SH2B3* in the pathophysiology of hypertension [111].

Together, these findings support the contribution of inflammation and immunity in human hypertension.

10.4 Renal Microangiopathic Disease

Thrombotic microangiopathy (TMA), a pathological entity observed in a diverse range of diseases, is characterized by thickening of the microvasculature wall, with intraluminal platelet thrombosis and obstruction of the vessel lumina, which leads to hypoperfusion and ischemia of the affected organ(s), especially the kidney [112]. Primary TMA etiologies include thrombotic thrombocytopenic purpura, Shiga toxin-mediated hemolytic uremic syndrome (HUS), and complement-mediated TMA, also known as atypical HUS (aHUS). The latter is typically caused by dysregulation of the complement alternative pathway due to genetic or acquired abnormalities [113]. TMA can also occur in the context of other disease processes, such as malignant hypertension [114], traditionally defined by the association of severe hypertension (diastolic blood pressure >120 mmHg) with advanced bilateral retinopathy. More modern definitions consider impairment to at least three different target organs, which is referred to as hypertension with multi-organ damage or hypertensive emergency [115]. Irrespective of the terms used, severe hypertension causes pressure natriuresis and consequent volume depletion, resulting in RAAS activation. Both activated RAAS and hypertension-induced shear stress lead to endothelial cell damage, which triggers the cascade of events culminating in TMA [116, 117]. There are clinical overlaps between malignant hypertension and aHUS. Indeed, malignant hypertension is highly prevalent (34–55%) in the setting of aHUS [118, 119], whereas among all cases of malignant hypertension, aHUS remains a marginal cause [120]. Adding further complexity to this scenario, a series of recent studies have identified pathogenic rare variants in genes responsible for complement alternative pathway regulation or anti-factor H antibodies in a subset of patients clinically diagnosed with TMA associated with malignant hypertension or hypertensive emergency [121–125], suggesting that these cases may in fact be reclassified as aHUS (Table 10.1). Nevertheless, not all patients with a clinical diagnosis of aHUS carry complement gene variants or anti-factor H antibodies [126]. Thus, it remains challenging to distinguish aHUS without genetic or acquired defects in the complement alternative pathway from malignant hypertension-associated TMA. Nonetheless, in the event of TMA and concomitant malignant

Table 10.1 Prevalence of pathogenic rare variants in genes responsible for complement alternative pathway regulation or anti-complement factor H antibodies in patients with TMA and concomitant malignant hypertension or hypertensive emergency

Study	Patients, *N*	Inclusion criteria	Patients with pathogenic rare complement gene variants, *n*/*N* (%)	Patients with anti-factor H antibodies, *n*/*N* (%)
Timmermans et al. (2018) [121]	17	Blood pressure ≥180/120 mmHg; impeding/progressive target organ dysfunction; TMA with pathologic features of severe hypertension in kidney biopsy	8/17 (47%)	NA
Larsen et al. (2018) [122]	100	Blood pressure >180/120 mmHg; pre-existing CKD; kidney biopsy showing arterial intimal edema or mucoid intimal hyperplasia in isolation without glomerular microthrombi, mesangiolysis or necrotizing arteritis/arteriolitis	0/100 (0%)	NA
Timmermans et al. (2020) [123]	26	Blood pressure ≥180/120 mmHg; impeding/progressive target organ dysfunction; TMA with pathologic features of severe hypertension in kidney biopsy	9/26 (35%)	NA
Zhang et al. (2020) [124]	50	Blood pressure ≥180/120 mmHg; pre-existing CKD; hypertensive retinopathy (grade III/IV); TMA features in kidney biopsy	8/20 (40%)[a]	NA
Chen et al. (2023) [125]	45	Blood pressure >180/120 mmHg; TMA features in kidney biopsy	3/45 (6.7%)	2/45 (4%)

CKD chronic kidney disease, *NA* not assessed, *TMA* thrombotic microangiopathy
[a]Twenty out of fifty patients were tested for complement gene variants

hypertension, some clinical and histological characteristics have been posited to suggest severe hypertension instead of aHUS as the underlying cause. These include male gender, age >45 years, history of hypertension and/or anti-hypertensive treatment discontinuation, rapid resolution of hematological TMA following strict blood pressure control, presence of left ventricular hypertrophy, and absence of glomerular thrombi in kidney biopsy [127]. In spite of the difficulties lying in differentiating aHUS from malignant hypertension-associated TMA, establishing a correct diagnosis is of utmost importance since the treatments of choice for these conditions vary considerably. The current standard of care for patients diagnosed with aHUS is complement component C5 blockade, whereas patients presenting with malignant hypertension or hypertension emergency are typically managed with blood pressure-lowering drugs [128, 129].

10.5 Conclusion

Hypertension is a common disorder encountered in patients with chronic kidney disease, and one of the leading causes of its progression. Here we have provided an in-depth overview of recent advances in our understanding of some of the multiple and intrinsically related processes underpinning the pathogenesis of hypertension and its attendant kidney end-organ damage. Such knowledge could eventually facilitate the development of novel treatments. In particular, accumulating data from rodent and human studies have highlighted cytokines and several immune cell types as critical mediators in the development and progression of hypertension which may be amenable to therapeutic targeting. The challenge is to design therapies able to target inflammatory and immune mechanisms that contribute to blood pressure elevation and hypertensive end-organ damage while sparing natural immune defenses.

References

1. Joyner MJ, Limberg JK. Blood pressure regulation: every adaptation is an integration? Eur J Appl Physiol. 2014;114:445–50.
2. Touyz RM, Rios FJ, Montezano AC, Neves KB, Eluwole O, Maseko MJ, et al. The vascular phenotype in hypertension. In: The vasculome. London: Academic Press; 2022. p. 327–42.
3. Schiffrin EL. How structure, mechanics, and function of the vasculature contribute to blood pressure elevation in hypertension. Can J Cardiol. 2020;36:648–58.
4. Vane JR, Anggård EE, Botting RM. Regulatory functions of the vascular endothelium. N Engl J Med. 1990;323:27–36.
5. Tare M, Parkington HC, Coleman HA, Neild TO, Dusting GJ. Hyperpolarization and relaxation of arterial smooth muscle caused by nitric oxide derived from the endothelium. Nature. 1990;346:69–71.
6. Konukoglu D, Uzun H. Endothelial dysfunction and hypertension. Adv Exp Med Biol. 2017;956:511–40.
7. Schiffrin EL, Pollock DM. Endothelin system in hypertension and chronic kidney disease. Hypertension. 2024;81:691–701.

8. Benigni A, Perico N, Remuzzi G. The potential of endothelin antagonism as a therapeutic approach. Expert Opin Investig Drugs. 2004;13:1419–35.
9. Ambrosino P, Bachetti T, D'Anna SE, Galloway B, Bianco A, D'Agnano V, et al. Mechanisms and clinical implications of endothelial dysfunction in arterial hypertension. J Cardiovasc Dev Dis. 2022;9:136.
10. Kishi S, Nagasu H, Kidokoro K, Kashihara N. Oxidative stress and the role of redox signalling in chronic kidney disease. Nat Rev Nephrol. 2024;20:101–19.
11. Dowsett L, Higgins E, Alanazi S, Alshuwayer NA, Leiper FC, Leiper J. ADMA: a key player in the relationship between vascular dysfunction and inflammation in atherosclerosis. J Clin Med. 2020;9:3026.
12. Janaszak-Jasiecka A, Płoska A, Wierońska JM, Dobrucki LW, Kalinowski L. Endothelial dysfunction due to eNOS uncoupling: molecular mechanisms as potential therapeutic targets. Cell Mol Biol Lett. 2023;28:21.
13. Landmesser U, Dikalov S, Price SR, McCann L, Fukai T, Holland SM, et al. Oxidation of tetrahydrobiopterin leads to uncoupling of endothelial cell nitric oxide synthase in hypertension. J Clin Invest. 2003;111:1201–9.
14. Hong HJ, Hsiao G, Cheng TH, Yen MH. Supplementation with tetrahydrobiopterin suppresses the development of hypertension in spontaneously hypertensive rats. Hypertension. 2001;38:1044–8.
15. Thida M, Earl J, Zhao Y, Wang H, Tse CS, Vickers JJ, et al. Effects of sepiapterin supplementation and NOS inhibition on glucocorticoid-induced hypertension. Am J Hypertens. 2010;23:569–74.
16. Larivière R, Thibault G, Schiffrin EL. Increased endothelin-1 content in blood vessels of deoxycorticosterone acetate-salt hypertensive but not in spontaneously hypertensive rats. Hypertension. 1993;21:294–300.
17. Sharifi AM, He G, Touyz RM, Schiffrin EL. Vascular endothelin-1 expression and effect of an endothelin ETA antagonist on structure and function of small arteries from stroke-prone spontaneously hypertensive rats. J Cardiovasc Pharmacol. 1998;31(Suppl 1):S309–12.
18. Moreau P, d'Uscio LV, Shaw S, Takase H, Barton M, Lüscher TF. Angiotensin II increases tissue endothelin and induces vascular hypertrophy: reversal by ET(a)-receptor antagonist. Circulation. 1997;96:1593–7.
19. Li JS, Larivière R, Schiffrin EL. Effect of a nonselective endothelin antagonist on vascular remodeling in deoxycorticosterone acetate-salt hypertensive rats. Evidence for a role of endothelin in vascular hypertrophy. Hypertension. 1994;24:183–8.
20. Amiri F, Virdis A, Neves MF, Iglarz M, Seidah NG, Touyz RM, et al. Endothelium-restricted overexpression of human endothelin-1 causes vascular remodeling and endothelial dysfunction. Circulation. 2004;110:2233–40.
21. Rautureau Y, Coelho SC, Fraulob-Aquino JC, Huo KG, Rehman A, Offermanns S, et al. Inducible human endothelin-1 overexpression in endothelium raises blood pressure via endothelin type a receptors. Hypertension. 2015;66:347–55.
22. Coelho SC, Berillo O, Caillon A, Ouerd S, Fraulob-Aquino JC, Barhoumi T, et al. Three-month endothelial human endothelin-1 overexpression causes blood pressure elevation and vascular and kidney injury. Hypertension. 2018;71:208–16.
23. Tostes RCA, Touyz RM, He G, Ammarguellat F, Schiffrin EL. Endothelin a receptor blockade decreases expression of growth factors and collagen and improves matrix metalloproteinase-2 activity in kidneys from stroke-prone spontaneously hypertensive rats. J Cardiovasc Pharmacol. 2002;39:892–900.
24. Muller DN, Mervaala EM, Schmidt F, Park JK, Dechend R, Genersch E, et al. Effect of bosentan on NF-kappaB, inflammation, and tissue factor in angiotensin II-induced end-organ damage. Hypertension. 2000;36:282–290.
25. Baltatu OC, Zaugg CE, Schumacher C, Louie P, Campos LA, Bader M. Avosentan is protective in hypertensive nephropathy at doses not causing fluid retention. Pharmacol Res. 2014;80:9–13.

26. Kappers MHW, van Esch JHM, Sluiter W, Sleijfer S, Danser AHJ, van den Meiracker AH. Hypertension induced by the tyrosine kinase inhibitor sunitinib is associated with increased circulating endothelin-1 levels. Hypertension. 2010;56:675–81.
27. Mirabito Colafella KM, Neves KB, Montezano AC, Garrelds IM, van Veghel R, de Vries R, et al. Selective ETA vs. dual ETA/B receptor blockade for the prevention of sunitinib-induced hypertension and albuminuria in WKY rats. Cardiovasc Res. 2020;116:1779–90.
28. Rajagopalan S, Kurz S, Münzel T, Tarpey M, Freeman BA, Griendling KK, et al. Angiotensin II-mediated hypertension in the rat increases vascular superoxide production via membrane NADH/NADPH oxidase activation. Contribution to alterations of vasomotor tone. J Clin Invest. 1996;97:1916–23.
29. Yoshizumi M, Kyotani Y, Zhao J, Nakahira K. Targeting the mitogen-activated protein kinase-mediated vascular smooth muscle cell remodeling by angiotensin II. Ann Transl Med. 2020;8:157.
30. Montezano AC, Nguyen Dinh Cat A, Rios FJ, Touyz RM. Angiotensin II and vascular injury. Curr Hypertens Rep. 2014;16:431.
31. Schreier B, Hünerberg M, Mildenberger S, Rabe S, Bethmann D, Wickenhauser C, et al. Deletion of the EGF receptor in vascular smooth muscle cells prevents chronic angiotensin II-induced arterial wall stiffening and media thickening. Acta Physiol (Oxf). 2018;222:e12996.
32. Schiffrin EL. Correction of remodeling and function of small arteries in human hypertension by cilazapril, an angiotensin I-converting enzyme inhibitor. J Cardiovasc Pharmacol. 1996;27(Suppl 2):S13–8.
33. Schiffrin EL, Park JB, Intengan HD, Touyz RM. Correction of arterial structure and endothelial dysfunction in human essential hypertension by the angiotensin receptor antagonist losartan. Circulation. 2000;101:1653–9.
34. Nishiyama A, Kim-Mitsuyama S. New approaches to blockade of the renin–angiotensin–aldosterone system: overview of regulation of the renin–angiotensin–aldosterone system. J Pharmacol Sci. 2010;113:289–91.
35. Lin H, Geurts F, Hassler L, Batlle D, Mirabito Colafella KM, Denton KM, et al. Kidney angiotensin in cardiovascular disease: formation and drug targeting. Pharmacol Rev. 2022;74:462–505.
36. Crowley SD, Gurley SB, Herrera MJ, Ruiz P, Griffiths R, Kumar AP, et al. Angiotensin II causes hypertension and cardiac hypertrophy through its receptors in the kidney. Proc Natl Acad Sci USA. 2006;103:17985–90.
37. Gurley SB, Riquier-Brison ADM, Schnermann J, Sparks MA, Allen AM, Haase VH, et al. AT1A angiotensin receptors in the renal proximal tubule regulate blood pressure. Cell Metab. 2011;13:469–75.
38. Chen D, Stegbauer J, Sparks MA, Kohan D, Griffiths R, Herrera M, et al. Impact of angiotensin type 1A receptors in principal cells of the collecting duct on blood pressure and hypertension. Hypertension. 2016;67:1291–7.
39. Stegbauer J, Chen D, Herrera M, Sparks MA, Yang T, Königshausen E, et al. Resistance to hypertension mediated by intercalated cells of the collecting duct. JCI Insight. 2017;2:e92720.
40. Giani JF, Janjulia T, Kamat N, Seth DM, Blackwell WLB, Shah KH, et al. Renal angiotensin-converting enzyme is essential for the hypertension induced by nitric oxide synthesis inhibition. J Am Soc Nephrol. 2014;25:2752–63.
41. Gonzalez-Villalobos RA, Janjoulia T, Fletcher NK, Giani JF, Nguyen MTX, Riquier-Brison AD, et al. The absence of intrarenal ACE protects against hypertension. J Clin Invest. 2013;123:2011–23.
42. Giani JF, Eriguchi M, Bernstein EA, Katsumata M, Shen XZ, Li L, et al. Renal tubular angiotensin converting enzyme is responsible for nitro-L-arginine methyl ester (L-NAME)-induced salt sensitivity. Kidney Int. 2017;91:856–67.
43. Kobori H, Harrison-Bernard LM, Navar LG. Urinary excretion of angiotensinogen reflects intrarenal angiotensinogen production. Kidney Int. 2002;61:579–85.

44. Kobori H, Alper AB, Shenava R, Katsurada A, Saito T, Ohashi N, et al. Urinary angiotensinogen as a novel biomarker of the intrarenal renin–angiotensin system status in hypertensive patients. Hypertension. 2009;53:344–50.
45. Park CH, Kim HW, Park JT, Chang TI, Yoo TH, Lee J, et al. Intrarenal renin–angiotensin system activation alters relationship between systolic blood pressure and progression of chronic kidney disease. Hypertension. 2023;80:1024–34.
46. Sommers SC, Relman AS, Smithwick RH. Histologic studies of kidney biopsy specimens from patients with hypertension. Am J Pathol. 1958;34:685–715.
47. Hughson MD, Gobe GC, Hoy WE, Manning RD, Douglas-Denton R, Bertram JF. Associations of glomerular number and birth weight with clinicopathological features of African Americans and whites. Am J Kidney Dis. 2008;52:18–28.
48. Crowley SD, Song YS, Lin EE, Griffiths R, Kim HS, Ruiz P. Lymphocyte responses exacerbate angiotensin II-dependent hypertension. Am J Physiol Regul Integr Comp Physiol. 2010;298:R1089–97.
49. Madhur MS, Elijovich F, Alexander MR, Pitzer A, Ishimwe J, Van Beusecum JP, et al. Hypertension: do inflammation and immunity hold the key to solving this epidemic? Circ Res. 2021;128:908–33.
50. Benson LN, Guo Y, Deck K, Mora C, Liu Y, Mu S. The link between immunity and hypertension in the kidney and heart. Front Cardiovasc Med. 2023;10:1129384.
51. Furusho T, Sohara E, Mandai S, Kikuchi H, Takahashi N, Fujimaru T, et al. Renal TNFα activates the WNK phosphorylation cascade and contributes to salt-sensitive hypertension in chronic kidney disease. Kidney Int. 2020;97:713–27.
52. Oosterhuis NR, Papazova DA, Gremmels H, Joles JA, Verhaar MC. T-cells contribute to hypertension but not to renal injury in mice with subtotal nephrectomy. BMC Nephrol. 2017;18:153.
53. De Ciuceis C, Amiri F, Brassard P, Endemann DH, Touyz RM, Schiffrin EL. Reduced vascular remodeling, endothelial dysfunction, and oxidative stress in resistance arteries of angiotensin II-infused macrophage colony-stimulating factor-deficient mice: evidence for a role in inflammation in angiotensin-induced vascular injury. Arterioscler Thromb Vasc Biol. 2005;25:2106–13.
54. Ko EA, Amiri F, Pandey NR, Javeshghani D, Leibovitz E, Touyz RM, et al. Resistance artery remodeling in deoxycorticosterone acetate-salt hypertension is dependent on vascular inflammation: evidence from m-CSF-deficient mice. Am J Physiol Heart Circ Physiol. 2007;292:H1789–95.
55. Wenzel P, Knorr M, Kossmann S, Stratmann J, Hausding M, Schuhmacher S, et al. Lysozyme M-positive monocytes mediate angiotensin II-induced arterial hypertension and vascular dysfunction. Circulation. 2011;124:1370–81.
56. Fehrenbach DJ, Mattson DL. Inflammatory macrophages in the kidney contribute to salt-sensitive hypertension. Am J Physiol Ren Physiol. 2020;318:F544–8.
57. Fehrenbach DJ, Abais-Battad JM, Dasinger JH, Lund H, Mattson DL. Salt-sensitive increase in macrophages in the kidneys of Dahl SS rats. Am J Physiol Ren Physiol. 2019;317:F361–74.
58. Huang L, Wang A, Hao Y, Li W, Liu C, Yang Z, et al. Macrophage depletion lowered blood pressure and attenuated hypertensive renal injury and fibrosis. Front Physiol. 2018;9:473.
59. Rudemiller NP, Patel MB, Zhang JD, Jeffs AD, Karlovich NS, Griffiths R, et al. C–C motif chemokine 5 attenuates angiotensin II-dependent kidney injury by limiting renal macrophage infiltration. Am J Pathol. 2016;186:2846–56.
60. Veiras LC, Shen JZY, Bernstein EA, Regis GC, Cao D, Okwan-Duodu D, et al. Renal inflammation induces salt sensitivity in male db/db mice through dysregulation of ENaC. J Am Soc Nephrol. 2021;32:1131–49.
61. Veiras LC, Bernstein EA, Cao D, Okwan-Duodu D, Khan Z, Gibb DR, et al. Tubular IL-1β induces salt sensitivity in diabetes by activating renal macrophages. Circ Res. 2022;131:59–73.
62. Lu X, Crowley SD. Actions of dendritic cells in the kidney during hypertension. Compr Physiol. 2022;12:4087–101.

63. Barbaro NR, Foss JD, Kryshtal DO, Tsyba N, Kumaresan S, Xiao L, et al. Dendritic cell Amiloride-sensitive channels mediate sodium-induced inflammation and hypertension. Cell Rep. 2017;21:1009–20.
64. Kirabo A, Fontana V, de Faria APC, Loperena R, Galindo CL, Wu J, et al. DC isoketal-modified proteins activate T cells and promote hypertension. J Clin Invest. 2014;124:4642–56.
65. Norlander AE, Madhur MS. Inflammatory cytokines regulate renal sodium transporters: how, where, and why? Am J Physiol Ren Physiol. 2017;313:F141–4.
66. Wen Y, Crowley SD. Renal effects of cytokines in hypertension. Adv Exp Med Biol. 2019;1165:443–54.
67. Xiao L, Kirabo A, Wu J, Saleh MA, Zhu L, Wang F, et al. Renal denervation prevents immune cell activation and renal inflammation in angiotensin II-induced hypertension. Circ Res. 2015;117:547–57.
68. Lu X, Rudemiller NP, Privratsky JR, Ren J, Wen Y, Griffiths R, et al. Classical dendritic cells mediate hypertension by promoting renal oxidative stress and fluid retention. Hypertension. 2020;75:131–8.
69. Lu X, Rudemiller NP, Wen Y, Ren J, Hammer GE, Griffiths R, et al. A20 in myeloid cells protects against hypertension by inhibiting dendritic cell-mediated T-cell activation. Circ Res. 2019;125:1055–66.
70. Shah KH, Shi P, Giani JF, Janjulia T, Bernstein EA, Li Y, et al. Myeloid suppressor cells accumulate and regulate blood pressure in hypertension. Circ Res. 2015;117:858–69.
71. Guzik TJ, Hoch NE, Brown KA, McCann LA, Rahman A, Dikalov S, et al. Role of the T cell in the genesis of angiotensin II induced hypertension and vascular dysfunction. J Exp Med. 2007;204:2449–60.
72. Mattson DL, Lund H, Guo C, Rudemiller N, Geurts AM, Jacob H. Genetic mutation of recombination activating gene 1 in Dahl salt-sensitive rats attenuates hypertension and renal damage. Am J Physiol Regul Integr Comp Physiol. 2013;304:R407–14.
73. De Miguel C, Guo C, Lund H, Feng D, Mattson DL. Infiltrating T lymphocytes in the kidney increase oxidative stress and participate in the development of hypertension and renal disease. Am J Physiol Ren Physiol. 2011;300:F734–42.
74. Liu Y, Rafferty TM, Rhee SW, Webber JS, Song L, Ko B, et al. CD8+ T cells stimulate Na-Cl co-transporter NCC in distal convoluted tubules leading to salt-sensitive hypertension. Nat Commun. 2017;8:14037.
75. Trott DW, Thabet SR, Kirabo A, Saleh MA, Itani H, Norlander AE, et al. Oligoclonal CD8+ T cells play a critical role in the development of hypertension. Hypertension. 2014;64:1108–15.
76. Benson LN, Liu Y, Deck K, Mora C, Mu S. IFN-γ contributes to the immune mechanisms of hypertension. Kidney360. 2022;3:2164–73.
77. Benson LN, Liu Y, Wang X, Xiong Y, Rhee SW, Guo Y, et al. The IFNγ-PDL1 pathway enhances CD8T-DCT interaction to promote hypertension. Circ Res. 2022;130:1550–64.
78. Zhang J, Patel MB, Griffiths R, Mao A, Song YS, Karlovich NS, et al. Tumor necrosis factor-α produced in the kidney contributes to angiotensin II-dependent hypertension. Hypertension. 2014;64:1275–81.
79. Zhang JD, Patel MB, Song YS, Griffiths R, Burchette J, Ruiz P, et al. A novel role for type 1 angiotensin receptors on T lymphocytes to limit target organ damage in hypertension. Circ Res. 2012;110:1604–17.
80. Madhur MS, Lob HE, McCann LA, Iwakura Y, Blinder Y, Guzik TJ, et al. Interleukin 17 promotes angiotensin II-induced hypertension and vascular dysfunction. Hypertension. 2010;55:500–7.
81. Norlander AE, Saleh MA, Kamat NV, Ko B, Gnecco J, Zhu L, et al. Interleukin-17A regulates renal sodium transporters and renal injury in angiotensin II-induced hypertension. Hypertension. 2016;68:167–74.
82. Kamat NV, Thabet SR, Xiao L, Saleh MA, Kirabo A, Madhur MS, et al. Renal transporter activation during angiotensin-II hypertension is blunted in interferon-γ−/− and interleukin-17A−/− mice. Hypertension. 2015;65:569–76.

83. Kleinewietfeld M, Manzel A, Titze J, Kvakan H, Yosef N, Linker RA, et al. Sodium chloride drives autoimmune disease by the induction of pathogenic TH17 cells. Nature. 2013;496:518–22.
84. Wu C, Yosef N, Thalhamer T, Zhu C, Xiao S, Kishi Y, et al. Induction of pathogenic TH17 cells by inducible salt-sensing kinase SGK1. Nature. 2013;496:513–7.
85. Norlander AE, Saleh MA, Pandey AK, Itani HA, Wu J, Xiao L, et al. A salt-sensing kinase in T lymphocytes, SGK1, drives hypertension and hypertensive end-organ damage. JCI Insight. 2017;2:e92801.
86. Amador CA, Barrientos V, Peña J, Herrada AA, González M, Valdés S, et al. Spironolactone decreases DOCA-salt-induced organ damage by blocking the activation of T helper 17 and the downregulation of regulatory T lymphocytes. Hypertension. 2014;63:797–803.
87. Barhoumi T, Kasal DA, Li MW, Shbat L, Laurant P, Neves MF, et al. T regulatory lymphocytes prevent angiotensin II-induced hypertension and vascular injury. Hypertension. 2011;57:469–76.
88. Katsuki M, Hirooka Y, Kishi T, Sunagawa K. Decreased proportion of Foxp3+ CD4+ regulatory T cells contributes to the development of hypertension in genetically hypertensive rats. J Hypertens. 2015;33:773–83.
89. Kasal DA, Barhoumi T, Li MW, Yamamoto N, Zdanovich E, Rehman A, et al. T regulatory lymphocytes prevent aldosterone-induced vascular injury. Hypertension. 2012;59:324–30.
90. Kassan M, Galan M, Partyka M, Trebak M, Matrougui K. Interleukin-10 released by CD4(+) CD25(+) natural regulatory T cells improves microvascular endothelial function through inhibition of NADPH oxidase activity in hypertensive mice. Arterioscler Thromb Vasc Biol. 2011;31:2534–42.
91. Taylor EB, Sasser JM, Maeda KJ, Ryan MJ. Expansion of regulatory T cells using low-dose interleukin-2 attenuates hypertension in an experimental model of systemic lupus erythematosus. Am J Physiol Ren Physiol. 2019;317:F1274–84.
92. Chen XH, Ruan CC, Ge Q, Ma Y, Xu JZ, Zhang ZB, et al. Deficiency of complement C3a and C5a receptors prevents angiotensin II-induced hypertension via regulatory T cells. Circ Res. 2018;122:970–83.
93. Mathis KW, Wallace K, Flynn ER, Maric-Bilkan C, LaMarca B, Ryan MJ. Preventing autoimmunity protects against the development of hypertension and renal injury. Hypertension. 2014;64:792–800.
94. Chan CT, Sobey CG, Lieu M, Ferens D, Kett MM, Diep H, et al. Obligatory role for B cells in the development of angiotensin II-dependent hypertension. Hypertension. 2015;66:1023–33.
95. Chen Y, Dale BL, Alexander MR, Xiao L, Ao M, Pandey AK, et al. Class switching and high-affinity immunoglobulin G production by B cells is dispensable for the development of hypertension in mice. Cardiovasc Res. 2021;117:1217–28.
96. Rauch M, Tussiwand R, Bosco N, Rolink AG. Crucial role for BAFF-BAFF-R signaling in the survival and maintenance of mature B cells. PLoS One. 2009;4:e5456.
97. Hamaguchi Y, Uchida J, Cain DW, Venturi GM, Poe JC, Haas KM, et al. The peritoneal cavity provides a protective niche for B1 and conventional B lymphocytes during anti-CD20 immunotherapy in mice. J Immunol. 2005;174:4389–99.
98. Youn JC, Yu HT, Lim BJ, Koh MJ, Lee J, Chang DY, et al. Immunosenescent CD8+ T cells and C–X–C chemokine receptor type 3 chemokines are increased in human hypertension. Hypertension. 2013;62:126–33.
99. Rodríguez-Iturbe B, Pons H, Quiroz Y, Gordon K, Rincón J, Chávez M, et al. Mycophenolate mofetil prevents salt-sensitive hypertension resulting from angiotensin II exposure. Kidney Int. 2001;59:2222–32.
100. Bravo Y, Quiroz Y, Ferrebuz A, Vaziri ND, Rodríguez-Iturbe B. Mycophenolate mofetil administration reduces renal inflammation, oxidative stress, and arterial pressure in rats with lead-induced hypertension. Am J Physiol Ren Physiol. 2007;293:F616–23.
101. Herrera J, Ferrebuz A, MacGregor EG, Rodriguez-Iturbe B. Mycophenolate mofetil treatment improves hypertension in patients with psoriasis and rheumatoid arthritis. J Am Soc Nephrol. 2006;17(Suppl 3):S218–25.

102. Urwyler SA, Ebrahimi F, Burkard T, Schuetz P, Poglitsch M, Mueller B, et al. IL (interleukin)-1 receptor antagonist increases Ang (angiotensin [1–7]) and decreases blood pressure in obese individuals. Hypertension. 2020;75:1455–63.
103. Ridker PM, Everett BM, Thuren T, MacFadyen JG, Chang WH, Ballantyne C, et al. Antiinflammatory therapy with canakinumab for atherosclerotic disease. N Engl J Med. 2017;377:1119–31.
104. Rothman AM, MacFadyen J, Thuren T, Webb A, Harrison DG, Guzik TJ, et al. Effects of interleukin-1β inhibition on blood pressure, incident hypertension, and residual inflammatory risk: a secondary analysis of CANTOS. Hypertension. 2020;75:477–82.
105. Dixon DL, Wohlford GF, Abbate A. Inflammation and hypertension: causal or not? Hypertension. 2020;75:297–8.
106. Levy D, Ehret GB, Rice K, Verwoert GC, Launer LJ, Dehghan A, et al. Genome-wide association study of blood pressure and hypertension. Nat Genet. 2009;41:677–87.
107. International Consortium for Blood Pressure Genome-Wide Association Studies, Ehret GB, Munroe PB, Rice KM, Bochud M, Johnson AD, et al. Genetic variants in novel pathways influence blood pressure and cardiovascular disease risk. Nature. 2011;478:103–9.
108. Siedlinski M, Jozefczuk E, Xu X, Teumer A, Evangelou E, Schnabel RB, et al. White blood cells and blood pressure: a Mendelian randomization study. Circulation. 2020;141:1307–17.
109. Keefe JA, Hwang SJ, Huan T, Mendelson M, Yao C, Courchesne P, et al. Evidence for a causal role of the SH2B3-β2M axis in blood pressure regulation. Hypertension. 2019;73:497–503
110. Huan T, Meng Q, Saleh MA, Norlander AE, Joehanes R, Zhu J, et al. Integrative network analysis reveals molecular mechanisms of blood pressure regulation. Mol Syst Biol. 2015;11:799.
111. Alexander MR, Hank S, Dale BL, Himmel L, Zhong X, Smart CD, et al. A single nucleotide polymorphism in SH2B3/LNK promotes hypertension development and renal damage. Circ Res. 2022;131:731–47.
112. Genest DS, Patriquin CJ, Licht C, John R, Reich HN. Renal thrombotic microangiopathy: a review. Am J Kidney Dis. 2023;81:591–605.
113. Noris M, Remuzzi G. Atypical hemolytic–uremic syndrome. N Engl J Med 2009;361:1676–87.
114. Cavero T, Auñón P, Caravaca-Fontán F, Trujillo H, Arjona E, Morales E, et al. Thrombotic microangiopathy in patients with malignant hypertension. Nephrol Dial Transplant 2023;38:1217–26.
115. Cremer A, Amraoui F, Lip GYH, Morales E, Rubin S, Segura J, et al. From malignant hypertension to hypertension-MOD: a modern definition for an old but still dangerous emergency. J Hum Hypertens. 2016;30:463–6.
116. Shibagaki Y, Fujita T. Thrombotic microangiopathy in malignant hypertension and hemolytic uremic syndrome (HUS)/thrombotic thrombocytopenic purpura (TTP): can we differentiate one from the other? Hypertens Res. 2005;28:89–95.
117. van den Born BJH, Koopmans RP, van Montfrans GA. The renin-angiotensin system in malignant hypertension revisited: plasma renin activity, microangiopathic hemolysis, and renal failure in malignant hypertension. Am J Hypertens. 2007;20:900–6.
118. Cavero T, Arjona E, Soto K, Caravaca-Fontán F, Rabasco C, Bravo L, et al. Severe and malignant hypertension are common in primary atypical hemolytic uremic syndrome. Kidney Int. 2019;96:995–1004.
119. El Karoui K, Boudhabhay I, Petitprez F, Vieira-Martins P, Fakhouri F, Zuber J, et al. Impact of hypertensive emergency and rare complement variants on the presentation and outcome of atypical hemolytic uremic syndrome. Haematologica. 2019;104:2501–11.
120. Rubin S, Cremer A, Boulestreau R, Rigothier C, Kuntz S, Gosse P. Malignant hypertension: diagnosis, treatment and prognosis with experience from the Bordeaux cohort. J Hypertens. 2019;37:316–24.
121. Timmermans SAMEG, Abdul-Hamid MA, Potjewijd J, Theunissen ROMFIH, Damoiseaux JGMC, Reutelingsperger CP, et al. C5b9 formation on endothelial cells reflects complement defects among patients with renal thrombotic Microangiopathy and severe hypertension. J Am Soc Nephrol. 2018;29:2234–43.

122. Larsen CP, Wilson JD, Best-Rocha A, Beggs ML, Hennigar RA. Genetic testing of complement and coagulation pathways in patients with severe hypertension and renal microangiopathy. Mod Pathol. 2018;31:488–94.
123. Timmermans SAMEG, Wérion A, Damoiseaux JGMC, Morelle J, Reutelingsperger CP, van Paassen P. Diagnostic and risk factors for complement defects in hypertensive emergency and thrombotic Microangiopathy. Hypertension. 2020;75:422–30.
124. Zhang Y, Yang C, Zhou X, Hu R, Quan S, Zhou Y, et al. Association between thrombotic microangiopathy and activated alternative complement pathway in malignant nephrosclerosis. Nephrol Dial Transplant. 2021;36:1222–33.
125. Chen X, Zhang X, Wang Y, Wang S, Zhao M. Genetic, clinical, and pathological study of patients with severe hypertension-associated renal microangiopathy. J Nephrol. 2023;36:2477–90.
126. Mele C, Remuzzi G, Noris M. Hemolytic uremic syndrome. Semin Immunopathol. 2014;36:399–420.
127. Fakhouri F, Frémeaux-Bacchi V. Thrombotic microangiopathy in aHUS and beyond: clinical clues from complement genetics. Nat Rev Nephrol. 2021;17:543–53.
128. Fakhouri F, Loirat C. Anticomplement treatment in atypical and typical hemolytic uremic syndrome. Semin Hematol. 2018;55:150–8.
129. van den Born BJH, Lip GYH, Brguljan-Hitij J, Cremer A, Segura J, Morales E, et al. ESC Council on hypertension position document on the management of hypertensive emergencies. Eur Heart J Cardiovasc Pharmacother. 2019;5:37–46.

Part VI

Cardiorenal Associations

CKD as a Cardiovascular Risk Factor

11

Fernando Martínez García
and Verónica Escudero Quesada

Abbreviations

ABPM	Ambulatory blood pressure monitoring
ACE	Angiotensin-converting enzyme
ADMA	Asymmetric dimethylarginine
ADN	Aortic depressor nerve
AGEs	Advanced glycation end-products
ALLHAT	Antihypertensive and Lipid-Lowering Treatment to Prevent Heart Attack Trial
apoB	Apolipoprotein B
ARB	Angiotensin II receptor blocker
ARV	Average real variability
AS	Arterial stiffness
baPWV	Brachial-ankle pulse wave velocity
BMI	Body mass index
BMM	Bone-mineral metabolism
BP	Blood pressure
BPV	Blood pressure variability
BRS	Baroreflex sensitivity

F. M. García (✉)
Hypertension Unit, Internal Medicine Department, Clinical University Hospital of Valencia, University of Valencia, Valencia, Spain

Cardiometabolic and Renal Research Group of the Research Institute of the Clinical Hospital of Valencia (INCLIVA), Valencia, Spain
e-mail: fermar23@uv.es; Fernando.Martinez-Garcia@uv.es

V. E. Quesada
Hypertension Unit; Nephrology Department, University Hospital Dr. Peset, Valencia, Spain

A. E. Berbari et al. (eds.), *Blood Pressure Disorders in Acute and Chronic Kidney Diseases*, Updates in Hypertension and Cardiovascular Protection,
https://doi.org/10.1007/978-3-031-81292-7_11

cIMT	Carotid intima-media thickness
CRIC	Chronic renal insufficiency cohort
CHF	Congestive heart failure
Ca	Calcium
CPPs	Calciprotein particles
CRP	C-reactive protein
CCB	Calcium channel blocker
CKD	Chronic kidney disease
CMERC-HI	Cardiovascular and Metabolic Diseases Etiology Research Center-High Impact
CV	Cardiovascular
CVE	Cardiovascular events
CVRFs	Cardiovascular risk factors
DBP	Diastolic blood pressure
DM	Diabetes mellitus
eGFR	Estimated glomerular filtration rate
ESH	European Society of Hypertension
FGF23	Fibroblast growth factor 23
FGFR	Fibroblast growth factor receptor
GH	Growth hormone
GLP-1	Glucagon-like peptide-1
GPx	Glutathione peroxidase
HBPM	Home blood pressure monitoring
HDL	High-density lipoprotein
HFP	High-frequency power
HMOD	Hypertension-mediated organ damage
HR	Heart rate
HTN	Hypertension
HR	Hazard ratio
IDL	Intermediate-density lipoprotein
IGF-1	Insulin growth factor-1
IL-6	Interleukin 6
IL-18	Interleukin 18
IR	Insulin resistance
iSGLT-2	Sodium-glucose co-transporter inhibitors
ISRNM	International Society of Renal Nutrition and Metabolism
LDL	Low-density lipoprotein
LFP	Low-frequency power
LVH	Left ventricular hypertrophy
MACE	Major adverse cardiovascular events
MBD	Mineral and bone disorder
MCS	Medial calcific sclerosis
MIA	Malnutrition-inflammation-atherosclerosis
MorStr	Morning surge
NADPH	Nicotinamide adenine dinucleotide phosphate

N/D	Night/day ratio
NF	Nocturnal fall
NLRP3	NOD-like receptor protein 3
NT-proBNP	N-Terminal pro-B-type natriuretic peptide
P	Phosphorus
PP	Pulse pressure
PEW	Protein-energy wasting
PTH	Parathyroid hormone
PWV	Pulse wave velocity
RAAS	Renin–angiotensin–aldosterone system
ROS	Reactive oxygen species
RSNA	Renal sympathetic nerve activity
RV	Residual variability
SBP	Systolic blood pressure
SD	Standard deviation
SieDip	Siesta dipping
SNA	Sympathetic nerve activity
SOD	Superoxide dismutase
TOD	Target organ damage
TMAO	Trimethylamine-N-oxide
TNF-α	Tumor necrosis factor-alpha
TR	Time rate
US	Uremic syndrome
VDR	Vitamin D receptor
VIM	Variability independent of the mean
VLFP	Very low-frequency power
VVV	Visit-to-visit variability
wSD	Weighed standard deviation

11.1 Introduction

11.1.1 General Background on CKD and Cardiovascular Risk

It is well-known that chronic kidney disease (CKD) patients die from cardiovascular diseases and not from renal causes [1, 2]. With the current use of new therapies that have demonstrated to slow the progression on renal deterioration, such as the sodium-glucose co-transporter inhibitors (iSGLT-2), the focused of our CKD patients must be on cardiovascular protection. In this sense, the recently published guidelines of the European Society of hypertension (ESH) [3] considered CKD patients as high or very high cardiovascular risk (Fig. 11.1).

Independently of the levels of blood pressure (BP), the presence of CKD permits to classify hypertension (HTN) as stage 2 or 3.

Hypertension disease staging	Other risk factors, HMOD, CVD or CKD	BP (mmHg) grading			
		High-normal SBP 130–139 DBP 85–89	Grade 1 SBP 140–159 DBP 90–99	Grade 2 SBP 160–179 DBP 100–109	Grade 3 SBP ≥ 180 DBP ≥ 110
Stage 1	No other risk factors[a]	Low risk	Low risk	Moderate risk	High risk
	1 or 2 risk factors	Low risk	Moderate risk	Moderate to high risk	High risk
	≥3 risk factors	Low to moderate risk	Moderate to high risk	High risk	High risk
Stage 2	HMOD, CKD grade 3, or diabetes mellitus	Moderate to high risk	High risk	High risk	Very high risk
Stage 3	Established CVD or CKD grade ≥4	Very high risk	Very high risk	Very high risk	Very high risk

Fig. 11.1 Cardiovascular risk according to grade and stage of hypertension. (Reproduced with permission [3])

Atherosclerosis is the most common type of arteriosclerosis in general and CKD patients, but CKD is probably, along with age, the most relevant factor for Mönckeberg's Arteriosclerosis or Medial Calcific Sclerosis (MCS).

Although the mechanisms associated with a higher risk of cardiovascular mortality are complex and not well understood, BP variability (BPV) and metabolic disturbances are two of the potential contributors to this risk.

In this chapter, the current evidence about how BP variability and metabolic disturbances in CKD may lead to CVD will be reviewed.

11.2 Circadian and Non-circadian BP Variability

11.2.1 Definitions, Patterns, and Diagnostic Approaches

Abnormal BP circadian patterns including non-dipper or riser are very common in CKD patients, thus the use of ambulatory blood pressure monitoring (ABPM) is strongly recommended in this high-risk population. This can be of interest beyond daytime BP, because nocturnal hypertension could be an independent risk factor for cardiovascular mortality in CKD population. Due to reproducibility issues, whenever possible the presence of an abnormal phenotype should be confirmed in a second ABPM in a few days or weeks [4, 5].

A typical ABPM with non-dipper pattern of a patient with advanced CKD is shown in Fig. 11.2.

Also, certain phenotypes such as masked hypertension [6] are more common in CKD patients. This hypertensive phenotype is characterized by normal office BP levels and elevated daytime BP levels (≥135/85 mmHg) in the ABPM. For instance, the prevalence of this phenotype on one study performed in Afro-Americans with hypertensive CKD was as high as 70% [7].

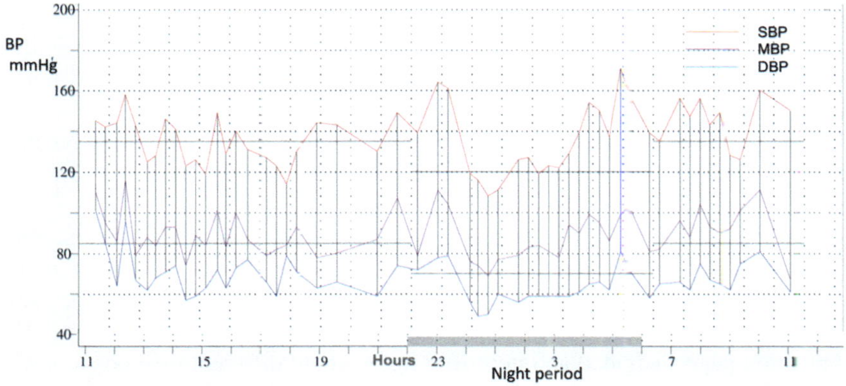

Fig. 11.2 Typical non-dipper pattern seen in ABPM of CKD patients. *BP* blood pressure, *SBP* systolic blood pressure, *MBP* mean arterial pressure, *DBP* diastolic blood pressure

Classically BP fluctuations or variability can be classified as a very short/short or mid-term/long-term [8]. This grade of variability can even be detected from beat to beat due to both physiological and external influences, such as changes in posture, emotional stress, and even the act of breathing itself. Daily shifts in BP stem from akin factors, including levels of physical exertion, sleep patterns, and changes in hormonal and sympathetic nervous system activity. Variations in BP over more extended periods, typically observed from one medical appointment to another over several months/years, result from factors like aging, medication adherence, and inaccuracies in BP measurements.

In patients with CKD, this BP variability, especially visit-to-visit variability (VVV), is highly relevant because not only is more frequent [9–11], but it also has been related with cardiovascular events and mortality in many studies [12–14].

A small Japanese study [15] tried to determine if the fluctuations in BP measured at home corresponded with those recorded during clinic visits, providing insights into managing hypertension in CKD patients.

The study involved 143 CKD patients who were monitored for BPV both at home and during clinic visits. Home BP measurements were taken every morning and evening for seven consecutive days, while clinic BP data were collected across approximately ten visits within a 24-month period. The results of the study revealed a significant but weak correlation between office BPV and home BPV. Specifically, the Coefficient of Variation (CV) of office SBP was significantly correlated with the mean and CV of both morning and evening SBP measured at home. This means that patients who experienced high BP variability at home tended to also show high variability during clinic visits [15].

Overall, their results suggest that while BP measurements at home can reflect the variability seen in clinical settings, they are not perfectly aligned. Several clinical variables were found to influence BPV. For instance, male gender, the number of antihypertensive drugs, urinary protein excretion, and changes in antihypertensive medications during the study period were significantly correlated with higher BP variability. This highlights the complex interplay between patient characteristics, medication regimens, and BP control [15].

The short-term BPV over 24 h may also be considered as a risk factor for cardiovascular events (CVE) or mortality on CKD, but the level of evidence is not as clear [16].

Although it does not specifically address BPV in CKD, there has been recently published a position paper on BPV by the Working Group on Blood Pressure Monitoring and Cardiovascular Variability [17].

This document titled "Blood pressure variability: methodological aspects, clinical relevance and practical indications for management" was published in the *Journal of Hypertension* in 2023 and provides a comprehensive review of the available evidence on BPV assessment methodology and its clinical applications [17]. The position paper included an interesting figure about different methods to evaluate BPV (Fig. 11.3) and a table showing the different types of BPV and the correspondent formulas (Table 11.1).

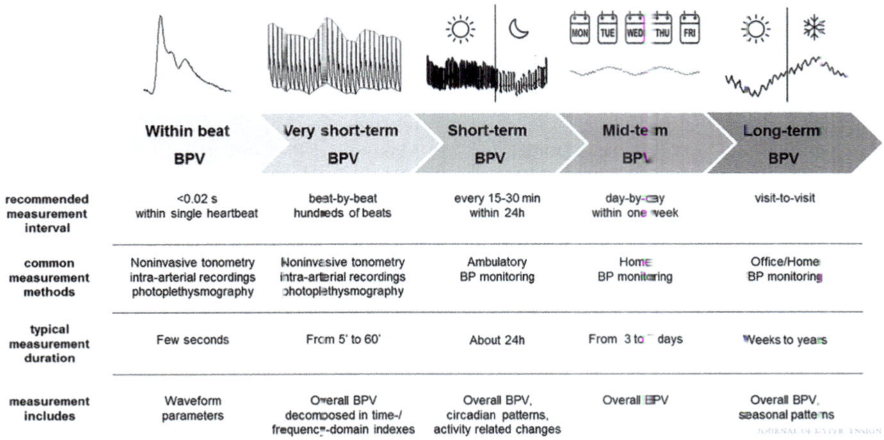

Fig. 11.3 Classification of BPV based on temporal frame of reference. *Key features of measurement methodology are summarized for each BPV subtype. "Overall" variability indicates total variance, including all components of BPV over a given time window. (Reproduced with permission [17])

Table 11.1 Type of BPV indices and their definition

Type of measurement/ time scale	Index [units]	Description/formula
Frequency domain (short-term and very short-term BPV)	HFP [$mmHg^2$] [18]	Integral of power spectrum P(f)[a] from 0.15 to 0.40 Hz
	LFP [$mmHg^2$]	Integral of power spectrum P(f) from 0.04 to 0.15 Hz
	VLFP [$mmHg^2$]	Integral of power spectrum P(f) from 0.003 to 0.04 Hz
	RV [$mmHg^2$] [19]	Sum of squared deviations from circadian pattern components
Complexity domain (short-term and very short-term BPV)	Self-similarity scale exponents [20]	Slopes α1 and α2 for small (<12 beats) and long (≥12 beats)blocks of BP segments
	Entropy [21]	Negative natural log of conditional probability of similar BP sequences
Dispersion (short, mid, and long-term BPV)	SD [mmHg] [22]	Standard deviation of BP readings
	CV [%]	$100 \times \frac{SD}{MeanBP}$
	SD_BP [mmHg]	Weighted SD during wake and sleep periods
	VIM [mmHg] [23]	Calculated as: $BP_{population} \times \left(\frac{SD_{BP}}{BP_{population}}\right)^x$
Sequence (short-, mid-, and long-term BPV)	ARV [mmHg] [24]	Average absolute difference between successive BP readings
	TR [mmHg/min] [25]	Rate of change in BP over time between readings

(continued)

Table 11.1 (continued)

Type of measurement/ time scale	Index [units]	Description/formula
Instability (short- and mid-term BPV)	Range [mmHg]	Difference between max and min BP readings
	Peak [mmHg]	Maximum BP recorded
	Trough [mmHg]	Minimum BP recorded
Patterns (short-term BPV)	Nocturnal fall [%]	Percent drop in BP from day to night
	N/D	Ratio of nighttime to daytime BP
	MorStr [mmHg] [26, 27]	Difference in morning BP from lowest nighttime reading
	SieDip [%] [28]	Percent BP reduction during daytime sleep vs awake BP
	PPF [mmHg] [29]	Drop in systolic BP post-lunch

Reproduced and modified with permission [17]

HFP high-frequency power, *LFP* low-frequency power, *VLFP* very-low-frequency power, *RV* residual variability, *SD* standard deviation, *CV* coefficient of variation, *SD_BP* weighted standard deviation, *VIM* variability independent of the mean, *ARV* average real variability, *TR* time rate, *NF* nocturnal fall, *N/D* night/day ratio, *MorStr* morning surge, *SieDip* siesta dipping, *PPF* postprandial fall

[a]P(f) represents the power spectrum of beat-by-beat BP values by Fast Fourier Transform or by autoregressive modelling

11.2.2 Mechanistic Insights

Many factors can affect the BP variability in CKD patients such as type 2 diabetes, male sex, obesity, and, as it was expected, the systolic BP levels [11]. The adherence or the lack of adherence as well as the impact of certain antihypertensive drugs although relevant is not well understood [10, 30]. Certain combination of drugs, such as the association of calcium channel blocker (CCB) with a thiazide-like diuretics, could reduce the BP variability, but this remains to be proven in clinical trials neither if their impact of this surrogate endpoint could reduce hard cardiovascular events [9, 10, 13, 31]. The article of Murphy et al. suggests that BP variability could be similar to other controversial markers in cardiovascular diseases, such as hyperhomocystenemia or hyperuricemia, which are not clear that its reduction can have an impact in cardiovascular disease [31].

The physiological mechanisms, which contribute to maintain the BP and its circadian pattern, are multiple and dysregulated in CKD patients. It is clear that the sympathetic tone with its own circadian rhythm and the sleep pattern/phases are the main responsible for BP variability although other factors such as the physical activity are of uttered importance [32, 33]. One piece of evidence is that the normal dipping BP pattern is reverse in night workers and vary in shift workers depending on the rest and activity hours [34–36].

Within the BP variability, other important contributor to cardiovascular events is the morning BP surge. This can be explained by the circadian pattern of cortisol being higher in early morning. Cortisol increases the sensitivity to catecholamines, and this can increase the vascular alpha-adrenergic tone and therefore lead to a BP

Table 11.2 Potential factors affecting BP variability

Modifiable	Non-modifiable	Mixed/other factors
Body mass index (BMI)	Age	Baroreflex sensitivity
Sodium intake	Gender	Arterial stiffness[a]
Smoking	Ethnicity	Seasonal variations[b]
Alcohol intake		Environmental factors[c]
Level of BP itself		Autonomic, humoral, and neural mechanisms[d]

[a]Arterial stiffness, while related to aging (thus potentially falling under non-modifiable), can also be influenced by lifestyle choices and medical treatment, placing it in the Mixed category

[b]Seasonal variations suggest an interplay between environmental factors and individual physiological responses, making it a mixed factor

[c]Environmental factors include a range of external conditions that can affect BP variability, such as temperature changes and altitude

[d]These mechanisms underline the complex regulation of BP involving various systems in the body, influenced by both genetic predispositions and lifestyle factors

rise [37, 38]. Also, the plasma renin activity and aldosterone levels seem to be higher at early hours [39].

The list of factors which can affect the BP variability is huge and can be classified as modifiable or not modifiable and are represented in Table 11.2.

It is clear that all of these factors also contribute to the abnormalities of BP variability usually seen in CKD patients.

In the following parts, some of the key factors contributing to BP variability in CKD will be analyzed.

11.2.2.1 Sodium and Fluid Retention

The relationship between sodium intake, fluid retention, and blood pressure variability in CKD is complex, with individual patient responses to sodium intake showing considerable variability. Sodium and fluid retention leading to hypervolemia is a primary factor for hypertension development in CKD, and salt restriction can reduce blood pressure levels and enhance the anti-proteinuric effect of renin–angiotensin–aldosterone system (RAAS) inhibitors in non-dialysis CKD patients [40]. However, the effectiveness of a low salt diet over the long term is mixed, potentially due to measurement bias, reverse epidemiology, and poor dietary adherence [40].

There is scarce information linking the grade of sodium intake with BPV on CKD. The Spirit Compliance Trial although only includes mild CKD patients is aimed to relate the sodium intake, estimated through 24-h urinary excretion, with BP variability SD and CV of ABPM measurements) and target organ damage (TOD) [41].

As it was demonstrated in a study of 119 patients with CKD and estimated glomerular filtration rate (eGFR) around 30 mL/min, the response of the mean arterial pressure to sodium intake was highly variable [42].

Taking into account the available data, we can assure that sodium and fluid retention is key factor to BP and BP variability, although is hardly to infer to what extent, due to the influence of the rest of potential contributors as well as the interindividual variability.

11.2.2.2 Baroreflex Abnormalities

The baroreflex mechanism, which is crucial in maintaining BP stability, undergoes significant alterations that contribute to increased BP variability [43–45].

In an interesting study performed by Tomiyama [44] in CKD secondary to glomerulonephritis, the baroreflex sensitivity (BRS) was reduced in patients with CKD specially in hypertensive patients compared to their normotensive counterparts. The BRS was assessed by the slope of the linear regression of the pulse interval on the rise in systolic blood pressure (SBP) with injection of phenylephrine or reduction by amyl nitrite inhalation. After saline infusion, there were two patients who developed hypertension, and this was in those with greater reduction of the BRS even when the increase on plasma volume was the same. This reduction in BRS associated with hypertension suggests a mechanistic link between impaired baroreflex function and elevated BP. The authors also found a positive correlation between BRS and motor nerve conduction velocity suggesting that uremic neuropathy may contribute to the impaired baroreflex function, providing a possible pathophysiological link between CKD and altered BP control. This experiment underscores the critical role of intact baroreflex function in preventing hypertension, even in the face of volume expansion, a common condition in CKD.

Other experimental study in rats by Salman et al. [43] demonstrates that in CKD, there is a deficit in both the afferent component of the baroreflex, evidenced by reduced gain and range of renal sympathetic nerve activity (RSNA) and heart rate (HR) barocurves, and the central regulation of RSNA and HR. This progressive impairment of both components is associated with marked dysfunction of the baroreflex pathway, correlating with structural remodeling of the aortic arch, a site critical for baroreceptor functionality.

Moreover, Johansson et al. [45] explored the impact of saline administration in normotensive CKD patients with varying levels of baroreflex sensitivity. The study found that patients with severely depressed baroreflex sensitivity experienced a significant increase in BP, resembling the hypertensive state observed in patients with naturally occurring CKD. This observation underscores the potential of impaired baroreflex function as an initiating factor for hypertension in CKD, further complicating the BP control in these patients and contributing to the disturbed BP variability.

11.2.2.3 Arterial Stiffness

Arterial stiffness (AS) has been identified as a key mechanism contributing to BPV in patients with CKD. This relationship is multifaceted, involving several pathophysiological processes that exacerbate cardiovascular risks.

One small study demonstrated that CKD patients showed a non-dipping pattern and lack of the diurnal variation in arterial stiffness as compared with controls and this could be related with the levels of endotelin-1 [46]. So arterial stiffness and non-dipping pattern are closely related in CKD patients [46].

Other prospective study across the spectrum of CKD was able to find an association between SBP variability from visit to visit with the progression in AS analyzed by means of the brachial-ankle (ba) pulse wave velocity (PWV) [47].

In the Japan Morning Surge-Home Blood Pressure (J-HOP study), several BP variability indexes coming from daily home blood pressure monitoring (HBPM) were analyzed [SD,CV, and ARV] and correlated with AS (estimated through the baPWV), and cardiac overload (estimated through levels of NT-proBNP) [48]. They found higher variability and cardiac overload in the group of higher than the median of baPWV [48].

As it has been discussed for a long time, it is difficult to say which come first, AS leading to an increase in BP variability or vice versa [49].

Other studies, although not specifically in CKD patients, pointed in the same direction showing a clear association between a composite index of SBP variability using the within-visit, 24-h and 7-day BPV, and the aortic stiffness with the use of the carotid-femoral PWV [50].

It is expected that those interventions able to reduce the stiffness of the arterial tree were also able to reduce the BP variability in CKD and potentially decrease cardiovascular events [51].

These findings collectively point to AS not only as a marker of vascular health but also as a potentially modifiable risk factor in CKD. The integration of measures to assess and ameliorate AS could therefore play a vital role in managing CKD and reducing the burden of cardiovascular disease within this population.

11.2.2.4 Oxidative Stress

The direct relationship between oxidative stress and BPV, specifically within the context of CKD, is a complex area of study. While the research provided does not explicitly link oxidative stress to BPV in CKD patients, we can infer potential connections based on known mechanisms.

Oxidative stress, characterized by an imbalance between the production of reactive oxygen species (ROS) and the body's ability to detoxify these reactive intermediates or repair the resulting damage, plays a crucial role in the pathophysiology of CKD. It contributes to the progression of kidney disease and is associated with several complications, including hypertension, atherosclerosis, inflammation, and anemia, especially in advanced stages of CKD [52, 53].

As it was shown in Table 11.2, several factors are related to BPV in CKD and oxidative stress can exacerbate these factors through various mechanisms. For example, oxidative stress is known to impair endothelial function, contributing to vascular stiffness and dysregulation of vascular tone, which can lead to fluctuations in blood pressure. Additionally, oxidative stress can influence the activity of the RAAS, further contributing to blood pressure variability [52, 54].

Given these connections, it's reasonable to speculate that interventions aimed at reducing oxidative stress might also impact blood pressure variability in CKD patients. However, direct studies focusing specifically on the link between oxidative stress and blood pressure variability in CKD population are limited. Future research in this area could provide valuable insights into potential therapeutic targets for managing both oxidative stress and BPV in CKD patients.

11.2.3 Clinical Implications

11.2.3.1 Association of BPV

Hypertension-Mediated Organ Damage (HMOD)

As it was commented above, BPV in CKD has been associated with hypertension-mediated organ damage (HMOD). For instance, in a recently published paper in 3442 non-dialysis CKD Chinese patients, 41.4% under antihypertensive treatment, short-term BPV, evaluated through the weighted SD (wSD) derived from ABPM, was associated with the presence of left ventricular hypertrophy (LVH), abnormal carotid intima-media thickness (cIMT), low eGFR, and albuminuria [55].

Although this type of cross-sectional study cannot establish causality between short-term BPV and the development of HMOD in CKD, and assessing the potential impact of antihypertensive drugs is challenging, it opens the door to well-designed prospective studies.

Renal Endpoints and Major Adverse Cardiovascular Events (MACE)

The most recent systematic review and meta-analysis examining the relationship between short-term BPV and the progression of CKD was published in 2023 by Yang et al. [56]. After applying the selected criteria, 23 studies focusing on the association between BPV and CKD progression were included with a total of 746,744 patients with CKD. Overall, the results of the meta-analysis seem to support that BPV is associated with a higher hazard ratio (HR) for CKD progression and the incidence of end-stage renal disease (ESRD). Regarding BPV, several metrics were selected including the VIM, the CV, the SD, and the ARV. These metrics were assessed primarily through 24-h ABPM, with some studies using office blood pressure monitoring (OBPM) or HBPM. For the selected studies, the renal outcomes were variable and included the progression of CKD stages, the development of ESRD, a decline in eGFR, or an increase in serum creatinine.

Like many meta-analyses, this study had considerable heterogeneity among the included studies, arising from variations in sample size, study design, blood pressure measurement techniques, and follow-up periods. These discrepancies could have impacted the study's results and conclusions. Additionally, there were methodological differences, with various blood pressure monitoring approaches and multivariate regression models, contributing to inconsistent findings across studies. The results also have limited generalizability because most studies were conducted in East Asian, North American, or European populations. Finally, many studies had small sample sizes, which could undermine the reliability and robustness of the meta-analysis results.

Despite these limitations, the chapter provides valuable evidence that high BPV is associated with poorer renal outcomes, particularly in terms of the incidence of ESRD, in the CKD population. These findings suggest that further well-designed prospective studies are necessary to validate the results and explore the therapeutic potential of BPV management in CKD patients.

An older meta-analysis, published by Li et al. (2020), also focused on visit-to-visit BPV as a potential risk factor for CKD [57]. This study included 14 cohort studies, with a total of 11,407,535 participants, highlighting that increased visit-to-visit BPV might be associated with CKD progression.

While both meta-analyses indicated that BPV could be associated with the progression of CKD, the meta-analysis by Li et al. primarily utilized the SD and CV as metrics to assess visit-to-visit systolic BPV and diastolic BPV.

The most recent meta-analysis by Yang et al. further expanded upon this, incorporating additional metrics such as the VIM and ARV, offering a broader perspective on BPV measures.

The meta-analysis by Li et al. also presented considerable heterogeneity due to additional factors like sample size, study design, and country of origin.

Despite these limitations, both meta-analysis [56, 57] concluded that high BPV is associated with poorer renal outcomes, suggesting that further well-designed prospective studies are necessary to explore this relationship in depth.

A visual representation of the two meta-analysis is shown in Fig. 11.4.

For the case of BPV and MACE risk, the most recent study in this regard was published in 2022 by Park et al. in 1575 Korean patients as part of the KNOW-CKD study [58]. Again, as it happened with softer cardiovascular endpoints, higher SBP variability during the first year of follow-up significantly correlated with an increased risk of MACE. Specifically, patients in the highest tertile of systolic BPV faced more than a twofold increase in MACE risk compared to those in the lowest tertile during a median of 4.2 years of follow-up. This relationship exhibited a dose-response characteristic, with progressively higher HR for the middle and highest tertiles of SBP variability.

Moreover, the association between systolic BPV and MACE was consistent across different metrics, including SD, CV, and VIM. Sensitivity analyses using

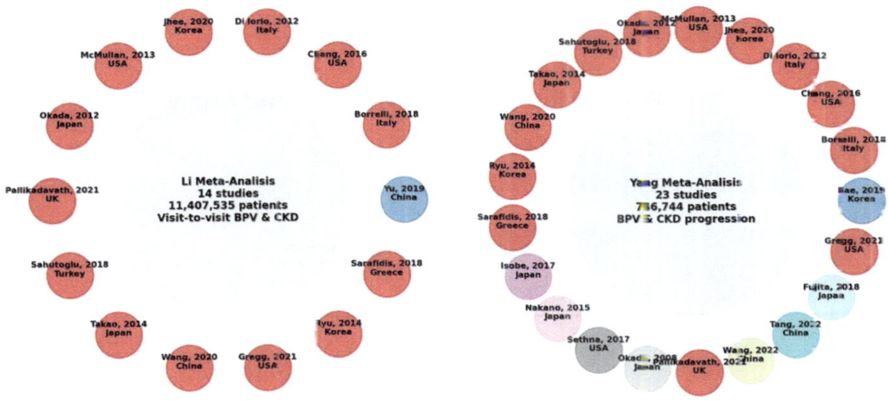

Fig. 11.4 More recent meta-analysis on BPV and renal endpoints. Red circles indicate overlapped studies between the two meta-analysis

alternative definitions of systolic BPV and multiple imputation for missing data, further support the robustness of the primary findings.

However, the study does face limitations, primarily its observational design which cannot establish causality definitively due to potential residual confounding. Additionally, the findings are based on a single ethnic group, which may limit the generalizability of the results to other populations. The study also did not employ 24-h ABPM, which could have provided more detailed insights into blood pressure patterns and variability. The strategy for assessment the systolic BPV in this study is shown in Fig. 11.5.

Overall, this research underscores the clinical importance of monitoring SBP variability in CKD patients, suggesting that maintaining stable blood pressure could be as crucial as controlling average blood pressure levels to mitigate cardiovascular risk.

In the same line, other recent study [59] also analyzed the impact of BPV on clinical outcomes in patients with heart failure (HF) and CKD over an average follow-up of 6.3 years. The study included 382 participants extracted from the Chronic Renal Insufficiency Cohort (CRIC), predominantly male (57.6%) with an average age of 60.2 years, and average eGFR of 39 mL/min/1.73 m^2 [59]. The researchers found that increases in baseline SBP and the CV of diastolic blood pressure (DBP) were significantly associated with an increase in primary CVE, renal events, and all-cause mortality. Interestingly, DBP CV demonstrated a nonlinear (J- or L-shaped) relationship with these outcomes using restricted cubic spline models, indicating that both high and low variability can be detrimental. Therefore, the results suggest a complex dynamic between BP regulation and clinical outcomes in this high-risk population. Again, it remains to be proved if stabilizing blood pressure fluctuations can lead to better CV outcomes in CKD. Also the relatively small sample size, considering the complexity of the diseases involved, might affect the statistical power and robustness of the conclusions [59].

The impact of short-term BPV on cardiovascular outcomes in patients with non-dialysis CKD has been analyzed in a retrospective study at Ningxia Medical

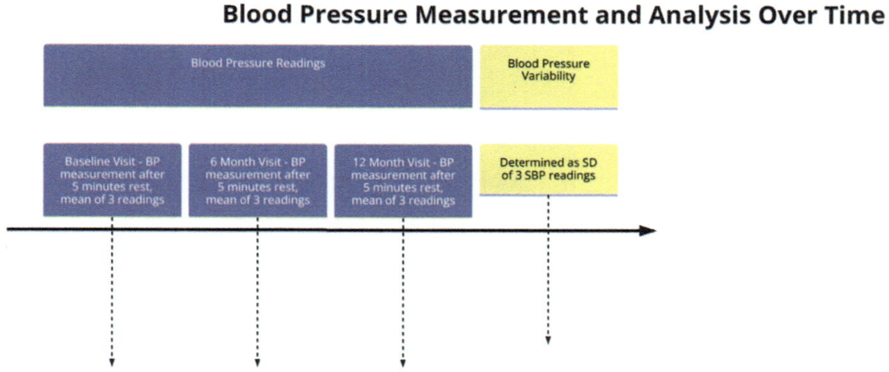

Fig. 11.5 Strategy for assessment the systolic BPV within the KNOWN-CKD study [58]

University [60]. The study involved 245 stage 1–4 CKD patients, investigating CV outcomes relative to BPV, which was calculated using several statistical measures such as SD and VIM. The authors found that higher short-term BPV was significantly linked to an increased risk of MACE, although it did not correlate with renal progression after full adjustments. These findings suggest that while BPV could be an independent cardiovascular risk factor, its impact on kidney disease progression in the non-dialysis CKD population may be limited [60].

Those patients in the higher BPV group based on the median 24-h systolic BP VIM had more risk of MACE comparing with those in the lower BPV group (HR 4.7, *p*-value 0.022) [60]. Multivariate analyses highlighted that high BMI, hyperkalemia, increased left ventricular end-diastolic diameter, and hypertension were significant independent risk factors for elevated BPV [60].

As it happened with many of these studies, the retrospective design and the potential confounding factors can limit the ability to establish causality, making it difficult to determine whether observed associations are truly indicative of direct relationships or are influenced by underlying variables not accounted for in the study.

In contrast to the study by Wang et al. [60], the CMERC-HI study [61] specifically addresses the relationship between BPV and the direct progression of kidney disease in a hypertensive cohort with initially normal kidney function. This study concludes that higher BPV is significantly associated with the development of adverse kidney outcomes. Over a median follow-up of 5.4 years among 1173 participants, those with higher systolic and diastolic BPV were found to have an increased risk of CKD progression. This association persisted even after adjusting for confounders such as mean BP, underscoring BPV as a potent independent risk factor for CKD [61]. These contrasting findings emphasize the complex role of BPV in renal health. Whereas Wang et al. [60] suggest that the direct implications of BPV on kidney function are minimal, the CMERC-HI study [61] robustly links BPV with a tangible progression in kidney disease.

Older studies, like the Jackson Heart Study [62] in African-American, highlighted that BPV might not independently predict cardiovascular risks beyond the baseline blood pressure levels and that BPV is primary influenced by higher MBP levels [62]. This evidence underscores the importance of lowering and controlling overall blood pressure as the primary goal, while treating BPV as a secondary consideration.

The topic of BPV as risk factor for CKD development or progression has also been evaluated within relevant clinical trials like the Antihypertensive and Lipid-Lowering Treatment to Prevent Heart Attack Trial (ALLHAT) [63]. Over 21,000 participants were monitored closely to evaluate how fluctuations in their BP from one medical visit to the next influenced their kidney function over time (onset of ESRD or a significant decline in eGFR). The study followed participants for an average of 3.5 years, measuring their BP at regular intervals and tracking their kidney function [63].

As it has happened in smaller and more recent studies, those individuals whose BP varied more significantly between visits were at a higher risk of experiencing severe renal complications. For instance, those in the highest quintile of BPV were more than twice as likely to develop serious renal issues compared to those in the lowest quintile, whose BP remained relatively stable. Specifically, the HR for the composite outcome of ESRD or a 50% decline in eGFR was 2.05 for the highest variability group compared to the lowest.

The methodology of the study was robust, utilizing data from multiple visits to ensure accuracy. BP was measured at 5–7 different times between 6 and 28 months after participants were randomized to receive one of three treatments: chlorthalidone, amlodipine, or lisinopril. By starting the measurements at the 6-month, the researchers aimed to avoid the initial BP changes that occur right after starting new medications, which could confound the results.

To confirm their findings, the researchers used several different statistical models and also examined alternative measures of BP variability, such as ARV and peak BP values. Consistently, higher BP variability was linked to worse kidney outcomes, even after adjusting for other factors that might influence kidney health, such as baseline eGFR, average BP levels, and the type of medication used.

Subgroup analyses reinforced the general findings, showing that the relationship between BP variability and renal outcomes held true across various segments of the population. This included individuals with different baseline levels of kidney function, those with or without diabetes, and those on different antihypertensive treatments. The consistency of these results across diverse groups strengthens the argument that BPV is a crucial factor in CKD progression [63].

The results of the extended study, up to 10.5 years after the initial BP variability assessment, merit some comment. While the trend of higher BP variability being associated with higher ESRD risk persisted, the statistical significance of this finding diminished over the extended period. This suggests that while BP variability is a significant short-to-medium-term risk factor, other factors may become more prominent over longer durations [63].

In summary, the ALLHAT study [63] provides compelling evidence that managing BP variability should be a key component of care for patients with CKD. The data indicates that stabilizing BP from one visit to the next could potentially slow the progression of kidney disease and reduce the risk of severe renal outcomes.

Knowledge Gap

Although antihypertensive treatments have the potential to lower all the different types of BPV, no study has ever addressed whether a treatment-related reduction of 24 h BP variability attenuates CV risk [64, 65]. Other drugs with BP and cardiovascular benefits, such as the iSGLT2, might also reduce BP variability but the scientific evidence is scarce [66, 67]. The same can be said for statins or glucagon-like peptide-1 (GLP-1) analogues although no study has specifically addressed the question of their effects on BPV [68, 69]. It is also difficult to isolate the potential benefit of BVP over the benefit by the overall reduction on BP levels [70, 71]. Probably, the majority of the antihypertensive drugs are able to reduce BPV albeit it can be difference among them as it has been shown in animal models [72]. CCBs like amlodipine and angiotensin II receptor blockers (ARBs) like olmesartan, especially when used in combination with other agents, have been shown to effectively reduce BPV

[70, 71]. This reduction is associated with better cardiovascular outcomes, including lower risks of stroke, heart failure, and overall mortality [17, 70], but it is still not clear if CCB can be better than others in this regard. The mechanisms behind these benefits include improved arterial compliance, reduced arterial stiffness, and enhanced autonomic regulation.

A recent study published by Gregg et al. on hypertension [73] investigated the effect of diuretics on BPV and its associations with cardiovascular outcomes The study included a large cohort of patients with CKD stages 1–5 and found consistent associations between higher BPV and increased cardiovascular risks across all stages. While diuretics were shown to attenuate the associations between high BPV and cardiovascular events, this effect was observed uniformly across the CKD spectrum, indicating no significant difference in the effect of diuretics between early and advanced CKD stages [73].

Another gap of knowledge is the lack of standardization among studies to measure or consider the presence of BPV beyond the expected normal physiological BPV. In this sense, daytime systolic SD BPV >15 mmHg, nocturnal systolic SD >12.2 mmHg, diastolic SD >7.9 mmHg, and systolic wSD >12.8 mmHg were proposed as markers of increased risk for cardiovascular events and death by the ESH position paper but only for the case of short-term BPV [17].

However, there are some issues to consider regarding short-term BPV. First, BP readings can vary significantly depending on the time of day and the devices used, leading to inconsistent results. Additionally, factors such as posture, physical activity, and diet can affect BP readings, making it challenging to assess BPV accurately based solely on these measurements.

Second, while there are positive associations between short-term BPV metrics and TOD or renal outcomes, most studies do not provide clear cutoff values for risk stratification. For instance, according to the European Society of Hypertension's position paper on BPV, specific thresholds for BPV metrics are proposed as markers for increased cardiovascular risk. However, these cutoffs are not universally accepted, and further research is necessary to determine their relevance to renal outcomes.

Third, short-term BPV only captures BP fluctuations within a 24-h period and does not account for long-term BPV. There is insufficient evidence to determine whether short-term or long-term BPV has a greater impact on kidney health, and additional research is needed to clarify this.

Lastly, the underlying mechanisms linking short-term BPV to kidney disease are not fully understood, which complicates the interpretation of study results. Despite recent studies showing an association between short-term BPV and kidney outcomes, more research is required to elucidate these mechanisms and to establish reliable predictive tools for clinical practice.

Overall, while short-term BPV shows promise as a prognostic tool for kidney disease, these unmet issues need to be addressed through further studies to enhance its clinical utility. For example, ARV, which averages the absolute differences between consecutive BP measurements, often shows a stronger association with clinical outcomes than SD or CV. In this case, the timing and order of BP measurements are crucial, especially in short-term BPV measured using 24-h ABPM [74].

The significance and comparative utility of short-term versus long-term BPV in CKD patients are not fully established. Mallamaci et al. [12] in a cohort of 402 CKD patients analyzed the relationship between these two types of BPV and the risk of death or CVE. The results indicated that long-term variability, but not short-term variability, was significantly associated with these outcomes. Specifically, an increase in long-term systolic BPV was linked to a higher risk of the composite endpoint of death or CVE. Conversely, short-term variability did not show a significant association with these outcomes when adjusted for other factors [12].

Interestingly, neither short-term nor long-term blood pressure variability significantly enhanced the prediction of risk when compared to a basic model using common clinical variables [12]. Thus, while long-term variability may be a more relevant factor for assessing risk in CKD patients, neither type of variability added substantial predictive value over traditional risk assessment methods. This suggests that while long-term variability may be a better indicator of risk, the overall utility of measuring blood pressure variability for predicting outcomes in CKD is limited.

Another unsolved issue regarding visit-to-visit BPV is if home BPV and office BPV can serve as alternative or complementary markers and its impact on CKD progression and cardiovascular outcomes [15].

As research continues to evolve, these findings underscore the importance of considering BPV as a plausible therapeutic target in CKD to optimize cardiovascular protection and patient outcomes.

11.3 Metabolic Disturbances in CKD

11.3.1 Role of Metabolic Disturbance in CKD

As it was commented in the first part of the chapter, CKD represents a situation of elevated CV risk, even in its milder stages being an independent CV risk factor (CVRF). This situation extends beyond the association with traditional CVRFs such as HTN and diabetes mellitus (DM), which are very common in these patients, many of whom are responsible for the onset of CKD itself. Furthermore, renal disease involves a series of non-traditional CVRFs, inherent to renal dysfunction [75], which gain increasing importance as the disease progresses. Among these factors are, for example, disturbances in bone-mineral metabolism (BMM), which are associated with cardiovascular calcifications and mortality, or inflammation and oxidative stress, crucial in the development of CVD in these patients. Thus, patients with CKD have a higher risk of experiencing a CV event and death than progressing to end-stage renal disease.

The spectrum of CVD varies according to the degree of renal dysfunction. In less advanced stages, atherosclerosis-related events predominate (affecting the arterial intima layer, leading to stenosis and obstructive phenomena), such as coronary artery disease, stroke, or peripheral arterial disease. As GFR decreases, non-atherosclerotic events gain importance, such as LVH, vascular calcifications, arrhythmias, or sudden cardiac death [76].

The prevalence of vascular calcification is exceedingly high in CKD and increases with the progressive decline of GFR [77, 78], being more severe and progressing faster than in the general population [78–80]. Part of the elevated CV risk in CKD is due to these calcifications, whose presence and progression are associated with a worse prognosis. There are two types of calcifications in the arterial wall, both present in CKD: intima layer calcification (atherosclerotic plaque calcification, an indicator of advanced atherosclerosis stages), typical in the aorta, coronaries, and other large elastic arteries [81], common in the general population; and media layer calcification (calcified arteriosclerosis or Mönckeberg's sclerosis), present in both large elastic arteries and especially in muscular resistance arteries [82] (typical in limb arteries), with less evidence of its association with inflammation compared to atherosclerosis, and associated with metabolic syndrome and diabetes, aging, or CKD, particularly with disturbances in calcium–phosphorus metabolism and the duration of hemodialysis [83]. Vascular calcification is now considered an active, regulated process involving various molecules.

AS is primarily caused by diffuse involvement in the arterial media layer. Calcification and arterial stiffness go hand in hand in the elevated CV risk of patients with CKD, with no clear boundaries between both processes. They are responsible for the reduction in arterial elasticity, elevation of pulse pressure (PP), and PWV [84]. Alterations in the viscoelastic properties or dimensions of the arterial wall interfere with the buffering function of the arteries (fundamental to protect the microcirculation), resulting in an increase in central BP that the heart has to confront, causing structural cardiac changes and being associated with LVH, congestive heart failure (CHF), and sudden death [85, 86].

11.3.2 Types of Metabolic Disturbances and Mechanisms Associated with CVD Risk

The progressive loss of renal mass and function leads to a decline in the kidneys' endocrine and exocrine functions, resulting in a series of complications, particularly in the more advanced stages of the disease, which are associated with CVD. The most relevant of these are:

- HTN and volume overload
- Anemia
- BMM disturbances, including hyperphosphatemia, hyperparathyroidism, and vitamin D deficiency
- Metabolic acidosis and hyperkalemia

However, even when controlling these abnormalities, the impact on reducing the CV mortality of these patients is not as significant, indicating the presence of other contributing factors to this elevated risk [75]. Among these other potential players, the following stand out:

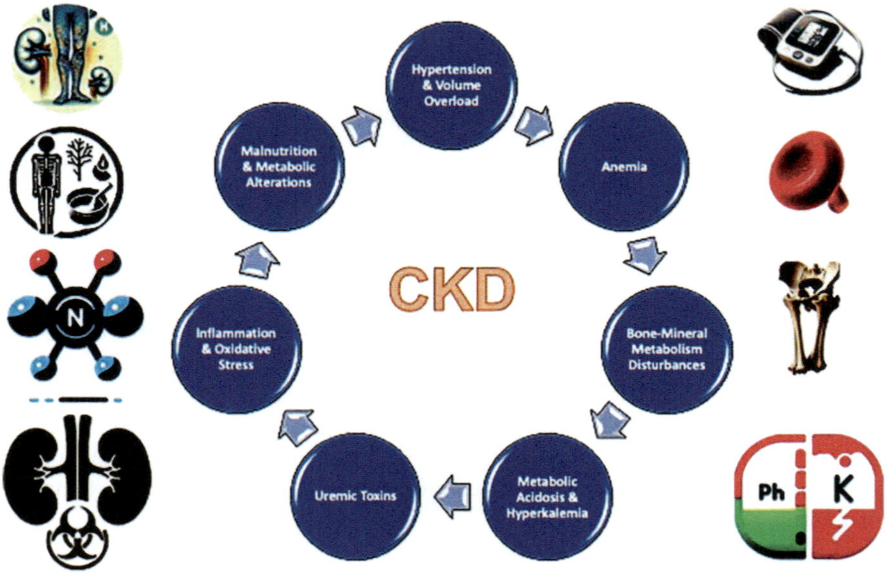
Hypertension
& Volume
Overload
Anemia
Bone-Mineral
Metabolism
Disturbances
Metabolic
Acidosis &
Hyperkalemia
Uremic Toxins
Inflammation
& Oxidative
Stress
Malnutrition
& Metabolic
Alterations
CKD
N
Ph
K

Fig. 11.6 Contributing factors to cardiovascular disease in CKD

- Uremic toxins
- Inflammation and oxidative stress

The contributing factors to cardiovascular disease in CKD are shown in Fig. 11.6. In the following sections, the main metabolic alterations involved in CVD associated with CKD will be reviewed.

11.3.2.1 Chronic Kidney Disease-Mineral and Bone Disorder (CKD-MBD)

This term, recommended by the KDIGO guidelines [78], encompasses all biochemical abnormalities, bone alterations (including bone turnover, mineralization, volume, linear growth, or strength), and extra-skeletal calcifications (including cardiovascular and other soft tissue calcifications). These changes arise due to disturbances in mineral homeostasis secondary to reduced renal function, as outlined by Torregrosa et al. [87] in the Spanish Nephrology Society's recommendations for managing CKD-MBD and described in the book "Brenner and Rector's The Kidney" by Yu et al. [88]. These alterations begin from the early stages of kidney disease and involve a tendency toward hypocalcemia, phosphorus (P) retention, and vitamin D deficiency, leading to elevated levels of parathyroid hormone (PTH) and fibroblast growth factor 23 (FGF23). The significance of CKD-MBD lies in its association with increased morbidity and mortality in these patients. Hyperphosphatemia is the most critical non-traditional cardiovascular risk factor associated with vascular calcification in patients with CKD and in the general population [89].

Key factors involved in renal regulation of P and calcium (Ca) include PTH, FGF23, Klotho, and 1,25-dihydroxyvitamin D (calcitriol). Calcitriol regulates intestinal absorption of Ca and P, renal tubular reabsorption of Ca, bone mobilization of Ca, and proliferation and differentiation of certain cell types; modulates the immune response; and affects the CV system. To perform its functions, it binds to its receptor (VDR), which is expressed in many tissues, primarily in the intestine, kidney, parathyroid, and bone [90]. Circulating calcitriol levels, which perform endocrine functions, originate from its renal synthesis through tubular hydroxylation of 25-hydroxyvitamin D (calcidiol) by the enzyme 1-alpha-hydroxylase. Calcitriol is also synthesized in other cells of the body for autocrine and paracrine functions, and this process is not hormonally regulated [87]. CKD is characterized by a deficiency and resistance to calcitriol, partly due to reduced expression of VDR [90].

FGF23 is a protein synthesized in bone osteocytes and osteoblasts, released into the blood, and functions as a hormone through activation of the FGF receptor (FGFR), requiring the co-receptor Klotho. Physiologically, it is secreted in response to phosphorus intake [91]. Its levels begin to rise in early stages of CKD, progressing as renal function worsens [90, 92, 93]. It functions at the renal level by increasing P excretion and decreasing calcitriol synthesis, and in the parathyroid gland by reducing PTH synthesis [90].

Klotho is a gene encoding a transmembrane protein (α-klotho) predominantly expressed in renal tubular cells, as well as in other tissues such as the parathyroid gland, brain, vascular tissue [94, 95], and osteocytes [96]. Discovered in 1997, it has been linked to longevity [94]. Klotho is the necessary co-receptor for FGF23 action through its binding to the FGFR, forming the FGF23–Klotho–FGFR complex [97, 98]. The extracellular domain of Klotho can be released from the membrane through proteases, being detectable in its soluble form in blood, urine, and cerebrospinal fluid [99]. Klotho exists in two forms, membrane-bound and soluble, with only the membrane-bound form functioning as a co-receptor for FGF23. The kidneys are likely the main source of soluble Klotho [94]. Soluble Klotho may have pleiotropic systemic effects independent of FGF23, such as inducing phosphaturia and tubular calcium reabsorption [98] and a probable role in vascular function and health [100].

A decline in Klotho levels has been linked to the onset of CVD [94]. In CKD, there is a deficiency of Klotho in all its forms from very early stages, with a multifactorial origin [97]: loss of renal mass, uremic toxins, ischemia, the RAAS, inflammation, or oxidative stress.

From early stages, renal function loss due to a decrease in functioning nephrons leads to reduced daily urinary P excretion, resulting in its retention [101] and a decrease in Klotho levels [98]. The decrease in urinary Klotho levels is probably the earliest detectable CKD-MBD alteration, noticeable in the earliest stages of CKD [98]. However, plasma P levels do not rise until advanced stages when the renal phosphaturic mechanisms of the residual nephrons are insufficient. The decrease in Klotho would produce resistance to FGF23 in organs (since it is the necessary co-receptor for its function), resulting in an increase in bone secretion of FGF23, which will exert its phosphaturic effect at the renal level (P excretion per nephron) to maintain plasma P levels within range, by increasing urinary fractional excretion of phosphorus or decreasing its tubular reabsorption in the proximal tubule, by reducing the expression of the tubular NaPi-II cotransporter [89, 102] as renal function worsens [101, 103]. Decreased in P tubular reabsorption are also observed from early stages of CKD, becoming significant from stage 3 [104]. FGF23, in turn, lowers PTH levels [91].

As eGFR decreases, calcitriol levels drop due to reduced availability of calcidiol at the tubular level [87] and decreased activity of 1-alpha-hydroxylase, caused by CKD itself and increased FGF23 [105] and hyperphosphatemia [106].

Circulating calcitriol activates bone secretion of FGF23, which in addition to decreasing 1-alpha-hydroxylase, increases 24-hydroxylase [107], which catabolizes both calcitriol and calcidiol. Since vitamin D induces the expression of the Klotho gene, vitamin D deficiency, as well as increased FGF23, contributes to decreased Klotho expression [98]. Calcitriol deficiency also causes hypocalcemia. Both processes, along with elevated P, stimulate PTH synthesis, leading to secondary hyperparathyroidism in CKD.

Elevated PTH acts on bone, increasing bone remodeling (releasing Ca but also P) and FGF23 secretion, and at the renal level by increasing phosphaturia (although the main burden of maintaining P homeostasis primarily falls on FGF23, which rises before PTH) [91], tubular reabsorption of Ca, and synthesis of calcitriol (thus increasing intestinal absorption of Ca but also P). With this rise in FGF23, the aim is to balance these excesses of P secondary to the process of trying to compensate for hypocalcemia, but in turn, FGF23 will lower calcitriol levels, worsening secondary hyperparathyroidism [108]. Additionally, as CKD progresses, vitamin D receptors in the parathyroid gland decrease, reducing the inhibition of vitamin D on PTH synthesis [87].

However, as CKD progresses and nephrons are lost, these compensatory mechanisms become overwhelmed and cease to be effective, leading to greater P retention and hyperphosphatemia, thus closing the cycle by producing a further increase in FGF23 and PTH, a decrease in calcitriol and Klotho [91].

Clinical Consequences of CKD-MBD

The increase in P excretion per nephron induces tubular damage and renal interstitial fibrosis [91]. Extracellular P at high concentrations is toxic to cells, inducing aging, endothelial damage, and renal injury [107, 109]. It forms insoluble nanoparticles with calcium and fetuin-A called calciprotein particles (CPPs) that can damage cells and may induce osteochondrogenic differentiation of vascular smooth muscle cells [90, 107, 109], directly contributing to cardiovascular calcifications and arterial stiffness [110, 111]. Elevated and overloaded P levels have been associated in many studies with vascular calcification, atherogenesis, parathyroid hyperplasia, loss of renal function and progression of CKD, AS, endothelial dysfunction, LVH, CVD, infections, decreased bone mass, fracture risk, and high mortality [89, 112–116], at any stage of CKD and in the general population. Therefore, MBD is considered an independent predictor of cardiovascular mortality [115, 117].

PTH has been related to the occurrence of many complications that occur in CKD [90], including hypertension, dyslipidemia, carbohydrate intolerance, LVH, left ventricular dysfunction, peripheral neuropathy, vascular calcification, and the entire spectrum of bone disease associated with CKD. As it happens with BP and risk of CHD, some studies have shown an association of very high or very low PTH levels (U-shaped curve) with mortality [118].

Also, the decrease in calcidiol and calcitriol has been associated with morbidity and mortality in CKD [119, 120].

Klotho deficiency is considered a state of premature aging, such that not only is it an early marker of renal damage, but it has also been associated with CKD progression, endothelial dysfunction, vascular calcification, uremic cardiomyopathy, and CHD [97, 121–124]. Reduced levels of soluble Klotho have shown independent predictive value for mortality [125] and have been associated with cardiovascular events [125] in the general population and in the CKD population. Therefore, klotho deficiency could be consider an independent predictor of complications and CV events in CKD [97, 126].

As it happens with klotho, FGF23, even from early stages of CKD, is also associated with increased cardiovascular risk, with independent predictive value for mortality, MACE, progression of CKD [127, 128], and increased vascular calcification [113].

In summary, CKD-MBD represents a complex interplay of metabolic, endocrine, and vascular alterations that begin in the early stages of CKD, contributing significantly to the morbidity and mortality of these patients. The identification and management of these alterations, including the correction of hyperphosphatemia, secondary hyperparathyroidism, vitamin D deficiency, and the evaluation of vascular calcifications, are fundamental in the comprehensive management of CV risk in CKD. Given their crucial roles in these processes, FGF23 Klotho, PTH, and calcitriol emerge as potential targets for therapeutic intervention.

11.3.2.2 Uremic Toxins

Uremic toxins are defined as those metabolites that accumulate in CKD due to a decrease in their clearance (and sometimes an increase in their production), affecting normal cellular and organ function, resulting in the so-called uremic syndrome (US) [129]. Their presence is associated with inflammation and oxidative stress, fundamental processes in the development of CVD in CKD patients [130]. US can be defined as the set of signs and symptoms derived from generalized organic dysfunction, due to alteration of multiple metabolic functions, which occurs in CKD as a result of the accumulation of uremic toxins [131]. The alteration of the intestinal flora observed in CKD leads to the production of some uremic toxins, which in turn have their absorption favored by the alteration of the intestinal epithelial barrier [106].

Endothelial dysfunction associated with CKD is very important in the development of atherosclerosis [132]. Atherosclerosis already begins in the early stages of CKD [76] and is characterized by an increase in oxidative stress, expression of pro-inflammatory and pro-thrombotic molecules, and a decrease in endothelial repair.

Uremic toxins could be involved in this endothelial damage [133], inducing inflammation and structural damage in endothelial cells and affecting their progenitors, as well as contributing to the pro-thrombotic state of the endothelium. Increasing data support the contribution of uremic toxins to the development and severity of CVD in CKD [130].

Uremic toxins are usually classified, based on their removal by dialysis, into [130]:

- Small water-soluble molecules (<500 Dalton): the prototype is urea. Easily removable by dialysis. Other toxins in this group are guanidines, oxalate, methylamines, polyamines, and purines.
- Protein-bound molecules: the prototype is Indoxyl sulfate. Difficult to remove by dialysis. Other toxins in this group are AGEs (advanced glycation end-products), cresols, indoles, and homocysteine.
- Middle molecules (≥500 Dalton): the prototype is β2-microglobulin. Removable by dialysis using membranes with large pores. Often expressed in response to other toxins. Other examples would be cytokines (IL-6, IL-18, TNF-α).

Small Water-Soluble Molecules

The main groups of molecules in this group that affect the largest number of systems in US are polyamines and guanidines. As individual toxins, the main ones involved would be urea and asymmetric dimethylarginine (ADMA), a type of guanidine [129]. The main consequences of the accumulation of this type of toxins are related to CVD, inflammation, and metabolic functions [129].

Urea is a marker of uremic retention and dialytic efficiency, with experimental data suggesting its possible association with endothelial damage [134], oxidative stress and inflammation [135], or insulin resistance [136], among others, but that has not been corroborated in clinical studies [137].

Guanidines are metabolites of the amino acid arginine. ADMA inhibits the synthesis of nitric oxide, leading to vasoconstriction. It also causes oxidative stress and aging of endothelial cells [138], preventing their repair [139]. ADMA has been linked to the development of hypertension, CVE and mortality [140, 141], renal fibrosis [142], and progression of kidney disease [143].

Trimethylamine-*N*-oxide (TMAO) (a methylamine) is a component of uremic biological fluids and may be associated with CVD [144]. However, fish, one of its main sources, is considered cardioprotective [145]. This apparent paradox suggests that the relationship between TMAO and cardiovascular health might be more complex than initially thought, warranting further investigation to clarify its role in CVD in the context of CKD.

Protein-Bound Molecules

This is a heterogeneous group of substances, most of which are produced in the gut [146]. The main group of these substances that affects the largest number of systems are the AGEs. As individual toxins, *p*-cresyl sulfate and indoxyl sulfate would be highlighted. The main consequences of the accumulation of this type of toxins are related to inflammation, metabolic functions, and cardiovascular damage [129].

AGEs are a group of compounds derived from the non-enzymatic glycation of proteins, lipids, and nucleic acids. In CKD, they accumulate due to decreased clearance and increased production by oxidative stress. The binding of these AGEs to their receptors leads to several processes, such as the induction of oxidative stress, inflammation, and reduction of nitric oxide, resulting in endothelial dysfunction, AS, vascular calcification, immune system dysregulation, and progression of atherosclerosis [147, 148]. AGEs also accumulate in the kidneys causing damage at this level [149] and, as a consequence, producing a greater accumulation of these products, closing a vicious circle.

p-Cresyl sulfate has shown in experimental studies to increase oxidative stress in leukocytes, exerting a pro-inflammatory effect. Additionally, in vascular wall cells, it releases endothelial microparticles as a marker of endothelial damage, induces oxidative stress in cardiomyocytes, favors their apoptosis, and leads to diastolic dysfunction [150]. Renal toxicity by *p*-cresyl sulfate has been observed at the level of tubular cells, including a decrease in Klotho production, activation of the RAAS, and expression of inflammatory cytokines, leading to kidney damage, fibrosis, and progression of CKD [150]. Clinically, it has been associated with CVE and mortality, both in dialysis and in earlier stages of CKD [151], progression of CKD [152] and pruritus in this disease [153]. It has been shown as the best independent predictor of cardiovascular and total mortality among all protein-bound uremic toxins [154].

Indoxyl sulfate is a metabolite of tryptophan. Experimental studies have observed the induction of glomerular sclerosis [155], with activation of the RAAS and suppression of Klotho synthesis, causing fibrosis [156, 157]. It has also been associated with endothelial dysfunction [158] and pro-fibrotic and pro-inflammatory effects in cardiac cells [159]. It may have implications in aortic calcification [160], PTH resistance [161], prothrombotic effect [162], or cognitive impairment [163]. Clinically, it has been seen associated with vascular damage and mortality in CKD [151, 164] and progression of CKD [152].

Medium Molecules

Unlike small molecules and protein-bound ones, which mostly originate from intestinal metabolism of food, most medium molecules are produced within the organism, as a reaction to other toxins or as compensatory mechanisms [129]. This group considers certain cytokines or PTH. The main consequences of the accumulation of these types of toxins are related to cardiovascular damage, inflammation, and fibrosis [129]. Some of these molecules are also implicated in protein energy wasting (PEW), a catabolic metabolic state of decreased body protein and energy reserves that CKD patients may suffer, primarily in advanced stages of the disease, and which is associated with morbidity and mortality [165]. The main toxins involved would be β2-microglobulin, ghrelin, leptin, PTH, IL-6, TNF-α, and FGF23 [129].

β2-Microglobulin is a component of the major histocompatibility complex class I and is one of the main constituents of amyloid deposits in the locomotor apparatus that occur in some dialysis patients. It could be related to the development of vascular disease [166] and cognitive impairment, and acts as an aging factor [167]. However, evidence is lacking to clarify its negative impact clinically, beyond renal amyloidosis and its role as a marker of clearance of medium molecules with dialysis [129].

11.3.2.3 Inflammation

CKD represents a state of chronic or recurrent systemic inflammation in the context of multiple factors, including oxidative stress [168]. For instance, ROS escaping from mitochondria, as a result of CKD and renal diseases affecting primarily the renal parenchyma such as glomerulonephritis or interstitial nephropathies, can activate the NLRP3 inflammasome (an intracellular multiprotein complex), initiating a cascade of pro-inflammatory cytokine activation [106]. Other implicated factors include the decrease in the clearance of pro-inflammatory cytokines and persistent immune stimulus (produced by metabolic acidosis, volume overload, and immune system dysfunction [106]), accumulation of uremic toxins, PEW, which appears to be both a cause and consequence of inflammation [169–171], gut dysbiosis, high incidence of infections (especially in dialysis) [172] and other comorbidities such as periodontal disease [173], factors associated with dialysis (such as exposure to dialyzer membranes, catheters, etc.) [172, 174] or maintaining a failed renal graft when returning to dialysis after a transplant [175].

Inflammation can be estimated by the determination of C-reactive protein (CRP), which is one of its most important markers. In dialysis patients, a sustained elevation of CRP has been observed in 30–60% of patients [176, 177].

An imbalance between endogenous oxidants and antioxidants, necessary for many physiological processes, leads to oxidative stress, which produces inflammation and contributes to vascular dysfunction [106]. Oxidative stress alters metabolism and produces oxidation of lipids, proteins, and nucleic acids, as well as damage at the cellular, tissue, and organ level [130]. CKD is characterized by an increase in oxidative stress, which also begins in the early stages of the disease and increases as it worsens. The involved factors are multiple and complex, but the existence of a basal inflammatory state and the associated factors discussed earlier could play a role [165]. Thus, inflammation and oxidative stress have a reciprocal relationship. In CKD, there is a high generation of ROS. The main mechanisms involved would be an increase in the activity of nicotinamide adenine dinucleotide phosphate (NADPH) oxidase, promoted among others by angiotensin II [178], xanthine oxidase (independent predictor of CV events in CKD with and without dialysis) [179], and mitochondrial dysfunction [106]. There is also a loss of antioxidants due to dietary restrictions, use of diuretics, the PEW syndrome, or intestinal malabsorption [180].

In addition to the malfunction of antioxidant agents, such as superoxide dismutases (SOD), glutathione peroxidase (GPx), or the alterations in trace elements like zinc or selenium [106], inflammation and oxidative stress play a pivotal role in the multi-organ damage caused by CKD [106]. For example, at the CV level, inflammation is considered one of the main mechanisms of atherosclerosis, which appears prematurely in CKD. Furthermore, it has been linked to atrial fibrillation, LVH, heart failure, insulin resistance, and PEW (possibly being the key element in the elevated mortality of CKD patients with this syndrome, especially in dialysis) [181] and with anemia and resistance to erythropoietin [169], potentially being a more important factor related to CV disease than LDL cholesterol [182] and one of the reasons for the high prevalence of atherosclerosis and CV morbidity and mortality in these patients [183]. Thus, the chronic elevation of CRP has been associated with endothelial dysfunction and atherosclerotic disease [184]. IL6 is considered one of the most important cytokines in the pathophysiology of inflammation in CKD [185]. Generally, the elevation of IL6 is associated with multiple pathological processes [186], including its association with atherosclerosis [187] and coronary calcification [188, 189], being one of the major risk factors for CV disease [190]. This elevation in IL6 not only correlates with these conditions but may also directly contribute to the onset and progression of cardiovascular disease in CKD patients [190].

11.3.2.4 Oxidative Stress

Oxidative stress contributes to cardiovascular damage by causing endothelial dysfunction, as an initial step toward HTN, arteriosclerosis, HF, and atherosclerosis [52, 191] through multiple mechanisms. Many markers of oxidative stress have shown their value as predictors of CVE, and even some studies with supplementation of antioxidant agents have shown promise in reducing CV risk in CKD [52, 192, 193]. It is considered one of the non-traditional risk factors for mortality in CKD [194].

Oxidative stress, as it happens with inflammation, also damage all renal structures: vasculature, glomeruli, tubules, and interstitium [106], and is involved in the progression of CKD [130]. For instance, oxidative stress promotes the contraction of vascular smooth muscle cells, worsens the synthesis of endothelial nitric oxide, induces phenotypic changes of mesangial cells toward fibroblasts and the synthesis of collagen and glomerular fibrosis, causes apoptosis of podocytes, dysfunction in tubular channels, etc. Additionally, renal regulatory mechanisms such as the tubulo-glomerular feedback, the myogenic reflex, or the RAAS are disrupted, complicating the correct maintenance of internal homeostasis as the normal management of hydroelectrolytic metabolism or acid-base balance does not function normally. In this scenario, the progression of CKD and its associated complications further exacerbate cardiovascular disease, perpetuating a cycle of worsening oxidative stress [106].

11.3.2.5 Protein-Energy Wasting (PEW) Syndrome

One of the most significant complications of CKD is the so-called MIA syndrome malnutrition–inflammation–atherosclerosis.

The importance of inflammation in CKD has been previously discussed

In 2009, the International Society of Renal Nutrition and Metabolism (ISRNM) recommended the term protein-energy wasting (PEW) syndrome to describe the nutritional situation characterized by a decline in protein and energy (primarily fats) reserves [195], affecting 28–54% of dialysis patients [196]. Unlike the general population, CKD patients, especially those on dialysis, with low weight, low blood pressure, and low total cholesterol levels have an increased incidence of CV events, a phenomenon known as reverse epidemiology [106]. Thus, overweight and obesity are associated with varying prognostic implications depending on the stage of CKD, indicating poor prognosis in stages 1–4 of the disease, yet appearing to confer a favorable prognosis in patients on hemodialysis [197]. PEW, one of the most potent predictors of total and CV mortality in CKD patients, could significantly influence this. Moreover, atherosclerosis develops markedly in patients with persistent inflammation and PEW, forming the MIA syndrome, whose components interact with each other, worsening and perpetuating the syndrome.

The pathogenesis of PEW is multifactorial. The most important causes implicated in malnutrition and PEW of these patients are shown in Table 11.3 [106, 198–200].

11.3.2.6 Insulin Resistance (IR), Hormonal, and Lipid Profile

IR can also contribute to CV risk through increased triglycerides, salt sensitivity, and the rise of uremic toxins like AGEs. Other hormonal alterations in CKD that

Table 11.3 Potential causes of the PEW syndrome

Condition	Description
Decreased intake and anorexia	Often due to loss of appetite from hormonal alterations (insulin, leptin), adipokines, inflammatory cytokines, accumulation of nitrogenous products, and uremic toxins. Also influenced by dietary restrictions, depression, sub-dialysis, or the inflammatory state
Malabsorption	Due to volume overload and thickening of the gastrointestinal mucosa
Gastroparesis	Common in CKD, it delays gastric emptying, impacting nutrient absorption and intake
Hypercatabolic state	Partly due to inflammation, contributing to increased metabolic rate and nutrient needs
Metabolic acidosis	Contributes to increased protein catabolism, resistance to many anabolic hormones, and increases the activity of catabolic corticosteroids
Oxidative stress and inflammation	Contributes to tissue damage and exacerbates metabolic imbalance in CKD
Acute and chronic comorbidities	Includes pulmonary diseases, heart failure, neoplasms, etc., which complicate management and can worsen nutritional status
Anemia	Leads to reduced oxygen transport to tissues, exacerbating fatigue and reducing physical capacity
Insulin resistance	Influenced by inflammation, oxidative stress, alterations in vitamin D metabolism, or metabolic acidosis, promoting lipid alterations such as lipolysis
Growth hormone (GH)–insulin growth factor-I (IGF-I) axis	Alterations present impacting protein synthesis and overall growth processes
Concurrent medication	Includes phosphate binders that worsen digestive absorption, affecting nutritional status
Protein loss during dialysis	Results in the loss of essential amino acids and proteins, aggravating malnutrition

may relate to increased CV disease include subclinical hypothyroidism and hypogonadism in males [165]. Another reason CKD is considered a situation of such high CV risk is due to its altered lipid profile, different from the dyslipidemia of the general population, with a higher atherogenic capacity [106, 201, 202]. It is characterized by quantitative and qualitative changes, in the context of an altered lipoprotein metabolism and oxidative stress. There is an increase in triglyceride levels due to a decrease in the catabolism of triglyceride-rich particles and an increase in their production, a decrease in HDL cholesterol levels which will also be altered and therefore dysfunctional, affecting reverse cholesterol transport, and variable levels of LDL cholesterol. Moreover, LDL particles tend to be smaller, denser, and therefore more atherogenic, with greater capacity to infiltrate the arterial intima and more susceptible to oxidation. An increase in IDL cholesterol levels and remnant chylomicrons, as well as a reduced apoC-II/apoC-III ratio, affecting the activity of lipoprotein-lipase, is also observed. The decrease in the catabolism of IDL and LDL particles would make them remain longer in the plasma, making their contained apolipoprotein B (apoB) more susceptible to changes by oxidation, carbamylation, and glycation. The triglycerides-cholesterol ratio contained in LDL and HDL particles is also increased. Levels of lipoprotein (a) are found to be higher, probably due to decreased renal clearance.

Given these complex alterations in lipid metabolism and their contribution to a heightened cardiovascular risk, it is essential for clinical management strategies in CKD patients to address these dyslipidemic profiles through targeted therapeutic approaches. These might include the use of statins or other lipid-lowering drugs, dietary interventions to manage carbohydrate metabolism and reduce triglyceride levels, and regular monitoring for hormonal imbalances that could exacerbate cardiovascular risks [203–205]. New drugs such as icosapent ethyl shows potential in reducing triglycerides effectively in patients with stage 3 chronic kidney disease who are at high cardiovascular disease risk [206]. This reduction is alongside improvements in other atherogenic and inflammatory parameters without adversely affecting low-density lipoprotein cholesterol levels. These findings underline icosapent ethyl's potential as a valuable addition to standard lipid-lowering therapies in managing elevated triglycerides at least in early stages of CKD [206]. Effective management of these metabolic disturbances is critical not only for slowing the progression of CKD but also for reducing the associated cardiovascular morbidity and mortality.

11.3.2.7 Metabolic Acidosis and Hyperkalemia

In CKD, various electrolyte disorders can occur, with hyperkalemia being among the most common and severe. Other conditions such as HF, diabetes, or treatments used in these conditions can interfere with renal mechanisms of potassium metabolism regulation, causing hyperkalemia [207]. Thus, the most significant risk factors for developing hyperkalemia are renal failure, DM, adrenal disease, and the use of angiotensin-converting enzyme (ACE) inhibitors, ARBs, or potassium-sparing diuretics [208]. The prevalence of hyperkalemia in CKD ranges from 14 to 20% [209].

Potassium is the principal intracellular cation. Its plasma concentration results from intake, elimination, and transcellular distribution. The primary route of elimination is renal, accounting for up to 80% of ingested potassium; up to 15% is eliminated via the intestines; and the remaining 5% through sweat. The kidney thus plays a fundamental role in potassium homeostasis. Several hormonal systems regulate its excretion, the most important being the RAAS and beta-adrenergic hormones, so drugs that interfere with these systems can cause potassium disorders [210]. With the decline in GFR, renal excretory mechanisms adapt, so in the absence of accompanying conditions, such as various drugs (nonsteroidal anti-inflammatory drugs, RAAS inhibitors, etc.), tissue lysis, or situations of hypoaldosteronism (like the hyporeninemic hypoaldosteronism that can occur in diabetes), hyperkalemia is not usually seen until CKD is very advanced, with GFR below 15 mL/min. The odds of hyperkalemia double for every 15 mL/min decrease in GFR [211].

Alterations in potassium concentration, both hypo and hyperkalemia, can cause alterations in cell membrane polarization leading to complications as severe as cardiac arrhythmias or sudden death [207]. Thus, the risk of adverse events related to potassium alterations (all-cause mortality, CV mortality, and end-stage renal disease) follows a U-shaped curve, with the lowest risk situated in the potassium range of 4–4.5 mmol/L [211]. Following a severe hyperkalemia episode, hyperkalemia can recur, and the evolution of potassium levels after such an event can predict mortality risk [212]. The most likely mechanism by which hyperkalemia could relate to mortality would be through the induction of lethal cardiac arrhythmias.

Metabolic acidosis is one of the complications of CKD, whose prevalence and severity increase as GFR decreases. Indeed, CKD is the main cause of chronic metabolic acidosis, as its function in maintaining acid-base balance fails [213]. It is caused by the dysfunction of the renal mechanism of ammonium and organic acids excretion and the decrease in bicarbonate reabsorption and production [214, 215]. The retained acids are buffered by bicarbonate in the extracellular fluid, by tissue buffers, and by bone, until renal failure is such that metabolic acidosis occurs. It usually begins to be observed with GFR below 40 mL/min [216]. Its significance lies in the cellular dysfunction that acid accumulation causes in many tissues. Thus, it has been associated with, bone demineralization, increased protein catabolism with loss of muscle mass, protein malnutrition, hypoalbuminemia, inflammation, alterations in insulin, leptin, and GH, worsening of secondary hyperparathyroidism, progression of CKD, deterioration of cardiac function, MACE, and increased mortality, among others [213, 216]. The use of bicarbonate could be associated with the reduction of cardiovascular events and mortality as well as the progression of CKD [215, 217]. By addressing acidosis, not only can the progression of CKD be potentially slowed, but also the quality of life for patients can be significantly improved by alleviating associated complications such as muscle wasting and bone disease [215, 217]. Similarly, managing potassium levels is crucial due to its strong correlation with cardiovascular health. Strategies to control hyperkalemia include dietary potassium restriction, the use of potassium-binding agents, and careful adjustment of medications that affect potassium levels, such as RAAS inhibitors. These interventions are vital to prevent the life-threatening complications of altered potassium levels, particularly the risk of cardiac arrhythmias, which can lead to sudden death [212].

11.3.3 Overview of Metabolic Disturbance in CKD

CKD represents a situation of high/very high CVD risk, being considered an independent CVRF. This is due to the confluence of a multitude of traditional and non-traditional CVRFs, inherent to kidney disease, resulting from the progressive loss of renal mass and function.

There is a higher risk in this population of suffering a mortal and non-mortal CV event than progressing to end stages of the disease.

Alterations in BMM are one of the complications of CKD most associated with morbidity and mortality. They are characterized by a tendency toward hypocalcemia, P retention, and vitamin D deficiency, with elevated PTH and FGF23 levels, decreased Klotho levels, bone disorders, and extra-skeletal calcifications.

The accumulation of uremic toxins in CKD is associated with inflammation, oxidative stress, and endothelial dysfunction, contributing to the development of CV damage.

CKD represents a state of chronic or recurrent systemic inflammation in the context of multiple factors, including oxidative stress, also characteristic of this disease from the early stages. Both processes, inflammation and oxidative stress, are highly involved in the CV damage of CKD and in the CKD progression. IL6 is considered one of the most important cytokines in CKD inflammation, potentially playing a causal role in CV damage.

PEW syndrome is one of the strongest predictors of total and CV mortality in patients with CKD, being associated with inflammation and atherosclerosis. Its origin is multifactorial. The dyslipidemia of CKD is highly atherogenic, characterized by an increase in triglycerides and lipoprotein (a), decrease in HDL-cholesterol levels, and variable levels of LDL-cholesterol, accompanied by qualitative alterations in all these particles making them more harmful.

Hyperkalemia is the most serious electrolyte disorder that can occur in CKD, due to its mortality risk. DM or cardiorenal protective treatments can promote its occurrence. CKD is the main cause of chronic metabolic acidosis, which is associated with cellular dysfunction at multiple levels, having been linked with CV events and mortality.

11.4 Conclusion

CKD markedly elevates cardiovascular risk through mechanisms such as BP circadian variability and various metabolic disturbances. These factors interplay to form a complex risk profile, necessitating comprehensive management strategies for CKD patients.

11.4.1 Blood Pressure Circadian/Non-circadian Variability

CKD patients frequently exhibit abnormal BP circadian patterns, such as non-dipping or nocturnal hypertension, which are associated with increased cardiovascular mortality. The use of ABPM is recommended to detect these abnormalities, as they often cannot be identified through office or home BP measurements alone. Abnormal BP patterns in CKD are influenced by several factors, including sodium retention, AS, and altered baroreflex sensitivity. These variations contribute to the overall cardiovascular risk by exacerbating conditions like LVH and atherosclerosis.

11.4.2 Metabolic Disturbances

Metabolic disturbances in CKD include dysregulation in BMM, leading to vascular calcifications, and conditions such as PEW syndrome, which are closely linked to systemic inflammation and oxidative stress. The CKD dyslipidemia, characterized by elevated triglycerides and altered lipoprotein profiles, significantly contributes to cardiovascular disease progression. Additionally, electrolyte imbalances like hyperkalemia and chronic metabolic acidosis further exacerbate the cardiovascular burden in CKD patients.

11.4.3 Clinical Implications and Future Directions

Understanding the dual impact of BPV and metabolic disturbances highlights the necessity for targeted therapeutic interventions. Optimizing BP control through regular monitoring and individualized treatment plans, along with addressing metabolic disturbances through dietary modifications and appropriate pharmacotherapy, can significantly reduce cardiovascular risk in CKD patients. Future research should focus on elucidating the precise mechanisms linking these factors to cardiovascular outcomes and developing robust predictive tools for better clinical management. Moreover, establishing uniform definitions, employing stringent methodology, and conducting rigorous clinical trials are crucial to definitively determine whether modifications of BPV or metabolic factors can reduce CVE in patients with CKD and to what extent.

Overall, the interplay between BP circadian variability and metabolic disturbances underscores the importance of a comprehensive approach in managing CKD to improve cardiovascular outcomes and enhance patient quality of life.

The summary of the chapter is graphically represented in Fig. 11.7.

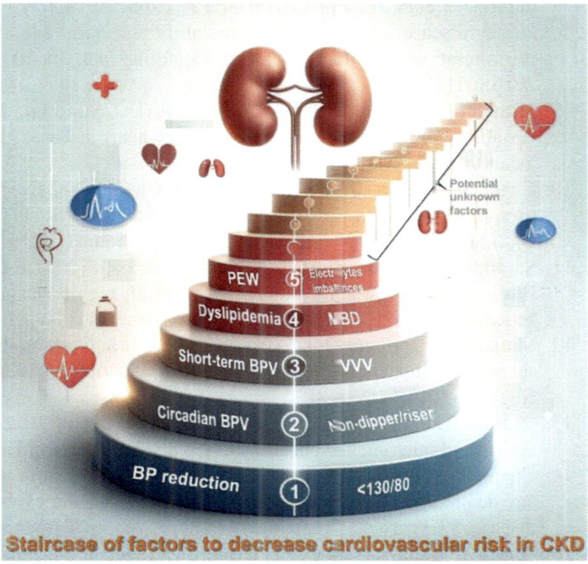

Fig. 11.7 Staircase to cardiovascular health: systematic strategies for reducing cardiovascular risk in chronic kidney disease

References

1. Tonelli M, Wiebe N, Culleton B, House A, Rabbat C, Fok M, et al. Chronic kidney disease and mortality risk: a systematic review. J Am Soc Nephrol. 2006;17:2034–47.
2. Sarnak MJ, Levey AS, Schoolwerth AC, Coresh J, Culleton B, Hamm LL, et al. Kidney disease as a risk factor for development of cardiovascular disease: a statement from the American Heart Association councils on kidney in cardiovascular disease, high blood pressure research, clinical cardiology, and epidemiology and prevention. Circulation. 2003;108:2154–69.
3. Mancia G, Kreutz R, Brunström M, Burnier M, Grassi G, Januszewicz A, et al. 2023 ESH guidelines for the management of arterial hypertension the task force for the management of arterial hypertension of the European Society of Hypertension Endorsed by the European renal association (ERA) and the International Society of Hypertension (ISH). J Hypertens. 2024;41:1874–2071.
4. Mancia G, Facchetti R, Bombelli M, Quarti-Trevano F, Cuspidi C, Grassi G. Short- and long-term reproducibility of nighttime blood pressure phenotypes and nocturnal blood pressure reduction. Hypertension. 2021;77:1745–55.
5. Mancia G, Facchetti R, Cuspidi C, Bombelli M, Corrao G, Grassi G. Limited reproducibility of MUCH and WUCH: evidence from the ELSA study. Eur Heart J. 2020;41:1565–71.
6. Pickering TG, Davidson K, Gerin W, Schwartz JE. Masked hypertension. Hypertension. 2002;40:795–6.
7. Pogue V, Rahman M, Lipkowitz M, Toto R, Miller E, Faulkner M, et al. Disparate estimates of hypertension control from ambulatory and clinic blood pressure measurements in hypertensive kidney disease. Hypertension. 2009;53:20–7.

8. Parati G, Ochoa JE, Bilo G, Agarwal R, Covic A, Dekker FW, et al. Hypertension in chronic kidney disease part 2: role of ambulatory and home blood pressure monitoring for assessing alterations in blood pressure variability and blood pressure profiles. Hypertension. 2016;67:1102–10.
9. Muntner P, Whittle J, Lynch AI, Colantonio LD, Simpson LM, Einhorn PT, et al. Visit-to-visit variability of blood pressure and coronary heart disease, stroke, heart failure, and mortality: a cohort study. Ann Intern Med. 2015;163:329–38.
10. Chang TI, Reboussin DM, Chertow GM, Cheung AK, Cushman WC, Kostis WJ, et al. Visit-to-visit office blood pressure variability and cardiovascular outcomes in SPRINT (Systolic Blood Pressure Intervention Trial). Hypertension. 2017;70:751–8.
11. Sarafidis PA, Ruilope LM, Loutradis C, Gorostidi M, De La Sierra A, De La Cruz JJ, et al. Blood pressure variability increases with advancing chronic kidney disease stage: a cross-sectional analysis of 16,546 hypertensive patients. J Hypertens. 2018;36:1076–85.
12. Mallamaci F, Tripepi G, D'Arrigo G, Borrelli S, Garofalo C, Stanzione G, et al. Blood pressure variability, mortality, and cardiovascular outcomes in CKD patients. Clin J Am Soc Nephrol. 2019;14:233–40.
13. Di Iorio B, Pota A, Sirico ML, Torraca S, Di Micco L, Rubino R, et al. Blood pressure variability and outcomes in chronic kidney disease. Nephrol Dial Transplant. 2012;27:4404–10.
14. Chang TI, Tabada GH, Yang J, Tan TC, Go AS. Visit-to-visit variability of blood pressure and death, end-stage renal disease, and cardiovascular events in patients with chronic kidney disease. J Hypertens. 2016;34:244–52.
15. Okada T, Wada T, Nagaoka Y, Kanno Y. Association between visit-to-visit clinic blood pressure variability and home blood pressure variability in patients with chronic kidney disease. Ren Fail. 2015;37:446–51.
16. Borrelli S, Garofalo C, Mallamaci F, Tripepi G, Stanzione G, Provenzano M, et al. Short-term blood pressure variability in nondialysis chronic kidney disease patients: correlates and prognostic role on the progression of renal disease. J Hypertens. 2018;36:2398–405.
17. Parati G, Bilo G, Kollias A, Pengo M, Ochoa JE, Castiglioni P, et al. Blood pressure variability: methodological aspects, clinical relevance and practical indications for management—a European Society of Hypertension position paper*. J Hypertens. 2023;41:527–44.
18. Bakkar NMZ, El-Yazbi AF, Zouein FA, Fares SA. Beat-to-beat blood pressure variability: an early predictor of disease and cardiovascular risk. J Hypertens. 2021;39:830–45.
19. Mancia G, Bombelli M, Facchetti R, Madotto F, Corrao G, Trevano FQ, et al. Long-term prognostic value of blood pressure variability in the general population: results of the Pressioni Arteriose Monitorate e Loro Associazioni study. Hypertension. 2007;49:1265–70.
20. Castiglioni P, Parati G, Di Rienzo M, Carabalona R, Cividjian A, Quintin L. Scale exponents of blood pressure and heart rate during autonomic blockade as assessed by detrended fluctuation analysis. J Physiol. 2011;589:355–69.
21. Gibson LE, Henriques TS, Costa MD, Davis RB, Mittleman MA, Mathur P, et al. Comparison of invasive and noninvasive blood pressure measurements for assessing signal complexity and surgical risk in cardiac surgical patients. Anesth Analg. 2020;130:1653–60.
22. Bilo G, Giglio A, Styczkiewicz K, Caldara G, Maronati A, Kawecka-Jaszcz K, et al. A new method for assessing 24-h blood pressure variability after excluding the contribution of nocturnal blood pressure fall. J Hypertens. 2007;25:2058–66.
23. Rothwell PM, Howard SC, Dolan E, O'Brien E, Dobson JE, Dahlöf B, et al. Prognostic significance of visit-to-visit variability, maximum systolic blood pressure, and episodic hypertension. Lancet. 2010;375:895–905.
24. Mena LJ, Felix VG, Melgarejo JD, Maestre GE. 24-hour blood pressure variability assessed by average real variability: a systematic review and meta-analysis. J Am Heart Assoc. 2017;6:e006895.
25. Manios E, Stamatelopoulos K, Tsivgoulis G, Barlas G, Koroboki E, Tsagalis G, et al. Time rate of blood pressure variation: a new factor associated with coronary atherosclerosis. J Hypertens. 2011;29:1109–14.

26. Kario K. Morning surge in blood pressure and cardiovascular risk: evidence and perspectives. Hypertension. 2010;56:765–73.
27. Stergiou GS, Mastorantonakis SE, Roussias LG. Morning blood pressure surge: the reliability of different definitions. Hypertens Res. 2008;31:1589–94.
28. Bursztyn M, Mekler J, Wachtel N, Ben-Ishay D. Siesta and ambulatory blood pressure monitoring comparability of the afternoon nap and night sleep. Am J Hypertens. 1994;7:217–21.
29. Tabara Y, Okada Y, Uetani E, Nagai T, Igase M, Kido T, et al. Postprandial hypotension as a risk marker for asymptomatic lacunar infarction. J Hypertens. 2014;32:1084–90.
30. Hong K, Muntner P, Kronish I, Shilane D, Chang TI. Medication adherence and visit-to-visit variability of systolic blood pressure in African Americans with chronic kidney disease in the AASK trial. J Hum Hypertens. 2016;30:73–8.
31. Murphy D, Drawz PE. Blood pressure variability in CKD: treatable or hypertension's homocysteine? Clin J Am Soc Nephrol. 2019;14:175–7.
32. Clark LA, Denby L, Pregibon D, Harshfield GA, Pickering TG, Blank S, et al. A quantitative analysis of the effects of activity and time of day on the diurnal variations of blood pressure. J Chronic Dis. 1987;40:671–81.
33. Somers VK, Dyken ME, Mark AL, Abboud FM. Sympathetic-nerve activity during sleep in normal subjects. N Engl J Med. 1993;328:303–7.
34. Sundberg S, Kohvakka A, Gordin A. Rapid reversal of circadian blood pressure rhythm in shift workers. J Hypertens. 1988;6:393–6.
35. Chau NP, Mallion JM, De Gaudemaris R, Ruche E, Siche JP, Pelen O, et al. Twenty-four-hour ambulatory blood pressure in shift workers. Circulation. 1989;80:341–7.
36. Sternberg H, Rosenthal T, Shamiss A, Green M. Altered circadian rhythm of blood pressure in shift workers. J Hum Hypertens. 1995;9:349–53.
37. Weitzman ED, Fukushima D, Nogeire C, Roffwarg H, Gallagher TF, Hellman L. Twenty-four hour pattern of the episodic secretion of cortisol in normal subjects. J Clin Endocrinol Metab. 1971;33:14–22.
38. Panza JA, Epstein SE, Quyyumi AA. Circadian variation in vascular tone and its relation to α-sympathetic vasoconstrictor activity. N Engl J Med. 1991;325:986–90.
39. Stern N, Sowers JR, McGinty D, Beahm E, Littner M, Catania R, et al. Circadian rhythm of plasma renin activity in older normal and essential hypertensive men: relation with inactive renin, aldosterone, cortisol and REM sleep. J Hypertens. 1986;4:543–50.
40. Borrelli S, Provenzano M, Gagliardi I, Michael A, Liberti M, De Nicola L, et al. Sodium intake and chronic kidney disease. Int J Mol Sci. 2020;21:4744.
41. Cai W, Lang M, Jiang X, Yu Q, Zhou C, Zou W, et al. Correlation among high salt intake, blood pressure variability, and target organ damage in patients with essential hypertension: study protocol clinical trial (SPIRIT compliant). Medicine (Baltimore). 2020;99:e19548.
42. Pathak CM, Ix JH, Anderson CAM, Woodell TB, Smits G, Persky MS, et al. Variation in sodium intake and intra-individual change in blood pressure in chronic kidney disease. J Ren Nutr. 2018;28:125–8.
43. Salman IM, Hildreth CM, Ameer OZ, Phillips JK. Differential contribution of afferent and central pathways to the development of baroreflex dysfunction in chronic kidney disease. Hypertension. 2014;63:804–10.
44. Tomiyama O, Shiigai T, Ideura T, Tomita K, Mito Y, Shinohara S, et al. Baroreflex sensitivity in renal failure. Clin Sci. 1980;58:21–7.
45. Johansson M, Gao S, Friberg P, Annerstedt M, Bergstrom G, Carlstrom J, et al. Reduced baroreflex effectiveness index in hypertensive patients with chronic renal failure. Am J Hypertens. 2005;18:995–1000.
46. Dhaun N, Moorhouse R, MacIntyre IM, Melville V, Oosthuyzen W, Kimmitt RA, et al. Diurnal variation in blood pressure and arterial stiffness in chronic kidney disease: the role of endothelin-1. Hypertension. 2014;64:296–304.
47. Park CH, Kim HW, Park JT, Chang TI, Yoo TH, Park SK, et al. Bidirectional association between SBP variability and arterial stiffness in patients with chronic kidney disease: findings from KNOW-CKD study. J Hypertens. 2023;41:90–8.

48. Ishiyama Y, Hoshide S, Kanegae H, Kario K. Increased arterial stiffness amplifies the association between home blood pressure variability and cardiac overload: the J-HOP study. Hypertension. 2020;75:1600–6.
49. Miyauchi S, Nagai M, Dote K, Kato M, Oda N, Kunita E, et al. Visit-to-visit blood pressure variability and arterial stiffness: which came first: the chicken or the egg? Curr Pharm Des. 2019;25:685–92.
50. Zhou TL, Henry RMA, Stehouwer CDA, Van Sloten TT, Reesink KD, Kroon AA. Blood pressure variability, arterial stiffness, and arterial remodeling: the Maastricht study. Hypertension. 2018;72:1002–10.
51. Townsend RR. Arterial stiffness in CKD: a review. Am J Kidney Dis. 2019;73:240–7.
52. Daenen K, Andries A, Mekahli D, Van Schepdael A, Jouret F, Bammens B. Oxidative stress in chronic kidney disease. Pediatr Nephrol. 2019;34:975–91.
53. Vida C, Oliva C, Yuste C, Ceprián N, Caro PJ, Valera G, et al. Oxidative stress in patients with advanced CKD and renal replacement therapy: the key role of peripheral blood leukocytes. Antioxidants. 2021;10:1155.
54. Dounousi E, Papavasiliou E, Makedou A, Ioannou K, Katopodis KP, Tselepis A, et al. Oxidative stress is progressively enhanced with advancing stages of CKD. Am J Kidney Dis. 2006;48:752–60.
55. Chen Z, Jiang X, Wu J, Lin L, Zhou Z, Li M, et al. Association between short-term blood pressure variability and target organ damage in non-dialysis patients with chronic kidney disease. BMC Nephrol. 2024;25:111.
56. Yang L, Li J, Wei W, Pu Y, Zhang L, Cui T, et al. Blood pressure variability and the progression of chronic kidney disease: a systematic review and meta-analysis. J Gen Intern Med. 2023;38:1272–81.
57. Li H, Xue J, Dai W, Chen Y, Zhou Q, Chen W. Visit-to-visit blood pressure variability and risk of chronic kidney disease: a systematic review and meta-analysis. PLoS One. 2020;15:e0233233.
58. Park CH, Kim HW, Joo YS, Park JT, Chang TI, Yoo T, et al. Association between systolic blood pressure variability and major adverse cardiovascular events in Korean patients with chronic kidney disease: findings from KNOW-CKD. J Am Heart Assoc. 2022;11:e025513.
59. Yuan Y, Liu M, Zhang S, Lin Y, Huang Y, Zhou H, et al. Effect of blood pressure index on clinical outcomes in patients with heart failure and chronic kidney disease. ESC Heart Fail. 2023;10:3330–9.
60. Wang G, Ma K, Ma Z, Guo X, Wang Y, Ma L, et al. Short-term blood pressure variability and outcomes in non-dialysis chronic kidney disease. Front Med. 2022;9:911205.
61. Jhee JH, Oh D, Seo J, Lee CJ, Chung MY, Park JT, et al. Short-term blood pressure variability and incident CKD in patients with hypertension: findings from the Cardiovascular and Metabolic Disease Etiology Research Center–High Risk (CMERC-HI) study. Am J Kidney Dis. 2023;81:384–93.
62. Tanner RM, Shimbo D, Dreisbach AW, Carson AP, Fox ER, Muntner P. Association between 24-h blood pressure variability and chronic kidney disease: a cross-sectional analysis of African Americans participating in the Jackson heart study. BMC Nephrol. 2015;16:84.
63. Whittle J, Lynch AI, Tanner RM, Simpson LM, Davis BR, Rahman M, et al. Visit-to-visit variability of BP and CKD outcomes: results from the ALLHAT. Clin J Am Soc Nephrol. 2016;11:471–80.
64. Bertera FM, Del Mauro JS, Lovera V, Chiappetta D, Héctor Polizio A, Alberto Taira C, et al. Acute effects of third generation β-blockers on short-term and beat-to-beat blood pressure variability in sinoaortic-denervated rats. Hypertens Res. 2013;36:349–55.
65. Frattola A, Parati G, Castiglioni P, Paleari F, Ulian L, Rovaris G, et al. Lacidipine and blood pressure variability in diabetic hypertensive patients. Hypertension. 2000;36:622–8.
66. Cherney DZ, Perkins BA, Soleymanlou N, Har R, Fagan N, Johansen O, et al. The effect of empagliflozin on arterial stiffness and heart rate variability in subjects with uncomplicated type 1 diabetes mellitus. Cardiovasc Diabetol. 2014;13:28.

67. Solini A, Giannini L, Seghieri M, Vitolo E, Taddei S, Ghiadoni L, et al. Dapagliflozin acutely improves endothelial dysfunction, reduces aortic stiffness and renal resistive index in type 2 diabetic patients: a pilot study. Cardiovasc Diabetol. 2017;16:138.
68. Ohara M, Kohata Y, Nagaike H, Koshibu M, Gima H, Hiromura M, et al. Association of glucose and blood pressure variability on oxidative stress in patients with type 2 diabetes mellitus and hypertension: a cross-sectional study. Diabetol Metab Syndr. 2019;11:29.
69. Baber U, Halperin JL. Variability in low-density lipoprotein cholesterol and cardiovascular risk. J Am Coll Cardiol. 2015;65:1549–51.
70. Omboni S, Kario K, Bakris G, Parati G. Effect of antihypertensive treatment on 24-h blood pressure variability: pooled individual data analysis of ambulatory blood pressure monitoring studies based on olmesartan mono or combination treatment. J Hypertens. 2018;36:720–33.
71. Kollias A, Stergiou GS, Kyriakoulis KG, Bilo G, Parati G. Treating visit-to-visit blood pressure variability to improve prognosis: is amlodipine the drug of choice? Hypertension. 2017;70:862–6.
72. Wang J, Shen F, Wang MW, Su DF. Effects of nine antihypertensive drugs on blood pressure variability in sinoaortic-denervated rats. Acta Pharmacol Sin. 2005;27:1013–7.
73. Gregg LP, Hedayati SS, Yang H, Van Buren PN, Banerjee S, Navaneethan SD, et al. Association of Blood Pressure Variability and Diuretics with Cardiovascular Events in patients with chronic kidney disease stages 1–5. Hypertension. 2021;77:948–59.
74. Hernandez MF, Chang TI. The need to reduce variability in the study of blood pressure variability. Am J Kidney Dis. 2023;81:379–81.
75. Liu M, Li XC, Lu L, Cao Y, Sun RR, Chen S, et al. Cardiovascular disease and its relationship with chronic kidney disease. Eur Rev Med Pharmacol Sci. 2014;18:2918–26.
76. Wanner C, Amann K, Shoji T. The heart and vascular system in dialysis. Lancet. 2016;388:276–84.
77. Temmar M, Liabeuf S, Renard C, Czernichow S, Esper NE, Shahapuni I, et al. Pulse wave velocity and vascular calcification at different stages of chronic kidney disease. J Hypertens. 2010;28:163–9.
78. Eckardt KU, Kasiske BL. Foreword. Kidney Int. 2009;76:S1–2.
79. Braun J, Oldendorf M, Moshage W, Heidler R, Zeitler E, Luft FC. Electron beam computed tomography in the evaluation of cardiac calcifications in chronic dialysis patients. Am J Kidney Dis. 1996;27:394–401.
80. Kestenbaum BR, Adeney KL, De Boer IH, Ix JH, Shlipak MG, Siscovick DS. Incidence and progression of coronary calcification in chronic kidney disease: the multi-ethnic study of atherosclerosis. Kidney Int. 2009;76:991–8.
81. Coll B, Betriu A, Martínez-Alonso M, Amoedo ML, Arcidiacono MV, Borras M, et al. Large artery calcification on dialysis patients is located in the intima and related to atherosclerosis. Clin J Am Soc Nephrol. 2011;6:303–10.
82. Adragao T, Pires A, Lucas C, Birne R, Magalhaes L, Goncalves M, et al. A simple vascular calcification score predicts cardiovascular risk in haemodialysis patients. Nephrol Dial Transplant. 2004;19:1480–8.
83. Lanzer P, Boehm M, Sorribas V, Thiriet M, Janzen J, Zeller T, et al. Medial vascular calcification revisited: review and perspectives. Eur Heart J. 2014;35:1515–25.
84. Schlieper G, Schurgers L, Brandenburg V, Reutelingsperger C, Floege J. Vascular calcification in chronic kidney disease: an update. Nephrol Dial Transplant. 2016;31:31–9.
85. Briet M, Boutouyrie P, Laurent S, London GM. Arterial stiffness and pulse pressure in CKD and ESRD. Kidney Int. 2012;82:388–400.
86. Chue CD, Townend JN, Steeds RP, Ferro CJ. Arterial stiffness in chronic kidney disease: causes and consequences. Heart. 2010;96:817–23.
87. Torregrosa JV, Bover J, Rodríguez Portillo M, González Parra E, Arenas MD, Caravaca F, et al. Recomendaciones de la Sociedad Española de Nefrología para el manejo de las alteraciones del metabolismo óseo-mineral en los pacientes con enfermedad renal crónica: 2021 (SEN-MM). Nefrologia. 2022;42:1–37.

88. AXÓN. Brenner and rector's the kidney, vol. 2. https://axon.es/ficha/libros/9780323532655/brenner-and-rector-s-the-kidney-2-vols-print-online.
89. Cannata-Andía JB, Martin KJ. The challenge of controlling phosphorus in chronic kidney disease. Nephrol Dial Transplant. 2016;31:541–7.
90. Evenepoel P, Rodriguez M, Ketteler M. Laboratory abnormalities in CKD-MBD: markers, predictors, or mediators of disease? Semin Nephrol. 2014;34:151–63.
91. Kuro-o M. The klotho proteins in health and disease. Nat Rev Nephrol. 2019;15:27–44.
92. Gutierrez O, Isakova T, Rhee E, Shah A, Holmes J, Collerone G, et al. Fibroblast growth factor-23 mitigates hyperphosphatemia but accentuates calcitriol deficiency in chronic kidney disease. J Am Soc Nephrol. 2005;16:2205–15.
93. Hruska KA, Seifert M, Sugatani T. Pathophysiology of the chronic kidney disease—mineral bone disorder. Curr Opin Nephrol Hypertens. 2015;24:303–9.
94. Donate-Correa J. Klotho in cardiovascular disease: current and future perspectives. World J Biol Chem. 2015;6:351–7.
95. Donate-Correa J, Mora-Fernández C, Martínez-Sanz R, Muros-de-Fuentes M, Pérez H, Meneses-Pérez B, et al. Expression of FGF23/KLOTHO system in human vascular tissue. Int J Cardiol. 2013;165:179–83.
96. Komaba H, Kaludjerovic J, Hu DZ, Nagano K, Amano K, Ide N, et al. Klotho expression in osteocytes regulates bone metabolism and controls bone formation. Kidney Int. 2017;92:599–611.
97. Hu MC, Kuro-o M, Moe OW. Klotho and chronic kidney disease. Contrib Nephrol. 2013;180:47–63.
98. John GB, Cheng CY, Kuro-o M. Role of klotho in aging, phosphate metabolism, and CKD. Am J Kidney Dis. 2011;58:127–34.
99. Olauson H, Vervloet MG, Cozzolino M, Massy ZA, Ureña Torres P, Larsson TE. New insights into the FGF23-klotho axis. Semin Nephrol. 2014;34:586–97.
100. Lewin E, Olgaard K. The vascular secret of klotho. Kidney Int. 2015;87:1089–91.
101. Craver L, Marco MP, Martinez I, Rue M, Borras M, Martin ML, et al. Mineral metabolism parameters throughout chronic kidney disease stages 1–5—achievement of K/DOQI target ranges. Nephrol Dial Transplant. 2007;22:1171–6.
102. Nitta K, Nagano N, Tsuchiya K. Fibroblast growth factor 23/klotho axis in chronic kidney disease. Nephron Clin Pract. 2014;128:1–10.
103. Slatopolsky E. The intact nephron hypothesis: the concept and its implications for phosphate management in CKD-related mineral and bone disorder. Kidney Int. 2011;79:S3–8.
104. Hong YA, Lim JH, Kim MY, Kim Y, Yang KS, Chung BH, et al. Assessment of tubular reabsorption of phosphate as a surrogate marker for phosphate regulation in chronic kidney disease. Clin Exp Nephrol. 2015;19:208–15.
105. Hasegawa H, Nagano N, Urakawa I, Yamazaki Y, Iijima K, Fujita T, et al. Direct evidence for a causative role of FGF23 in the abnormal renal phosphate handling and vitamin D metabolism in rats with early-stage chronic kidney disease. Kidney Int. 2010;78:975–80.
106. Podkowińska A, Formanowicz D. Chronic kidney disease as oxidative stress- and inflammatory-mediated cardiovascular disease. Antioxidants. 2020;9:752.
107. Kuro-o M. Phosphate and klotho. Kidney Int. 2011;79:S20–3.
108. Rodríguez M, López I, Muñoz J, Aguilera-Tejero E, Almaden Y. FGF23 and mineral metabolism, implications in CKD-MBD. Nefrologia. 2012;32:275–8.
109. Kuro-o M. A phosphate-centric paradigm for pathophysiology and therapy of chronic kidney disease. Kidney Int Suppl. 2013;3:420–6.
110. Paloian NJ, Giachelli CM. A current understanding of vascular calcification in CKD. Am J Physiol Ren Physiol. 2014;307:F891–900.
111. Kendrick J, Ix JH, Targher G, Smits G, Chonchol M. Relation of serum phosphorus levels to ankle brachial pressure index (from the Third National Health and Nutrition Examination Survey). Am J Cardiol. 2010;106:564–8.
112. Hruska K, Mathew S, Lund R, Fang Y, Sugatani T. Cardiovascular risk factors in chronic kidney disease: does phosphate qualify? Kidney Int. 2011;79:S9–13.

113. Adeney KL, Siscovick DS, Ix JH, Seliger SL, Shlipak MG, Jenny NS, et al. Association of serum phosphate with vascular and valvular calcification in moderate CKD. J Am Soc Nephrol. 2009;20:381–7.
114. Foley RN, Collins AJ, Herzog CA, Ishani A, Kalra PA. Serum phosphorus levels associate with coronary atherosclerosis in young adults. J Am Soc Nephrol. 2009;20:397–404.
115. Block GA, Klassen PS, Lazarus JM, Ofsthun N, Lowrie EG, Chertow GM. Mineral metabolism, mortality, and morbidity in maintenance hemodialysis. J Am Soc Nephrol. 2004;15:2208–18.
116. Betriu A, Martinez-Alonso M, Arcidiacono MV, Cannata-Andia J, Pascual J, Valdivielso JM, et al. Prevalence of subclinical atheromatosis and associated risk factors in chronic kidney disease: the NEFRONA study. Nephrol Dial Transplant. 2014;29:1415–22.
117. Uribarri J. Phosphorus metabolism and management in chronic kidney disease: phosphorus homeostasis in normal health and in chronic kidney disease patients with special emphasis on dietary phosphorus intake. Semin Dial. 2007;20:295–301.
118. Floege J, Kim J, Ireland E, Chazot C, Drueke T, De Francisco A, et al. Serum iPTH, calcium and phosphate, and the risk of mortality in a European haemodialysis population. Nephrol Dial Transplant. 2011;26:1948–55.
119. Drechsler C, Verduijn M, Pilz S, Dekker FW, Krediet RT, Ritz E, et al. Vitamin D status and clinical outcomes in incident dialysis patients: results from the NECOSAD study. Nephrol Dial Transplant. 2011;26:1024–32.
120. Wolf M, Shah A, Gutierrez O, Ankers E, Monroy M, Tamez H, et al. Vitamin D levels and early mortality among incident hemodialysis patients. Kidney Int. 2007;72:1004–13.
121. Hu MC, Shi M, Zhang J, Quiñones H, Griffith C, Kuro-o M, et al. Klotho deficiency causes vascular calcification in chronic kidney disease. J Am Soc Nephrol. 2011;22:124–36.
122. Xie J, Yoon J, An SW, Kuro-o M, Huang CL. Soluble klotho protects against uremic cardiomyopathy independently of fibroblast growth factor 23 and phosphate. J Am Soc Nephrol. 2015;26:1150–60.
123. Hu MC, Kuro-o M, Moe OW. αKlotho and vascular calcification: an evolving paradigm. Curr Opin Nephrol Hypertens. 20141;23:331–9.
124. Navarro-González JF, Donate-Correa J, Muros De Fuentes M, Pérez-Hernández H, Martínez-Sanz R, Mora-Fernández C. Reduced Klotho is associated with the presence and severity of coronary artery disease. Heart. 2014;100:34–40.
125. Semba RD, Cappola AR, Sun K, Bandinelli S, Dalal M, Crasto C, et al. Plasma Klotho and mortality risk in older community-dwelling adults. J Gerontol A Biol Sci Med Sci. 2011;66A:794–800.
126. Memmos E, Sarafidis P, Pateinakis P, Tsiantoulas A, Faitatzidou D, Giamalis P, et al. Soluble Klotho is associated with mortality and cardiovascular events in hemodialysis. BMC Nephrol. 2019;20:217.
127. Kendrick J, Cheung AK, Kaufman JS, Greene T, Roberts WL, Smits G, et al. FGF-23 associates with death, cardiovascular events, and initiation of chronic dialysis. J Am Soc Nephrol. 2011;22:1913–22.
128. Ott SM, Moe SM, Drüeke TB. The authors reply. Kidney Int. 2010;78:1186.
129. Vanholder R, Pletinck A, Schepers E, Glorieux G. Biochemical and clinical impact of organic uremic retention solutes: a comprehensive update. Toxins. 2018;10:33.
130. Wojtaszek E, Oldakowska-Jedynak U, Kwiatkowska M, Glogowski T, Malyszko J. Uremic toxins, oxidative stress, atherosclerosis in chronic kidney disease and kidney transplantation. Oxidative Med Cell Longev. 2021;2021:6651367.
131. Nigam SK, Bush KT. Uraemic syndrome of chronic kidney disease: altered remote sensing and signalling. Nat Rev Nephrol. 2019;15:301–16.
132. Valdivielso JM, Rodríguez-Puyol D, Pascual J, Barrios C, Bermúdez-López M, Sánchez-Niño MD, et al. Atherosclerosis in chronic kidney disease: more, less, or just different? Arterioscler Thromb Vasc Biol. 2019;39:1938–66.
133. Cunha RSD, Santos AF, Barreto FC, Stinghen AEM. How do uremic toxins affect the endothelium? Toxins. 2020;12:412.

134. Ok E, Basnakian AG, Apostolov EO, Barri YM, Shah SV. Carbamylated low-density lipoprotein induces death of endothelial cells: a link to atherosclerosis in patients with kidney disease. Kidney Int. 2005;68:173–8.
135. D'Apolito M, Du X, Pisanelli D, Pettoello-Mantovani M, Campanozzi A, Giacco F, et al. Urea-induced ROS cause endothelial dysfunction in chronic renal failure. Atherosclerosis. 2015;239:393–400.
136. Koppe L, Nyam E, Vivot K, Manning Fox JE, Dai XQ, Nguyen BN, et al. Urea impairs β cell glycolysis and insulin secretion in chronic kidney disease. J Clin Invest. 2016;126:3598–612.
137. Vanholder R, Glorieux G, Eloot S. Once upon a time in dialysis: the last days of K*t*/*V*? Kidney Int. 2015;88:460–5.
138. Scalera F, Borlak J, Beckmann B, Martens-Lobenhoffer J, Thum T, Täger M, et al. Endogenous nitric oxide synthesis inhibitor asymmetric dimethyl L-arginine accelerates endothelial cell senescence. Arterioscler Thromb Vasc Biol. 2004;24:1816–22.
139. Wojciak-Stothard B, Torondel B, Tsang LYF, Fleming I, Fisslthaler B, Leiper JM, et al. The ADMA/DDAH pathway is a critical regulator of endothelial cell motility. J Cell Sci. 2007;120:929–42.
140. Zoccali C, Bode-Böger SM, Mallamaci F, Benedetto FA, Tripepi G, Malatino LS, et al. Plasma concentration of asymmetrical dimethylarginine and mortality in patients with end-stage renal disease: a prospective study. Lancet. 2001;358:2113–7.
141. Shafi T, Hostetter TH, Meyer TW, Hwang S, Hai X, Melamed ML, et al. Serum asymmetric and symmetric dimethylarginine and morbidity and mortality in hemodialysis patients. Am J Kidney Dis. 2017;70:48–58.
142. Mihout F, Shweke N, Bigé N, Jouanneau C, Dussaule J, Ronco P, et al. Asymmetric dimethylarginine (ADMA) induces chronic kidney disease through a mechanism involving collagen and TGF-β1 synthesis. J Pathol. 2011;223:37–45.
143. Eiselt J, Rajdl D, Racek J, Vostrý M, Rulcová K, Wirth J. Asymmetric dimethylarginine and progression of chronic kidney disease—a 1-year follow-up study. Kidney Blood Press Res. 2014;39:50–7.
144. Wang Z, Klipfell E, Bennett BJ, Koeth R, Levison BS, DuGar B, et al. Gut flora metabolism of phosphatidylcholine promotes cardiovascular disease. Nature. 2011;472:57–63.
145. Griffin JL, Wang X, Stanley E. Does our gut microbiome predict cardiovascular risk? A review of the evidence from metabolomics. Circ Cardiovasc Genet. 2015;8(1):187–91.
146. Schepers E, Glorieux G, Vanholder R. The gut: the forgotten organ in uremia? Blood Purif. 2010;29:130–6.
147. Stinghen AEM, Massy ZA, Vlassara H, Striker GE, Boullier A. Uremic toxicity of advanced glycation end products in CKD. J Am Soc Nephrol. 2016;27:354–70.
148. Taki K, Takayama F, Tsuruta Y, Niwa T. Oxidative stress, advanced glycation end product, and coronary artery calcification in hemodialysis patients. Kidney Int. 2006;70:218–24.
149. Schinzel R, Münch G, Heidland A, Sebekova K. Advanced glycation end products in end-stage renal disease and their removal. Nephron. 2001;87:295–303.
150. Gryp T, Vanholder R, Vaneechoutte M. Glorieux G p-cresyl sulfate. Toxins. 2017;9:52.
151. Lin CJ, Wu V, Wu PC, Wu CJ. Meta-analysis of the associations of p-cresyl sulfate (PCS) and indoxyl sulfate (IS) with cardiovascular events and all-cause mortality in patients with chronic renal failure. PLoS One. 2015;10:e0132589.
152. Wu IW, Hsu KH, Lee CC, Sun CY, Hsu HJ, Tsai CJ, et al. P-Cresyl sulphate and indoxyl sulphate predict progression of chronic kidney disease. Nephrol Dial Transplant. 2011;26:938–47.
153. Wang CP, Lu YC, Tsai IT, Tang WH, Hsu CC, Hung WC, et al. Increased levels of total *p*-cresylsulfate are associated with pruritus in patients with chronic kidney disease. Dermatology. 2016;232:363–70.
154. Glorieux G, Vanholder R, Van Biesen W, Pletinck A, Schepers E, Neirynck N, et al. Free *p*-cresyl sulfate shows the highest association with cardiovascular outcome in chronic kidney disease. Nephrol Dial Transplant. 2021;36:998–1005.

155. Niwa T, Ise M. Indoxyl sulfate, a circulating uremic toxin, stimulates the progression of glomerular sclerosis. J Lab Clin Med. 1994;124:96–104.
156. Sun CY, Chang SC, Wu MS. Uremic toxins induce kidney fibrosis by activating intrarenal renin–angiotensin–aldosterone system associated epithelial-to-mesenchymal transition. PLoS One. 2012;7:e34026.
157. Sun CY, Chang SC, Wu MS. Suppression of klotho expression by protein-bound uremic toxins is associated with increased DNA methyltransferase expression and DNA hypermethylation. Kidney Int. 2012;81:640–50.
158. Faure V, Dou L, Sabatier F, Cerini C, Sampol J, Berland Y, et al. Elevation of circulating endothelial microparticles in patients with chronic renal failure. J Thromb Haemost. 2006;4:566–73.
159. Lekawanvijit S, Adrahtas A, Kelly DJ, Kompa AR, Wang BH, Krum H. Does indoxyl sulfate, a uraemic toxin, have direct effects on cardiac fibroblasts and myocytes? Eur Heart J. 2010;31:1771–9.
160. Adijiang A, Goto S, Uramoto S, Nishijima F, Niwa T. Indoxyl sulphate promotes aortic calcification with expression of osteoblast-specific proteins in hypertensive rats. Nephrol Dial Transplant. 2008;23:1892–901.
161. Iwasaki-Ishizuka Y, Yamato H, Nii-Kono T, Kurokawa K, Fukagawa M. Downregulation of parathyroid hormone receptor gene expression and osteoblastic dysfunction associated with skeletal resistance to parathyroid hormone in a rat model of renal failure with low turnover bone. Nephrol Dial Transplant. 2005;20:1904–11.
162. Chitalia VC, Shivanna S, Martorell J, Balcells M, Bosch I, Kolandaivelu K, et al. Uremic serum and solutes increase post-vascular interventional thrombotic risk through altered stability of smooth muscle cell tissue factor. Circulation. 2013;127:365–76.
163. Bobot M, Thomas L, Moyon A, Fernandez S, McKay N, Balasse L, et al. Uremic toxic blood–brain barrier disruption mediated by AhR activation leads to cognitive impairment during experimental renal dysfunction. J Am Soc Nephrol. 2020;31:1509–21.
164. Barreto FC, Barreto DV, Liabeuf S, Meert N, Glorieux G, Temmar M, et al. Serum indoxyl sulfate is associated with vascular disease and mortality in chronic kidney disease patients. Clin J Am Soc Nephrol. 2009;4:1551–8.
165. Chmielewski M, Carrero JJ, Stenvinkel P, Lindholm B. Metabolic abnormalities in chronic kidney disease that contribute to cardiovascular disease, and nutritional initiatives that may diminish the risk. Curr Opin Lipidol. 2009;20:3–9.
166. Wilson AM, Kimura E, Harada RK, Nair N, Narasimhan B, Meng XY, et al. β2-microglobulin as a biomarker in peripheral arterial disease: proteomic profiling and clinical studies. Circulation. 2007;116:1396–403.
167. Smith LK, He Y, Park JS, Bieri G, Snethlage CE, Lin K, et al. β2-microglobulin is a systemic pro-aging factor that impairs cognitive function and neurogenesis. Nat Med. 2015;21:932–7.
168. Himmelfarb J, Stenvinkel P, Ikizler TA, Hakim RM. The elephant in uremia: oxidant stress as a unifying concept of cardiovascular disease in uremia. Kidney Int. 2002;62:1524–38.
169. Qureshi AR, Alvestrand A, Divino-Filho JC, Gutierrez A, Heimbürger O, Lindholm B, et al. Inflammation, malnutrition, and cardiac disease as predictors of mortality in hemodialysis patients. J Am Soc Nephrol JASN. 2002;13(Suppl 1):S28–36.
170. Kalantar-Zadeh K, Kopple JD. Relative contributions of nutrition and inflammation to clinical outcome in dialysis patients. Am J Kidney Dis. 2001;38:1343–50.
171. Kalantar-Zadeh K. Recent advances in understanding the malnutrition–inflammation–cachexia syndrome in chronic kidney disease patients: what is next? Semin Dial. 2005;18:365–9.
172. Banerjee T, Kim SJ, Astor B, Shafi T, Coresh J, Powe NR. Vascular access type, inflammatory markers, and mortality in incident hemodialysis patients: the choices for healthy outcomes in caring for end-stage renal disease (CHOICE) study. Am J Kidney Dis. 2014;64:954–61.
173. Kshirsagar AV, Moss KL, Elter JR, Beck JD, Offenbacher S, Falk RJ. Periodontal disease is associated with renal insufficiency in the atherosclerosis risk in communities (ARIC) study. Am J Kidney Dis. 2005;45:650–7.

174. Cappelli G, Tetta C, Canaud B. Is biofilm a cause of silent chronic inflammation in haemodialysis patients? A fascinating working hypothesis. Nephrol Dial Transplant. 2005;20:266–70.
175. López-Gómez JM, Pérez-Flores I, Jofré R, Carretero D, Rodríguez-Benitez P, Villaverde M, et al. Presence of a failed kidney transplant in patients who are on hemodialysis is associated with chronic inflammatory state and erythropoietin resistance. J Am Soc Nephrol. 2004;15:2494–501.
176. Yeun JY, Levine RA, Mantadilok V, Kaysen GA. C-reactive protein predicts all-cause and cardiovascular mortality in hemodialysis patients. Am J Kidney Dis. 2000;35:469–76.
177. Zoccali C, Benedetto FA, Mallamaci F, Tripepi G, Fermo I, Focà A, et al. Inflammation is associated with carotid atherosclerosis in dialysis patients. J Hypertens. 2000;18:1207–13.
178. Griendling KK, Minieri CA, Ollerenshaw JD, Alexander RW. Angiotensin II stimulates NADH and NADPH oxidase activity in cultured vascular smooth muscle cells. Circ Res. 1994;74:1141–8.
179. Gondouin B, Jourde-Chiche N, Sallee M, Dou L, Cerini C, Loundou A, et al. Plasma xanthine oxidase activity is predictive of cardiovascular disease in patients with chronic kidney disease, independently of uric acid levels. Nephron. 2015;131:167–74.
180. Tbahriti HF, Kaddous A, Bouchenak M, Mekki K. Effect of different stages of chronic kidney disease and renal replacement therapies on oxidant-antioxidant balance in uremic patients. Biochem Res Int. 2013;2013:1–6.
181. Menon V, Wang X, Greene T, Beck GJ, Kusek JW, Marcovina SM, et al. Relationship between C-reactive protein, albumin, and cardiovascular disease in patients with chronic kidney disease. Am J Kidney Dis. 2003;42:44–52.
182. Ridker PM, Rifai N, Rose L, Buring JE, Cook NR. Comparison of C-reactive protein and low-density lipoprotein cholesterol levels in the prediction of first cardiovascular events. N Engl J Med. 2002;347:1557–65.
183. Zebrack JS, Anderson JL, Beddhu S, Horne BD, Bair TL, Cheung A, et al. Do associations with C-reactive protein and extent of coronary artery disease account for the increased cardiovascular risk of renal insufficiency? J Am Coll Cardiol. 2003;42:57–63.
184. Kalantar-Zadeh K. Inflammatory marker mania in chronic kidney disease: pentraxins at the crossroad of universal soldiers of inflammation. Clin J Am Soc Nephrol. 2007;2:872–5.
185. Stenvinkel P, Barany P, Heimbürger O, Pecoits-Filho R, Lindholm B. Mortality, malnutrition, and atherosclerosis in ESRD: what is the role of interleukin-6? Kidney Int. 2002;61:S103–8.
186. Jones SA, Fraser DJ, Fielding CA, Jones GW. Interleukin-6 in renal disease and therapy. Nephrol Dial Transplant. 2015;30:564–74.
187. Friedrich B, Alexander D, Janessa A, Häring HU, Lang F, Risler T. Acute effects of hemodialysis on cytokine transcription profiles: evidence for C-reactive protein-dependency of mediator induction. Kidney Int. 2006;70:2124–30.
188. Rho YH, Chung CP, Oeser A, Solus J, Asanuma Y, Sokka T, et al. Inflammatory mediators and premature coronary atherosclerosis in rheumatoid arthritis. Arthritis Care Res. 2009;61:1580–5.
189. Ramadan MM, Mahfouz EM, Gomaa GF, El-Diasty TA, Alldawi L, Ikrar T, et al. Evaluation of coronary calcium score by multidetector computed tomography in relation to endothelial function and inflammatory markers in asymptomatic individuals. Circ J. 2008;72:778–85.
190. Spoto B, Mattace-Raso F, Sijbrands E, Leonardis D, Testa A, Pisano A, et al. Association of IL-6 and a functional polymorphism in the IL-6 gene with cardiovascular events in patients with CKD. Clin J Am Soc Nephrol. 2015;10:232–40.
191. Di Meo S, Reed TT, Venditti P, Victor VM. Role of ROS and RNS sources in physiological and pathological conditions. Oxidative Med Cell Longev. 2016;2016:1–44.
192. Boaz M, Smetana S, Weinstein T, Matas Z, Gafter U, Iaina A, et al. Secondary prevention with antioxidants of cardiovascular disease in endstage renal disease (SPACE): randomised placebo-controlled trial. Lancet. 2000;356:1213–8.
193. Rassaf T, Rammos C, Hendgen-Cotta UB, Heiss C, Kleophas W, Dellanna F, et al. Vasculoprotective effects of dietary cocoa flavanols in patients on hemodialysis: a double-blind, randomized, placebo-controlled trial. Clin J Am Soc Nephrol. 2016;11:108–18.

194. Rapa SF, Di Iorio BR, Campiglia P, Heidland A, Marzocco S. Inflammation and oxidative stress in chronic kidney disease—potential therapeutic role of minerals, vitamins and plant-derived metabolites. Int J Mol Sci. 2019;21:263.
195. Fouque D, Kalantar-Zadeh K, Kopple J, Cano N, Chauveau P, Cuppari L, et al. A proposed nomenclature and diagnostic criteria for protein–energy wasting in acute and chronic kidney disease. Kidney Int. 2008;73:391–8.
196. Carrero JJ, Thomas F, Nagy K, Arogundade F, Avesani CM, Chan M, et al. Global prevalence of protein-energy wasting in kidney disease: a meta-analysis of contemporary observational studies from the international society of renal nutrition and metabolism. J Ren Nutr. 2018;28:380–92.
197. Kalantar-Zadeh K, Kuwae N, Wu DY, Shantouf RS, Fouque D, Anker SD, et al. Associations of body fat and its changes over time with quality of life and prospective mortality in hemodialysis patients. Am J Clin Nutr. 2006;83:202–10.
198. Wright M, Woodrow G, O'Brien S, Armstrong E, King N, Dye L, et al. Cholecystokinin and leptin: their influence upon the eating behaviour and nutrient intake of dialysis patients. Nephrol Dial Transplant. 2004;19:133–40.
199. Muscaritoli M, Molfino A, Chiappini MG, Laviano A, Ammann T, Spinsanti P, et al. Anorexia in hemodialysis patients: the possible role of des-acyl ghrelin. Am J Nephrol. 2007;27:360–5.
200. Kosmas CE, Silverio D, Tsomidou C, Salcedo MD, Montan PD, Guzman E. The impact of insulin resistance and chronic kidney disease on inflammation and cardiovascular disease. Clin Med Insights Endocrinol Diabetes. 2018;11:1179551418792257.
201. Mathew RO, Rosenson RS, Lyubarova R, Chaudhry R, Costa SP, Bangalore S, et al. Concepts and controversies: lipid management in patients with chronic kidney disease. Cardiovasc Drugs Ther. 2021;35:479–89.
202. Ferro CJ, Mark PB, Kanbay M, Sarafidis P, Heine GH, Rossignol P, et al. Lipid management in patients with chronic kidney disease. Nat Rev Nephrol. 2018;14:727–49.
203. Upadhyay A, Earley A, Lamont JL, Haynes S, Wanner C, Balk EM. Lipid-lowering therapy in persons with chronic kidney disease: a systematic review and meta-analysis. Ann Intern Med. 2012;157:251.
204. Kochan Z, Szupryczynska N, Malgorzewicz S, Karbowska J. Dietary lipids and dyslipidemia in chronic kidney disease. Nutrients. 2021;13:3138.
205. Elewa U, Fernández-Fernández B, Mahillo-Fernández I, Martin-Cleary C, Sanz AB, Sanchez-Niño MD, et al. PCSK 9 in diabetic kidney disease. Eur J Clin Investig. 2016;46:779–86.
206. Vijayaraghavan K, Szerlip HM, Ballantyne CM, Bays HE, Philip S, Doyle RT, et al. Icosapent ethyl reduces atherogenic markers in high-risk statin-treated patients with stage 3 chronic kidney disease and high triglycerides. Postgrad Med. 2019;131:390–6.
207. Collins AJ, Pitt B, Reaven N, Funk S, McGaughey K, Wilson D, et al. Association of serum potassium with all-cause mortality in patients with and without heart failure, chronic kidney disease, and/or diabetes. Am J Nephrol. 2017;46:213–21.
208. Hunter RW, Bailey MA. Hyperkalemia: pathophysiology, risk factors and consequences. Nephrol Dial Transplant. 2019;34(Supplement 3):iii2–11.
209. Gilligan S, Raphael KL. Hyperkalemia and hypokalemia in CKD: prevalence, risk factors, and clinical outcomes. Adv Chronic Kidney Dis. 2017;24:315–8.
210. de Sequera OP, Alcázar Arroyo R, Albalate RM. Trastornos del potasio. Hipopotasemia e hiperpotasemia Nefrología al día. http://www.nefrologiaaldia.org/es-articulo-613
211. Kovesdy CP, Matsushita K, Sang Y, Brunskill NJ, Carrero JJ, Chodick G, et al. Serum potassium and adverse outcomes across the range of kidney function: a CKD prognosis consortium meta-analysis. Eur Heart J. 2018;39:1535–42.
212. Gorriz JL, D'Marco L, Pastor-González A, Molina P, Gonzalez-Rico M, Puchades MJ, et al. Long-term mortality and trajectory of potassium measurements following an episode of acute severe hyperkalaemia. Nephrol Dial Transplant. 2022;37:522–30.
213. Kraut JA, Madias NE. Adverse effects of the metabolic acidosis of chronic kidney disease. Adv Chronic Kidney Dis. 2017;24:289–97.

214. Alcázar Arroyo R, Albalate Ramón M, de Sequera Ortíz P. Trastornos del metabolismo ácido-base. Nefrología al día. http://www.nefrologiaaldia.org/es-articulo-403.
215. Cheng YL, Huang SC, Ho MY, Li YR, Yen CL, Chen KH, et al. Effect of sodium bicarbonate on cardiovascular outcome and mortality in patients with advanced chronic kidney disease. Front Pharmacol. 2023;14:1146668.
216. KDIGO Guidelines. Chapter 3: management of progression and complications of CKD. Kidney Int Suppl. 2013;3:73–90.
217. The UBI Study Group, Di Iorio BR, Bellasi A, Raphael KL, Santoro D, Aucella F, et al. Treatment of metabolic acidosis with sodium bicarbonate delays progression of chronic kidney disease: the UBI study. J Nephrol. 2019;32:989–1001.

Hypertension-Induced Renal Structural Changes in Chronic Kidney Disease

12

Kidney Alterations in Malignant and in Resistant Hypertension

Liffert Vogt, Joris J. T. H. Roelofs, and Peter W. de Leeuw

12.1 Introduction

Nearly 200 years ago, the English physician Richard Bright discovered that patients who had died of nephrosclerosis associated with oedema, uraemic symptoms, and proteinuria not only exhibited granular and shrunken kidneys at autopsy but enlarged hearts as well [1]. Some 80 years later, Volhard and Fahr described the renal lesions in "Bright's disease" in greater detail and attributed those to "vasospastic" renal ischemia [2]. Volhard also introduced routine blood pressure measurements in his clinic and was able to distinguish two types of high blood pressure which he called "roter und blasser Hochdruck" (red and white hypertension). In retrospect, this may have reflected primary or essential hypertension in patients with a red-bluish complexion and malignant hypertension, characterized by extreme vasoconstriction and paleness, respectively. It soon became clear that hypertension was the link between the renal and cardiac abnormalities in Bright's disease.

L. Vogt
Department of Internal Medicine, section Nephrology, Amsterdam University Medical Center, University of Amsterdam, Amsterdam, The Netherlands
e-mail: l.vogt@amsterdamumc.nl

Joris J. T. H. Roelofs
Department of Pathology, Amsterdam University Medical Center, University of Amsterdam, Amsterdam, The Netherlands
e-mail: j.j.roelofs@amsterdamumc.nl

P. W. de Leeuw (✉)
Department of Medicine, Maastricht University Medical Center, Maastricht, The Netherlands
e-mail: p.deleeuw@maastrichtuniversity.nl

A. E. Berbari et al. (eds.), *Blood Pressure Disorders in Acute and Chronic Kidney Diseases*, Updates in Hypertension and Cardiovascular Protection,
https://doi.org/10.1007/978-3-031-81292-7_12

The years after World War II have seen an explosion in hypertension research, particularly with respect to the role of the kidney. In this regard, a great deal of attention has been directed toward renal structural changes in various forms of hypertension. At the same time, this raised the virtually unsolvable question whether alterations in renal morphology are primary and a potential cause of the elevated pressure, or the result of damage due to the hypertensive process.

Most investigators now agree that in patients with chronic kidney disease (CKD), regardless of its origin, hypertension is a secondary phenomenon. Even though such patients may have been diagnosed once with primary (essential) hypertension, the question remains whether they truly had primary hypertension when the alleged hypertension-induced renal damage progresses to end-stage kidney disease (ESKD). In the present chapter, we will elaborate on the structural changes and their etiology in specific hypertensive phenotypes, including malignant and treatment-resistant hypertension.

12.2 Epidemiology of Chronic Kidney Disease, Attributable to Hypertension

Based on the widely recommended 2024 Clinical Practice Guideline for the Evaluation and Management of Chronic Kidney Disease, CKD is defined as an estimated glomerular filtration rate (eGFR) <60 mL/min/1.73 m^2 and/or the presence of albuminuria [i.e., urine albumin-to-creatinine ratio (ACR) >3 mg/mmol] for a period of more than 3 months [3]. While there are wide geographic variations in CKD, in high income countries hypertension and diabetes are the most frequent causes of CKD, especially in the elderly. According to the National Kidney Foundation, approximately one in five adults in the USA with high blood pressure may have CKD [4]. In populations with a high prevalence of diabetes and hypertension, it can, however, be difficult to distinguish hypertension from diabetes as a cause of CKD. In other countries, other causes of CKD may be as frequent as hypertension and diabetes (e.g., glomerular disease in East Asia) or coexist with them, complicating the epidemiology of true hypertension-caused CKD [3]. In a recent multi-ethnic European cohort study, the contribution of hypertension to the burden of CKD across ethnic groups highly varied and was different between men and women. In the multi-ethnic HELIUS study, including over 20,000 participants of various origin living in the city of Amsterdam, the age-adjusted prevalence of CKD attributable to hypertension strongly outweighed other CKD risk factors like diabetes, obesity, and smoking [5]. Overall, the population attributable fractions were 33% in women vs 55% in men, with higher fractions in the South-Asian and African subgroups (up to about 45% in women and about 60% in men with these ethnic backgrounds). The overall contribution of diabetes to CKD was 2.5 lower as compared to hypertension, a finding that underscores the crucial impact of hypertension on CKD [5].

12.3 Hypertensive Nephropathy

Hypertensive nephropathy or hypertensive chronic kidney disease refers to the condition where chronic hypertension leads to chronic damage to the kidneys Arteriosclerosis is observed in arcuate and larger arteries, characterized by the presence of fibrous thickening in the intima layer (Fig. 12.1a). Interlobular arteries manifest fibro-elastic thickening in the intima layer and may harbor lipid-laden macrophages. The extent of intimal thickening in arteries is closely associated with changes occurring in arterioles. The media layer in small arteries and/or arterioles may exhibit thickening, indicative of hypertrophy, hyperplasia, or remodeling. Arteriolar hyalinosis and intramural deposition of opaque-glassy matter derived from vascular matrix and plasma-derived proteins (Fig. 12.1b) are usually present [6].

As a result of these changes, the vascular luminal diameter decreases which leads to relative glomerular ischemia (Fig. 12.1c). This, in turn, is thought to lead to stimulation of juxtaglomerular cells, hypersecretion of renin, and hence a further elevation of blood pressure. In addition, enhanced renal vasoconstriction (mediated, among other peptides, by endothelin I and angiotensin II) will cause ischemic

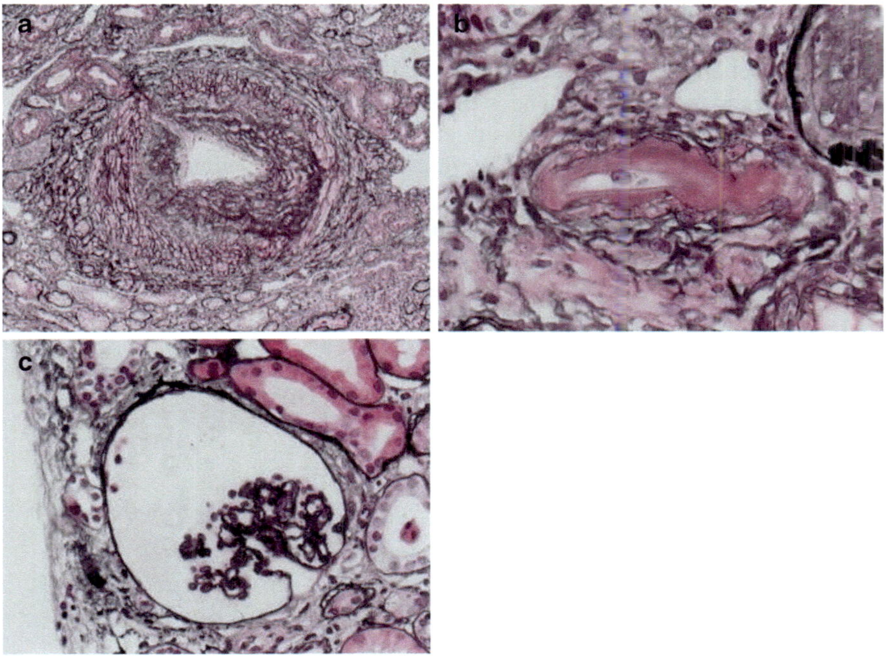

Fig. 12.1 Histopathological characteristics of hypertensive nephropathy. (**a**) Interlobular artery with severe concentric fibrous intimal thickening. (**b**) Arteriolar hyalinosis. (**c**) Glomerular ischemia, characterized by deflation of the glomerular tuft and wrinkling of the glomerular basement membrane. Jones' methenamine silver staining; original magnification ×20. (Source: Department of Translational Pathology. Amsterdam University Medical Center)

glomerular atrophy and finally obliteration of glomeruli. This sets into motion a vicious cycle between renal damage and hypertension.

Arterionephrosclerosis yields two distinct types of glomerular alterations: ischemic glomeruli and solidified glomerulosclerosis. Ischemic glomeruli exhibit wrinkling of the capillary basement membrane and tuft retraction, resulting in an apparent enlargement of Bowman's space (Fig. 12.1c). Over time, the entire glomerular tuft deflates and withdraws toward the vascular pole, while collagen deposits fill up the empty Bowman's spaces [7]. These abnormalities are depicted in Fig. 12.2a. As shown in Fig. 12.2b, solidified glomeruli are characterized by an augmentation of the mesangial matrix, leading to global consolidation (sclerosis) of the glomerular tuft, extending up to Bowman's capsule, without collagenization of Bowman's space [8]. In addition, kidneys from patients with hypertension-associated kidney disease may reveal focal and segmental glomerulosclerosis (FSGS) lesions. These lesions typically localize either in the glomerular perihilar region or exhibit a nondescript (FSGS-NOS) morphology and are frequently accompanied by glomerulomegaly, which is characteristic of secondary-adaptive FSGS.

Of note, the abovementioned morphological changes are not specific for hypertensive damage. Several conditions display comparable pathologic changes. These include both normal and accelerated aging, diabetes, and the spectrum of thrombotic microangiopathies of any cause such as cocaine-associated nephropathy and the antiphospholipid syndrome.

Aging leads to identical changes as observed in hypertension, including glomerular ischemic wrinkling and subsequent obsolescence, interstitial fibrosis, tubular atrophy, arterial intimal thickening, and arteriolar hyalinosis [9]. However, the solidified form of glomerulosclerosis is usually not a feature of aging. Also, extensive arterial medial thickening is usually absent in non-hypertensive aged subjects.

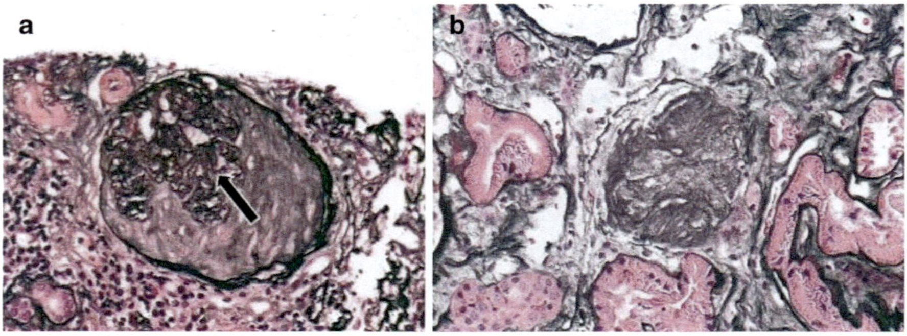

Fig. 12.2 Glomerular obsolescence in hypertension. (**a**) Globally sclerosed glomerulus of ischemic origin, with retraction and sclerosis of the capillary tuft (arrow), accompanied by collagenization of Bowman's space. (**b**) Globally solidified glomerulus. Jones' methenamine silver staining; original magnification ×20. (Source: Department of Translational Pathology, Amsterdam University Medical Center)

12.3.1 Low Nephron Numbers Are Related to Hypertension

Over the past decades, several studies have found that hypertensive patients have lower nephron numbers than normotensives. Keller and coworkers, for instance, compared the number and volume of glomeruli in 10 middle-aged hypertensive patients and 10 normotensive subjects matched for age, sex, and body size [10]. All these individuals had died in accidents. The hypertensives appeared to have approximately half the number of glomeruli with a two to threefold greater volume than the controls. However, while low nephron endowment is associated with intimal hyperplasia and glomerulosclerosis, the association of a low nephron number and hypertension is not a universally finding [11]. As reviewed by Kanzaki and colleagues, a variety of genetic and metabolic factors may also be involved in nephron loss [12]. Moreover, any association between low nephron numbers and hypertension still does not tell us anything about what came first. Indeed, low nephron numbers may either be the cause of low gestational age or low birthweight leading to hypertension in later life, or the consequence of chronic damage from whatever cause to the kidney with loss of nephrons.

Regardless of its cause, a lower nephron number in young hypertensive patients may not affect GFR per se. In contrast to normotensive people, GFR may even increase in response to stress or high salt consumption [13]. Glomerular hypertrophy (Fig. 12.3), disturbed autoregulation, and activation of the renin–angiotensin system are believed to contribute to the alleged hyperfiltrating state in the early stages of hypertension. These structural and hemodynamic changes, together with loss of the endothelial barrier function, elicit the development of albuminuria. Indeed, in the above-mentioned multi-ethnic HELIUS population study, albuminuria was attributable to hypertension in most of the participants, presumably because the mean age in this cohort was just above 40 years [5]. Sustained hypertension may, however, lead to loss of GFR. Due to damage of the renal vasculature, the loss of proportionate autoregulatory vasoconstriction in response to high systemic

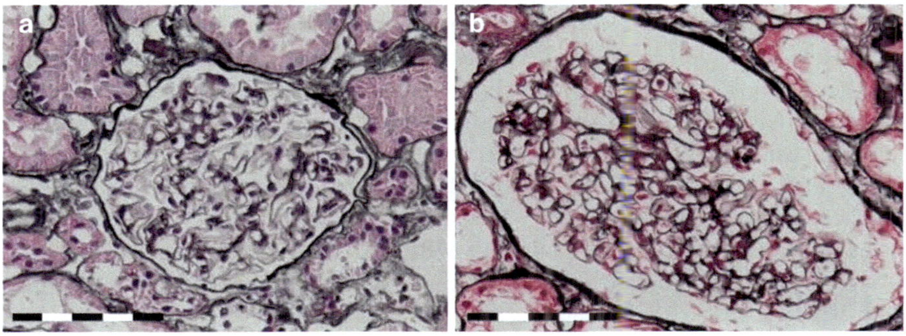

Fig. 12.3 Glomerular hypertrophy in early-stage hypertensive nephropathy. (**a**) Normal sized glomerulus of a normotensive subject. (**b**) Glomerular hypertrophy. Black and white scale bars represent 100 µm. Jones' methenamine silver staining; original magnification ×40. (Source: Department of Translational Pathology, Amsterdam University Medical Center)

arterial pressure translates into the development of glomerulosclerosis, increased protein loss into the urine space, tubulointerstitial damage, and, subsequently, progressive loss of functional nephrons.

Thus, a low nephron number, loss of autoregulation, glomerular hyperfiltration damage, arteriolosclerosis in preglomerular arteries (including myo-intimal proliferation and hyalinosis), and ultimately glomerulosclerosis due to ischemia and solidification all represent the spectrum of structural changes from the time of being at risk for hypertension to sustained uncontrolled hypertension.

12.3.2 CKD Caused by Hypertension or Hypertension Caused by CKD

Although it is widely accepted that hypertension may lead to functional and structural kidney damage, in many patients with hypertension the exact cause of CKD cannot be ascertained with certainty. However, given the high costs and risks associated with specialized diagnostic testing such as kidney biopsy, invasive imaging studies, and/or genetic testing, the clinician will order such tests only when another cause for CKD than hypertension is considered. Specifically, advanced CKD at a relatively young age, progressive kidney function decline, severe albuminuria, and presence of hematuria are reasons for further investigation.

Overactivity of the adrenergic system frequently accompanies CKD, and this may cause blood pressure to go up, regardless of the underlying renal pathology. As muscle sympathetic activity progressively increases with deterioration of eGFR [14] and renal denervation can reduce blood pressure without significant effects on kidney function [15], it may well be that neurally mediated hypertension is, at least in part, secondary to CKD. However, it is currently unknown what the impact of sympathetic overactivity is on morphological changes within the kidney. Therefore, it remains possible that the sympathetic system first causes intrarenal abnormalities, for instance via increased vasoconstriction with ensuing ischemia. At the time that CKD and hypertension develop, it may not be possible anymore to separate the effects of the sympathetic system from those by the kidney itself.

Likewise, we do not know to what extent inflammatory and immune pathways and gut dysbiosis, which have recently been implicated as possible causes of hypertension in CKD [16], are cause or consequence of merely a permissive factor in the pathogenesis of hypertension in CKD.

It should be stressed that the risk of kidney failure (defined as the need for kidney replacement therapy, being either dialysis or kidney transplantation) due to sustained hypertension is low. Although the MRFIT study with an average follow-up of 16-years and comprising 332,544 men, 35–57 years of age, observed a graded relation between both systolic and diastolic blood pressure and the risk of end-stage kidney disease due to any cause, the absolute risk remained below 3.5% [17]. Only in patients with stage 4 hypertension (systolic blood pressure ≥210 mmHg and/or diastolic blood pressure ≥120 mmHg at baseline), the absolute risk difference was about 25 per 1000 patients in comparison to individuals with an optimal blood pressure, i.e., systolic <120 mmHg and diastolic <80 mmHg. In this regard, though, we cannot exclude the possibility that this severe form of hypertension reflects a different hypertensive phenotype.

12.4 Malignant Hypertension

The classic definition of malignant hypertension consists of severe hypertension and acute microvascular complications, including grade III or IV hypertensive retinopathy [18]. The incidence of malignant hypertension and related renal complications is higher in people of Sub-Saharan descent than in Europeans [19]. The definition of a hypertensive emergency, which often fulfills the definition of malignant hypertension, includes any situation where very high BP values are associated with acute hypertension-mediated organ damage that requires immediate BP reduction [20]. If left untreated, the 5-year survival rate is less than 5%—reflecting its malignant prognosis—because of stroke, myocardial infarction, congestive heart failure, and end-stage kidney disease [21]. While kidney failure has almost the greatest impact on the risk of death in patients with malignant hypertension, this occurs independently of traditional risk factors such as excessive smoking, dyslipidemia, and poor BP control and mainly strikes people below 45 years of age [21]. The clinical characteristics of this hypertensive phenotype, therefore, strongly suggest that renal involvement in this condition differs substantially from that in essential hypertension. Indeed, the latter leads to kidney function decline over time in conjunction with diabetes and other cardiovascular risk factors and comorbidities. Moreover, in patients with malignant hypertension, secondary causes can be found in up to 20–40%. Most often, these consist of renal parenchymal disease or renal artery stenosis, whereas endocrine causes appear to be rare [20].

12.4.1 Thrombotic Microangiopathy Is a Hallmark of Kidney Involvement

Various pathophysiological mechanisms contribute to the development and maintenance of malignant hypertension. Pronounced activation of the renin–angiotensin system, often induced or exacerbated by microvascular damage, is frequently observed. Hyperactivity of the sympathetic nervous system and increased vasopressin levels, secondary to medullary ischemia, further contribute to microvascular injury. Experimental models have shown that the onset of acute hypertensive micro-angiopathy is preceded by enhanced renal vasoconstriction and microvascular injury, ultimately triggering renin–angiotensin system activation.

The histopathological manifestations associated with malignant hypertension resemble those of thrombotic microangiopathy (TMA), with or without actual thrombosis. The typical lesions of TMA include fibrinoid alterations occurring in both glomeruli and renal arterioles, concomitant with fragmented erythrocytes. Renal arterioles and small arteries display intimal thickening often with a striking mucoid appearance, resulting in significant constriction of their lumen. Additionally, thrombotic occlusion of the lumen may be present (Fig. 12.4).

The hallmark lesion of malignant hypertension is fibrinoid necrosis of blood vessels and is characterized by the presence of eosinophilic, granular material within the media layer. Thrombus formation frequently occurs in conjunction with necrotic areas, culminating in complete occlusion of the vessel. Fragmented red blood cells

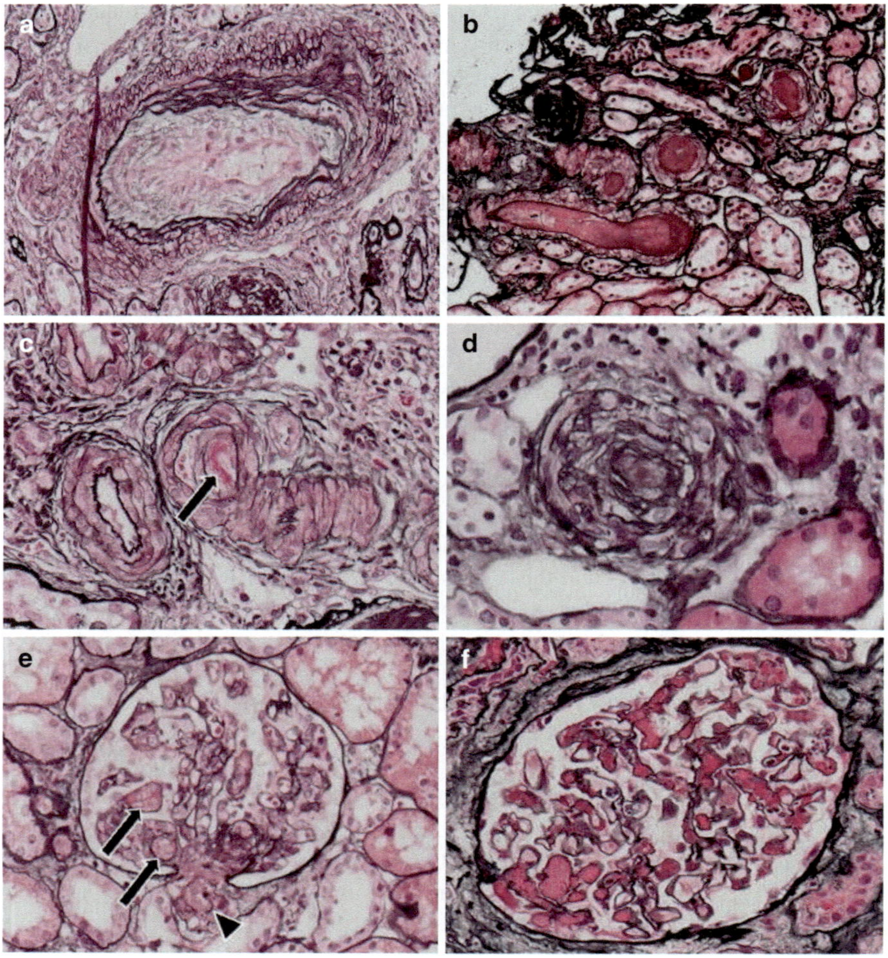

Fig. 12.4 TMA in malignant hypertension. (**a**) Middle-sized artery with severe acute endothelial separation with intimal mucoid degeneration. (**b**) Arterioles with complete occlusion of the lumens by fibrin thrombi (arrows). (**c**) Arteriole with endothelial cell swelling, entrapment of red blood cells and fibrinoid necrosis (arrow). (**d**) Chronic arteriolar TMA, characterized by onion-skin type intimal fibrosis. (**e**) Glomerulus with endothelial cell swelling, intracapillary fibrin microthrombi (arrows) and hilar thrombosis (arrowhead). (**f**) Glomerulus with severe congestion ("glomerular paralysis"). Jones' methenamine silver staining; original magnifications ×20 (**a**, **b**) and ×40 (**c**–**f**). (Source: Department of Translational Pathology, Amsterdam University Medical Center)

are commonly observed either within the thickened intima or the vessel wall (Fig. 12.4).

During the chronic phase of injury which develops because of severe hypertension, intimal thickening extends extensively along the vessels' length, inducing significant constriction of the lumen. These chronic and irreversible alterations, usually described as "onion-skin thickening" of the vessel wall, lead to ischemia and subsequent kidney failure.

Glomerular changes in malignant hypertension can manifest themselves as acute or chronic conditions. The acute alterations are focal in nature and encompass segmental fibrinoid necrosis of the capillary wall, and occasionally mesangiolysis, which is characterized by the loss of mesangial cells and variable dissolution of mesangial matrix. Swelling of endothelial cells in arterioles and capillaries may occlude the lumen. Furthermore, fibrin-platelet thrombi, accompanied by fragments of red blood cells, may be present. Some glomeruli may exhibit collapse and wrinkling of the tuft (Fig. 12.1), while others primarily display intense congestion with dilation of the capillaries, a phenomenon often described as "glomerular paralysis" (Fig. 12.4f).

12.4.2 Structural Changes Related to Primary Kidney Diseases

Given that malignant hypertension commonly stems from renovascular disease (e.g., renal artery stenosis, polyarteritis nodosa, and Takayasu arteritis) or primary parenchymal disease (e.g., glomerulonephritis, tubulointerstitial nephritis, systemic sclerosis, hemolytic-uremic syndrome, or systemic lupus erythematosus nephritis), an array of renal pathological findings, beyond intima hyperplasia and hyalinosis, and thrombotic microangiopathy, can be observed. However, due to the high risks associated with performing kidney biopsies in the setting of severely elevated blood pressure, the literature describing such renal structural changes primarily relies on case reports and small cohorts.

Isolated malignant hypertension and renovascular disease may induce such abnormalities as ischemic wrinkling, periglomerular fibrosis, and even acute tubular necrosis. Conversely, malignant hypertension resulting from primary glomerular disease often presents with features which are diagnostic for the glomerulopathy or glomerulonephritis at hand. One frequently reported primary glomerular disease associated with malignant hypertension is IgA nephropathy [22].

12.5 Renal Abnormalities in Resistant Hypertension

Treatment-resistant hypertension (TRH) is defined as a blood pressure that remains above 140/90 mmHg despite optimal use of three antihypertensive medications of different classes, including a diuretic. Admittedly, the term "resistant" is not very helpful as there may not be true resistance or unresponsiveness to medication. Often the condition is better called difficult-to-treat hypertension. The diagnosis of TRH requires at least the exclusion of white-coat hypertension and lack of adherence. In case pseudo-resistance due to, for instance, non-adherence cannot be completely excluded, the term apparent TRH (aTRH) is in vogue.

The exact epidemiology of a TRH is not well known. Estimates vary from less than 10% to almost 20%, depending on the population studied [23, 24]. Data from the Chronic Renal Insufficiency Cohort (CRIC) study, an observational study in almost 4000 patients with CKD, indicate that in this population the prevalence of aTRH may be as high as 40% [25]. In this study, treatment-resistant patients were more often older, male, of African descent, and they had higher body mass index and systolic blood pressures. The prevalence of aTRH increased with worsening of kidney function from 22.3% in those with an estimated glomerular filtration rate (eGFR) >60 mL/min/1.73 m^2 to 54.2% in patients with an eGFR below 30 mL/min/1.73 m^2. Comparable results were obtained in the population-based Reasons for Geographic and Racial Differences in Stroke (REGARDS) study [26]. In that study in more than 10,000 individuals, the prevalence of aTRH increased proportionally to the decline in renal function and the increase in the urinary albumin-to-creatinine ratio. Additionally, patients with CKD were found to have aTRH twice as often as those without CKD.

Potentially curable causes of treatment resistance in patients with CKD are primary aldosteronism and renal artery stenosis both of which may have an impact on nephron mass and inflammatory processes within the kidney. Lifestyle factors also play a role. Besides obesity, excess salt intake is associated with treatment resistance. In line with this, an early trial of sodium restriction in 20 hypertensive stage 3–4 CKD patients demonstrated a statistically significant fall in blood pressure of 10/4 mmHg [27]. According to the investigators, a substantial proportion of these patients exhibited apparent TRH.

12.6 Hypertension and End-Stage Kidney Disease

According to the 2021 annual report of the European Renal Association registry, hypertension was identified as the primary cause of kidney replacement therapy dependency in 15% of incident end-stage kidney disease patients [28]. Among individuals aged over 65 years, this incidence rose to nearly 20%. Remarkably, hypertension emerged as the second most prevalent cause of ESKD. Despite these statistics, it is improbable that essential hypertension was the primary instigator of ESKD (vide supra). Malignant hypertension, usually prevalent among younger individuals, cannot explain the ESKD incidence either, rendering hypertension as one of the leading causes of ESKD even more puzzling.

Diagnosing an underlying renal cause at this stage of chronic kidney disease (CKD) poses significant challenges and offers limited clinical insights. When ESKD develops, kidney size has importantly decreased, and taking biopsies from small kidneys entails significant risks of bleeding complications. Additionally, renal pathology from biopsies often lacks specificity, typically revealing an atrophic cortex with obsolescent glomeruli, areas of interstitial fibrosis and tubular atrophy,

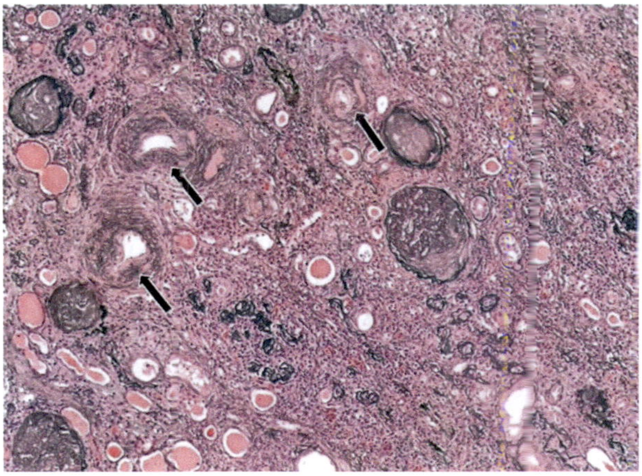

Fig. 12.5 End-stage kidney in hypertension. Complete loss of functional renal parenchyma, characterized by numerous globally sclerosed glomeruli, and extensive areas of interstitial fibrosis and tubular atrophy, accompanied by interstitial lymphoplasmacytic resorption infiltrate. Several thick-walled arterioles with intimal hyalinosis are present (arrows). Jones' methenamine silver staining, original magnifications ×10. (Source: Department of Translational Pathology, Amsterdam University Medical Center)

scattered interstitial chronic inflammatory cell infiltrates, and thick-walled arteries and arterioles (Fig. 12.5). Despite these challenges, further examination of renal biopsies occasionally uncovers primary kidney disease, such as immune complex or complement mediated glomerular disease, identified by immune fluorescence or other ancillary techniques.

12.7 Concluding Remarks

Despite more than a century of research, the relationship between chronic kidney disease and hypertension in humans is still not fully understood. It remains elusive, for instance, whether hypertension is the cause or the consequence of CKD or that it is just a permissive factor in its development. Additionally, it is unclear which factor is most deleterious for the kidney, the mechanical force of an elevated blood pressure or the noxious action of humoral factors such as angiotensin II, endothelin, and many others. Paradoxically, scientific progress in this area is hampered by technological advances. The development of new techniques that allow non-invasive evaluation of kidney function like, for instance, BOLD MRI precludes obtaining tissue material. The sequence of events at the molecular level will, therefore, continue to be a black box as a "side-effect"' of improved imaging techniques. Studies in animals will not help as the abnormalities in humans evolve over a much longer time scale than can ever be achieved under experimental conditions.

The emerging role of clinical genetics in chronic kidney disease, however, presents promising diagnostic opportunities, notably through next-generation sequencing (NGS). With this technique, we may obtain significant results in patients with CKD of unknown etiology, including those with hypertension-related nephropathy [29]. Depending on factors such as age, healthcare setting, ethnicity, and geography, NGS diagnostic yield ranges from 17 to 50%. By elucidating primary causes and pathogenic pathways, NGS enables reevaluation of diagnoses, particularly regarding hypertensive nephropathy. The most prominent example is the association between apolipoprotein L1 (APOL1) renal-risk variants and glomerulosclerosis in African Americans [30]. This condition leads to a form of secondary hypertension which may be mistakenly held for primary hypertension. Mechanisms of APOL1 risk variant protein-mediated renal toxicity are actively under investigation. Ongoing clinical trials explore targeted therapies, including APOL1 small molecule inhibitors, APOL1 antisense oligonucleotides, and inhibitors of APOL1-associated inflammatory pathways, all showing promising preliminary results [31].

References

1. Bright R. Tabular view of the morbid appearances in 100 cases connected with albuminous urine. Guys Hosp Rep. 1836;1:380–402.
2. Volhard F, Fahr T. Die Brightsche Krankheit. Klinik, Pathologie und Atlas. Berlin: Springer; 1914.
3. Kidney Disease: Improving Global Outcomes (KDIGO) CKD Work Group. KDIGO. Clinical practice guideline for the evaluation and Management of Chronic Kidney Disease. Kidney Int. 2024;2024(105):S117–314.
4. Centers for Disease Control and Prevention. Chronic kidney disease in the United States, 2021. Atlanta: Centers for Disease Control and Prevention; 2021.
5. Vosters TG, Kingma FM, Stel VS, van den Born BH, Huisman BJMV, van Ittersum FJ, et al. Sex differences in CKD risk factors across ethnic groups. Nephrol Dial Transplant. 2024;39:1194–7.
6. Fogo A, Breyer JA, Smith MC, Cleveland WH, Agodoa L, Kirk KA, AASK Pilot Study Investigators, et al. Accuracy of the diagnosis of hypertensive nephrosclerosis in African Americans: a report from the African American Study of Kidney Disease (AASK) Trial. Kidney Int. 1997;51:244–52.
7. Haas M, Seshan SV, Barisoni L, Amann K, Bajema IM, Becker JU, et al. Consensus definitions for glomerular lesions by light and electron microscopy: recommendations from a working group of the Renal Pathology Society. Kidney Int. 2020;98:1120–34.
8. Marcantoni C, Ma LJ, Federspiel C, Fogo AB. Hypertensive nephrosclerosis in African Americans versus Caucasians. Kidney Int. 2002;62:172–80.
9. Glassock RJ. The aging kidney: more pieces to the puzzle. Mayo Clin Proc. 2011;86:271–2.
10. Keller G, Zimmer G, Mall G, Ritz E, Amann K. Nephron number in patients with primary hypertension. N Engl J Med. 2003;348:101–8.
11. Hoy WE, Bertram JF, Denton RD, Zimanyi M, Samuel T, Hughson MD. Nephron number, glomerular volume, renal disease and hypertension. Curr Opin Nephrol Hypertens. 2008;17:258–65.
12. Kanzaki G, Tsuboi N, Haruhara K, Koike K, Ogura M, Shimizu A, et al. Factors associated with a vicious cycle involving a low nephron number, hypertension and chronic kidney disease. Hypertens Res. 2015;38:633–41.
13. Schmieder RE, Veelken R, Schobel H, Dominiak P, Mann JF, Luft FC. Glomerular hyperfiltration during sympathetic nervous system activation in early essential hypertension. J Am Soc Nephrol. 1997;8:893–900.

14. Grassi G, Quarti-Trevano F, Seravalle G, Arenare F, Volpe M, Furiani S, et al. Early sympathetic activation in the initial clinical stages of chronic renal failure. Hypertension. 2011;57:846–51.
15. Schmieder RE. Renal denervation: where do we stand and what is the relevance to the nephrologist? Nephrol Dial Transplant. 2022;37:638–44.
16. Altamura S, Pietropaoli D, Lombardi F, Del Pinto R, Ferri C. An overview of chronic kidney disease pathophysiology: the impact of gut Dysbiosis and Oral disease. Biomedicines. 2023;11:3033.
17. Klag MJ, Whelton PK, Randall BL, Neaton JD, Brancati FL, Ford CE, et al. Blood pressure and end-stage renal disease in men. N Engl J Med. 1996;334:13–8.
18. Lip GY, Beevers M, Beevers DG. Complications and survival of 315 patients with malignant-phase hypertension. J Hypertens. 1995;13:915–24.
19. van den Born BJ, Koopmans RP, Groeneveld JO, van Montfrans GA. Ethnic disparities in the incidence, presentation and complications of malignant hypertension. J Hypertens. 2006;24:2299–304.
20. van den Born BH, Lip GYH, Brguljan-Hitij J, Cremer A, Segura J, Morales E, et al. ESC Council on hypertension position document on the management of hypertensive emergencies. Eur Heart J Cardiovasc Pharmacother. 2019;5:37–46.
21. Amraoui F, Van Der Hoeven NV, Van Valkengoed IG, Vogt L, Van Den Born BJ. Mortality and cardiovascular risk in patients with a history of malignant hypertension: a case-control study. J Clin Hypertens (Greenwich). 2014;16:122–6.
22. Subias R, Botey A, Darnell A, Montoliu J, Revert L. Malignant or accelerated hypertension in IgA nephropathy. Clin Nephrol. 1987;27:1–7.
23. Dybiec J, Krzemińska J, Radzioch E, Szlagor M, Wronka M, Młynarska E, et al. Advances in the pathogenesis and treatment of resistant hypertension. Int J Mol Sci. 2023;24:12911.
24. Shalaeva EV, Messerli FH. What is resistant arterial hypertension? Blood Press. 2023;32:2185457.
25. Thomas G, Xie D, Chen HY, Anderson AH, Appel LJ, Bodana S, et al. Prevalence and prognostic significance of apparent treatment resistant hypertension in chronic kidney disease: report from the chronic renal insufficiency cohort study. Hypertension. 2016;67:387–96.
26. Tanner RM, Calhoun DA, Bell EK, Bowling CB, Gutiérrez OM, Irvin MR, et al. Prevalence of apparent treatment-resistant hypertension among individuals with CKD. Clin J Am Soc Nephrol. 2013;8:1583–90.
27. McMahon EJ, Bauer JD, Hawley CM, Isbel NM, Stowasser M, Johnson DW, et al. A randomized trial of dietary sodium restriction in CKD. J Am Soc Nephrol. 2013;24:2096–103.
28. Boerstra BA, Boenink R, Astley ME, Bonthuis M, Abd ElHafeez S, Arribas Monzón F, et al. The ERA registry annual report 2021: a summary. Clin Kidney J. 2024;17:sfad281.
29. de Haan A, Eijgelsheim M, Vogt L, Knoers NVAM, de Borst MH. Diagnostic yield of next-generation sequencing in patients with chronic kidney disease of unknown etiology. Front Genet. 2019;10:1264.
30. Robinson TW, Freedman BI. The impact of APOL1 on chronic kidney disease and hypertension. Adv Chronic Kidney Dis. 2019;26:131–6.
31. Friedman DJ, Ma L, Freedman BI. Treatment potential in APOL1-associated nephropathy. Curr Opin Nephrol Hypertens. 2022;31:442–8.

13 Diagnostic Approaches in Hypertension and Chronic Kidney Disease Renal Markers in Evaluation and Follow-Up of Hypertension and Classical and Modern Imaging Techniques in Evaluation of BP Disorders

Michel Burnier, Wendy Brito Rodriguez, and Menno Pruijm

13.1 Introduction

Hypertension and chronic kidney diseases (CKD) are two intrinsically associated clinical conditions [1–4]. This is due in part to the fact that hypertension is both a cause and a consequence of CKD and that both conditions increase significantly with age and hence coexist in many patients. Thus, hypertension is recognized as a strong determinant of worse renal and cardiovascular outcomes in CKD patients, and CKD directly affects the management of hypertensive patients, for example during optimization of drug therapies [5]. Indeed, several drugs are eliminated by the kidneys and their prescription deserves particular attention in patients with reduced renal function.

The recent guidelines for the management of hypertension in adults published by the European Society of Hypertension have clearly defined which markers should be measured in the evaluation of hypertension-mediated organ damages and in the diagnosis and follow-up processes of hypertensive patients' management [6]. To assess kidney damages induced by hypertension, three main renal parameters are recommended, e.g., the estimation of glomerular filtration rate (GFR), the quantification of albuminuria, and the measurement of renal resistive indices (RRI). These

M. Burnier (✉)
Faculty of Biology and Medicine, University of Lausanne, Lausanne, Switzerland

Hypertension Research Foundation, Saint-Légier, Switzerland
e-mail: michel.burnier@netplus.ch

W. B. Rodriguez · M. Pruijm
Service of Nephrology and Hypertension, Department of Medicine, Centre Hospitalier Universitaire Vaudois (CHUV), Lausanne, Switzerland

A. E. Berbari et al. (eds.), *Blood Pressure Disorders in Acute and Chronic Kidney Diseases*, Updates in Hypertension and Cardiovascular Protection,
https://doi.org/10.1007/978-3-031-81292-7_13

recommendations are based on their sensitivity to changes, reproducibility and operator independence, time to changes, and mainly the prognostic value of their changes. Indeed, all three parameters have been shown to be significant predictors of the risk of cardiovascular mortality and mortality and adverse renal outcomes [7–9].

In this chapter, one shall review the various biochemical and radiological methods that can be used to assess these markers of kidney involvement in hypertensive patients based on the most recent developments.

13.2 Renal Markers in Evaluation and Follow-Up of Hypertension

13.2.1 Glomerular Filtration Rate (GFR)

Glomerular filtration is the main kidney function, and the determination of GFR is accepted as the best way to assess kidney function whatever the circumstances (clinical practice, epidemiological studies, research). However, a precise assessment of GFR is rather difficult because GFR can only be measured indirectly using markers and methods that are either more accurate but not convenient to use (inulin, iohexol…) or convenient in clinical practice but less accurate and reproducible (formula based on creatinine or cystatin C) because of the intrinsic characteristics of the markers.

In clinical practice, the easiest and cheapest way of assessing kidney function remains the determination of creatinine in blood or eventually a creatinine clearance based on a 24-h urine collection. However, it is now well recognized that these two approaches do not provide an accurate and reproducible assessment of GFR. Serum creatinine alone is an insensitive marker of renal impairment because a major reduction in kidney function can occur before creatinine rises in blood. Indeed, correlations between serum creatinine and measured GFR have consistently shown that patients may lose almost half of their kidney function with no significant change in blood creatinine or creatinine variations within the normal range as illustrated in Fig. 13.1 [10]. Regarding the use of 24-h creatinine clearance, its validity is also limited by the problems associated with the quality of 24-h urine collections. In addition, one has to remember that creatinine clearance is not only determined by the filtration of creatinine, but also by its tubular secretion, which can increase to up to 50% when kidney function is impaired or in some specific groups of patients such as those suffering from obesity.

13.2.1.1 Measured GFR

In order to be more accurate, glomerular filtration rate can be either *measured* (mGFR) using exogenous markers such as inulin, iohexol, iothalamate, or ^{51}Cr-EDTA or *estimated* (eGFR) using endogenous substances such as creatinine or cystatin or the combination of both. Today, mGFR is still considered the reference standard for the assessment of kidney function. To this purpose, exogenous markers

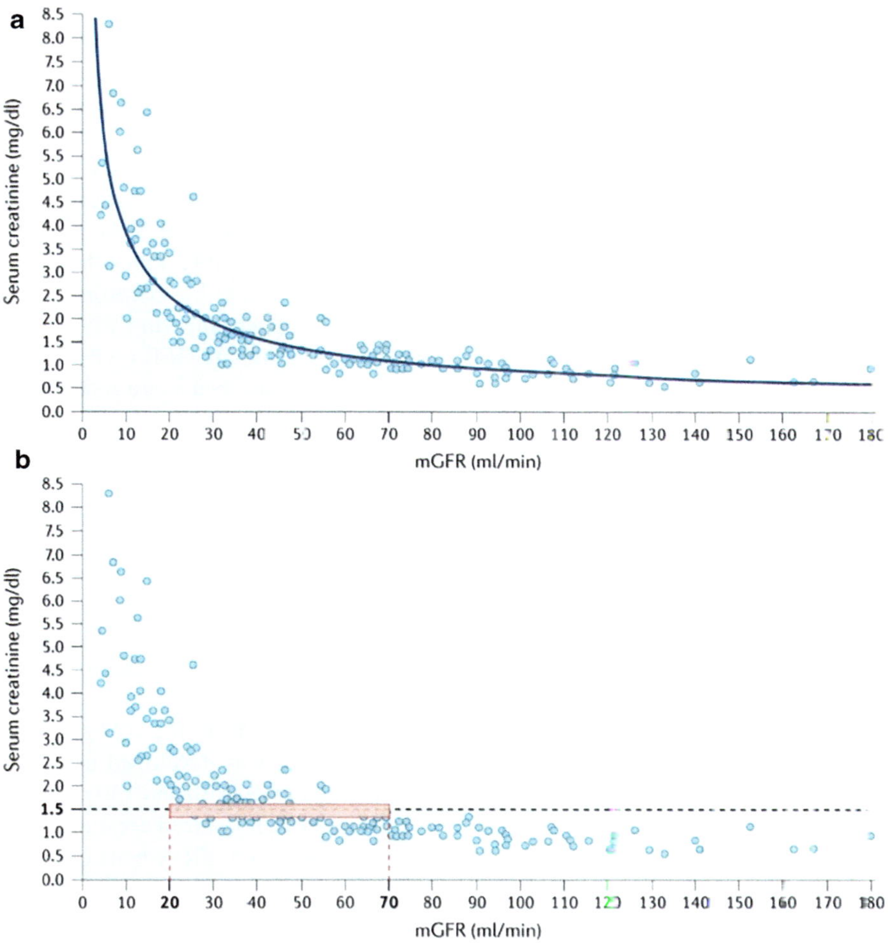

Fig. 13.1 Relation between serum creatinine and measured GFR (from ref. [10] with permission). The bar indicates that eGFR can vary substantially without significant changes in serum creatinine

must be used, which are not metabolized by the kidneys, are freely filtered through glomeruli and neither secreted nor reabsorbed at the tubular level. For several decades, the urinary clearance of inulin during a continuous intravenous infusion of inulin was used as the reference method. Later, other methodological approaches have been implemented using a single injection of the exogenous marker and several consecutive blood samplings to calculate GFR based on the blood decay of the injected marker. In a review and meta-analysis of published studies using inulin clearance as the reference, most of these methods were considered as sufficiently accurate to measure GFR [11]. However, the classical endogenous creatinine clearance, commonly used in practice, was found to be inaccurate with strong evidence, the problem being the quality of 24 h urine collections.

The use of mGFR methods is limited by their cost and their relative complexity as they need to be performed in an organized structure, which is incompatible with clinical practice. Therefore, mGFR remains restricted to specialized facilities. For example, mGFR is regularly measured in drug development when assessing the pharmacokinetic or pharmacodynamic profile of new drugs according to the recommendations of American and European authorities [12]. This is particularly relevant to investigate the pharmacological alterations that could occur in patients with abnormal kidney function. Moreover, except for inulin, several of these markers might still either overestimate (iothalamate) or underestimate GFR (Iohexol, EDTA) because of a possible tubular secretion (iothalamate), a possible reabsorption or protein binding (Iohexol, EDTA), or an incomplete bladder emptying when urine collections are needed. For these reasons, equations to estimate GFR (eGFR) have been developed which do not need any urine collection and hence are much more convenient to be used by practitioners. These equations use endogenous markers such as creatinine or cystatin C or the combination of both.

13.2.1.2 Estimated GFR Using Creatinine

The search for accurate and simple ways of assessing GFR has started in the mid-1950s but the first widely used equation was developed by Cockcroft and Gault (CG) and published in 1976 [13]. Since then, more than 70 equations have been proposed to estimate GFR. Table 13.1 shows the characteristics of some of the most commonly used equations including the very recent ones based on cystatin C alone or in combination with creatinine.

The Cockroft–Gault equation was used until the early years of the 2000s. It integrated serum creatinine, age, body weight, and sex and was developed using the data from 249 men with creatinine clearances ranging between 30 and 130 mL/min. The major issue with this equation is the lack of use of standardized creatinine values leading to inaccurate results (10–20% overestimation of GFR) when compared to more recent formulas or to mGFR. Moreover, the impact of body weight was too important causing important mis-estimation in patients with undernutrition or overweight/obesity. Today, this equation has been abandoned.

The Modification of Diet in Renal Disease (MDRD) equation was introduced in 1999 based on the data of 585 patients with GFR of 25–55 mL/min/1.73 m^2 enrolled in the trial [14]. The original MDRD equation had six variables: age, sex, race, creatinine, urea, and albumin, but later, urea and albumin were dropped without affecting the accuracy of the equation. As no patient with a GFR above 60 mL/min was enrolled in the study, the MDRD equation was found to be less accurate in patients with normal kidney function and more accurate in patients with reduced kidney function. Thus, the equation's results are considered unreliable in patients with GFRs >60 mL/min/1.73 m^2. For this reason, this equation was progressively abandoned and replaced by the CKP-EPI equations.

The Chronic Kidney Disease Epidemiology Collaboration (CKD-EPI) equation, published in 2009, was developed to circumvent the limitations of the MDRD equation, e.g., the limited precision and the systematic mis-estimation of GFR at higher levels [15]. Variables included in the CKD-EPI equation were log serum creatinine

Table 13.1 Various formulas developed over years to estimate glomerular filtration rate

Name	Age	Gender/markers	eGFR equation
Cockcroft–Gault [13]	≥18		GFR = [(140 − age) × weight/SCr] × 0.85 if female
MDRD [14]	≥18		$GFR = 175 \times SCr^{-1.154} \times age^{-0.203}$ (×0.742 if female) (×1.212 if black)
CKD-EPI (2009) [15]	≥18	Female	GFR = SCr ≤0.7 mg/dL: $144 \times (SCr/0.7)^{-0.329} \times 0.9929^{age}$ (×1.159 if black)
			GFR = SCr >0.7 mg/dL: $144 \times (SCr/0.7)^{-1.209} \times 0.9929^{age}$ (×1.159 if black)
		Male	GFR = SCr ≤0.9 mg/dL: $141 \times (SCr/0.9)^{-0.411} \times 0.9929^{age}$ (×1.159 if black)
			GFR = SCr >0.9 mg/dL: $141 \times (SCr/0.9)^{-1.209} \times 0.9929^{age}$ (×1.159 if black)
CKD-EPIcrea (2021) [16]	≥18	Female	SCr ≤0.70 $GFR = 143 \times (SCr/0.70)^{0.241} \times 0.9938^{Age} \times 1.012$
			SCr >0.70 $GFR = 143 \times (SCr/0.70)^{-1.200} \times 0.9938^{Age} \times 1.012$
		Male	SCr ≤0.90 $GFR = 142 \times (SCr/0.90)^{-0.302} \times 0.9938^{Age}$
			SCr >0.90 $GFR = 142 \times (SCr/0.90)^{-1.200} \times 0.9938^{Age}$
EKFC (2021) [17]	2–40 year		SCr/Q <1: $107.3 \times (SCr/Q)^{-0.322}$ or SCr/Q ≥1: $107.3 \times (SCr/Q)^{-1.132}$
	>40 year	*Q* values found in refs [17, 18].	SCr/Q <1: $107.3 \times (SCr/Q)^{-0.322} \times 0.990^{(\text{age in years} - 40)}$ SCr/Q ≥1: $07.3 \times (SCr/Q)^{-1.132} \times 0.990^{(\text{age in years} - 40)}$
CKD-EPIcysC (2012) [19]			cysC ≤0.8 $eGFR = 133 \times (cysC/0.8)^{-0.499} \times 0.996^{Age}$ (×0.932 if female)
			cysC >0.8 $eGFR = 133 \times (cysC/0.8)^{-1.328} \times 0.996^{Age}$ (×0.932 if female)
CAPA eq. (2014) [20]			$eGFR = 130 \times (cys\ C)^{-1.069} \times age^{-0.117}$–7
CKD-EPIScysC (2021) [16]	≥18	ScysC ≤0.80	$GFR = 133 \times (SCysC/0.80)^{-0.499} \times 0.9962^{Age}$ (×0.932 if female)
		ScysC >0.80	$GFR = 133 \times (SCysC/0.80)^{-1.328} \times 0.9962^{Age}$ (×0.932 if female)
CKD-EPIcrea/cysC (2021) [16]	≥18		$GFR_{cr\text{-}cys} = 135 \times \min(S_{cr}/\kappa, 1)^{\alpha} \times \max(S_{cr}/\kappa, 1)^{-0.544} \times \min(S_{cys}/0.8, 1)^{-0.323} \times \max(S_{cys}/0.8, 1)^{-0.778} \times 0.9961^{Age}$ (×0.963 if female) Where $\kappa = 0.7$ (females) or 0.9 (males); $\alpha = -0.219$ (female) or −0.144 (male) $\min(S_{cr}/\kappa, 1)$ is the minimum of S_{cr}/κ or 1.0; $\max(S_{cr}/\kappa, 1)$ is the maximum of S_{cr}/κ or 1.0

(continued)

Table 13.1 (continued)

Name	Age	Gender/markers	eGFR equation
EKFC (2023) [21]	FAS	No sex and race	$GFR = 107.3/[\text{biomarker}/Q]^{\alpha} \times [0.990^{(\text{Age}-40)}$ if age >40 years
			$\alpha = 0.322$ when biomarker/Q is less than 1 and $\alpha = 1.132$ when biomarker/Q is 1 or more
Berlin Initiative Study [22]	≥70	Creatinine	$GFR = 3736 \times \text{creatinine}^{-0.87} \times \text{age}^{-0.95}$ (×0.82 if female)
Berlin Initiative Study [22]	≥70	Creatinine/cystatinC	$GFR = 767 \times \text{cystatin C}^{-0.61} \times \text{creatinine}^{-0.40} \times \text{age}^{-0.57}$ (×0.87 if female)
FAScysC (2017) [23]	<70 year	QcysC = 0.95	$GFR = 107.3/(\text{ScysC}/\text{QcysC}) \times 0.988^{(\text{Age}-40)}$ when age >40
	≥70 year	QcysC = 0.82	$GFR = 107.3/(\text{ScysC}/\text{QcysC}) \times 0.988^{(\text{Age}-40)}$ when age >40

cysC cystatin C, *Crea* creatinine, *MDRD* modification of diet in renal disease, *EKFC* European Kidney Function Consortium, *CKD* chronic kidney disease, *EPI* epidemiology, *FAS* full age spectrum [modeled as a two-slope linear spline with sex-specific knots at 62 μmol/L (0.7 mg/dL) for women and 80 μmol/L (0.9 mg/dL) in men], sex, race and age. The new formula was developed using the data of 5504 subjects and validated internally and externally using the data of respectively 2750 and 3896 people. The CKD-EPI 2009 equation was found to be more accurate than the MDRD equation and to have a lower bias particularly among patients with a GFR greater than 60 mL/min/1.73 m^2. Yet, precision remained limited. Today, CKD-EPI has remained the most widely used and most accurate equation based on creatinine for the estimation of GFR in both clinical practice and epidemiologic studies, and its use is recommended by most current nephrology guidelines, at least until 2021. One of the limitations of this equation is the lack of validation in patients older than 70 years, the mean age of the subjects enrolled in the initial study being 47–50 years of age, and a poor representation of some communities (Hispanic and Asian).

More recently, concerns have been raised regarding the inclusion of race among parameters used to calculate CKD-EPI in 2009, considering that race is a social and not a biologic construct. Therefore, new equations have been developed, which do not include race, based on creatinine or cystatin C and the combination of both [16]. One important issue when adapting equation to race in creatinine-based equation is to take in consideration the fact that muscle mass and meat intake may differ significantly among ethnic groups, and this can have a major impact on the mean level of serum creatinine in populations, as creatinine is produced by muscles and is influenced by meat intake as well. The new CKD-EPI 2021 formulas have been found to introduce some inaccuracies, but these latter were considered adequate for clinical decisions in most circumstances. Indeed, the age and sex equations based on creatinine underestimated measured GFR in Black participants and overestimated mGFR in non-Black participants. When considering the creatinine-based new formula, these inaccuracies could lead to differences in CKD prevalence and GFR stages in the United States as well as in Europe [16, 24]. As will be discussed below, these biases were markedly minimized using cystatin C in the equation. In young adult subjects (<30 years), CKD-EPICr formulas tend to overestimate GFR and the new 2021 equation does not perform better than the 2009 equation. When assessed for its utility in Europe, it was concluded that CKD-EPICr 2021 performed worse than the CKD-EPI 2009 in White Europeans, and provided no or limited performance gains in Black European and Black African populations [13, 25, 26]. In this respect, new equations have been further developed and validated by the European Kidney Function Consortium (EKFC) for White Europeans and Black Africans or Black Europeans, with the potential advantage of being used throughout the age spectrum [17]. In the EKFC creatinine-based equation, the serum creatinine level was rescaled, i.e., the serum creatinine level was divided by the median serum creatinine level among healthy persons to control for variation related to differences in age, sex, or race [17]. When compared to the CKD-EPI 2021 the EKFC equation presented the best performance in the whole age range in the European and African populations [17, 18].

13.2.1.3 Estimated GFR Using Cystatin C

Cystatin C is a 13-kDa cysteine proteinase inhibitor protein produced by all nucleated cells at a steady rate. It is freely filtered by the kidney with near-complete reabsorption and catabolism in the proximal tubule, and thus no significant urinary excretion. Cystatin-C levels are less affected by non-GFR variations related to age, sex, body composition, nutritional status, and race than serum creatinine. However, cystatin C levels are influenced by thyroid diseases, corticosteroid treatments, and the level of inflammation (CRP) [27].

Cystatin C is an independent predictor of morbidity and mortality in a variety of populations: cystatin C has been associated with progression to end-stage kidney disease and mortality in patients with diabetes, CKD, acute kidney diseases, and on dialysis. Rising cystatin C values are associated with the development and progression of cardiovascular diseases, independent of renal function and other cardiovascular risk factors [27]. Cystatin-C has been found to be a more accurate measure of kidney function than serum creatinine and creatinine-based formulas used to calculate eGFR in different patient populations. Cystatin-C captures earlier, more subtle changes in kidney function, which makes its use suitable to identify patients with early impaired function, i.e., when serum creatinine is in the upper normal or mildly elevated range. However, cystatin C has a low availability because of higher costs than creatinine. Hence, the cost-effectiveness and clinical relevance of a wider use in clinical practice remain to be determined.

An eGFR calculation based on cystatin C was proposed in 2012 with the first equation using either cystatin C alone or in combination with creatinine [19]. Across the range of estimated GFRs from 15 to 120 mL/min/1.73 m^2, the cystatin C equation and the creatinine equation were similar in terms of both bias and accuracy. Adding race into the equation did not improve the cystatin C equation. However, the equation combining creatinine and cystatin C had greater precision and accuracy and resulted in a more accurate classification of measured GFR as less than 60 mL/min/1.73 m^2, the threshold proposed by guidelines to define CKD. The cystatin-based equations were further improved over time with the calibration and improvement of cystatin C assays [20]. In addition, a cystatin-based full-age-spectrum equation (FAScysC) for estimating GFR for healthy and kidney-diseased subjects of all ages was developed [23]. The FAScysC equation performed as well as CKD-EPIcysC and the FAS-combi equation was also equal to the combined CKD-EPI equation. In older adults, FAS cysC was actually superior to CKD-EPIcysC and so was the equation combining creatinine and cystatine [23]. The EKFC also developed a cystatin C-based equation to estimate GFR without including sex and race. In cohorts from Europe, the United States, and Africa, this equation appeared to improve the accuracy of GFR assessment over that of commonly used equations [21].

Taken together, this summary shows that developing a very accurate equation to estimate GFR is a very difficult task, which is still ongoing. Newer equations tend to avoid the use of race as an equation parameter, and with the use of cystatin C, the use of the sex variable can also be omitted. According to the most recent developments, an equation including both creatinine and cystatin would be the most accurate approach, but this is, once again, limited by the price of cystatin measurement, and the added value may not be uniform among geographical areas of the world. Regarding the impact of age, some equations can cover the entire adult age spectrum from 18 to more than 70 years [23]. Yet, some specific equations have been developed for older patients such as those proposed by the Berlin Initiative Study group [22], based on creatinine or the combination of creatinine and cystatin C.

Globally, even though there is no perfect equation available so far, the topic remains important because an accurate estimation of GFR is essential to adequately assess the prevalence of kidney disease according to the various CKD stages in different populations, and to guide preventive therapeutic strategies in the management of CKD patients. In this context, excellent reviews discussing the current situation and the future developments of the determination of GFR in various circumstances have been published by Levey et al. [12] and Delanaye et al. [25].

13.2.2 Albuminuria

Normal urine contains either no or negligible amounts of albumin. Thus, the presence of albuminuria is a marker of kidney damage. Therefore, since 2002, the definition of CKD is based on five levels of GFR and also on three levels of albuminuria [28]. Guidelines recommend the measurement of the albumin/creatinine ratio (ACR) in untimed urine samples. The three levels of ACR are <3, 3–30, and >30 in mg/mol or <30, 30–300, and >300 in mg/g. In 2010, the CKD Prognosis Consortium evaluated the association of albuminuria with all-cause and cardiovascular mortality from the data of 14 studies and a total of 105,872 subjects. Their analysis clearly showed that the ACR is associated linearly with all-cause and cardiovascular mortality independently of GFR [7] suggesting that ACR is not only a risk marker for kidney diseases. More recently, in a retrospective analysis of 114 cohorts including more than 27 million individuals from the general population, lower eGFR and more severe ACR were each independently associated with increased rate of adverse outcomes, including kidney failure requiring replacement therapy, all-cause mortality, cardiovascular mortality, acute kidney injury, any hospitalization, coronary heart disease, stroke, heart failure, atrial fibrillation, and peripheral artery disease [9]. One important finding is that changes in ACR are associated with a significant reduction in the risk of mortality and kidney disease progression. The association between treatment effects on early changes in albuminuria and treatment effects on clinical endpoints and surrogate endpoints was analyzed using the data from 41 randomized clinical trials (29,979 patients) [29]. In this meta-analysis, each 30% decrease in geometric mean albuminuria versus control was associated with an average 27% lower risk of a clinical endpoint, and the association was stronger in patients with baseline albuminuria >30 mg/g. Whether a low baseline ACR was associated with an increased risk of poor cardiovascular and renal outcomes remained unclear. A similar observation was reported regarding the risk of end-stage kidney disease in observational studies that assessed CKD progression in the context of increased albuminuria [30]. In a post hoc analysis of the ONTARGET and TRANSCEND trials, Schmieder et al. assessed whether improvement or deterioration of albuminuria over time in patients with differing changes in glucose and BP changed their cardiovascular risk [31]. Data on mortality, cardiovascular, and renal outcomes were available from 22,984 high-risk patients, mostly hypertensive, followed for 56 months. Improvements in albuminuria at 2 years were associated with a lower risk of all-cause and cardiovascular mortality and of cardiovascular and renal events. Interestingly, in these trials, albuminuria over time was better than the glucose status and BP control in predicting mortality and both cardiovascular and renal outcomes. In 2022, Pasternak et al. [32] performed a population-based study of adults with incidence moderate to severe CKD to analyze the 5-year probability of a CKD regression, progression, or death across albuminuria categories after correction for baseline characteristics [32]. As expected, the probability of CKD regression was highest in patients pertaining to the lowest category of albuminuria (A1) and even lower in those patients combining a low ACR and an eGFR >60 mL/min/1.73 m^2. These data thus confirmed the prognostic role of albuminuria in the management of patients with moderate to severe CKD.

13.2.3 Other Markers of Kidney Disease Associated with Hypertension

In addition to markers of glomerular filtration rate and glomerular lesions, there are also kidney tubule biomarkers that may be used to evaluate either tubular cells dysfunction such as α1-microglobulin or uromodulin, or tubule injury such as kidney injury molecule 1 (KIM1), epidermal growth factor (EGF) or interleukin 18 (IL-18), or even the repair process [human cartilage glycoprotein 39 (YKL-40)] or inflammation [monocyte chemoattractant protein 1 (MCP1)]. These biomarkers may be of interest to monitor more accurately the kidney tubule involvement in the pathogenesis of hypertension [33], in particular salt-sensitive hypertension, but also the role of these markers in assessing the risk of developing hypertension or poor cardiovascular and renal outcomes. At last, these biomarkers can help in the evaluation of the kidney response to treatments in CKD patients and in hypertension [33]. Thus, in a subgroup of patients having participated in the Action to Control Cardiovascular Risk in Diabetes BP (ACCORD-BP) trial, the changes in eGFR observed in the intensive group did not always associate with the changes in injury marker levels [34]. However, in participants of the CARDIA study (Coronary Artery Risk Development in Young Adults) with a mean age of 45 years and without hypertension at baseline, the risk of developing incident hypertension after 9.9 years of follow-up was lower in subjects of the higher tertile of epidermal growth factor (EGF) in both Black and White participants. EGF was the only biomarker associated with 10-year systolic and diastolic blood pressure changes. Ikeme et al. [35] have investigated the association of clinical risk factors with specific kidney tubule biomarkers in a subgroup of patients with an eGFR <60 mL/min/1.73 m^2 having participated in the Systolic Blood Pressure Intervention Trial (SPRINT). In this analysis, higher age (9 years), male gender, Black race, and a high systolic BP were associated with significant differences in biomarkers indicating either higher levels of tubulointerstitial inflammation and repair or a worse tubule resorptive function or a higher level of tubulointerstitial inflammation and repair. These data suggested that clinical and demographic characteristics, such as race, sex, and elevated SBP, are associated with unique profiles of tubular damages in patients with reduced kidney function.

Among tubular biomarkers, uromodulin is perhaps the one with the greater potential to become a reliable marker of renal risk in hypertension as reviewed recently [36]. Uromodulin is the most abundant protein secreted in the urine. It is produced by the tubular cells of the thick ascending limb (90%) and the distal convoluted tubules (10%). Uromodulin is also secreted into the kidney interstitium and enters the blood at a much lower concentration than in the urine (~1000-fold less). Uromodulin plays an important role in water homeostasis and urine concentration and in the regulation of several ion excretions (potassium, calcium, and magnesium). Studies have also demonstrated that uromodulin is involved in sodium homeostasis and hence blood pressure regulation [37, 38]. The interest of uromodulin as a renal biomarker relies in the fact that uromodulin is expressed and released only within the kidney. One study has actually shown that uromodulin is a marker of kidney mass in living kidney donors and in the general population [39]. Therefore, several studies have investigated the predictive value of uromodulin as an outcome biomarker in kidney transplantation, acute kidney diseases, CKD, and cardiovascular diseases [36]. Thus, higher levels of uromodulin have been associated with a lower risk of developing end-stage kidney disease (ESKD) and conversely low urinary uromodulin levels have been associated with more rapid decline in kidney function progression toward ESKD as well as a higher risk of mortality and poor cardiovascular outcome [40–42]. In the general population, Ponte et al. reported that each 1-mg genetically predicted urinary uromodulin/g creatinine was associated with a 1 mL/min lower eGFR, an increased odd of having CKD (−6%), and higher systolic and diastolic BP values [43]. These effects were mediated in part by direct effects of uromodulin and GFR-mediated effects. In the general population, subjects with higher uromodulin levels had higher 24-h diastolic blood pressure, eGFR, and 24-h urinary sodium and potassium excretion than those with low levels of uromodulin [44]. In addition, the association of 24-h systolic and diastolic blood pressures with 24-h sodium excretion varied according to 24-h levels of uromodulin levels as shown in Fig. 13.2. Yet, in a subset of 157 subjects randomized to the control diet of the Dietary Approaches to Stop Hypertension (DASH)-Sodium trial who were assigned to three sodium diets (low, medium, and high) in random order, higher urine uromodulin levels were not associated with a greater increase in blood pressure in response to high salt intake [45]. More recently, an increased risk of developing hypertension has been reported in a two-sample Mendelian randomization (MR) analysis [46]. In this study, six datasets based on the UK Biobank and the International Consortium for Blood Pressure (ICBP) served as outcomes with a large sample of hypertension (n = 46,188), systolic blood pressure (SBP, n = 1,194,020), and diastolic blood pressure (DBP, n = 1,194,020).

Based on information available today regarding the associations of uromodulin with CKD and cardiovascular risk in hypertension, uromodulin might become an

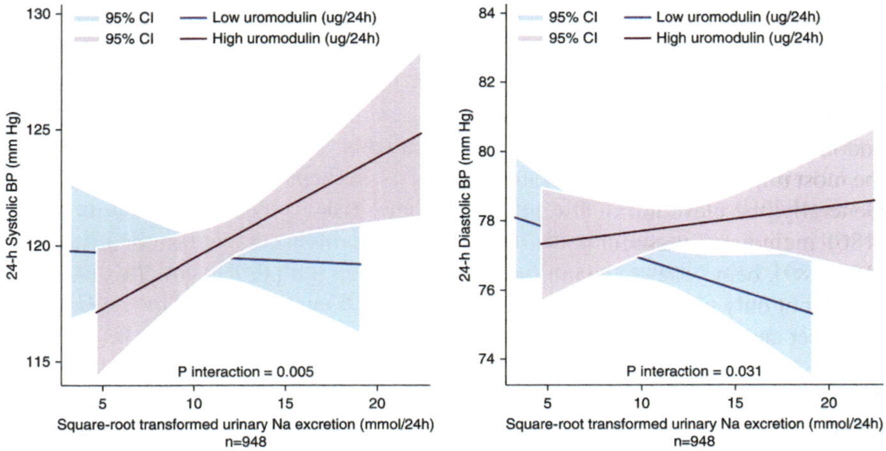

Fig. 13.2 Association of 24-h systolic BP and diastolic BP with 24-h sodium excretion in 948 individuals with high or low 24-h uromodulin levels. (From ref. [44] with permission)

interesting new kidney biomarker for the hypertensive population. Yet, there is still missing information, mainly regarding the changes in uromodulin upon blood pressure control using antihypertensive drug therapies. Uromodulin levels could also serve as a marker enabling to identify patients who could respond to some drug therapies such as loop diuretics. Thus, hypertensive patients with some uromodulin-increasing allele may respond better to loop diuretics. A prospective study testing this hypothesis is ongoing (UMOD study) [47].

13.3 Classical and Modern Renal Imaging Techniques in the Evaluation of BP Disorders

13.3.1 Kidney Ultrasound

Over the last decades, the role of kidney ultrasound in hypertensive patients has rapidly increased. This is illustrated by the place reserved for kidney ultrasound in the guidelines of the European Society of Hypertension (ESH). Whereas the 2013 ESH guidelines reserved its use to patients with suspected renal artery stenosis (RAS) [48], the 2018 and 2023 ESH guidelines integrated kidney ultrasound as one of the key procedures in the work-up of hypertensive patients with impaired renal function, albuminuria, or suspected secondary hypertension (level of evidence: IIB) [6, 49]. The 2018 and 2023 guidelines also acknowledged the importance of the Renal Resistive Index (RRI), a parameter that can be measured with high reproducibility in the Doppler mode. The ESH 2023 guidelines confirm the importance of kidney ultrasound in the assessment of hypertension-mediated organ damage (HMOD), and also briefly discuss the emerging role of contrast-enhanced ultrasound [6]. The emerging role of ultrasound in the field of nephrology and hypertension is basically due to the development of new techniques and improvements in the resolution of images. Besides, the size of the equipment has largely decreased: the first devices used in the 1970s had the size of an oversized refrigerator, whereas nowadays, modern devices are composed of a probe with a wireless connection to a random smartphone. These point-of-care devices allow bedside evaluation 24 h a day, without side effects and excellent image quality. Basic principles, indications, and future developments are discussed in this section.

13.3.1.1 Basic Principles

The probe of each sonography device contains crystals that transmit high-frequency soundwaves (usually between 3 and 20 MHz) into the human body. The reflected waves are captured by the same crystals, and their characteristics allow the reconstruction of the underlying structures. B-mode ultrasound expresses the intensity and time interval of the reflected waves in brightness and results in the classic gray-scaled image. The Doppler mode can measure the direction and speed of moving structures (blood), as they lead to a phase-shift of the sound waves. The direction is expressed in color (in general, red: toward the probe, blue: away from the probe), and the speed in cm/s or m/s. The speed of blood in the main renal arteries is usually between 60 and 180 cm/s and decreases to 20–30 cm/s in renal segmentary and interlobar arteries [50]. The speed increases during cardiac contraction and decreases during diastole, resulting in a Doppler curve with typical features that will be discussed in more detail below. Duplex combines Doppler and B-mode in the same image. In contrast-enhanced ultrasound (CEUS), a contrast product composed of non-nephrotoxic microbubbles is injected into the circulation [51]. The microbubbles are composed of an inert gas and a phospholipid shell. They have the size of human red blood cells and therefore remain intra-vascular; they are not filtered by kidneys but rapidly eliminated by the liver and lungs. CEUS improves visualization of the aorta and renal arteries and provides detailed information on intra-renal blood flow. Some examples of the different techniques are shown in Fig. 13.3.

13.3.1.2 Indications and Use of the Different Ultrasound Techniques

B-Mode Ultrasound

Ultrasonography of the kidneys plays an essential part in the clinical work-up of every patient with newly discovered acute or chronic kidney disease. In patients with both acute kidney injury and chronic kidney disease, B-mode ultrasound can identify an obstructive cause (hydronephrosis, bladder distention, urogenital tumors) and provide information on kidney size and structure, whereas Doppler or CEUS mode can identify renal infarction, arterial occlusion, or venous thrombosis. The timely detection of arterial occlusion is especially important in patients who have undergone endovascular repair of an aortic aneurysm with placement of branched prostheses that cover the renal arteries, as they are at high risk of uni-or bilateral occlusion.

As mentioned above, the role of kidney ultrasound in patients with hypertension was initially reserved for those with suspected renal artery stenosis, but with the

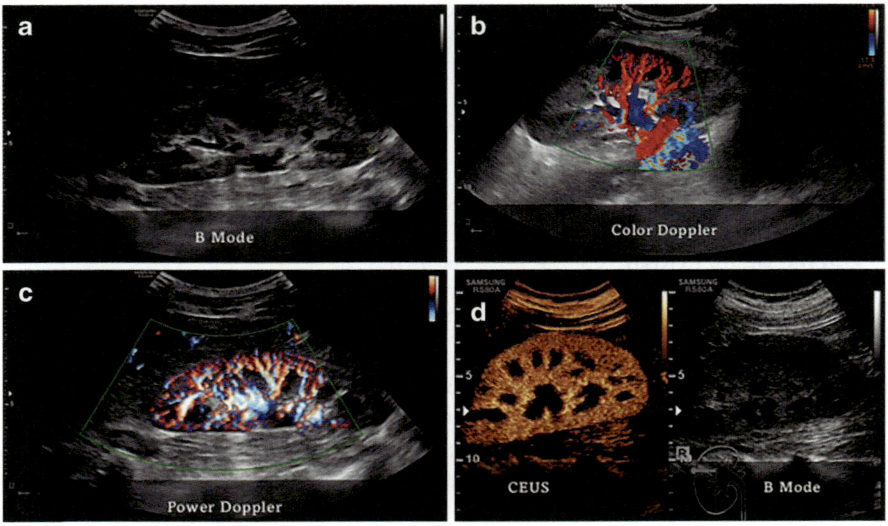

Fig. 13.3 Examples of different ultrasound techniques. (**a**) Conventional B-mode image of a normal right kidney; (**b**) color Doppler ultrasound, showing renal segmentary and interlobar arteries in red; (**c**) power Doppler mode depicting not only segmentary and interlobar, but also interlobular arteries; (**d**) contrast-enhanced ultrasound providing detailed information on the cortical microvasculature. (Personal data)

accumulation of data on the diagnostic and prognostic potential of the Renal Resistive Index, kidney ultrasound has become an integral part of the assessment of HMOD [52].

Doppler Ultrasound of the Kidneys and the Renal Resistive Index
The Renal Resistive Index (RRI) is a unitless ratio between maximum and minimum blood velocities that can be easily measured with Doppler/Duplex ultrasound at the level of segmentary arteries and defined as [(Peak Systolic Velocity-Diastolic Velocity)/Peak Systolic Velocity]. In general, the average of three segmentary arteries is provided separately for each kidney. By definition, the RRI is between 0 and 1. Small studies in the general population have shown that RRI is on average <0.7. A large study of 726 subjects of European descent found that RRI remains stable until the age of 40, but sharply increases hereafter [53]. Besides, women had higher RRI values than men in this study.

Patients with CKD have significantly higher RRI values than controls. This is possibly linked to an increased amount of interstitial fibrosis in these patients, which compresses the intra-renal blood vessels and thus leads to higher peak velocities. However, it may also refer to unaccounted differences in systemic factors such as the degree of arteriosclerosis [54, 55]. Indeed, RRI is influenced not only by intrarenal but also (and probably foremost) by systemic factors such as pulse pressure, systolic blood pressure, heart rate, and aortic pulse wave velocity as an indirect marker of the degree of systemic atherosclerosis [56]. This probably explains why the RRI is often increased in hypertensive patients and will decrease once blood pressure control is improved [57]. The role of systemic factors was also illustrated in an elegant study of 321 renal allograft recipients by Naesens et al. [58]. In their study, the RRI was not associated with histological features of the renal allograft, but merely with recipient factors such as recipient age.

Although the exact mechanisms and factors that influence RRI are still the subject of research, the prognostic value of RRI has been demonstrated in many studies and patient groups. In a cohort of 311 patients with CKD of mixed origin (diabetes, hypertension, glomerulonephritis) and a follow-up of 2 years, an RRI ≥0.7 was an independent risk factor for worsening renal function, defined as a decrease in eGFR of ≥20 mL/min/1.73 m^2 or the need for renal replacement therapy [59]. RRI had a sensitivity of 68% and a specificity of 69% to predict adverse renal outcome. Similar results were found in an Italian study that included 157 CKD patients with type 2 diabetes [60]. In this study, patients with an RRI ≥0.8 had a two to three times higher risk of a yearly decline of their renal function with ≥3 mL/min/1.73 m^2.

Of interest, in a prospective study of 426 patients with essential hypertension but no previous cardiovascular disease, Doi and colleagues reported that RRI was an independent predictor of the primary composite outcome that included all-cause death, myocardial infarction, stroke, congestive heart failure, aortic dissection, and end-stage renal failure [8]. Considering the aforementioned associations, it is not always possible to disentangle the role of renal factors from systemic factors in the prognostic information provided by RRI in these studies. Nevertheless, RRI is easily and rapidly measured during a conventional kidney ultrasound in any patient with CKD.

Assessment of the RRI also provides important information on the probability of an underlying unilateral renal artery stenosis, defined as a narrowing of the lumen of the renal artery of at least 50%. As such, a difference in RRI of ≥0.05 between two kidneys is one of the indirect ultrasound criteria of renal artery stenosis (RAS). The RRI is lower in the stenotic kidney, probably due to lower perfusion pressure [61].

Spectral analysis of the waveforms acquired while assessing the RRI in each kidney also allows the measurement of two other indirect criteria: prolonged acceleration time (AT) and index (AI). As flow is dampened in the stenotic kidney, Doppler curves are dampened (flatter), peak systolic velocity is reached later, and thus AT (the interval measured in seconds between the onset of the wave and the initial systolic peak) and AI (the upstroke of the systolic peak adjusted to the transmitted frequency) are prolonged. An acceleration time ≥0.08 s and an acceleration index ≥300 cm/s^2 are in favor of the diagnosis of RAS [62] (see Table 13.2). The dampened aspect of the curves is called tardus parvus (see Fig. 13.4 for different Doppler patterns). Nevertheless, alterations of these indirect criteria occur mostly when the renal stenosis is severe (>75%), and the absence of indirect criteria does not exclude the presence of RAS. Reported sensitivity and specificity of the AT were, respectively, 80% and 88%, and of the AI 74% and 85% in a systematic review that included 88 studies and 8147 patients with proven RAS [63].

Table 13.2 Direct and indirect Doppler ultrasound criteria for the diagnosis of renal artery stenosis

Blood flow parameter	Renal artery stenosis (≥60%)	Sensitivity	Specificity
Direct criteria			
Peak systolic velocity	≥200 cm/s	85%	92%
Renal-aortic ratio (RAR)	≥3.5	78%	89%
Indirect criteria			
Resistive index difference	≥5% (Δ0.40 – 0.50)		
Acceleration time	≥0.08 s	80%	88%
Acceleration index	≥300 cm/s^2	74%	85%

Direct criteria are measured in the renal artery, whereas indirect criteria are measured in the segmentary arteries in the kidneys

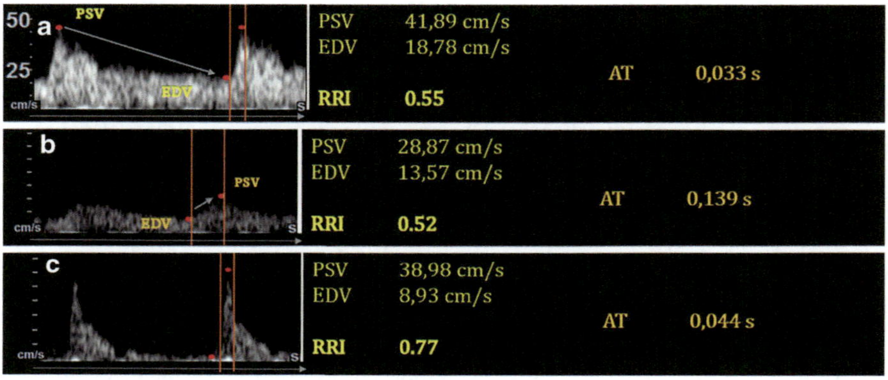

Fig. 13.4 Examples of Doppler curves according to the clinical situation. (**a**) Normal Doppler curve; (**b**) dampened Doppler spectrum with prolonged acceleration time [AT, the time interval (in seconds) between the orange lines, corresponding to the onset of the wave and the peak systolic velocity (PSV)], as well as reduced PSV and RRI in case of severe renal artery stenosis (tardus parvus pattern); (**c**) increased RRI as encountered in patients with CKD and/or essential hypertension. (Personal data)

Assessment of the RRI has not only diagnostic but also some prognostic potential in patients with RAS. The landmark study performed by Radermacher et al. [64] reported that an RRI >0.8 reliably identified patients with RAS in whom revascularization of the renal artery did not improve blood pressure or renal survival. However, others did not confirm the predictive potential of RRI in this context [65]. Today, most experts agree that the decision to revascularize the renal artery should not be based on Doppler criteria, but on a combination of clinical and radiological parameters [66].

Doppler Ultrasound of the Renal Arteries

Doppler ultrasound of the renal arteries is essentially performed to screen for renal artery stenosis. Doppler ultrasound of the renal arteries is also indicated to assess the patency of the renal arteries, for example after the placement of (branched)

endovascular stents [67] or in patients with aortic dissection. Depending on the population, RAS is present in approximately 2–5% of all patients with essential hypertension [6], but its prevalence increases to 10–30% in patients with coronary artery disease and to 20–40% in patients with resistant hypertension [68]. Atherosclerotic disease accounts for 90% of cases with documented RAS, and fibromuscular dysplasia (FMD) for 10%, but the prevalence of FMD may be higher as this disease is possibly under-diagnosed [69, 70].

RAS should be suspected in any patient with resistant hypertension, especially when there is a sudden onset of severe hypertension in patients >50 years, an abdominal bruit, recurrent flash pulmonary edema, or an increase in serum creatinine of 30–50% after the introduction of a blocker of the renin–angiotensin system [68, 70].

According to the 2023 ESH guidelines, renal artery Doppler/Duplex ultrasound is the first-choice screening test in patients with suspected RAS [6]. This approach is supported by the excellent sensitivity (91–94%) and specificity (82–91%) obtained with this technique, a result that is close to the performance obtained with CT angiography or magnetic resonance angiography [71].

Parameters that are measured are the peak systolic velocity (PSV) of blood flow in the proximal, medium, and distal parts of the left and right renal arteries and the aorta (see Fig. 13.5 for an example). A PSV ≥180 cm/s in any part of the renal artery or a renal-aortic PSV ratio (RAR) ≥3.5 is considered as direct criteria for the presence of an RAS, with a sensitivity and specificity of respectively 85% and 92% for PSV, and 78% and 89% for RAR [63].

Disadvantages of the technique remain its operator-dependent nature and limited feasibility in obese patients. Besides, the medium part of the renal artery is often difficult to visualize due to the interposition of bowel loops. This is a particular problem for FMD, as the stenotic lesions are often located in this segment. Therefore, the European consensus paper states that Duplex ultrasound of the renal arteries is the first-choice exam to screen for FMD, but CTA or MRA should be performed in order to confirm positive Duplex findings, or to exclude the disease in patients with negative Duplex findings but high clinical suspicion [72].

Contrast-Enhanced Ultrasound of the Kidneys and Renal Arteries
Contrast-enhanced ultrasound (CEUS) can overcome some of the shortcomings of Doppler ultrasound, as the injected contrast product increases the ultrasonic signal, and thus the visibility of the renal arteries in obese subjects. The degree of renal artery stenosis is not expressed as the degree of acceleration in blood flow with this technique, but as the ratio between the diameter of the stenotic part and the normal portion of the renal artery distal of the stenosis. This ratio is expressed as a percentage. Claudon et al. were the first to report that the accuracy to detect an RAS increased from 64 to 84% in 198 patients with CEUS as compared to Doppler ultrasound [68]. More recently, similar results were obtained in 60 patients with mild CKD [eGFR 66 (min 48–max 85) mL/min/1.73 m^2, age 64.4 18 years, 31.7% DM], and a suspected RAS. Sensitivity was 94.7% and specificity 84% in this Chinese study, and no side effects occurred [73]. Of interest, the technique also correctly

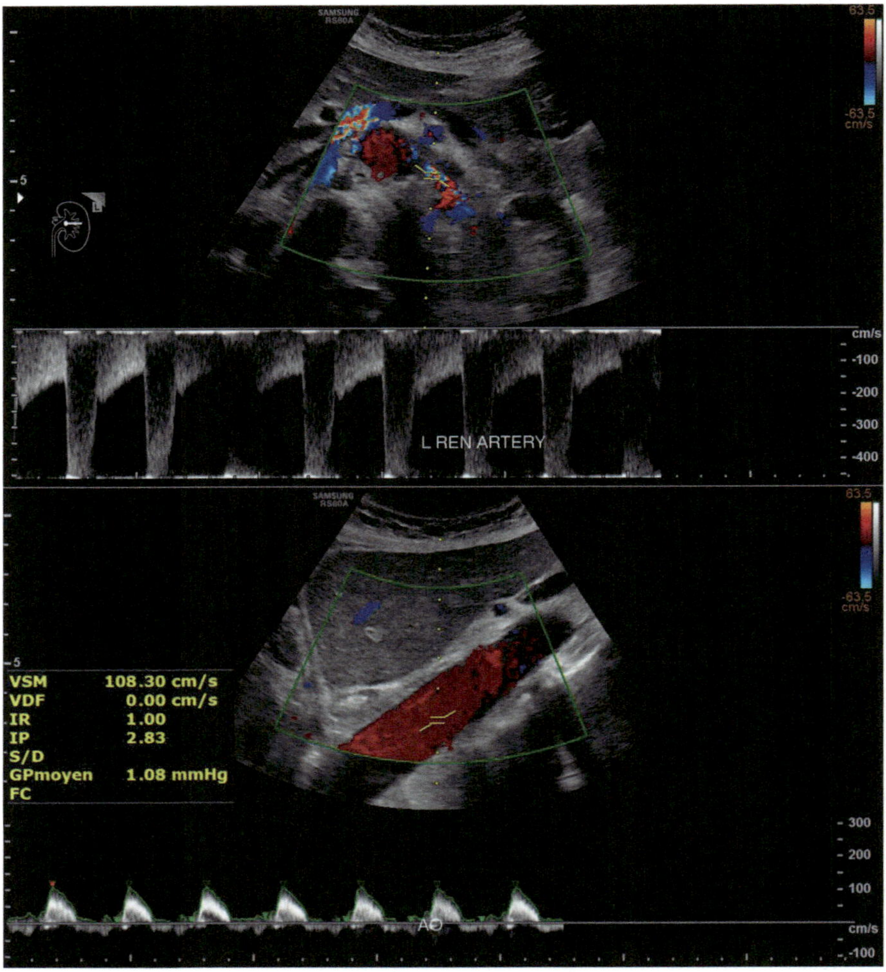

Fig. 13.5 Example of severe stenosis of the left renal artery, with peak systolic velocity (PSV) of blood flow >300 cm/s in the proximal part of left renal artery, and a normal blood velocity in the longitudinal axis of the aorta (bottom figure; PSV = VSM = 108 cm/s, renal-aortic ratio >3.5). (Personal data)

diagnosed lesions compatible with Takayasu arteritis, a common cause of renal artery stenosis in China, and present in 12/60 patients of this study [73]. Yet, the number of studies remains too limited to draw conclusions about the definite place of CEUS in RAS diagnosis and follow-up. Nevertheless, results are promising and more studies will certainly follow.

During the same exam, CEUS of the kidneys can be performed; CEUS provides excellent resolution, and is a well-established method to classify renal cysts, a common finding in patients with arterial hypertension. CEUS offers a valuable alternative to CT and MRI, especially in patients with hypertension and CKD. due to the limitations of iodinated or gadolinium-based contrast products in these patients. Both arterial hypertension and CKD are characterized histologically by a vascular rarefaction, and CEUS represents an excellent method to depict not only large, but also small intra-renal blood vessels. Intra-renal micro-perfusion can be quantified based on the brightness and temporal characteristics of the injected microbubbles. Recent studies have shown that CEUS-assessed cortical perfusion is indeed lower in patients with hypertension and/or CKD as compared to age- and sex-matched controls [74–77]. Further studies should now explore whether CEUS-assessed cortical micro-perfusion has a real added value for the prediction of adverse renal outcomes in hypertensive patients with or without CKD.

13.3.1.3 Future Developments

The widespread use of CEUS is limited by the expertise needed for this technique. Besides, costly contrast products have to be injected and may result in allergic reactions. The so-called microvascular imaging technique may overcome these issues by using Doppler algorithms and filters to suppress noise caused by motion artifacts [78, 79]. With this approach, small intra-renal blood vessels are depicted in detail without contrast product. Microvascular imaging offers a quality close to CEUS for kidney imaging, but the visibility of the main renal arteries is not improved with this technique.

Ultrasound shear-wave elastography is a validated method to assess liver fibrosis, which has shown promise for the assessment of fibrosis in kidneys. Interstitial fibrosis is the most important histological factor to predict adverse renal outcome in CKD patients, and a non-invasive marker is definitively needed. Fibrosis assessment is also important in the field of hypertension, in particular in renal artery stenosis. The optimal management of RAS remains debated, notably whether surgical or endovascular revascularization should be performed. Randomized studies comparing stenting versus medical therapy did not show any benefit for revascularization-stenting, but studies have—among others—been criticized for erroneous patient selection [80]. A key question remains the viability of the parenchyma of the post-stenotic kidney, as revascularization is less useful in case of advanced, irreversible kidney fibrosis. The use of elastography for assessment of kidney fibrosis could be one approach enabling to improve the patients' selection. However, so far, this technique has been investigated mainly in patients with a kidney graft, because of the superficial location of the transplant [81, 82].

13.3.2 MRI of the Kidneys

13.3.2.1 Magnetic Resonance Angiography (MRA) with Gadolinium

It is well established that gadolinium-enhanced MRA has a very high sensitivity and specificity to detect renal artery stenosis that is similar to computed tomographic angiography (CTA) [83, 84]. This is especially the case in obese patients, as the performance of ultrasound is suboptimal in these patients. MRA also provides excellent assessment of accessory renal arteries. However, the high costs and low availability of the technique have limited its clinical use. Besides, the risk of nephrogenic systemic fibrosis (NSF) is also a drawback. For these reasons, many centers prefer the use of CTA, despite the risk of iodinated contrast-associated acute kidney injury. However, the number of reported cases of NSF has rapidly decreased since the use of gadodiamide and other gadolinium-based category I. Contrast products with a linear ligand have been largely abandoned. These products have been replaced by category II products such as gadobutrol that contain cyclic ligand and that can also be used in patients with advanced CKD [85]. Besides, the number of MRI devices increases rapidly, at least in developed countries, leading to easier access and possibly more widespread use of MRA in the future.

13.3.2.2 Emerging MRI Techniques

The field of MRI is evolving quickly, and techniques that were so far limited to research might be integrated in the clinic in the near future. These techniques offer possibilities to measure hemodynamic parameters such as per-kidney cortical and medullary blood flow, but also provide information on structural or metabolic aspects such as the degree of fibrosis, oxygenation, and sodium handling. None of these techniques needs the administration of IV contrast products. Therefore, exams can be repeated safely several times. Thanks to shorter acquisition protocols, different MRI techniques can be combined and performed within one MRI session (called multiparametric MRI). In light of the ongoing debate on the optimal treatment of patients with renal artery stenosis, an MRI assessment of the degree of perfusion, oxygenation, and fibrosis is clearly of interest, as this may be helpful to identify those patients that may benefit from revascularization. The following paragraphs provide a brief description of the major techniques and their main results in the field of hypertension.

Phase-Contrast MRI

Phase-contrast (PC) MRI can measure blood flow velocity separately in the left and right renal artery by applying bipolar magnetic gradients that induce phase shift differences between the spins of moving protons in blood versus static protons in surrounding tissues. The phase shift differences are proportional to the speed of blood in the vessel of interest. The diameter of the renal artery is measured simultaneously, thus enabling computation of the single-kidney renal blood flow (sk-RBF) and global RBF [86]. PC-MRI-assessed RBF corresponds well to PAH-based RBF measurements, although the number of included individuals was low in the validation studies (between 8 and 14). In hypertensive patients, Schoenberg et al. reported that PC-MRI had a sensitivity of 100% and a specificity of 93% to distinguish those patients with no RAS from those with an RAS >50% [87, 88], but another research group found a rather poor correlation between PC-MRI-assessed RBF and the presence of RAS [89], underlining technical difficulties that may be met with this technique. Binkert et al. assessed whether PC-MRI could predict clinical success (defined as a reduction in BP of >15% and/or a reduction in creatinine of >20%) of percutaneous transluminal angioplasty (PTA) in patients with RAS. A combination of PC-MRI and MRI-assessed renal volume had a sensitivity of 91% and specificity of 67% to predict clinical success; those with normal renal volume and reduced flow had the best outcome [90]. These findings still await confirmation but underline the potential of PC-MRI, especially in combination with other MR techniques.

Arterial Spin Labeling (ASL) MRI

ASL MRI is a sophisticated subtraction technique that uses magnetically labeled water protons in blood to quantify (without the use of contrast product) cortical and medullary perfusion of each kidney, expressed as mL/100 g/min [91]. The technique is sensitive to movement and breathing artifacts and is rather time-consuming. Therefore, the number of studies performed in the field of hypertension is limited. In a study of seven renal transplant patients with a documented RAS, Li and colleagues reported that ASL MRI-assessed perfusion was lower as compared to controls and improved after PTA [92]. Arterial spin-labeling is suited for longitudinal studies. For example, Prasad et al. showed in a study of 41 patients with diabetic CKD and 13 matched controls that ASL MRI-assessed cortical perfusion is an independent predictor of the yearly decline in eGFR [93]. ASL MRI is also a very interesting tool to assess whether drugs induce short-term changes in cortical or medullary perfusion. Haddock et al. performed ALS MRI before and up to 12 min after the IV injection of furosemide (20 mg) in nine healthy volunteers, and demonstrated that cortical nor medullary perfusion changed, whereas medullary oxygenation (measured with BOLD-MRI) increased [94]. In a study with a similar design, Laursen et al. found that the administration of the SGLT2-inhibitor dapagliflozin increased cortical oxygenation, without changing renal perfusion (ASL) or global blood flow (measured with PC-MRI) in patients with type 1 diabetes with albuminuria [95]. In healthy subjects, however, no change in renal oxygenation was observed in response to empagliflozin [96]. These studies demonstrate the potential of MRI in drug research, especially when multiparametric MRI is performed.

Blood Oxygenation Level-Dependent (BOLD) MRI

BOLD-MRI allows the estimation of both cortical and medullary tissue oxygenation by using the paramagnetic properties of deoxyhemoglobin that shortens the relaxation times of T2* weighted images. The higher the local deoxyHb levels, the shorter T2* relaxation times, the higher the decline rate R2*. Hence, a high local R2* value corresponds to low oxygenation, and vice versa [97, 98].

Without surprise, BOLD-MRI has been extensively used in the field of hypertension and particularly in patients with atherosclerotic RAS, as RAS is the classic example of ischemic kidney disease.

The research group of the Mayo Clinic led by Stephen Textor has been very active in this field, and was the first to show that R2* is indeed increased in patients with severe (>90%) RAS, but not in those with less severe stenosis [99]. They also demonstrated that the acute response to IV furosemide can be used as a non-invasive test to assess the viability of kidney parenchyma. In those with severe RAS and reduced kidney volume, there was only a small or no decrease in medullary R2* levels after furosemide, whereas those with moderate RAS or no stenosis had large changes in medullary R2*.

In addition, stenting of the renal artery reduced R2* values of the stenotic kidney, and increased the R2* change after furosemide [100]. More recently, the same research group demonstrated that the infusion of autologous mesenchymal stem cells without angioplasty also leads to a decrease in R2* of the stenotic kidney, corresponding to an increase in oxygenation [101]. These changes occurred in parallel with improvements in multidetector CT-assessed perfusion and reductions in inflammatory markers.

Several (small) studies have shown that patients with an RAS and high cortical or medullary R2* values and preserved renal volume have a better outcome after revascularization than those with lower values, suggesting that BOLD-MRI is an interesting tool to select patients who will have a favorable outcome after revascularization [102]. Thus, BOLD-MRI may help to predict outcome after angioplasty.

In hypertensive patients without RAS and healthy controls, BOLD-MRI has mainly been used to study the effects of drugs or nutrition. Among the drugs that increase BOLD MRI-assessed oxygenation are inhibitors of the renin-angiotensin system and SGLT2-inhibitors [103], whereas angiotensin-II infusion and iodinated contrast products decrease oxygenation [98]. Of note, a high salt intake reduces medullary oxygenation, both in hypertensive patients and controls [104].

BOLD-MRI has been criticized, as it is a simplification to state that this technique measures renal tissue oxygenation. Indeed, R2* values are influenced by many factors. The major drawback is the bias induced by the partial volume effect. BOLD-MRI measures R2* values voxel per voxel (a voxel is the smallest part of the MR image) and assumes that the blood volume within each voxel doesn't change over time. However, in case of interstitial edema, reduced arterial blood flow, or venous congestion, this may not be the case. For example, the furosemide-induced decrease in R2* is basically not only due to the decrease in oxygen-consuming sodium reabsorption in Henle's loops but also due to changes in the partial volume, as the swelling of the tubules will lead to a reduction of relative blood volume per voxel.

A new technique that needs the injection of ferumoxytol has recently been proposed to overcome this problem and will certainly lead to interesting results in the future [105].

Diffusion MRI

Diffusion-weighted (DW) MRI quantifies the motion of water in the tissue over time, by acquiring images with different weighing factors called *b* values. The movement of water and microcirculation is expressed as the apparent diffusion coefficient (ADC), the outcome variable [97]. DW MRI provides information on the micro-structure of kidney tissue, in particular the degree of fibrosis. As such, it has been demonstrated in humans that ADC values correlate inversely with the degree of fibrosis at kidney biopsy, both in transplant and native kidneys [106, 107]. Most studies have focused on CKD patients and shown its prognostic potential [106]. One study has been performed in 20 patients with suspected RAS; in this study, the degree of RAS correlated strongly and inversely with ADC values, and ADC values were significantly lower in kidneys with arterial stenosis than in kidneys of patients without RAS [108]. Whether DW MRI can be of help in the selection of RAS patients that may benefit from revascularization remains to be determined.

13.4 Conclusion

The herein described MRI techniques offer possibilities to obtain detailed and unique information on renal perfusion, metabolism, and structure in hypertensive patients with and without CKD. The techniques can be combined with one another, and also with classic MR techniques such as MRA. However, several factors limit thus far their implementation in the clinic. The required scanning times are long; in many countries, there is a low availability of MR scanners, costs are high, and local expertise is lacking to acquire and analyze images. Besides, more data on their diagnostic and prognostic potential are needed before these techniques can be proposed for wider clinical use. In hypertensive patients, their first application will probably be in the field of renal artery stenosis.

References

1. Lee H, Kwon SH, Jeon JS, Noh H, Han DC, Kim H. Association between blood pressure and the risk of chronic kidney disease in treatment-naïve hypertensive patients. Kidney Res Clin Pract. 2022;41:31–42. https://doi.org/10.23876/j.krcp.21.099.
2. Sim JJ, Shi J, Kovesdy CP, Kalantar-Zadeh K, Jacobsen SJ. Impact of achieved blood pressures on mortality risk and end-stage renal disease among a large, diverse hypertension population. J Am Coll Cardiol. 2014;64:588–97. https://doi.org/10.1016/j.jacc.2014.04.065.
3. Hsu CY, McCulloch CE, Darbinian J, Go AS, Iribarren C. Elevated blood pressure and risk of end-stage renal disease in subjects without baseline kidney disease. Arch Intern Med. 2005;165:923–8. https://doi.org/10.1001/archinte.165.8.923.
4. Tozawa M, Iseki K, Iseki C, Kinjo K, Ikemiya Y, Takishita S. Blood pressure predicts risk of developing end-stage renal disease in men and women. Hypertension. 2003;41:1341–5. https://doi.org/10.1161/01.HYP.0000069699.92349.8C.
5. Burnier M, Damianaki A. Hypertension as cardiovascular risk factor in chronic kidney disease. Circ Res. 2023;132:1050–63. https://doi.org/10.1161/CIRCRESAHA.122.321762.
6. Mancia G, Kreutz R, Brunstrom M, Burnier M, Grassi G, Januszewicz A, et al. 2023 ESH guidelines for the management of arterial hypertension the task force for the management of arterial hypertension of the European Society of Hypertension: endorsed by the International Society of Hypertension (ISH) and the European Renal Association (ERA). J Hypertens. 2023;41:1874–2071. https://doi.org/10.1097/HJH.0000000000003480.
7. Chronic Kidney Disease Prognosis C, Matsushita K, van der Velde M, Astor BC, Woodward M, Levey AS, de Jong PE, et al. Association of estimated glomerular filtration rate and albuminuria with all-cause and cardiovascular mortality in general population cohorts: a collaborative meta-analysis. Lancet. 2010;375:2073–81. https://doi.org/10.1016/S0140-6736(10)60674-5.
8. Doi Y, Iwashima Y, Yoshihara F, Kamide K, Hayashi S, Kubota Y, et al. Renal resistive index and cardiovascular and renal outcomes in essential hypertension. Hypertension. 2012;60:770–7. https://doi.org/10.1161/hypertensionaha.112.196717.
9. Grams ME, Coresh J, Matsushita K, Ballew SH, Sang Y, Surapaneni A, et al. Estimated glomerular filtration rate, albuminuria, and adverse outcomes: an individual-participant data meta-analysis. JAMA. 2023;330:1266–77. https://doi.org/10.1001/jama.2023.17002.

10. Porrini E, Ruggenenti P, Luis-Lima S, Carrara F, Jimenez A, de Vries APJ, et al. Estimated GFR: time for a critical appraisal. Nat Rev Nephrol. 2019;15:177–90. https://doi.org/10.1038/s41581-018-0080-9.
11. Soveri I, Berg UB, Bjork J, Elinder CG, Grubb A, Mejare I, Group SGR, et al. Measuring GFR: a systematic review. Am J Kidney Dis. 2014;64:411–24. https://doi.org/10.1053/j.ajkd.2014.04.010.
12. Levey AS, Coresh J, Tighiouart H, Greene T, Inker LA. Measured and estimated glomerular filtration rate: current status and future directions. Nat Rev Nephrol. 2020;16:51–64. https://doi.org/10.1038/s41581-019-0191-y.
13. Cockcroft DW, Gault MH. Prediction of creatinine clearance from serum creatinine. Nephron. 1976;16:31–41. https://doi.org/10.1159/000180580.
14. Levey AS, Bosch JP, Lewis JB, Greene T, Rogers N, Roth D, Modification of Diet in Renal Disease Study Group. A more accurate method to estimate glomerular filtration rate from serum creatinine: a new prediction equation. Ann Intern Med. 1999;130:461–70. https://doi.org/10.7326/0003-4819-130-6-199903160-00002.
15. Levey AS, Stevens LA, Schmid CH, Zhang YL, Castro AF 3rd, Feldman HI, et al. A new equation to estimate glomerular filtration rate. Ann Intern Med. 2009;150:604–12. https://doi.org/10.7326/0003-4819-150-9-200905050-00006.
16. Inker LA, Eneanya ND, Coresh J, Tighiouart H, Wang D, Sang Y, et al. New creatinine- and cystatin C-based equations to estimate GFR without race. N Engl J Med. 2021;385:1737–49. https://doi.org/10.1056/NEJMoa2102953.
17. Pottel H, Björk J, Courbebaisse M, Couzi L, Ebert N, Eriksen BO, et al. Development and validation of a modified full age spectrum creatinine-based equation to estimate glomerular filtration rate: a cross-sectional analysis of pooled data. Ann Intern Med. 2021;174:183–91. https://doi.org/10.7326/m20-4366.
18. Delanaye P, Vidal-Petiot E, Björk J, Ebert N, Eriksen BO, Dubourg L, et al. Performance of creatinine-based equations to estimate glomerular filtration rate in White and black populations in Europe, Brazil and Africa. Nephrol Dial Transplant. 2023;38:106–18. https://doi.org/10.1093/ndt/gfac241.
19. Inker LA, Schmid CH, Tighiouart H, Eckfeldt JH, Feldman HI, Greene T, et al. Estimating glomerular filtration rate from serum creatinine and cystatin C. N Engl J Med. 2012;367:20–9. https://doi.org/10.1056/NEJMoa1114248.
20. Grubb A, Horio M, Hansson LO, Bjork J, Nyman U, Flodin M, et al. Generation of a new cystatin C-based estimating equation for glomerular filtration rate by use of 7 assays standardized to the international calibrator. Clin Chem. 2014;60:974–86. https://doi.org/10.1373/clinchem.2013.220707.
21. Pottel H, Bjork J, Rule AD, Ebert N, Eriksen BO, Dubourg L, et al. Cystatin C-based equation to estimate GFR without the inclusion of race and sex. N Engl J Med. 2023;388:333–43. https://doi.org/10.1056/NEJMoa2203769.
22. Schaeffner ES, Ebert N, Delanaye P, Frei U, Gaedeke J, Jakob O, et al. Two novel equations to estimate kidney function in persons aged 70 years or older. Ann Intern Med. 2012;157:471–81. https://doi.org/10.7326/0003-4819-157-7-201210020-00003.
23. Pottel H, Delanaye P, Schaeffner E, Dubourg L, Eriksen BO, Melsom T, et al. Estimating glomerular filtration rate for the full age spectrum from serum creatinine and cystatin C. Nephrol Dial Transplant. 2017;32:497–507. https://doi.org/10.1093/ndt/gfw425.
24. Fu EL, Coresh J, Grams ME, Clase CM, Elinder CG, Paik J, et al. Removing race from the CKD-EPI equation and its impact on prognosis in a predominantly White European population. Nephrol Dial Transplant. 2023;38:119–28. https://doi.org/10.1093/ndt/gfac197.
25. Delanaye P, Cavalier E, Pottel H, Stehlé T. New and old GFR equations: a European perspective. Clin Kidney J. 2023;16:1375–83. https://doi.org/10.1093/ckj/sfad039.
26. Fu EL, Levey AS, Coresh J, Grams ME, Faucon AL, Elinder CG, et al. Accuracy of GFR-estimating equations based on creatinine, cystatin C or both in routine care. Nephrol Dial Transplant. 2024;39:694–706. https://doi.org/10.1093/ndt/gfad219.
27. Benoit SW, Ciccia EA, Devarajan P. Cystatin C as a biomarker of chronic kidney disease: latest developments. Expert Rev Mol Diagn. 2020;20:1019–26. https://doi.org/10.1080/14737159.2020.1768849.

28. Group KCW. KDIGO 2012 clinical practice guideline for the evaluation and management of chronic kidney disease. Kidney Int Suppl. 2013;3:1–150.
29. Heerspink HJL, Greene T, Tighiouart H, Gansevoort RT, Coresh J, Simon AL, et al. Change in albuminuria as a surrogate endpoint for progression of kidney disease: a meta-analysis of treatment effects in randomised clinical trials. Lancet Diabetes Endocrinol. 2019;7:128–39. https://doi.org/10.1016/s2213-8587(18)30314-0.
30. Coresh J, Heerspink HJL, Sang Y, Matsushita K, Arnlov J, Astor BC, et al. Change in albuminuria and subsequent risk of end-stage kidney disease: an individual participant-level consortium meta-analysis of observational studies. Lancet Diabetes Endocrinol. 2019;7:115–27. https://doi.org/10.1016/S2213-8587(18)30313-9.
31. Schmieder RE, Schutte R, Schumacher H, Böhm M, Mancia G, Weber MA, et al. Mortality and morbidity in relation to changes in albuminuria, glucose status and systolic blood pressure: an analysis of the ONTARGET and TRANSCEND studies. Diabetologia. 2014;57:2019–29. https://doi.org/10.1007/s00125-014-3330-9.
32. Pasternak M, Liu P, Quinn R, Elliott M, Harrison TG, Hemmelgarn B, et al. Association of Albuminuria and Regression of chronic kidney disease in adults with newly diagnosed moderate to severe chronic kidney disease. JAMA Netw Open. 2022;5:e2225821. https://doi.org/10.1001/jamanetworkopen.2022.25821.
33. Johnson RJ, Herrera-Acosta J, Schreiner GF, Rodriguez-Iturbe B. Subtle acquired renal injury as a mechanism of salt-sensitive hypertension. N Engl J Med. 2002;346:913–23. https://doi.org/10.1056/NEJMra011078.
34. Nadkarni GN, Chauhan K, Rao V, Ix JH, Shlipak MG, Parikh CR, et al. Effect of intensive blood pressure lowering on kidney tubule injury: findings from the ACCORD trial study participants. Am J Kidney Dis. 2019;73:31–8. https://doi.org/10.1053/j.ajkd.2018.07.016
35. Ikeme JC, Katz R, Muiru AN, Estrella MM, Scherzer R, Garimella PS, et al. Clinical risk factors for kidney tubule biomarker abnormalities among hypertensive adults with reduced eGFR in the SPRINT trial. Am J Hypertens. 2022;35:1006–13. https://doi.org/10.1093/ajh/hpac102.
36. Mary S, Boder P, Padmanabhan S, McBride MW, Graham D, Delles C, et al. Role of uromodulin in salt-sensitive hypertension. Hypertension. 2022;79:2419–29. https://doi.org/10.1161/hypertensionaha.122.19888.
37. Graham LA, Padmanabhan S, Fraser NJ, Kumar S, Bates JM, Raffi HS, et al. Validation of uromodulin as a candidate gene for human essential hypertension. Hypertension. 2014;63:551–8. https://doi.org/10.1161/HYPERTENSIONAHA.113.01423.
38. Trudu M, Janas S, Lanzani C, Debaix H, Schaeffer C, Ikehata M, et al. Common noncoding UMOD gene variants induce salt-sensitive hypertension and kidney damage by increasing uromodulin expression. Nat Med. 2013;19:1655–60. https://doi.org/10.1038/nm.3384.
39. Pivin E, Ponte B, de Seigneux S, Ackermann D, Guessous I, Ehret G, et al. Uromodulin and nephron mass. Clin J Am Soc Nephrol. 2018;13:1556–7.
40. Steubl D, Block M, Herbst V, Nockher WA, Schlumberger W, Kemmner S, et al. Urinary uromodulin independently predicts end-stage renal disease and rapid kidney function decline in a cohort of chronic kidney disease patients. Medicine (Baltimore). 2019;98:e15808. https://doi.org/10.1097/md.0000000000015808.
41. Steubl D, Buzkova P, Garimella PS, Ix JH, Devarajan P, Bennett MR, et al. Association of serum uromodulin with ESKD and kidney function decline in the elderly: the cardiovascular health study. Am J Kidney Dis. 2019;74:501–9. https://doi.org/10.1053/j.ajkd.2019.02.024.
42. Steubl D, Schneider MP, Meiselbach H, Nadal J, Schmid MC, Saritas T, et al. Association of serum uromodulin with death, cardiovascular events, and kidney failure in CKD. Clin J Am Soc Nephrol. 2020;15:616–24. https://doi.org/10.2215/cjn.11780919.
43. Ponte B, Sadler MC, Olinger E, Vollenweider P, Bochud M, Padmanabhan S, et al. Mendelian randomization to assess causality between uromodulin, blood pressure and chronic kidney disease. Kidney Int. 2021;100:1282–91. https://doi.org/10.1016/j.kint.2021.08.032.
44. Ponte B, Pruijm M, Ackermann D, Olinger E, Youhanna S, Vogt B, et al. Uromodulin, salt, and 24-h blood pressure in the general population. Clin J Am Soc Nephrol. 2021;16:787–9.

45. Bakhoum CY, Anderson CAM, Juraschek SP, Rebholz CM, Appel LJ, Miller ER, et al. The relationship between urine uromodulin and blood pressure changes: the DASH-sodium trial. Am J Hypertens. 2021;34:154–6. https://doi.org/10.1093/ajh/hpaa140.
46. You R, Chen L, Xu L, Zhang D, Li H, Shi X, Zheng Y. High level of uromodulin increases the risk of hypertension: a Mendelian randomization study. Front Cardiovasc Med. 2021;8:736001. https://doi.org/10.3389/fcvm.2021.736001.
47. McCallum L, Brooksbank K, McConnachie A, Aman A, Lip S, Dawson J, et al. Rationale and design of the genotype-blinded trial of torasemide for the treatment of hypertension (BHF UMOD). Am J Hypertens. 2021;34:92–9. https://doi.org/10.1093/ajh/hpaa166.
48. Mancia G, Fagard R, Narkiewicz K, Redon J, Zanchetti A, Bohm M, et al. 2013 ESH/ESC guidelines for the management of arterial hypertension: the task force for the management of arterial hypertension of the European Society of Hypertension (ESH) and of the European Society of Cardiology (ESC). J Hypertens. 2013;31:1281–357. https://doi.org/10.1097/01.hjh.0000431740.32696.cc.
49. Williams B, Mancia G, Spiering W, Agabiti Rosei E, Azizi M, Burnier M, et al. 2018 ESC/ESH guidelines for the management of arterial hypertension: the task force for the management of arterial hypertension of the European Society of Cardiology and the European Society of Hypertension: the task force for the management of arterial hypertension of the European Society of Cardiology and the European Society of Hypertension. J Hypertens. 2018;36:1953–2041. https://doi.org/10.1097/HJH.0000000000001940.
50. Al-Katib S, Shetty M, Jafri SM, Jafri SZ. Radiologic assessment of native renal vasculature: a multimodality review. Radiographics. 2017;37:136–56. https://doi.org/10.1148/rg.2017160060.
51. Dietrich CF, Averkiou M, Nielsen MB, Barr RG, Burns PN, Calliada F, et al. How to perform contrast-enhanced ultrasound (CEUS). Ultrasound Int Open. 2018;4:E2–15. https://doi.org/10.1055/s-0043-123931.
52. Tsioufis C, Andrikou I, Pruijm M, Ponte B, Sarafidis P, Koureas A, et al. Should renal color Doppler ultrasonography be a routine test in newly diagnosed hypertensive patient? J Hypertens. 2018;36:16–22. https://doi.org/10.1097/hjh.0000000000001508.
53. Ponte B, Pruijm M, Ackermann D, Vuistiner P, Eisenberger U, Guessous I, et al. Reference values and factors associated with renal resistive index in a family-based population study. Hypertension. 2014;63:136–42. https://doi.org/10.1161/hypertensionaha.113.02321.
54. Bige N, Levy PP, Callard P, Faintuch JM, Chigot V, Jousselin V, et al. Renal arterial resistive index is associated with severe histological changes and poor renal outcome during chronic kidney disease. BMC Nephrol. 2012;13:139. https://doi.org/10.1186/1471-2369-13-139.
55. O'Neill WC. Renal resistive index: a case of mistaken identity. Hypertension. 2014;64:915–7. https://doi.org/10.1161/hypertensionaha.114.04183.
56. Hashimoto J, Ito S. Central pulse pressure and aortic stiffness determine renal hemodynamics: pathophysiological implication for microalbuminuria in hypertension. Hypertension. 2011;58:839–46. https://doi.org/10.1161/hypertensionaha.111.177469.
57. Ogata C, Kamide K, Suzuki Y, Sasaki O, Kubota Y, Sato H, et al. Evaluation of intrarenal hemodynamics by Doppler ultrasonography for renoprotective effect of angiotensin receptor blockade. Clin Nephrol. 2005;64:352–7. https://doi.org/10.5414/cnp64352.
58. Naesens M, Heylen L, Lerut E, Claes K, De Wever L, Claus F, et al. Intrarenal resistive index after renal transplantation. N Engl J Med. 2013;369:1797–806. https://doi.org/10.1056/NEJMoa1301064.
59. Sugiura T, Wada A. Resistive index predicts renal prognosis in chronic kidney disease. Nephrol Dial Transplant. 2009;24:2780–5. https://doi.org/10.1093/ndt/gfp121.
60. Nosadini R, Velussi M, Brocco E, Abaterusso C, Carraro A, Piarulli F, et al. Increased renal arterial resistance predicts the course of renal function in type 2 diabetes with microalbuminuria. Diabetes. 2006;55:234–9.
61. Drelich-Zbroja A, Jargiello T, Drelich G, Lewandowska-Stanek H, Szczerbo-Trojanowska M. Renal artery stenosis: value of contrast-enhanced ultrasonography. Abdom Imaging. 2004;29:518–24. https://doi.org/10.1007/s00261-003-0125-8.

62. Zachrisson K, Herlitz H, Lonn L, Falkenberg M, Eklof H. Duplex ultrasound for identifying renal artery stenosis: direct criteria re-evaluated. Acta Radiol. 2017;58:176–82. https://doi.org/10.1177/0284185116641345.
63. Williams GJ, Macaskill P, Chan SF, Karplus TE, Yung W, Hodson EM, et al. Comparative accuracy of renal duplex sonographic parameters in the diagnosis of renal artery stenosis: paired and unpaired analysis. AJR Am J Roentgenol. 2007;188:798–811. https://doi.org/10.2214/AJR.06.0355.
64. Radermacher J, Chavan A, Bleck J, Vitzthum A, Stoess B, Gebel MJ, et al. Use of Doppler ultrasonography to predict the outcome of therapy for renal-artery stenosis. N Engl J Med. 2001;344:410–7. https://doi.org/10.1056/NEJM200102083440603.
65. Garcia-Criado A, Gilabert R, Nicolau C, Real MI, Muntana X, Blasco J, et al. Value of Doppler sonography for predicting clinical outcome after renal artery revascularization in atherosclerotic renal artery stenosis. J Ultrasound Med. 2005;24:1641–7. https://doi.org/10.7863/jum.2005.24.12.1641.
66. Parikh SA, Shishehbor MH, Gray BH, White CJ, Jaff MR. SCAI expert consensus statement for renal artery stenting appropriate use. Catheter Cardiovasc Interv. 2014;84:1163–71. https://doi.org/10.1002/ccd.25559.
67. Zierler RE. Duplex ultrasound follow-up after fenestrated and branched endovascular aneurysm repair (FEVAR and BEVAR). Semin Vasc Surg. 2020;33:60–4. https://doi.org/10.1053/j.semvascsurg.2020.05.006.
68. Calhoun DA, Jones D, Textor S, Goff DC, Murphy TP, Toto RD, et al. Resistant hypertension: diagnosis, evaluation, and treatment: a scientific statement from the American Heart Association Professional Education Committee of the Council for High Blood Pressure Research. Circulation. 2008;117:e510–26. https://doi.org/10.1161/CIRCULATIONAHA.108.189141.
69. Persu A, Canning C, Prejbisz A, Dobrowolski P, Amar L, Chrysochou C, et al. Beyond atherosclerosis and fibromuscular dysplasia: rare causes of renovascular hypertension. Hypertension. 2021;78:898–911. https://doi.org/10.1161/hypertensionaha.121.17004.
70. Sarafidis PA, Theodorakopoulou M, Ortiz A, Fernandez-Fernández B, Nistor I, Schmieder R, et al. Atherosclerotic renovascular disease: a clinical practice document by the European Renal Best Practice (ERBP) board of the European Renal Association (ERA) and the Working Group Hypertension and the Kidney of the European Society of Hypertension (ESH). Nephrol Dial Transplant. 2023;38:2835–50. https://doi.org/10.1093/ndt/gfad095.
71. Hicks CW, Clark TWI, Cooper CJ, de Bhailis AM, De Carlo M, Green D, et al. Atherosclerotic renovascular disease: a KDIGO (Kidney Disease: Improving Global Outcomes) Controversies Conference. Am J Kidney Dis. 2022;79:289–301. https://doi.org/10.1053/j.ajkd.2021.06.025.
72. Persu A, Giavarini A, Touze E, Januszewicz A, Sapoval M, Azizi M, et al. European consensus on the diagnosis and management of fibromuscular dysplasia. J Hypertens. 2014;32:1367–78. https://doi.org/10.1097/HJH.0000000000000213.
73. Li T, Mao Y, Zhao B, Wang H, Ren J, Ma N, et al. Value of contrast-enhanced ultrasound for diagnosis and follow-up of renal artery stenosis in patients with chronic kidney disease. Abdom Radiol (NY). 2022;47:1853–61. https://doi.org/10.1007/s00261-022-03457-w.
74. Garessus J, Brito W, Loncle N, Vanelli A, Hendriks-Balk M, Wuerzner G, et al. Cortical perfusion as assessed with contrast-enhanced ultrasound is lower in patients with chronic kidney disease than in healthy subjects but increases under low salt conditions. Nephrol Dial Transplant. 2022;37:705–12. https://doi.org/10.1093/ndt/gfab001.
75. Ulpiano Trillig A, Damianaki A, Hendriks-Balk M, Brito W, Garessus J, Burnier M, et al. Determinants of renal micro-perfusion as assessed with contrast-enhanced ultrasound in healthy males and females. J Clin Med. 2023;12:4141. https://doi.org/10.3390/jcm12124141.
76. Damianaki A, Hendriks-Balk M, Brito W, Polychronopoulou E, Theiler K, Maillard M, et al. Contrast enhanced ultrasonography reveals a lower cortical perfusion and a decreased renal flow reserve in hypertensive patients. Nephrol Dial Transplant. 2024;39:242–50. https://doi.org/10.1093/ndt/gfad158.

77. Hendriks-Balk MC, Damianaki A, Polychronopoulou E, Brito W, Pruijm M, Wuerzner G. Contrast-enhanced ultrasonography enables the detection of a cold pressor test-induced increase in renal microcirculation in healthy participants. Front Cardiovasc Med. 2022;9:899327. https://doi.org/10.3389/fcvm.2022.899327.
78. Yoo J, Je BK, Choo JY. Ultrasonographic demonstration of the tissue microvasculature in children: microvascular ultrasonography versus conventional color Doppler ultrasonography. Korean J Radiol. 2020;21:146–58. https://doi.org/10.3348/kjr.2019.0500.
79. Yoo J, Je BK, Choo JY. Erratum: ultrasonographic demonstration of the tissue microvasculature in children: microvascular ultrasonography versus conventional color Doppler ultrasonography. Korean J Radiol. 2020;21:509. https://doi.org/10.3348/kjr.2020.0208.
80. Van der Niepen P, Rossignol P, Lengelé JP, Berra E, Sarafidis P, et al. Renal artery stenosis in patients with resistant hypertension: stent it or not? Curr Hypertens Rep. 2017;19:5. https://doi.org/10.1007/s11906-017-0703-8.
81. Klinkhammer BM, Boor P. Kidney fibrosis: emerging diagnostic and therapeutic strategies. Mol Asp Med. 2023;93:101206. https://doi.org/10.1016/j.mam.2023.101206.
82. Kim TM, Ahn H, Cho JY, Han A, Min SI, Ha J, et al. Prediction of acute rejection in renal allografts using shear-wave dispersion slope. Eur Radiol. 2024;34:4527–37. https://doi.org/10.1007/s00330-023-10492-8.
83. Vasbinder GB, Nelemans PJ, Kessels AG, Kroon AA, de Leeuw PW, van Engelshoven JM. Diagnostic tests for renal artery stenosis in patients suspected of having renovascular hypertension: a meta-analysis. Ann Intern Med. 2001;135:401–11. https://doi.org/10.7326/0003-4819-135-6-200109180-00009.
84. Wang L, Zhu L, Li G, Zhang Y, Jiang Y, Shui B, et al. Gadolinium-enhanced magnetic resonance versus computed tomography angiography for renal artery stenosis: a systematic review and meta-analysis. J Formos Med Assoc. 2021;120:1171–8. https://doi.org/10.1016/j.jfma.2021.01.007.
85. Clingan MJ, Zhang Z, Caserta MP, Cox KL, Gupta V, Baumgarten DA, et al. Imaging patients with kidney failure. Radiographics. 2023;43:e220116. https://doi.org/10.1148/rg.220116.
86. Villa G, Ringgaard S, Hermann I, Noble R, Brambilla P, Khatir DS, et al. Phase-contrast magnetic resonance imaging to assess renal perfusion: a systematic review and statement paper. MAGMA. 2020;33:3–21. https://doi.org/10.1007/s10334-019-00772-0.
87. Schoenberg SO, Knopp MV, Londy F, Krishnan S, Zuna I, Lang N, et al. Morphologic and functional magnetic resonance imaging of renal artery stenosis: a multireader tricenter study. J Am Soc Nephrol. 2002;13:158–69. https://doi.org/10.1681/asn.V131158.
88. Schoenberg SO, Knopp MV, Bock M, Kallinowski F, Just A, Essig M, et al. Renal artery stenosis: grading of hemodynamic changes with cine phase-contrast MR blood flow measurements. Radiology. 1997;203:45–53. https://doi.org/10.1148/radiology.203.1.9122415.
89. de Haan MW, van Engelshoven JM, Houben AJ, Kaandorp DW, Kessels AG, Kroon AA, et al. Phase-contrast magnetic resonance flow quantification in renal arteries: comparison with ^{133}Xenon washout measurements. Hypertension. 2003;41:114–8. https://doi.org/10.1161/01.hyp.0000047466.98321.9d.
90. Binkert CA, Debatin JF, Schneider E, Hodler J, Ruehm SG, Schmidt M, et al. Can MR measurement of renal artery flow and renal volume predict the outcome of percutaneous transluminal renal angioplasty? Cardiovasc Interv Radiol. 2001;24:233–9. https://doi.org/10.1007/s00270-001-0005-y.
91. Odudu A, Nery F, Harteveld AA, Evans RG, Pendse D, Buchanan CE, et al. Arterial spin labelling MRI to measure renal perfusion: a systematic review and statement paper. Nephrol Dial Transplant. 2018;33:ii15–21. https://doi.org/10.1093/ndt/gfy180.
92. Li X, Wang W, Cheng D, Yu Y, Wu Q, Ni X, et al. Perfusion and oxygenation in allografts with transplant renal artery stenosis: evaluation with functional magnetic resonance imaging. Clin Transplant. 2022;36:e14806. https://doi.org/10.1111/ctr.14806.
93. Prasad PV, Li LP, Thacker JM, Li W, Hack B, Kohn O, et al. Cortical perfusion and tubular function as evaluated by magnetic resonance imaging correlates with annual loss in renal function in moderate chronic kidney disease. Am J Nephrol. 2019;49:114–24. https://doi.org/10.1159/000496161.

94. Haddock B, Larsson HBW, Francis S, Andersen UB. Human renal response to furosemide simultaneous oxygenation and perfusion measurements in cortex and medulla. Acta Physiol (Oxf). 2019;227:e13292. https://doi.org/10.1111/apha.13292.
95. Laursen JC, Sondergaard-Heinrich N, de Melo JML, Haddock B, Rasmussen IKB Safavimanesh F, et al. Acute effects of dapagliflozin on renal oxygenation and perfusion in type 1 diabetes with albuminuria: a randomised, double-blind, placebo-controlled crossover trial. EClinicalMedicine. 2021;37:100895. https://doi.org/10.1016/j.eclinm.2021.100895.
96. Zanchi A, Burnier M, Muller ME, Ghajarzadeh-Wurzner A, Maillard M, Loncle N, et al Acute and chronic effects of SGLT2 inhibitor empagliflozin on renal oxygenation and blood pressure control in nondiabetic normotensive subjects: a randomized, placebo-controlled trial. J Am Heart Assoc. 2020;9:e016173. https://doi.org/10.1161/jaha.119.016173.
97. Caroli A, Pruijm M, Burnier M, Selby NM. Functional magnetic resonance imaging of the kidneys: where do we stand? The perspective of the European COST action PARENCHIMA. Nephrol Dial Transplant. 2018;33:ii1–3. https://doi.org/10.1093/ndt/gfy181.
98. Pruijm M, Mendichovszky IA, Liss P, Van der Niepen P, Textor SC, Lerman LO, et al. Renal blood oxygenation level-dependent magnetic resonance imaging to measure renal tissue oxygenation: a statement paper and systematic review. Nephrol Dial Transplant. 2018;33:ii22–8. https://doi.org/10.1093/ndt/gfy243.
99. Gloviczki ML, Glockner JF, Crane JA, McKusick MA, Misra S, Grande JP, et al. Blood oxygen level-dependent magnetic resonance imaging identifies cortical hypoxia in severe renovascular disease. Hypertension. 2011;58:1066–72. https://doi.org/10.1161/HYPERTENSIONAHA.111.171405.
100. Herrmann SM, Saad A, Eirin A, Woollard J, Tang H, McKusick MA, et al. Differences in GFR and tissue oxygenation, and interactions between stenotic and contralateral kidneys in unilateral atherosclerotic renovascular disease. Clin J Am Soc Nephrol. 2016;11:458–69. https://doi.org/10.2215/CJN.03620415.
101. Abumoawad A, Saad A, Ferguson CM, Eirin A, Herrmann SM, Hickson LJ, et al. In a phase 1a escalating clinical trial, autologous mesenchymal stem cell infusion for renovascular disease increases blood flow and the glomerular filtration rate while reducing inflammatory biomarkers and blood pressure. Kidney Int. 2020;97:793–804. https://doi.org/10.1016/j.kint.2019.11.022.
102. Pruijm M, Milani B, Burnier M. Blood oxygenation level-dependent MRI to assess renal oxygenation in renal diseases: progresses and challenges. Front Physiol. 2016;7:667. https://doi.org/10.3389/fphys.2016.00667.
103. Hesp AC, Schaub JA, Prasad PV, Vallon V, Laverman GD, Bjornstad P, et al. The role of renal hypoxia in the pathogenesis of diabetic kidney disease: a promising target for newer renoprotective agents including SGLT2 inhibitors? Kidney Int. 2020;98:579–89. https://doi.org/10.1016/j.kint.2020.02.041.
104. Pruijm M, Hofmann L, Maillard M, Tremblay S, Glatz N, Wuerzner G, et al. Effect of sodium loading/depletion on renal oxygenation in young normotensive and hypertensive men. Hypertension. 2010;55:1116–22. https://doi.org/10.1161/HYPERTENSIONAHA.109.149682.
105. Prasad PV, Li LP, Hack B, Leloudas N, Sprague SM. Quantitative blood oxygenation level dependent magnetic resonance imaging for estimating intra-renal oxygen availability demonstrates kidneys are hypoxemic in human CKD. Kidney Int Rep. 2023;8:1057–67. https://doi.org/10.1016/j.ekir.2023.02.1092.
106. Berchtold L, Crowe LA, Combescure C, Kassaï M, Aslam I, Legouis D, et al. Diffusion-magnetic resonance imaging predicts decline of kidney function in chronic kidney disease and in patients with a kidney allograft. Kidney Int. 2022;101:804–13. https://doi.org/10.1016/j.kint.2021.12.014.
107. Caroli A, Schneider M, Friedli I, Ljimani A, De Seigneux S, Boor P, et al. Diffusion-weighted magnetic resonance imaging to assess diffuse renal pathology: a systematic review and statement paper. Nephrol Dial Transplant. 2018;33:ii29–40. https://doi.org/10.1093/ndt/gfy163.
108. Yildirim E, Kirbas I, Teksam M, Karadeli E, Gullu H, Ozer I. Diffusion-weighted MR imaging of kidneys in renal artery stenosis. Eur J Radiol. 2008;65:148–53. https://doi.org/10.1016/j.ejrad.2007.03.007.

Part VII

Therapeutic Approaches

Treatment of Hypertension in Acute Kidney Injury

14

Jelena Kos, Ana Jelaković, Vedran Premužić,
Ivana Vuković Brinar, and Bojan Jelaković

14.1 Introduction

14.1.1 Acute Kidney Injury (AKI): Definition and Classification

Acute kidney injury (AKI), a frequent heterogenic state that accompanies 20% emergency hospital admissions, is associated with various adverse short- and long-term outcomes and subsequent increased heath care expenditure [1–3]. Contemporary diagnosis of AKI is brought by consensus definition from KDIGO guidelines, and it is based on serum creatinine (SCr) rise and/or decrease in urine output [4]. AKI is a broad and complex clinical entity, more akin to a syndrome than single disease. AKI does not have a single etiological origin, but rather a combination of multiple interweaving etiological points, both intrarenal and extra-renal, all combining into multiple clinical conditions resulting in a syndrome comprising of both direct injury and impairment of function. In simpler terms, AKI represents a sudden loss of kidney function that happens over a period of up to 7 days [5–8]. Considering that AKI represents a complex clinical entity, multiple classification systems were devised in order to simplify definition and classification of AKI. Most popular are Risk, Injury, Failure, Loss, End-stage System (RIFLE) devised by Bellomo et al. and Acute Kidney Injury Networks (AKIN)-modified RIFLE classification system by Mehta et al. Both systems provide invaluable tool to identify hospitalized patients with

J. Kos · A. Jelaković · V. Premužić
Department of Nephrology, Arterial Hypertension, Dialysis and Transplantation, University Hospital Centre Zagreb, Zagreb, Croatia

I. V. Brinar · B. Jelaković (✉)
Department of Nephrology, Arterial Hypertension, Dialysis and Transplantation, University Hospital Centre Zagreb, Zagreb, Croatia

School of Medicine, University of Zagreb, Zagreb, Croatia

A. E. Berbari et al. (eds.), *Blood Pressure Disorders in Acute and Chronic Kidney Diseases*, Updates in Hypertension and Cardiovascular Protection,
https://doi.org/10.1007/978-3-031-81292-7_14

increased risk of unfavorable outcomes, including the need for renal replacement therapy (RTT) and death (Tables 14.1 and 14.2) [5, 9, 10]. AKI is linked with a number of significant consequences, both while undergoing treatment in the hospital and in out-patient care. Although recovery in the hospital setting is possible, mortality and morbidity remain high, despite timely treatment [8]. Complications in hospital setting include fluid overload, electrolyte and acid-base abnormalities, and innate immune system impairment leading to infections [7, 8].

14.1.1.1 Distinguishing Prerenal Azotaemia and Acute Kidney Injury

KDIGO definition of AKI fails to discriminate presumed AKI due to renal hemodynamic changes from real AKI, especially acute tubular injury [11]. AKI without SCr changes is described as subclinical AKI [12]. In acute state, there is usually 48–72-h lag in SCr elevation. During that time, patient may be exposed to various nephrotoxic agents leading to further damage [12]. In previously unaffected kidneys, remaining nephrons enter hyperfiltration state, masking and compensating ongoing injury, which is called renal reserve [13]. Finally, SCr concentrations may stay relatively stable despite AKI due to low creatinine production in bed-ridden acutely ill patient and masked by dilution from i.v. fluid administration [12]. Conceptional model describing limitations of using SCr to define AKI is shown in Table 14.3 [12]. SCr-based AKI definition has many limitations; it lacks the accuracy for a diagnosis of structural kidney injury and it provides no information on AKI etiology, prognosis, molecular pathways, or response to treatment [12].

Table 14.1 RIFLE criteria for acute kidney injury, modified from Bellomo et al. [9]

	RIFLE criteria	
	SCr	Urine output
Risk	↑ sCr × 1.5	<0.5 mL/kg/h in 6 h
Injury	↑ sCr × 2	<0.5 mL/kg/h in 12 h
Failure	↑ sCr × 3 OR ≥44.21 μmol/L if baseline sCr ↑ >353.68 μmol/L	<0.3 mL/kg/h in 24 h OR anuria in 12 h
Loss	Total loss of renal function for more than 4 weeks	
End stage	Development of end-stage renal disease	

SCr serum creatinine

Table 14.2 AKIN criteria for acute kidney injury, modified from Mehta et al. [10]

	AKIN criteria	
	Serum creatinine	Urine output
Stage 1	↑ SCr × 1.5 OR ↑ ≥26.52 μmol/L in SCr	<0.5 mL/kg/h in 6 h
Stage 2	↑ SCr × 2	<0.5 mL/kg/h in 12 h
Stage 3	↑ SCr × 3 OR ↑ ≥44.21 μmol/L if baseline SCr >353.68 μmol/L	<0.3 mL/kg/h in 24 h OR anuria in 12 h

Patients who receive renal replacement therapy meet Stage 3 criteria regardless of the stage they are in at the time of receiving renal replacement therapy

Table 14.3 Limitations of serum creatinine-based AKI definition

		Structural kidney injury	
		No damage	Damage
SCr-based AKI	No	**A.** No kidney injury	**B.** "Subclinical AKI"[a]
	Yes	**C.** "Hemodynamic AKI"[b]	**D.** Clinical AKI

Adopted from [12]

[a]Renal reserve; SCr kinetics; decreased SCr production

[b]Pre-renal, azotaemia; hepatorenal syndrome; cardiorenal syndrome, RAAS inhibition

14.1.1.2 Tubular Biomarkers in Acute Kidney Injury

Proximal tubules are often the primary site of nephrotoxic and ischemic kidney injuries but remain clinically silent until advanced stage. Tubulointerstitial damage and fibrosis are prognostic for kidney disease progression and end-stage kidney disease (ESKD) [14]. Search for more specific and sensitive biomarkers of kidney tubular injury is in the focus of interest last decades [15]. After tubule injury, various proteins and enzymes can be detected in the urine due to proximal tubular dysfunction or direct tubular damage. Hence, there are two groups of proteins that could serve as potential tubular biomarkers: (1) proteins that appear in urine because of inadequate absorption of freely filtered low molecular weight (LMW) proteins: cystatin C (Cys C), β2 microglobulin, α1-microglobulin, retinol-binding proteins, clear cell protein, etc.; (2) proteins that are released in urine after direct epithelial cell damage - lysosomal enzymes: *N*-acetyl-β-D-glycosaminidase (NAG); brush border enzymes: gamma-glutamyl transferase, alkaline phosphatase, neutral endopeptidase; and cytosolic proteins: α-glutathione-*S*-transferase (α-GST). Proteins that appear in the urine can be constitutive—proteins/enzymes that are normally present in tubular epithelial cells or tubule lumen after filtration, but are not normally excreted in the urine in significant concentrations (α-GST, cystatin C); and inducible—proteins and enzymes that are not normally found in tubular epithelial cells and urine, but their synthesis is induced by tubular damage [e.g. kidney injury molecule-1—(KIM-1)]. KIM-1 is a transmembrane glycoprotein expressed by proximal tubular cells in response to kidney injury [15]. In various animal models of toxic and ischemic AKI, KIM-1 was significantly better in prediction and early detection of AKI compared to traditional markers [16]. In patients who underwent cardiac surgery, KIM-1 was a good predictor of the subsequent AKI [17]. In a study that compared nine biomarkers of kidney injury (KIM-1, HGF, IP-10, NGAL, NAG, IL-18, VEGF cystatin C, total proteins) in comparison to traditional markers (creatinine and eGFR), it has been shown that all novel biomarkers identify AKI earlier than traditional markers [18]. The sensitivity and specificity for diagnosis of AKI were significantly greater by combining the urinary levels of KIM-1, NGAL, HGF, and total protein [18]. KIM-1, NAG, HGF, and VEGF predicted death and/or need for RRT with KIM-1 showing superiority compared to other biomarkers. NGAL is expressed in the lung, gastrointestinal tract, liver, and kidney and is significantly induced in epithelial cells in response to injury, inflammation, and neoplastic transformation [19]. In animal model, urinary NGAL levels rise within 2 h of renal ischemia-reperfusion injury [20]. Urine and serum NGAL levels were elevated within 2 h after cardiac surgery in children with subsequent postoperative AKI [21]. In meta-analysis of 19 studies, urinary NGAL showed excellent performance for prediction of AKI (summary ROC curve of 0.837; 95% CI, 0.762–0.906) [22]. HGF was discovered as a protein with mitogenic properties for differentiated hepatocytes [23]. HGF is expressed in tissues of mesodermal origin, while its c-met receptor is expressed in epithelial cells including the liver and kidney [24–26]. L-FABP is a protein expressed in the proximal tubular epithelial cells [27]. The L-FABP gene is upregulated in hypoxic stress such as kidney ischemia-reperfusion injury with markedly elevated urinary excretion of L-FABP correlating with severity of ischemic tubular injury [28, 29]. TIMP-2 and insulin-like growth factor binding protein-7 (IGFBP7) are biomarkers of G1 cell cycle arrest of the renal tubular epithelial cell during ischemic or septic AKI [30, 31]. Kashani et al. evaluated the diagnostic value of biomarkers for early detection of AKI and found that AUC-ROC of urine TIMP-2 multiplied by urine IGFBP7 ([TIMP-2] *[IGFBP7]) was 0.80, which is superior to that of other biomarkers including NGAL, KIM-1, IL-18 as well as urine TIMP-2 and urine IGFBP7 independently [31]. The kit that measures these two biomarkers in urine is commercially available [32]. UMOD, also known as Tamm-Horsfall protein, is a glycoprotein produced by epithelial cells of the thick ascending limb of Henle. In physiological conditions, it is the most abundant protein in the urine. Studies have shown that UMOD is a direct marker of the amount of intact tubular cells and may represent a biomarker of tubular mass and renal function [33]. Early after kidney injury many different inflammatory pathways are activated, and many inflammatory mediators can be detected in urine. One of these mediators is interleukin-18 (IL-18). After kidney transplantation, increased urinary IL-18 was found in patients with acute tubular necrosis [34]. In patients with AKI after cardiopulmonary bypass, increased urinary IL-18 levels may be detected over the first 4–6 h, earlier than SCr but slower than that observed in other urinary biomarkers such as NGAL [35]. Urinary IL-18 might be useful to predict clinical outcomes including mortality and RRT in intensive care unit (ICU) population [36]. Studies on kidney injury biomarkers in patients in ICU have identified a considerable proportion of patients (15–20%) with positive biomarkers of tubular injury (KIM-1 and NGAL) in the absence of eGFR decline [37–39]. Such patients are considered to have subclinical AKI [26]. ICU patients with subclinical AKI are at two- to threefold increased risk of RRT or death compared to patients with negative tubular biomarkers and preserved eGFR [37, 38]. Patients with both elevated tubular biomarkers and SCr had the worst prognosis with need for RRT or death 15.5–17.5% [37, 38]. Urinary biomarkers could help distinguish between hemodynamical changes reflected in acute eGFR decline versus intrinsic kidney damage. In the SPRINT study, intensive blood pressure (BP) control reduced risk for CV outcomes but associated with more AKI [40]. Despite eGFR decline in intensive BP group, there was no increase in levels of urinary tubular biomarkers including KIM-1, NGAL, IL-18, which suggests that eGFR decline is due to hemodynamic changes rather than intrinsic kidney injury [41]. However, baseline concentrations of urinary KIM-1 and monocyte chemoattractant protein-1 (MCP-1) were associated with incident CKD during follow-up suggesting that urinary biomarkers could identify subset of patients with subclinical kidney damage who are at increased risk of eGFR decline [42]. In summary, many novel kidney injury biomarkers predict AKI earlier than traditional markers such as SCr and eGFR. However, kidney injury biomarkers still have not been widely implemented in routine clinical practice. Studies performed on kidney injury biomarkers are very heterogeneous with different definitions of AKI, heterogeneous populations, various causes of AKI, different outcomes, etc., that make comparison of the results difficult. So far there is no single biomarker that would be highly specific and sensitive for any cause of AKI. That is why biomarker panels are now in focus of research not only for AKI in general but also for specific subtypes of AKI according to underlying etiology and the site of kidney injury. Finding which biomarkers fit which type of AKI might help to conduct less heterogeneous clinical trials, and the results of such studies would provide accurate results on biomarker performance in specific AKI settings. Implementation of kidney injury biomarkers in clinical practice would identify patients at high risk of developing AKI and patients at risk for AKI progression and need for RRT. They would also help differentiate between different etiologies of AKI and guide the therapeutic approach.

Box 14.1 Acute Kidney Injury (AKI)

AKI is a frequent heterogenic state that accompanies 20% emergency hospital admissions associated with various adverse short- and long-term outcomes and subsequent increased heath care expenditure.

AKI is a broad and complex clinical entity, more alike to a syndrome than single disease.

KDIGO definition of AKI fails to discriminate presumed AKI due to renal hemodynamic changes from real AKI, especially acute tubular injury. Serum creatinine-based AKI definition has many limitations.

Proximal tubules are often the primary site of nephrotoxic and ischemic kidney injuries but remain clinically silent until advanced stage. So far, there is no single biomarker that would be highly specific and sensitive for any cause of AKI.

AKI without serum creatinine changes is described as subclinical AKI.

14.1.2 Acute Kidney Injury, Arterial Hypertension, Cardiovascular and ESKD Risk

Causes of AKI are heterogeneous and many of acute conditions are not associated with elevated BP (e.g. sepsis, hypovolemia due to any cause) [1]. In developed countries with aging population more causes of AKI are related to high BP: heart failure hospitalization with development of cardiorenal syndrome, nephrotoxicity of radiocontrast, drugs or chemotherapeutics in CKD patient, cardiac and noncardiac surgery in elderly, frail, and multimorbid patients. The declining kidney function in a rapid matter is associated with an increased risk for CV disease regardless of prior CKD [43]. Kidney pressure control system increases body fluid volume when the pressure falls (or decreases the volume when the pressure rises) which is the dominant method of establishing long-term pressure control [44]. Therefore, elevation of BP can reflect a subtle kidney injury as well, or better than elevation in SCr levels [45]. Hsu et al. reported the independent association of AKI, in patients without prior AH, with an increased risk of developing elevated BP levels within the first 180 days post-discharge with higher risk when greater severity of AKI was present [45]. AH prevalence in CKD is predominant, yet the data on prevalence of AH in AKI are very scarce. AH is an independent risk factor for AKI. In a meta-analysis, the incidence of AKI among general population cohort was 0.6–2%, while in hypertensive individuals, it was 14.5% [46]. There is large quantity of observational AKI trials, but not many are focused on AH treatment during hospital treatment of AKI. CKD is associated with 18-fold increase in CV risk, but data on AKI and CV risk are limited. There are reports showing that AKI is strongly associated with an increase in risk of CV mortality and morbidity [8, 47]. Odutayo et al. showed that AKI is associated with increased risk of major CV events and mortality, congestive heart failure, acute myocardial infarction, as well as stroke [47]. Interestingly, the same study showed that severity of AKI increased the risk of chronic heart failure but not the risk of myocardial infarction [45, 47]. In addition to these findings, a study published by Hsu et al. showed that an episode of AKI during hospitalization is an independent risk factor for later development of AH up to 2 years of follow-up [45]. These two studies provide a possible connection between AKI and subsequent increase in adverse CV events, with proposed pathophysiological mechanism being disruption of hemodynamic due to incidental AH during and after AKI or exacerbation of preexisting AH [45]. All these findings only reaffirm the statement that continuous and multifaceted follow-up is needed in patients that survived AKI [8, 45, 47]. Progression from AKI to acute kidney disease (ACD), CKD, and ESKD represent a combination of short-term and long-term outcomes of AKI. Different potential mechanisms have been proposed to explain both pathogenesis of AKI and post-AKI kidney impairment including mitochondrial dysfunction, cell death, inflammation, and chronic hypoxia, with maladaptive repair mechanism in AKI leading to progression into CKD. Existing injury caused by AKI increases oxidative stress and fibrosis, leading to induction of kidney hypertrophy and glomerulosclerosis, which further contributes to the progression of CKD but also to appearance of recurring AKI episodes [8, 48, 49]. Up until now, outcomes of AKI in patients with various underlying conditions were put aside in favor of clinical improvement. However, a study by Su et al. showed that 15.6–40% of patients that ever developed AKI progressed to AKD, a transitional step toward CKD and ESKD [49]. A study by Coca et al. also showed that AKI survivors have an increased risk of progression to CKD, ESKD, and other adverse outcomes including CV disease and congestive heart failure, decompensated liver disease, malignancies, and acute coronary syndrome, while Wu et al. showed that AKI contributes to cardiac dysfunction including coronary events [8, 50, 51]. In effort to stall the progression of AKI into CKD and ESKD, it is of vital importance to provide long-term care for AKI survivors in the form of both inpatient and outpatient (post-discharge) care [8].

Box 14.2 AKI, Blood Pressure, and Arterial Hypertension

In developed countries with aging population more causes of AKI are related to high BP: heart failure hospitalization, cardiorenal syndrome, nephrotoxicity of radiocontrast, drugs, surgery in elderly, frail and multimorbid patient.

The data on prevalence of arterial hypertension in AKI are very scarce.

Arterial hypertension is an independent risk factor for AKI.

In normotensive patients, there is an independent association of AKI with an increased risk of developing arterial hypertension post-discharge.

AKI is strongly associated with an increase in risk of CV mortality and morbidity, as well as progression to CKD/ESKD.

14.2 Target Blood Pressure and Risk for Acute Kidney Injury with Intensive BP Reduction

The landmark Systolic BP Intervention Trial (SPRINT study) on intensive BP reduction dramatically changed hypertension management in the past 5 years [52]. Participants randomized to intensive BP treatment (SBP <120 mmHg) had increased risk for AKI compared to standard treatment in unadjusted model (HR 1.83; 95% CI 1.43–2.33; $p < 0.001$) [53]. Modified KDIGO AKI definition was used in SPRINT trial based solely on SCr levels since urine output was not recorded. Participants in SPRINT trial who experienced AKI had a significantly higher risk of the primary CV outcome (HR 2.38; 95% CI 1.7–3.32, $p < 0.001$) and death from any cause (HR 3.43; 95% CI 2.38–4.94, $p < 0.001$) [53]. Even though major events of AKI in SPRINT trial were mild, authors conclude that for kidney disease, intensive BP reduction may not provide benefit [53]. However, in post-hoc analysis, the possibility of reverse causality where CV disease contributes to occurrence of AKI and hence to CV morbidity and all-cause mortality cannot be excluded. One must keep in mind that the SPRINT trial was not designed to determine the effect of AKI on CV events and death, and overall incidence of AKI was small [54]. The most common reasons for AKI in SPRINT trial were dehydration and intravascular volume depletion followed by hypotension [55]. Most AKI in SPRINT was by KDIGO classification characterized as stage I, and 90% recovered to base line kidney function during the trial [55]. As mentioned before, it is likely that most AKI in SPRINT were hemodynamic changes without structural changes in kidney function, and without long-term follow-up of SPRINT trial participants, it is not possible to derive final conclusion [12]. Studies on kidney biomarkers and findings of ACCORD BP trial support this hypothesis [42, 56]. In another post-hoc analysis of SPRINT trial, early eGFR decline >20% did not attenuate the CV or mortality benefits in intensive BP control group [57]. The SPRINT trial cohort is still the largest group of CKD patient studied primarily for CV outcomes. In SPRINT trial, 29% of examinees had

CKD and 19% had mild albuminuria (ACR 70 mg/g) [58]. The incidence rate of eGFR decline >40% (as a surrogate of ESKD) was much higher in albuminuric examinees (1.74 vs. 1.17); however, absolute risk differences for intensive versus standard BP arms in those with and without albuminuria did not differ ($p = 0.609$) [58]. High baseline albuminuria was the major eGFR decline risk factor [58]. CV events and all-cause mortality were reduced in intensive BP reduction arm regardless of albuminuria. Similar observation was observed when comparing SPRINT population and diabetic population in ACCORD BP study [59]. However, SPRINT study terminated early and there were only few kidney failure events. In AASK and MDRD study with longer follow-up, higher prevalence of advanced CKD stages and higher albuminuria at baseline, intensive BP target tend to be beneficial on CKD progression, especially in those with albuminuria [60, 61]. Yet, these and other CKD studies failed to detect beneficial effect of intensive BP reduction on CV events and mortality [60–62]. These studies were not designed and not powered enough to detect CV outcomes. The ACCORD BP study, in which the diabetic patients with similar CV risk as in SPRINT were enrolled, in failed to find significant benefits of intensive BP lowering on the primary CV outcome (HR 0.88; CI 95%, 0.73–1.06; $p = 0.55$) and even showed the non-significant increase in the risk for all-cause mortality [56]. However, careful post-hoc analysis taking only standard and not intensive glycemic controlled patient into account revealed reduced CV event rate in intensive BP arm, yet smaller than in SPRINT [59]. SPRINT trial post-hoc analysis also detected clear attenuation in benefit of intensive BP reduction in linear correlation with descending eGFR [63]. CV event rate was lower in CKD participants among intensive BP arm in SPRINT, but this cumulative event curves were visible after approximately 2 years, compared with <6 months among non-CKD participants [63]. A lag effect of CV intervention in CKD is one of the reasons why CV protection of RAAS blockade was never proven in this population [64].

Box 14.3 Blood Pressure Level and Risk for AKI in Hypertensive Patients

Even though major events of AKI in SPRINT trial were mild, it was concluded that for kidney disease, intensive BP reduction may not provide benefit. However, in post-hoc analysis, the possibility of reverse causality where CV disease contributes to occurrence of AKI and hence to CV morbidity and all-cause mortality cannot be excluded.

SPRINT trial post-hoc analysis detected clear attenuation in benefit of intensive BP reduction in linear correlation with descending eGFR.

One must keep in mind that the SPRINT trial was not designed to determine the effect of AKI.

Most AKI in SPRINT were hemodynamic changes without structural changes in kidney function.

In AASK and MDRD study with longer follow-up, higher prevalence of advanced CKD stages and higher albuminuria at baseline, intensive BP target tend to be beneficial on CKD progression, especially in those with albuminuria.

14.3 Preferred Antihypertensive Drugs in Acute Kidney Injury

It is common knowledge that the healthy kidneys could autoregulate renal blood flow across a wide range of systemic BP, including low BP targets set in SPRINT and ACCORD BP trials. However, different antihypertensive drugs may impair kidney's ability to autoregulate blood flow, especially in case of structural damage. Clinicians cannot be aware of such changes based solely on SCr and ACR (e.g., tubular impairment, low total nephron count, subclinical renal artery stenosis). While waiting for appropriate biomarkers to reach clinical practice, practicing clinician should not be forced to choose between CV and renal protection. Meanwhile, based on SPRINT cohort, on-line tool is developed to facilitate the decision whether particular patient could benefit from intensive BP treatment or is on higher risk of adverse event. Of note, authors tested only AKI model in predicting renal failure and albuminuria attributed to BP medication. For other renal outcomes (doubling SCr, decrease of eGFR >20%, SCr >280 μmol/L), the discrimination performance was poor [65]. Nevertheless, this risk prediction can be used to support decision-making and allows easy checking of the risk levels associated with different treatment strategies. It is speculated that substantial drop of systemic BP could lead to renal ischemia and structural damage [66]. There are two major question among many others: (1) the strategy of using RAAS inhibition during AKI and (2) whether using loop diuretics harm or improve outcome in AKI patient.

14.3.1 Using RAAS Inhibitors During and After AKI

Animal study on hypertensive rat models showed that renal autoregulation is disabled when dual RAAS blockade is administered [67]. Under RAAS blockade, smooth muscle cells of the renal arterioles adopt endocrine phenotype that diminishes their contractility (myogenic-mesenchymal transformation) [68]. RAAS inhibitors (RAASi) are the cornerstone of CV protection and renal preservation in CKD, yet there are concerns the RAASi can cause recurrent AKI in acute illness [66]. Some observational studies excluded patients with heart failure, and others include only men or do not distinguish between previous users of RAASi and new users of RAASi after AKI [66–70]. From a large general population in Stockholm data base, utilization of RAASi after AKI stage 2 or 3 was assessed [71]. The primary outcome was composite of myocardial infarction, stroke, and all-cause mortality, and the secondary outcome was recurrent AKI. Because previously mentioned studies have contradictory results, risk of heart failure hospitalization and risk of CKD progression were tertiary outcomes. Median age was 78 years and most of participants were older than 80 years. Compared with continuing RAASi, stopping this medication was associated with increased risk of death, myocardial infarction, and stroke but with a similar risk of recurrent AKI [71]. From Taiwan National Insurance cohort, 8558 hypertensive patients with AKI stage 3 (requiring RRT) and follow-up for 4.4 years were analyzed regarding antihypertensives usage after AKI

[72]. The ACEI/ARB users were associated with a reduced risk of progression to ESKD necessitating maintenance dialysis (adjusted HR 0.95; 95% CI 0.90–1.01; $p = 0.06$) and all-cause mortality (adjusted HR 0.93; 95% CI 0.87–0.98; $p = 0.011$). The protective effects of RAASi were more profound in the higher dose group [72].

14.3.2 Diuretics and Acute Kidney Injury

Animal studies have suggested that loop diuretics might decrease the tubular reabsorption and metabolic demand, but distal tubular delivery of sodium leads to activation of RAAS and sympathetic nervous system with adverse outcomes [73]. Since oliguric AKI has far worse prognosis then non-oliguric AKI, loop diuretics are widely used in high doses to increase urine output or to reverse oliguric to non-oliguric AKI. In meta-analysis of RCT on the use of furosemide to prevent or to treat AKI, furosemide failed to reduce the risk of requiring RRT (RR 102, 95% CI, 090–1.16, $p = 0.73$) and hospital mortality (RR 1.12, 95% CI 0.93–1.34, $p = 0.23$) [74]. Loop diuretics can increase urine output without improving eGFR and overall renal function. A transient increase in urine output has the potential to delay the diagnosis of underlying causes of AKI (hypovolemia, sepsis, urinary tracts obstruction) [74]. Loop diuretics lead to aciduria, which facilitates UMOD, casts formation in AKI, and methemoglobin cast formation in severe intravascular hemolysis as seen in malignant hypertension with endothelial destruction or in aHUS [75]. Loop diuretics have major systemic effects; high doses of loop diuretic (as given in acute heart failure) lead to hypovolemia and increase peripheral vasoconstriction that poses more afterload burden to failing myocardia [76]. In acute heart failure, rapid systolic BP reduction (even in hypertensive patient) within first 6 h of admission predisposes patients for AKI [76]. Positive fluid balance is an independent risk factor for AKI and mortality [77]. It is uncertain whether positive fluid balance is an epiphenomenon or causal in AKI, but it is certain that loop diuretics should not be used to prevent or to treat AKI, except in the management of volume overload [74]. Spironolactone, a weak class diuretic, but powerful drug to prevent renal fibrosis and renal vasoconstriction by decreasing oxidative stress and upregulation of eNOS expression, has the potential to ameliorate renal fibrosis in AKI and hence prevent CKD [78]. Although RCTs for malignant AH with AKI are missing, there is reasonable physiological argument to use ACEi/ARBs as well as mineralocorticoid receptor antagonist in hypertensive crisis accompanied with AKI [79].

Box 14.4 AKI and Antihypertensive Drugs

Just a few of observational trials on AKI were focused on hypertension treatment during hospital treatment of AKI.

Two most frequent and important concerns are (1) the strategy of using RAAS inhibition during AKI and (2) whether using loop diuretics harm or improve outcome in AKI patient.

Compared with continuing RAAS inhibition, stopping this medication was associated with increased risk of death, myocardial infarction, and stroke but with a similar risk of recurrent AKI (Stockholm data base). The ACEI/ARB users were associated with a reduced risk of progression to ESKD (Taiwan National Insurance cohort).

In a meta-analysis of RCT on the use of furosemide to prevent or to treat AKI, furosemide failed to reduce the risk of requiring RRT and hospital mortality.

14.4 Comorbidities, Blood Pressure, and Acute Kidney Injury

14.4.1 Heart Failure and Acute Kidney Injury

Patients suffering from both acute and chronic heart failure are at greater risk of AKI, with more than half of all hospitalized heart failure patients having some degree of renal function impairment with up to 35% of cases being severe [80]. AKI is a common and frequent finding in heart failure patients mainly caused by decrease in renal perfusion and venous congestion paired with endothelial dysfunction, neurohormonal activation, and inflammation as contributing factors [81]. A study by Metra et al. showed that baseline kidney impairment, NYHA class, reduced ejection fraction, and diuretic dose in some cases act as independent risk factors for worsening renal function [80]. All these findings point that kidney impairment of any kind, in both in-hospital and out-hospital setting, is associated with poor outcome, increased length of hospital stay, decreased quality of life, increased mortality rate and treatment cost [80–82]. Considering the frequency of AKI and other forms of renal impairment in heart failure patients, more meticulous and careful monitoring of these patients is required [81]. ***Acute decompensated heart failure (ADHF)*** is a life-threating condition that requires prompt and adequate treatment. Current ESC guidelines recommend aggressive BP reduction of 25% immediately after admission to reduce cardiac preload and afterload [83]. AKI is a serious complication during ADHF treatment and there is no established evidence regarding optimal BP reduction, particularly in hypertensive ADHF patient [76]. In a retrospective analysis, hypertensive ADHF patients (systolic BP >140 mmHg on admission) were divided into two groups: AKI within first 48 h and non-AKI ADHP patients [76].

Systolic BP-fall beyond 25% in first 6 h was independent predictor of AKI in hypertensive patients. One year after the acute event, AKI group had higher rate of CV death and HF rehospitalizations [76]. The continuous relationship between systolic BP-fall and OR for AKI showed positive linear correlation. Aggressive BP reduction at least in the first 6 h after ADHF admission did not reduce in-hospital death or shorten the duration of in-hospital stay [76]. In 2021, KDIGO guidelines recommend that "adults with high BP and CKD be treated to a target systolic BP of <120 mmHg, when tolerated, using a standardized office BP" [84]. This recommendation was based solely on one RCT—the SPRINT study—and renal implications and AKI risk are discussed in the beginning of this chapter. Since recommendation published, nephrology community has many safety concerns for overall clinical applicability of these recommendations [86]. Short-term follow-up of both SPRINT and ACCORD BP does not warrant long-term renal stability in frail and multimorbid, polypharmacy-prone CKD patient [85]. Of note is that KDIGO guidelines are an outliner among international guidelines for BP target in CKD [85]. Most studies in CKD patients showed J-shaped curve relationship between BP target and CV morbidity and mortality. There is no evidence that BP <130/70 mmHg could improve renal outcomes and there are reasonable concerns for unintentional reduction of renal function with lower BP targets, leading to increased CV risk [86].

14.4.2 Acute Kidney Injury and Arterial Hypertension in the Setting of Sepsis

In the ICU setting, >50% of patients develop AKI, which greatly contributes to overall mortality of ICU patients. One of the main causes of AKI in this setting is sepsis, a syndrome comprised of various physiologic, pathologic, and biochemical aberrations brought about by infection, or more simply put, a life-threatening organ dysfunction brought on by dysregulated host response to infection [87–89]. Acting as an independent risk factor for mortality in hospitalized patients with sepsis, it is imperative to control AKI by maintaining adequate renal function via optimization of BP, which presents a unique challenge in the case of sepsis [88, 89]. To maintain optimal renal perfusion, hemodynamic control must be accomplished through prevention of hypoperfusion of kidneys and optimization of BP. However, ameliorating BP in hope of preventing kidney injury presents a challenge, considering lack of consensus on most favorable mean arterial pressure (MAP) [88, 89]. Studies by Dewitte et al. and Zhao et al. have shown that patients with prior history of AH benefit from higher MAP values, i.e., 70–85 mmHg instead of usual 65–75 mmHg in patients without prior AH [88, 89]. Additionally, Zhao et al. also recommend that diastolic BP range should be around 54–62 mmHg in patients with chronic AH instead of 50–60 mmHg as is recommended in patients with AKI without AH [89]. MAP 70–80 mmHg was related to considerably higher eGFR, although there was no effect on the ability of the kidneys to concentrate urine, indicating no effect on tubular function [88, 89].

14.4.3 Postoperative Acute Kidney Injury

AKI is considered one of the most common and serious postsurgical complications, with rates ranging from 3 to 43% affecting the outcomes and mortality rates after otherwise successful surgical procedures. AH is the most common comorbidity among patients undergoing surgery, and according to some reports, hypertensive levels of BP can be found in as many as 26.5% patients in perioperative period [90]. Patients with AH are especially prone to development of AKI, often leading to ICU treatment early in recovery to prevent adverse outcomes. Considering that AKI greatly contributes to negative postsurgical outcomes, ranging from fatal CV incidents and myocardial infarction to overall mortality rate within 5 years, a need for prediction models that can be used to identify and evaluate high-risk patients has arisen [91–96]. One such prediction model was devised by authors Liu et al. who through rigorous selection of potential variables came up with a model comprised of 13 variables with specific coefficients (Table 14.4) aimed at predicting a possibility of AKI developing in postsurgical patients [91]. However, the authors also pointed out that further need for evaluation and additional studies are needed before this model can be applied with sufficient scientific validation. Nevertheless, it remains a useful tool for predicting a complication with far-reaching consequences and potentially fatal outcome [91]. There is a gap in current guidelines regarding perioperative management of AH in high-risk population for developing postoperative AKI. In a retrospective cohort study on hospitalized non-cardiac surgery patient after propensity matching, two comparable groups of more than 2000 patient each were formed (receiving vs not receiving RAASi in perioperative period) [97]. Those receiving RAAS inhibitors had a lower incidence of postoperative AKI (7.53% for the RASI group vs. 9.87% for the non-RASI group, adjusted OR 0.68, 95% CI:

Table 14.4 Overview of variables used for prediction model for predicting postoperative acute kidney injury in hypertensive patients, modified according to Liu et al. [91]

Variables
Estimated glomerular filtration rate
Neutrophil-to-lymphocyte ratio
Thrombin time
Serum potassium
Presence of pulmonary infection
Age
Uric acid
Serum albumin
Aspartate amino transferase
Total cholesterol
Gender
Prothrombin time
Hemoglobin

0.57–0.82). The observed frequency of all-cause death was not significantly different [97]. The mechanisms of postoperative AKI are perioperative hypotension, increased renovascular resistance, reduced renal blood flow leading to increased oxidative stress, endothelial dysfunction, and inflammatory response with tubular cell necrosis [97]. There is increased RAAS activation during any type of surgery, thus RAAS inhibition could improve renal perfusion by blocking RAAS activity. The logistic regression analysis showed that preoperative use of RAAS inhibitors reduced the risk of postoperative AKI, diuretics increased the risk of postoperative AKI, and calcium channel blockers (CCB) had no significant effect on postoperative AKI [97]. In study designed to assess the effect of withholding RAASi on the day of surgery, the authors observed that continuing or withholding RAASi had no effect on the occurrence of postoperative AKI [98]. The data on beta-blockers and AKI are lacking, but there is evidence that beta-blocker use may be associated with increased risks of perioperative MACEs and all-cause mortality in patients with uncomplicated AH [99]. While AH is a more common cause of AKI in surgical settings, AH can also be associated with post-operative AKI and possible progression to CKD leading to further complications due to impaired kidney function [96]. In order to prevent postoperative complications linked to impaired kidney function, timely and precise management of BP is warranted.

14.4.4 Acute Kidney Injury and Arterial Hypertension Associated with Use of Contrast

AKI after administrating contrast medium, also known as contrast-induced acute kidney injury (CI-AKI), is one of the most frequent adverse effects of the contrast media in total, causing an increase in length of hospital stay, mortality, and morbidity [5, 100]. CI-AKI is mostly caused by iodinated contrast media, but non-iodine contrast media can also sporadically induce CI-AKI [5]. CI-AKI accounts for around 10% of all hospital-acquired renal failure [101]. Considering that there are no adequate and effective ways of neither preventing nor curing CI-AKI, significant efforts have been made to successfully identify potential risk factors so that measures can be taken in order to prevent CI-AKI [100]. Considering that AH by itself present a risk factor for AKI and progressive kidney disease including CKD and ESKD, it has been shown that it can also act as a risk factor for CI-AKI, increasing the risk up to two times [46, 100]. In the effort to prevent CI-AKI, a study by Yin et al. followed 2666 hypertensive patients who received contrast medium in their final analysis, and the results showed that a duration of more than 3 days and normal dose of either 5 mg amlodipine or 2.5 mg levamlodipine daily before contrast administration resulted in better outcomes with regard to prevention of CI-AKI [100].

14.4.5 Acute Kidney Injury and Arterial Hypertension in the Setting of Scleroderma

Scleroderma, also known as systemic sclerosis, is a complex, multifaceted, immune-mediated rheumatic disease with fibrosis of skin and internal organs, as well as vasculopathy as hallmark manifestations [102]. With around 1 in 10,000 people being affected with systemic sclerosis, it is an uncommon disease with complex interactions between equally complex set of risk factors, including environmental, genetic, and epigenetic factors [102]. Clinical manifestations of systemic sclerosis are multiple and various, ranging from gastroesophageal reflux, Raynaud's phenomenon, inflammatory skin disease, swollen fingers and joints, fatigue and exhaustion, and different organ-based manifestations that include lung fibrosis, AH, gastrointestinal manifestations, and renal failure paired with thrombotic microangiopathy [102]. One specific complication of systemic sclerosis is scleroderma renal crisis, a major organ-based manifestation presenting with features of thrombotic microangiopathy, malignant hypertension, and oligo/anuric AKI [102, 103]. Scleroderma renal crisis can be found in roughly 4–6% of all scleroderma patients. The pathogenesis remains a mystery, with suggested mechanisms being proliferation of the vascular intima with subsequent narrowing of lumen and reduction in blood flow, vascular hyperreactivity, and activity of RAAS and decreased renal perfusion, in particular in the renal cortex [103]. The treatment comprises zealous and assertive control of BP through use of ACEi preferably intravenous, despite AKI and the need for RRT. RAAS inhibition in setting of scleroderma renal crisis should be continued and overtly combined with other antihypertensive drugs and RRT [103]. The use of ACEi as a preventive measure against scleroderma renal crisis is debated mostly based on poor evidence from one study with a few patients and questionable results [104].

14.4.6 Acute Kidney Injury and Arterial Hypertension as Manifestations of Thrombotic Microangiopathies

Elevated BP may cause various clinical consequences, one of worse being thrombotic microangiopathies (TMA), clinical entities characterized by microangiopathic hemolytic anemia, thrombocytopenia and end-organ damage, usually of renal type [105]. There is a pathophysiological link between AH and end-organ damage in TMA, and endothelium and vascular smooth muscles play a key role in the regulation of vascular tone. Endothelial dysfunction can cause alterations in vascular tone, leading to BP changes. These changes are responsible for damaging the endothelium, furthering endothelial dysfunction, which in turn, combined with neurohormonal activation and inflammation and play a mediating role in impairment of renal function. Given that endothelium dysfunction plays a key role in both AH and TMA, it is possible that one condition perpetuates the other. Malignant hypertension, a severe form of AH followed by acute multi-organ ischemic complications, usually results in TMA [81, 105, 106]. Both TMA and malignant hypertension can perpetuate AKI, and it is important to closely follow patients with unstable AH that can potentially be characterized as malignant, as well as closely follow for signs of potential microangiopathy (appearance of schistocytes in peripheral blood smears, platelet consumption and elevated lactic dehydrogenase levels, paired with oliguria) [105, 106]. Out of all TMAs, hemolytic uremic syndrome (HUS), more specifically atypical hemolytic uremic syndrome (aHUS), is more commonly associated with AH and AKI [105]. Thrombotic thrombocytopenic purpura (TTP) can resemble TMA with renal involvement. Distinguishing between TMA/aHUS and thrombotic thrombocytopenic purpura (TTP), is of high importance for the choice of therapeutic approach. Plasmapheresis is beneficial in TTP while TMA/aHUS best responds to complement blockade, specifically C5 component blockade being therapy of choice [106, 107].

Box 14.5 AKI in Subgroups of Patients and Blood Pressure

In patients with acute heart failure, systolic BP-fall beyond 25% in first 6 h was independent predictor of AKI in hypertensive patients.

In hospitalized patients with sepsis, it is imperative to control AKI by maintaining adequate renal function via optimization of BP.

Septic patients with prior history of arterial hypertension benefit from higher MAP values.

Arterial hypertension is the most common comorbidity among persons undergoing surgery, and hypertensive patients are especially prone to development of AKI.

There is a gap in current guidelines regarding perioperative management of arterial hypertension in high-risk population for developing postoperative AKI.

Preoperative use of RAAS inhibitors reduced the risk of postoperative AKI, diuretics increased the risk of postoperative AKI, and CCB had no significant effect on postoperative AKI. The data on beta-blockers and AKI are lacking, but there is evidence that beta-blocker use may be associated with increased risks of perioperative MACEs and all-cause mortality in patients with uncomplicated AH.

14.5 Renal Replacement Therapy in AKI Patients with Arterial Hypertension

Renal replacement therapy, mostly continuous methods or intermittent hemodialysis, is the primary therapy for oliguric AKI patients, and it might be considered when diuretic resistance occurs. In patients with chronic heart failure and a prolonged decrease of renal blood flow, the sensitivity to diuretics is greatly reduced [108]. Continuous renal-replacement therapy (CRRT) has become the most used therapy for AKI patients. Through continuous and slow fluid removal and blood purification, CRRT achieves the goal of stabilizing blood circulation and reduces the mortality of these patients [109]. Studies reported better therapeutic effects in patients with heart failure and AKI treated with CRRT than in patients treated with routine hemodialysis treatment [110]. Compared with routine hemodialysis treatment, CRRT can more gradually and effectively remove fluid which stabilizes hemodynamic status of patients. At the same time, it regulates fluid balance through continuous and slow blood purification, with no deleterious effects on the CV system [111]. Routine hemodialysis and its prolonged duration can influence hemodynamic state with hypotensive episodes and target organ damage of the brain, heart, and kidneys decreasing blood flow and increasing risk for arrhythmias [112]. The additional adsorption of inflammatory markers as well as small- and medium-size molecular toxins by CRRT hemofilters can additionally improve circulatory status of these patients [113]. Volume overload and its association with fatal CV events in hemodialyzed patients were reported in previous studies. Zoccali et al. showed the increased risk for mortality of 26% in patients with baseline volume overload and when compared to patients without volume overload [114]. The results were similar when pre-hemodialysis systolic BP was analyzed as well. Cumulative volume overload after the first year of hemodialysis was also associated with increased mortality with the highest risks at of pre-hemodialysis systolic BP <130 and >160 mmHg. Failure to reach the prescribed target weight and the end of hemodialysis session was also associated with increased CV mortality [115]. Strict and personalized ultrafiltration by which volume overload could be avoided and BP could be better controlled has been recognized since the inception of dialysis [116]. This can be easily extrapolated to intensive-care unit's patients with AKI. In critically ill patients with cardiogenic and septic shock, adequate fluid resuscitation is essential to the restoration of cardiac output, systemic BP, and renal perfusion [117, 118]. When fluid overload is refractory to medical therapy, CRRT should be administered especially due to hemodynamic instability and multiple organ failure in these patients. The optimal RRT for patients with AKI and fluid overload has not been defined yet and there is still an ongoing debate. Choice of the initial modality needs to be based on the availability of resources, local expertise, the individual needs of the patients, and finally on patient's hemodynamic status. It is reported that slower fluid removal and better fluid balance control when compared to intermittent hemodialysis result in more hemodynamic stability avoiding large fluctuations and fluid shifts [119]. It is still not yet fully explained which CRRT modality is advantageous. Continuous veno-venous hemofiltration (CVVH) allows meticulous control of fluid balance by providing continuous fluid, electrolyte, and toxin clearance while continuous veno-venous hemodiafiltration (CVVHDF) with its two methods of clearance, diffusion and convection, may provide better clearance of middle molecular weight solutes like cytokines compared with diffusive modalities [120]. Therefore, in septic patients with AKI, CVVHDF is probably the most suitable one. Slow continuous ultrafiltration (SCUF) is a type of CRRT usually performed with lower blood flow rates and ultrafiltration rates between 100 and 300 mL/h according to fluid balance necessities. It is mostly prescribed in patients with fluid overload without AKI or with low-grade AKI in cardiothoracic and cardiological intensive care units. The ultimate goal is to preserve tissue perfusion, optimizing fluid balance by effectively removing fluid without compromising the kidney and heart function.

Box 14.6 Renal Replacement Therapy in AKI Patients with Arterial Hypertension

Studies reported better therapeutic effects in patients with heart failure and AKI treated with CRRT than in patients treated with routine hemodialysis.

The optimal RRT for patients with AKI and fluid overload has not been defined yet and there is still an ongoing debate.

Slow continuous ultrafiltration (SCUF) is prescribed in patients with fluid overload without AKI or with low-grade AKI. The goal is to preserve tissue perfusion, optimizing fluid balance by effectively removing fluid without compromising the kidney and heart function.

References

1. Hoste EA, Bagshaw SM, Bellomo R, Cely CM, Colman R, Cruz DN, et al. Epidemiology of acute kidney injury in critically ill patients: the multinational AKI-EPI study. Intensive Care Med. 2015;41:1411–23.
2. Zeng X, McMahon GM, Brunelli SM, Bates DW, Waikar SS. Incidence, outcomes, and comparisons across definitions of AKI in hospitalized individuals. Clin J Am Soc Nephrol. 2014;9:12–20.
3. Hobson C, Ozrazgat-Baslanti T, Kuxhausen A, Thottakkara P, Efron PA, Moore FA, et al. Cost and mortality associated with postoperative acute kidney injury. Ann Surg. 2015;261:1207–14.
4. KDIGO Clinical Practice Guideline for the Diagnosis. Evaluation, prevention, and treatment of chronic kidney disease-mineral and bone disorder (CKD-MBD). Kidney Int Suppl. 2009;113:S1–130.
5. Kidney Disease: Improving Global Outcomes (KDIGO) Acute Kidney Injury Work Group. KDIGO clinical practice guideline for acute kidney injury. Kidney Int. 2012;2(1):1–138. https://kdigo.org/wp-content/uploads/2016/10/KDIGO-2012-AKI-Guideline-English.pdf
6. McCullough JW, Renner B, Thurman JM. The role of the complement system in acute kidney injury. Semin Nephrol. 2013;33(6):543–56.
7. Singbartl K, Kellum JA. AKI in the ICU: definition, epidemiology, risk stratification, and outcomes. Kidney Int Suppl. 2012;81(9):819–25.
8. Alwagdani A, Awad AS, Abdel-Rahman EM. Optimum post-discharge Care of Acute Kidney Injury (AKI) survivors. J Clin Med. 2022;11(21):6277.
9. Bellomo R, Ronco C, Kellum JA, Mehta RL, Palevsky P. Acute renal failure—definition, outcome measures, animal models, fluid therapy and information technology needs: the Second International Consensus Conference of the Acute Dialysis Quality Initiative (ADQI) Group. Crit Care. 2004;8(4):R204–12.
10. Mehta RL, Kellum JA, Shah SV, Molitoris BA, Ronco C, Warnock DG, et al. Acute kidney injury network: report of an initiative to improve outcomes in acute kidney injury. Crit Care. 2007;11(2):R31.
11. Chen TK, Parikh CR. Management of presumed acute kidney injury during hypertensive therapy: stay calm and carry on? Am J Nephrol. 2020;51(2):108–15.
12. Moledina DG, Parikh CR. Phenotyping of acute kidney injury: beyond serum creatinine. Semin Nephrol. 2018;38(1):3–11.
13. Palsson R, Waikar SS. Renal functional reserve revisited. Adv Chronic Kidney Dis. 2018;25(3):e1–8.

14. Nath KA. Tubulointerstitial changes as a major determinant in the progression of renal damage. Am J Kidney Dis. 1992;20(1):1–17.
15. Han WK, Bailly V, Abichandani R, Thadhani R, Bonventre JV. Kidney injury molecule-1 (KIM-1): a novel biomarker for human renal proximal tubule injury. Kidney Int. 2002;62(1):237–44.
16. Vaidya V, Ozer J, Dieterle F, Collings F, Ramirez V, Troth S, et al. Kidney injury molecule-1 outperforms traditional biomarkers of kidney injury in preclinical biomarker qualification studies. Nat Biotechnol. 2010;28(5):478–85.
17. Han W, Wagener G, Zhu Y, Wang S, Lee H. Urinary biomarkers in the early detection of acute kidney injury after cardiac surgery. Clin J Am Soc Nephrol. 2009;4:873–82.
18. Vaidya V, Waikar S, Ferguson M, Collings F, Sunderland K, Gioules C, et al. Urinary biomarkers for sensitive and specific detection of acute kidney injury in humans. Clin Transl Sci 2008;1(3):200–8.
19. Soni SS, Cruz D, Bobek I, Chionh CY, Nalesso F, Lentini P, et al. NGAL: a biomarker of acute kidney injury and other systemic conditions. Int Urol Nephrol. 2010;42:141–50
20. Mishra J, Ma Q, Prada A, Mitsnefes M, Zahedi K, Yang J, et al. Identification of neutrophil gelatinase-associated lipocalin as a novel early urinary biomarker for ischemic renal injury. J Am Soc Nephrol. 2003;14:2534–43.
21. Mishra J, Dent C, Tarabishi R, Mitsnefes MM, Ma Q, Kelly C, et al. Neutrophil gelatinase-associated lipocalin (NGAL) as a biomarker for acute renal injury after cardiac surgery. Lancet. 2005;365:1231–8.
22. Haase M, Bellomo R, Devarajan P, Schlattmann P, Haase-Fielitz A. Accuracy of neutrophil gelatinase-associated lipocalin (NGAL) in diagnosis and prognosis in acute kidney injury: a systematic review and meta-analysis. Am J Kidney Dis. 2009;54(6):1012–24.
23. Nakamura T, Nawa K, Ichihara A. Partial purification and characterization of hepatocyte growth factor from serum of hepatectomized rats. Biochem Biophys Res Commun. 1984;122:1450–9.
24. Nakamura H, Tashiro K, Nakamura T, Shiokawa K. Molecular cloning of Xenopus HGF cDNA and its expression studies in Xenopus early embriogenesis. Mech Dev. 1995;49:123–31.
25. Yang X, Park M. Expression of the hepatocyte growth factor/scatter factor receptor tyrosine kinase is localized to epithelia in the adult mouse. Lab Investig. 1995;73:483–91.
26. Kawaida K, Matsumoto K, Shimazu H, Nakamura T. Hepatocate growth factor prevents acute renal failure and accelerates renal regeneration in mice. Proc Natl Acad Sci USA. 1994;91:4357–61.
27. Maatman RG, van de Westerlo EM, van Kuppevelt TH, Veerkamp JH. Molecular identification of the liver- and the heart-type fatty acid-binding proteins in human and rat kidney. Use of the reverse transcriptase polymerase chain reaction. Biochem J. 1992;288(Pt 1):285–90.
28. Kamijo A, Sugaya T, Hikawa A, Okada M, Okumura F, Yamanouchi M, et al. Urinary excretion of fatty acid-binding protein reflects stress overload on the proximal tubules. Am J Pathol. 2004;165(4):1243–55.
29. Negishi K, Noiri E, Doi K, Maeda-Mamiya R, Sugaya T, Portilla D, et al. Monitoring of urinary L-type fatty acid-binding protein predicts histological severity of acute kidney injury. Am J Pathol. 2009;174(4):1154–9.
30. Price PM, Safirstein RL, Megyesi J. The cell cycle and acute kidney injury. Kidney Int. 2009;76(6):604–13.
31. Kashani K, Al-Khafaji A, Ardiles T, Artigas A, Bagshaw SM, Bell M, et al. Discovery and validation of cell cycle arrest biomarkers in human acute kidney injury. Crit Care. 2013;17(1):R25. https://doi.org/10.1186/cc12503.
32. Food and Drug Administration. Letter to astute medical. 2014. http://www.accessdata.fda.gov/cdrh_docs/pdf13/den130031.pdf.
33. Steubl D, Block M, Herbst V, Nockher WA, Schlumberger W, Satanovskij R, et al. Plasma uromodulin correlates with kidney function and identifies early stages in chronic kidney disease patients. Medicine. 2016;95:e3011.

34. Parikh CR, Jani A, Melnikov VY, Faubel S, Edelstein CL. Urinary interleukin-18 is a marker of human acute tubular necrosis. Am J Kidney Dis. 2004;43:405–14.
35. Parikh CR, Mishra J, Thiessen-Philbrook H, Dursun B, Ma Q, Kelly C, et al. Urinary IL-18 is an early predictive biomarker of acute kidney injury after cardiac surgery. Kidney Int. 2006;70:199–203.
36. Siew ED, Ikizler TA, Gebretsadik T, Shintani A, Wickersham N, Bossert F, et al. Elevated urinary IL-18 levels at the time of ICU admission predict adverse clinical outcomes. Clin J Am Soc Nephrol. 2010;5:1497–505.
37. Haase M, Devarajan P, Haase-Fielitz A, Bellomo R, Cruz DN, Wagener G, et al. The outcome of neutrophil gelatinase-associated lipocalin-positive subclinical acute kidney injury: a multicenter pooled analysis of prospective studies. J Am Coll Cardiol. 2011;57:1752–61.
38. Nickolas TL, Schmidt-Ott KM, Canetta P, Forster C, Singer E, Sise M, Elger A, et al. Diagnostic and prognostic stratification in the emergency department using urinary biomarkers of nephron damage: a multicenter prospective cohort study. J Am Coll Cardiol. 2012;59:246–55.
39. Haase M, Kellum JA, Ronco C. Subclinical AKI—an emerging syndrome with important consequences. Nat Rev Nephrol. 2012;8:735–9.
40. Cheung AK, Rahman M, Reboussin DM, Craven TE, Greene T, Kimmel PL, SPRINT Research Group, et al. Effects of intensive BP control in CKD. J Am Soc Nephrol. 2017;28:2812–23.
41. Malhotra R, Craven T, Ambrosius WT, Killeen AA, Haley WE, Cheung AK, SPRINT Research Group, et al. Effects of intensive BP lowering on kidney tubule injury in CKD: a longitudinal subgroup analysis in SPRINT. Am J Kidney Dis. 2019;73(1):21–30.
42. Zhang WR, Craven TE, Malhotra R, Cheung AK, Chonchol M, Drawz P, SPRINT Research Group, et al. Kidney damage biomarkers and incident chronic kidney disease during BP reduction: a case–control study. Ann Intern Med. 2018;169(9):610–8.
43. Shlipak MG, Katz R, Kestenbaum B, Siscovick D, Fried L, Newman A, et al. Rapid decline of kidney function increases cardiovascular risk in the elderly. J Am Soc Nephrol. 2009;20:2625–30.
44. Guyton AC. BP control—special role of the kidneys and body fluids. Science. 1991;252(5014):1813–6.
45. Hsu CY, Hsu RK, Yang J, Ordonez JD, Zheng S, Go AS. Elevated BP after AKI. J Am Soc Nephrol. 2016;27(3):914–23.
46. Xu X, Nie S, Liu Z, Chen C, Xu G, Zha Y, et al. Epidemiology, and clinical correlates of AKI in Chinese hospitalized adults. Clin J Am Soc Nephrol. 2015;10:1510–8.
47. Odutayo A, Wong CX, Farkouh M, Altman DG, Hopewell S, Emdin CA, et al. AKI and long-term risk for cardiovascular events and mortality. J Am Soc Nephrol. 2017;28(1):377–87.
48. Zuk A, Bonventre JV. Recent advances on acute kidney injury and its consequences and impact on chronic kidney disease. Curr Opin Nephrol Hypertens. 2019;28(4):397–405.
49. Su CC, Chen JY, Chen SY, Shiao CC, Neyra JA, Matsuura R, et al. Outcomes associated with acute kidney disease: a systematic review and meta-analysis. eClinicalMedicine. 2022;55:101760.
50. Coca SG, Singanamala S, Parikh CR. Chronic kidney disease after acute kidney injury: a systematic review and meta-analysis. Kidney Int. 2013;81(5):442–8.
51. Wu VC, Wu CH, Huang TM, Wang CY, Lai CF, Shiao CC, et al. Long-term risk of coronary events after AKI. J Am Soc Nephrol. 2014;25(3):595–605.
52. Wright JT Jr, Williamson JD, Whelton PK, Snyder JK, Sink KM, Rocco MV, SPRINT Research Group, et al. A randomized trial of intensive versus standard blood-pressure control. N Engl J Med. 2015;373(22):2103–16.
53. Dieter BP, Daratha KB, McPherson SM, Short R, Alicic RZ, Tuttle KR. Association of acute kidney injury with cardiovascular events and death in systolic blood pressure intervention trial. Am J Nephrol. 2019;49(5):359–67.
54. Thomas G, Schold JD. Blood pressure control, acute kidney injury, and cardiovascular events: separating the chaff from the wheat. Am J Nephrol. 2019;49(5):356–8.

55. Rocco MV, Sink KM, Lovato LC, Wolfgram DF, Wiegmann TB, Wall BM, SPRINT Research Group, et al. Effects of intensive blood pressure treatment on acute kidney injury events in the systolic blood pressure intervention trial (SPRINT). Am J Kidney Dis. 2018;71(3):352–61.
56. Nadkarni GN, Chauhan K, Rao V, Ix JH, Shlipak MG, Parikh CR, et al. Effect of intensive blood pressure lowering on kidney tubule injury: findings from the ACCORD trial study participants. Am J Kidney Dis. 2019;73(1):31–8.
57. Beddhu S, Shen J, Cheung AK, Kimmel PL, Chertow GM, Wei G, et al. Implications of early decline in eGFR due to intensive BP control for cardiovascular outcomes in SPRINT. J Am Soc Nephrol. 2019;30(8):1523–33.
58. Chang AR, Kramer H, Wei G, Boucher R, Grams ME, Berlowitz D, SPRINT Research Group, et al. Effects of intensive blood pressure control in patients with and without albuminuria: post hoc analyses from SPRINT. Clin J Am Soc Nephrol. 2020;15(8):1121–8.
59. Beddhu S, Greene T, Boucher R, Cushman WC, Wei G, Stoddard G, et al. Intensive systolic blood pressure control and incident chronic kidney disease in people with and without diabetes mellitus: secondary analyses of two randomised controlled trials. Lancet Diabetes Endocrinol. 2018;6:555–63.
60. Appel LJ, Wright JT Jr, Greene T, Agodoa LY, Astor BC, Bakris GL, AASK Collaborative Research Group, et al. Intensive blood-pressure control in hypertensive chronic kidney disease. N Engl J Med. 2010;363:918–29.
61. Klahr S, Levey AS, Beck GJ, Caggiula AW, Hunsicker L, Kusek JW, Modification of Diet in Renal Disease Study Group, et al. The effects of dietary protein restriction and blood-pressure control on the progression of chronic renal disease. N Engl J Med. 1994;330:877–84.
62. Ruggenenti P, Perna A, Loriga G, Ganeva M, Ene-Iordache B, Turturro M, REIN-2 Study Group, et al. Blood-pressure control for renoprotection in patients with non-diabetic chronic renal disease (REIN-2): multicentre randomised controlled trial. Lancet. 2005;365:939–46.
63. Hu AH, Chang TI. SPRINT-A kidney-centric narrative review: recent advances in hypertension. Hypertension. 2021;78(4):946–54.
64. Ruiz-Hurtado G, Sarafidis P, Fernández-Alfonso MS, Waeber B, Ruilope LM. Global cardiovascular protection in chronic kidney disease. Nat Rev Cardiol. 2016;13(10):603–8.
65. Venäläinen MS, Klén R, Mahmoudian M, Raitakari OT, Elo LL. Easy-to-use tool for evaluating the elevated acute kidney injury risk against reduced cardiovascular disease risk during intensive blood pressure control. J Hypertens. 2020;38:511–8.
66. Sequeira-Lopez MLS, Gomez RA. Preserving kidney health during intensive blood pressure control. Nat Rev Nephrol. 2018;14(9):537–8.
67. Moniwa N, Varagic J, Ahmad S, VonCannon JL, Simington SW, Wang H, et al. Hemodynamic and hormonal changes to dual renin–angiotensin system inhibition in experimental hypertension. Hypertension. 2013;61:417–24.
68. Brar S, Ye F, James MT, Hemmelgarn B, Klarenbach S, Pannu N, Interdisciplinary Chronic Disease Collaboration. Association of angiotensin-converting enzyme inhibitor or angiotensin receptor blocker use with outcomes after acute kidney injury. JAMA Intern Med. 2018;178(12):1681–90.
69. Hsu CY, Liu KD, Yang J, Glidden DV, Tan TC, Pravoverov L, et al. Renin–angiotensin system blockade after acute kidney injury (AKI) and risk of recurrent AKI. Clin J Am Soc Nephrol. 2020;15:26–34.
70. Siew ED, Parr SK, Abdel-Kader K, Perkins AM, Greevy RA Jr, Vincz AJ, et al. Renin–angiotensin aldosterone inhibitor use at hospital discharge among patients with moderate to severe acute kidney injury and its association with recurrent acute kidney injury and mortality. Kidney Int. 2021;99(5):1202–12.
71. Janse RJ, Fu EL, Clase CM, Tomlinson L, Lindholm B, van Diepen M, et al. Stopping versus continuing renin–angiotensin-system inhibitors after acute kidney injury and adverse clinical outcomes: an observational study from routine care data. Clin Kidney J. 2022;15:1109–19.
72. Yang CY, Liu JS, Tseng WC, Tsai MT, Lin MH, Kao ZK, et al. Effect of renin–angiotensin–aldosterone system blockade on long-term outcomes in postacute kidney injury patients with hypertension. Crit Care Med. 2020;48(12):e1185–93.

73. Singh P, Ricksten SE, Bragadottir G, Redfors B, Nordquist L. Renal oxygenation and haemodynamics in acute kidney injury and chronic kidney disease. Clin Exp Pharmacol Physiol. 2013;40:138–47.
74. Ho KM, Power BM. Benefits and risks of furosemide in acute kidney injury. Anaesthesia. 2010;65(3):283–93.
75. Bosch X, Poch E, Grau JM. Rhabdomyolysis and acute kidney injury. N Engl J Med. 2009;361:62–72.
76. Arao Y, Sawamura A, Nakatochi M, Okumura T, Kato H, Oishi H, et al. Early blood pressure reduction by intravenous vasodilators is associated with acute kidney injury in patients with hypertensive acute decompensated heart. Circ J. 2019;23(83):1883–90.
77. Grams ME, Estrella MM, Coresh J, Brower RG, Liu KD, National Heart, Lung, and Blood Institute Acute Respiratory Distress Syndrome Network. Fluid balance, diuretic use, and mortality in acute kidney injury. Clin J Am Soc Nephrol. 2011;6:966–73.
78. Sánchez-Pozos K, Barrera-Chimal J, Garzón-Muvdi J, Pérez-Villalva R, Rodríguez-Romo R, Cruz C, et al. Recovery from ischemic acute kidney injury by spironolactone administration. Nephrol Dial Transplant. 2012;27:3160–9.
79. Watanabe K, Hamada T, Shimada K, Fujimaru T, Ito Y, Nagahama M, et al. Efficacy of renin–angiotensin–aldosterone system blockades for acute phase hypertensive emergencies in patient complicating severe acute kidney injury. CEN Case Rep. 2022;11(1):105–9.
80. Metra M, Nodari S, Parrinello G, Bordonali T, Bugatti S, Danesi R, et al. Worsening renal function in patients hospitalised for acute heart failure: clinical implications and prognostic significance. Eur J Heart Fail. 2008;10(2):188–95.
81. Damman K, Jaarsma T, Voors AA, Navis G, Hillege HL, Van Veldhuisen DJ. Both in- and out-hospital worsening of renal function predict outcome in patients with heart failure: results from the coordinating study evaluating outcome of advising and counseling in heart failure (COACH). Eur J Heart Fail. 2009;11(9):847–54.
82. Shirakabe A, Hata N, Kobayashi N, Shinada T, Tomita K, Tsurumi M, et al. Prognostic impact of acute kidney injury in patients with acute decompensated heart failure. Circ J. 2013;77(3):687–96.
83. Ponikowski P, Voors AA, Anker SD, Bueno H, Cleland JGF, Coats AJS, ESC Scientific Document Group, et al. 2016 ESC guidelines for the diagnosis and treatment of acute and chronic heart failure: the task force for the diagnosis and treatment of acute and chronic heart failure of the European Society of Cardiology (ESC) developed with the special contribution of the Heart Failure Association (HFA) of the ESC. Eur Heart J. 2016;37:2129–200.
84. Cheung AK, Chang TI, Cushman WC, Furth SL, Hou FF, Ix JH, et al. Executive summary of the KDIGO 2021 clinical practice guideline for the management of blood pressure in chronic kidney disease. Kidney Int. 2021;99:559–69.
85. Dasgupta I, Zoccali C. Is the KDIGO systolic blood pressure target <120 mmHg for chronic kidney disease appropriate in routine clinical practice? Hypertension. 2022;79(1):4–11.
86. Robles NR, Hernandez-Gallego R, Fici F, Grassi G. Does a blood pressure J curve exist for patients with chronic kidney disease? J Clin Hypertens (Greenwich). 2017;19(8):764–70.
87. Singer M, Deutschman CS, Seymour CW, Shankar-Hari M, Annane D, Bauer M, et al. The third international consensus definitions for sepsis and septic shock (Sepsis-3). JAMA. 2016;315(8):801–10.
88. Dewitte A, Labat A, Duvignaud PA, Bouche G, Joannes-Boyau O, Ripoche J, et al. High mean arterial pressure target to improve sepsis-associated acute kidney injury in patients with prior hypertension: a feasibility study. Ann Intensive Care. 2021;11(1):139. https://doi.org/10.1186/s13613-021-00925-2.
89. Zhao L, Fan Y, Wang Z, Wei Z, Zhang Y, Li Y, et al. The BP targets in sepsis patients with acute kidney injury: an observational cohort study of multiple ICUs. Front Immunol. 2022;13:1060612.
90. Sapkota S, Sherpa M, Bhattarai B. Incidence of hypertension in patients undergoing surgery at Dhulikhel Hospital-Kathmandu University Hospital. Kathmandu Univ Med J (KUMJ). 2011;9:40–3.

91. Liu X, Ye Y, Mi Q, Huang W, He T, Huang P, et al. A predictive model for assessing surgery-related acute kidney injury risk in hypertensive patients: a retrospective cohort study. PLoS One. 2016;11(11):1–15.
92. Guangyu Y, Jingfeng L, Xing L, Hong Y, Yao L. Cardio- and cerebrovascular outcomes of postoperative acute kidney injury in noncardiac surgical patients with hypertension. Front Pharmacol. 2021;12:696456.
93. Kandler K, Jensen ME, Nilsson JC, Møller CH, Steinbrüchel DA. Acute kidney injury is independently associated with higher mortality after cardiac surgery. J Cardiothorac Vasc Anesth. 2014;28:1448–52.
94. Najjar M, Salna M, George I. Acute kidney injury after aortic valve replacement: incidence, risk factors and outcomes. Expert Rev Cardiovasc Ther. 2015;13(3):301–15.
95. Pickering JW, James MT, Palmer SC. Acute kidney injury and prognosis after cardiopulmonary bypass: a meta-analysis of cohort studies. Am J Kidney Dis. 2015;65(2):283–93.
96. Shaw AD, Khanna AK, Smischney NJ, Shenoy AV, Boero IJ, Bershad M, et al. Intraoperative hypotension is associated with persistent acute kidney disease after noncardiac surgery: a multicentre cohort study. Br J Anaesth. 2022;129(1):13–21.
97. Xu N, Long Q, He T, Liu X, Dai H, Lu Y, et al. Association between preoperative renin–angiotensin system inhibitor use and postoperative acute kidney injury risk in patients with hypertension. Clin Nephrol. 2018;89(6):403–14.
98. Vijay A, Grover A, Coulson TG, Myles PS. Perioperative management of patients treated with angiotensin-converting enzyme inhibitors and angiotensin II receptor blockers: a quality improvement audit. Anaesth Intensive Care. 2016;44:346–52.
99. Jørgensen ME, Hlatky MA, Køber L, Sanders RD, Torp-Pedersen C, Gislason GH, et al. β-Blocker-associated risks in patients with uncomplicated hypertension undergoing noncardiac surgery. JAMA Intern Med. 2015;175(12):1923–31.
100. Yin WJ, Zhou LY, Li DY, Xie YL, Wang JL, Zuo SR, et al. Protective effects of amlodipine pretreatment on contrast-induced acute kidney injury and overall survival in hypertensive patients. Front Pharmacol. 2020;11:44.
101. Nash K, Hafeez A, Hou S. Hospital-acquired renal insufficiency. Am J Kidney Dis. 2002;39(5):930–6.
102. Denton CP, Khanna D. Systemic sclerosis. Lancet. 2017;390:1685–99.
103. Mouthon L, Bérezné A, Bussone G, Noël LH, Villiger PM, Guillevin L. Scleroderma renal crisis: a rare but severe complication of systemic sclerosis. Clin Rev Allergy Immunol. 2011;40(2):84–91.
104. Hudson M, Baron M, Tatibouet S, Furst DE, Khanna D, International Scleroderma Renal Crisis Study Investigators. Exposure to ACE inhibitors prior to the onset of scleroderma renal crisis-results from the international scleroderma renal crisis survey. Semin Arthritis Rheum. 2014;43(5):666–72.
105. Mathew RO, Nayer A, Asif A. The endothelium as the common denominator in malignant hypertension and thrombotic microangiopathy. J Am Soc Hypertens. 2016;10(4):352–9.
106. Nzerue C, Oluwole K, Adejorin D, Paueksakon P, Fremont R, Akatue R, et al. Malignant hypertension with thrombotic microangiopathy and persistent acute kidney injury (AKI). Clin Kidney J. 2014;7(6):586–9.
107. Fakhouri F, Zuber J, Frémeaux-Bacchi V, Loirat C. Haemolytic uraemic syndrome. Lancet. 2017;390(10095):681–96.
108. Cappannoli L, Scacciavillani R, Rocco E, Perna F, Narducci ML, Vaccarella M, et al. Cardiac contractility modulation for patient with refractory heart failure: an updated evidence-based review. Heart Fail Rev. 2021;26(2):227–35.
109. Tandukar S, Palevsky PM. Continuous renal replacement therapy: who, when, why, and how. Chest. 2019;155(3):626–38.
110. Zhang M, Li J. Continuous renal replacement therapy for hypertension complicated by refractory Heart failure: an analysis of safety and nursing highlights. Comput Math Methods Med. 2022;2022:7951744.

111. Yoon J, Kim Y, Kym D, Hur J, Yim H, Cho YS, et al. Subgroup analysis of continuous renal replacement therapy in severely burned patients. PLoS One. 2017;12(11):e0189057.
112. Zhou X, Zhao C, Feng X, Samanta A, Lin YN, Chen J, et al. Continuous renal replacement therapy for haemodynamic collapse and rhabdomyolysis induced by pheochromocytoma crisis. ESC Heart Fail. 2016;3(4):282–7.
113. Bellavia D, Iacovoni A, Scardulla C, Moja L, Pilato M, Kushwaha SS, et al. Prediction of right ventricular failure after ventricular assist device implant: systematic review and meta-analysis of observational studies. Eur J Heart Fail. 2017;19(7):926–46.
114. Zoccali C, Moissl U, Chazot C, Mallamaci F, Tripepi G, Arkossy O, et al. Chronic fluid overload and mortality in ESRD. J Am Soc Nephrol. 2017;28:2491–7.
115. Movilli E, Camerini C, Gaggia P, Zubani R, Feller P, Poiatti P, et al. Magnitude of end-dialysis overweight is associated with all-cause and cardiovascular mortality: a 3-year prospective study. Am J Nephrol. 2013;37:370–7.
116. Scribner BH, Buri R, Caner JE, Hegstrom R, Burnell JM. The treatment of chronic uremia by means of intermittent hemodialysis: a preliminary report. Trans Am Soc Artif Intern Organs. 1960;6:114–22.
117. Prowle JR, Echeverri JE, Ligabo EV, Ronco C, Bellomo R. Fluid balance and acute kidney injury. Nat Rev Nephrol. 2010;6(2):107–15.
118. Levy MM, Artigas A, Phillips GS, Rhodes A, Beale R, Osborn T, et al. Outcomes of the surviving sepsis campaign in intensive care units in the USA and Europe: a prospective cohort study. Lancet Infect Dis. 2012;12(12):919–24.
119. Kidney Disease Improving Global Outcomes (KDIGO) Working Group Section. 5: Dialysis interventions for treatment of AKI. Kidney Int Suppl. 2012;2(1):89–115.
120. Wan L, Bagshaw SM, Langenberg C, Saotome T, May C, Bellomo R. Pathophysiology of septic acute kidney injury: what do we really know? Crit Care Med. 2008;36:S198–203.

Treatment of Hypertension in Chronic Kidney Disease

15

Josep Redon

15.1 Introduction

The relationship between hypertension (HTN) and kidney damage has been well known since Bright's observations in the late nineteenth century. The fact that HTN is a cause of impaired renal function and that its deterioration leads to stable hypertension is a binomial of great clinical significance; chronic kidney disease (CKD) is not only a consequence of hypertension but also contributes to hypertension. Furthermore, hypertension in CKD is often uncontrolled and resistant to treatment, and its presence increases the risk of mortality [1] (Fig. 15.1). It is therefore of great clinical importance to know when, how and what is the best treatment in patients with CKD to reduce the consequences of uncontrolled hypertension and slow the progressive decline in renal function towards end-stage renal disease (ESRD), as well as to reduce CV events and mortality. It is believed that the best treatment to prevent the development of CKD is the treatment of hypertension. In addition, HTN in CKD creates a vicious circle as it contributes to the progression of CKD and high cardiovascular risk in this patient population [2].

This chapter provides an overview of how HTN causes kidney damage, the mechanisms of HTN in CKD, blood pressure targets and the best management approach.

J. Redon (✉)
INCLIVA Health Research Institute, University of Valencia, Valencia, Spain
e-mail: josep.redon@uv.es

A. E. Berbari et al. (eds.), *Blood Pressure Disorders in Acute and Chronic Kidney Diseases*, Updates in Hypertension and Cardiovascular Protection,
https://doi.org/10.1007/978-3-031-81292-7_15

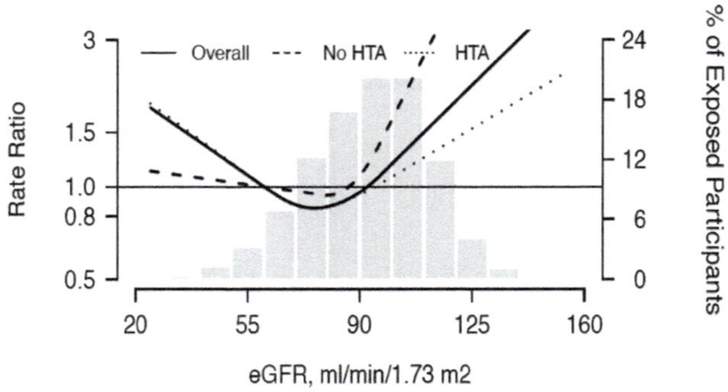

Fig. 15.1 Impact of HTN on mortality risk through eGFR in a population of 52,007 with CV risk from an Electronic Health Recording of the general population. While hypertensives have an increased risk below 55 mL/min/1.73 m^2, patients without HTN do not have an increased risk [1]

15.2 Mechanisms of HTN-Induced Renal Damage

The traditional view of the relationship between HTA and renal damage has been that HTN causes glomerular ischaemia and hypoperfusion by progressive luminal narrowing in preglomerular arteries and arterioles. Ischaemia may result from structural narrowing due to atheromatous disease or malignant HTN or from exaggerated functional afferent vasoconstriction as seen in some subgroups of hypertensive patients [3, 4].

Based on experimental animal models of HTN, glomerular capillary hypertension and hyper perfusion, rather than hypoperfusion, are the important factors leading to glomerular damage and progressive loss of renal function. According to this hypothesis, the increase in afferent arteriolar resistance is part of a compensatory mechanism to prevent the transmission of increased preglomerular pressure to the capillary network. This autoregulatory response is mediated by two mechanisms, a myogenic reflex and a mechanism whereby increased sodium delivery in the distal tubule triggers a vasoconstrictor response of the afferent arteriole. If either of these mechanisms is impaired, the increased systemic pressure is transmitted unhindered to the glomerular and peritubular capillaries [5].

Increased glomerular capillary pressure leads to an increase in single nephron GFR, transglomerular passage of proteins and influx of proteins and other macromolecules into the mesangium. Activation of mesangial cells, which is thought to increase the production of cytokines and growth factors, results in increased glomerular hypertension leading to glomerular sclerosis [6]. In addition, increased protein flux across the mesangium may lead to increased trans-glomerular passage of protein into the urinary tract, thereby increasing urinary protein excretion. Increased protein transport into the urinary tract leads to excessive protein reabsorption by the proximal tubule with subsequent tubulointerstitial damage [7].

Further interstitial damage can result from increased pressure in the peritubular capillary due to impaired autoregulatory mechanisms. This process is more evident in the nephrons of the deeper juxtamedullary regions of the kidney. An increase in blood pressure has been shown to increase peritubular capillary and interstitial pressure in this region. The increased interstitial pressure is in turn transmitted throughout the renal parenchyma, including the cortex. The three main consequences are (1) passive retardation of sodium chloride reabsorption due to paracellular back leakage of sodium across the tight junction complexes of the proximal tubule (hence the development of a state of SLT-dependent hypertension); (2) induction of ischaemia in the surrounding tubules and interstitium and (3) restriction of blood flow to the more distal vasa recta supplying the medulla and consequent medullary ischaemia [8, 9].

Mechanisms leading to renal parenchymal fibrosis play an important role in the decline of renal function [10, 11]. Hypertension increases the mesenchymal transition of epithelial [12] and endothelial [13] cells. Cells involved in this process respond to stimuli that alter polarity and adhesion by lacking cell–cell junctions and promoting fibrosis.

Finally, the persistence of elevated blood pressure during the night means that the physiological fall in blood pressure is absent or reduced. In the supine position, the activity of the mediators controlling preglomerular tone, mainly sympathetic and renin–angiotensin activities is reduced, with easier transmission of high pressure to the pericapillary glomerulus and tubule. This triggers mechanisms leading to renal tissue damage as the burden of high BP is maintained over time, increasing the impact on vascular, glomerular and interstitial structures. An additional and sometimes competing possibility is that blunted nocturnal BP fall is not only a cause but also a consequence of renal abnormalities, as sustained high BP levels may be required to overcome reduced availability of sodium excretion and/or high vascular resistance [14]. Figure 15.2 summarises the mechanisms of HTN-induced renal injury.

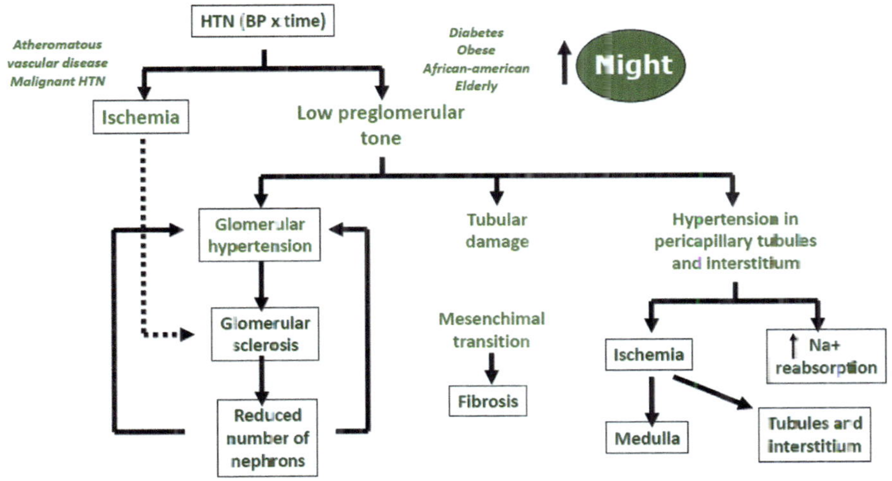

Fig. 15.2 Mechanisms of hypertension-induced kidney damage

15.3 Mechanisms of Hypertension in Chronic Kidney Disease

The pathogenesis of hypertension in patients with CKD is multifactorial and often resistant to treatment due to its complexity [2]. Given the importance of the kidney in maintaining the homeostasis of the body and the relevance of BP, it is not difficult to consider that when the kidney is damaged, there are several mechanisms that contribute to maintaining elevated BP [15]. We will consider each of these separately, although their relevant interactions will be mentioned.

15.3.1 Sodium Sensitivity and Sodium/Water Retention

Hypertension in CKD is a salt-sensitive condition with an impaired pressure-natriuresis curve, characterised by Na^+ retention leading to an increase in extracellular fluid volume [16, 17]. Although impaired pressure natriuresis depends on hemodynamic factors, the distal nephron plays an important role in salt sensitivity, being stimulated by the renin–angiotensin system and aldosterone secretion, which is partly responsible for the increase in potassium levels. In addition, sodium reabsorption is stimulated in the presence of proteinuria, although Na+ reabsorption does not appear to be relevant in the absence of nephrotic syndrome [18]. Sodium retention causes volume-dependent and -independent HTN, including vascular stiffness and increased central sympathetic outflow [19].

Recent studies have shown that part of the salt load accumulates in the interstitial space of the skin in a non-osmotic association with glycosaminoglycans and lymphatic vessels [20]. Although this mechanism appears to be relevant to sodium homeostasis, a causal link between skin sodium and hypertension is still lacking.

15.3.2 Sympathetic Nervous System

Sympathetic overactivity has been observed in patients with CKD and increases with reduced eGFR [21] and has been implicated in the progression of CKD. Mechanisms implicated in progression include increased central sympathetic outflow [22] generated by signals from the kidney and the influx of high levels of angiotensin II [23]. Renal sympathetic activation decreases renal blood flow and increases renin levels with consequent activation of the RAAS and stimulation of tubular sodium reabsorption [24]. All these elements contribute to the maintenance of elevated blood pressure and to the nocturnal rise in blood pressure [25]. The identification of a new player in SNS overactivity, renalase, opens up new scenarios for the future. This is an amine oxidase that metabolises catecholamines involved in the regulation of cardiac function, renal damage and blood pressure. Secreted in the glomerulus and renal tubule, blood levels are inversely proportional to GFR and overactivity of SNS in CKD could be derived from abnormalities in the renalase pathway [15].

15.3.3 Renin–Angiotensin–Aldosterone System

The renin–angiotensin–aldosterone system (RAAS) is activated in patients with CKD. Activation reduces blood flow in the peritubular capillaries downstream of the sclerosed glomeruli, increasing renin secretion and consequently angiotensin II, which (a) directly causes vasoconstriction with an increase in vascular resistance and blood pressure; (b) increases aldosterone, which promotes sodium reabsorption in the proximal tubule; and (c) the reduced number of glomeruli must increase systemic pressure to maintain glomerular perfusion [26].

15.3.4 Vascular Changes

The vascular tree is constantly exposed to a variety of hormones, uremic toxins and other factors that cause dysfunction and structural damage and increase blood pressure. These include endothelial dysfunction, alteration of NO signalling and the effects of prostanoids, endothelin signalling and the uremic state. The consequence of such an adverse scenario is an increase in peripheral resistance and vascular stiffness [27].

15.3.5 Metabolic Disturbance

Some of the metabolic derangements associated with reduced renal function in maintaining electrolyte and mineral metabolite levels also contribute to the elevation and maintenance of high blood pressure [28]. These include increased calcium phosphate products, hyperphosphataemia, decreased 1,25(OH)2D synthesis, decreased ionised magnesium and alpha-glucoproteins, and secondary hyperparathyroidism [29]. These conditions lead to endothelial dysfunction and vascular stiffness. Another mechanism is the level of fibroblast growth factor 23 (FGF23), which regulates phosphate homeostasis. Advances in experimental and clinical research have described links between FGF23 and hemodynamic and cardiovascular changes that may affect blood pressure. These include direct and indirect mechanistic links between the FGF23–Klotho axis, vitamin D and the RAAS. Excess FGF23 and insufficient Klotho availability cross-talk with the RAAS and modulate Na reabsorption, blood volume, oxidative stress and mineral metabolism homeostasis [30].

Figure 15.3 summarises the mechanisms of HTN-induced renal injury.

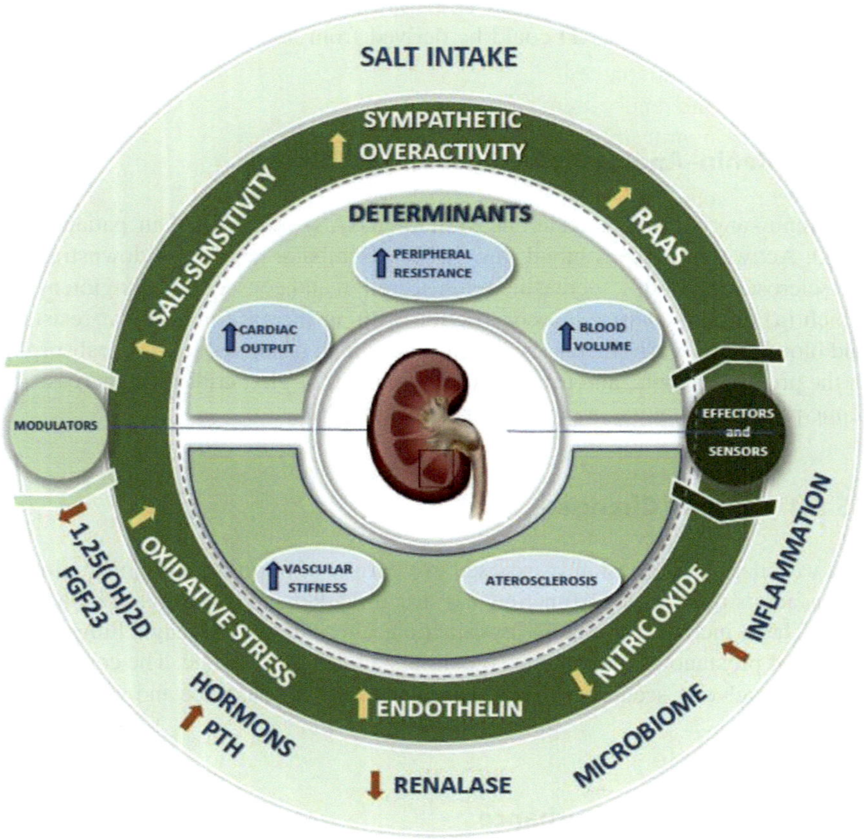

Fig. 15.3 Mechanisms of CKD that increase hypertension. (**a**) Determinants, (**b**) effectors, and (**c**) modulators

15.4 Hypertension in CKD: Key Features

Hypertension in patients with CKD is characterised by altered circadian variability with a blunted fall in BP during sleep, maintenance of elevated nocturnal BP, a non-dipping pattern and resistance to treatment.

The non-dipping pattern is present in a large proportion of patients with CKD, increases as GFR declines and is associated with a higher prevalence of other organ damage, mainly left ventricular hypertrophy, and a higher risk of cardiovascular events, progression to ESRD and mortality [31]. Many years ago, a non-dipping pattern in adolescents with type 1 diabetes was a predictor of the development of diabetic nephropathy [32]. Subsequent studies have shown that nocturnal BP in patients with CKD is associated with a higher risk of cardiovascular events [33, 34] and progression of renal damage [35].

In a recent study, the Chinese Cohort Study of Chronic Kidney Disease (C-STRIDE), 73% of patients had elevated nocturnal HTN, with systolic HTN being the most common, followed by nocturnal diastolic HTN. Their impact on cardiovascular and renal events was recorded and showed that those without nocturnal HTN had a significantly lower risk compared to those with nocturnal HTN. While nocturnal diastolic HTN was associated with a slightly increased risk compared to normotensive subjects, systolic HTN was associated with a higher risk of CV events. Elevated nocturnal systolic and diastolic blood pressure increased not only the risk of CV events but also the risk of renal events [31].

Together with increased nocturnal BP, CKD often has a resistant hypertension phenotype [36]. Several studies support the high prevalence of apparent treatment-resistant hypertension in CKD patients, 29% [37], 40% [38]. The prevalence increases with GFR decline from 34% in stage 3a to 42% in stage 3b, 52% in stage 4 and 60% in those with stage 5 [39].

15.5 Blood Pressure Goals

Treatment of hypertension is essential to reduce the rate of progression of CKD, the cardiovascular risk associated with hypertension, and mortality. However, the therapeutic target for BP reduction has been controversial for decades, as too much BP reduction may worsen the rate of progression of CKD [40]. A landmark article published many years ago was the Modification of Diet in Renal Disease Study MDRD [41]. In this study, patients with CKD were randomised to a normal or low protein diet and to usual or intensive blood pressure lowering. The study found that in non-diabetic patients with CKD, the low blood pressure group had a faster decline in glomerular filtration rate during the first 4 months after randomisation and a slower decline thereafter. In addition, those who had more proteinuria at baseline had a significantly slower rate of decline in GFR. Years later, during long follow-up, it was found that patients with a low target BP of 126/77 mmHg had a greater slowing of progression to ESRD compared to patients with a less demanding BP reduction [42].

The African American Study of Kidney Disease and Hypertension Study Group (AASK) randomised trial [43] found that intensive blood pressure control had no effect on progression of kidney disease (130/78 vs 141/85 mmHg), but there was a differential effect in those with baseline proteinuria, with the lowest BP having a greater beneficial effect [44].

More recently, the SPRINT trial reported the effect of intensive SBP reduction, <120 mmHg compared with <140 mmHg, in a high-risk non-diabetic population. A significant reduction in cardiovascular events and mortality was observed, but there was also an increase in acute renal failure or injury [45]. Analysis of enrolled patients with hypertensive CKD showed that the intensive arm reduced the rates of cardiovascular events and all-cause mortality, but no detrimental effect on the main renal outcome was observed [46]. In contrast, there was an increase in incident CKD with intensive SBP lowering, although significant reductions in cardiovascular events and mortality were observed [47]. It should be noted that the patients enrolled were poorly representative of the CKD population under nephrology care [48].

The beneficial effect on mortality was also seen in a meta-analysis of 18 randomised control trials with 15,924 participants with CKD who potentially met the inclusion criteria. From a baseline of 148 mmHg, blood pressure fell to 132 mmHg in the more intensive group and to 140 mmHg in the less intensive group. A 14.0% lower risk of all-cause mortality was observed in those achieving the lowest blood pressure levels [49].

Recently, the Kidney Disease Improving Global Outcomes 2021 (KDIGO) Clinical Practice Guideline for the Management of Blood Pressure in Chronic Kidney Disease in Patients Not on Dialysis presented an update on BP targets in patients with CKD [50]. Based mainly on data from SPRINT, a systolic BP target of less than 120 mmHg using standardised office BP measurement was proposed on the basis that this target is associated with lower mortality, although the benefit in terms of renal function remains unclear. The KDIGO recommendation recognises that there are some limitations, including lack of evidence in diabetic nephropathy and in patients over 60 years of age. There is no question that the <120 mmHg target is associated with more adverse effects, mainly electrolyte changes and reduced eGFR. Information is also more limited for stage 4–5 CKD and diabetic nephropathy, and the guideline also expresses concern about the lack of solid information.

Given the available information, a target of <130/80 mmHg seems reasonable, but individualised treatment should be considered in the presence of albuminuria. If a more stringent target of <120 mmHg is implemented, potential adverse effects should be closely monitored.

Two other aspects of targets require attention. The first is the fact that some of the drugs used to reduce BP in CKD, RAAS blockers and SGLT2i, induce a functional reduction in GFR by reducing the filtration fraction, with consequent protection against glomerular damage despite the initial reduction in GFR. After starting treatment with these drugs, a decrease in GFR of up to 30% can be considered functional and treatment should be maintained.

Secondly, renal protection has always been assessed by GFR and/or albuminuria. The assessment of tubular markers has emerged as a potential to better assess the impact of treatment on renal injury. Several approaches have been used to assess tubular damage, ranging from the urine-plasma ratio for novel endogenous measures of tubular secretion to a mixture of different tubular elements reflecting tubular injury/repair (NGAL, IL-18 and YKL-40), tubular injury/fibrosis (KIM-1 and MCP-1), tubular reabsorption (A1M and B2M) and tubular reserve/mineral metabolism (UMOD, FGF-23 and PTH). In SPRINT CKD patients, several approaches to the relevance of tubular markers have been made. Bullen describes that worse tubular secretion was associated with a greater risk of adverse events, specifically progression of renal damage [51], the risk of progressive eGFR decline and the incidence of acute kidney injury [52], all independent of eGFR and albuminuria. Interestingly, two markers of tubular reabsorption, A1M and B2M, do not increase tubular marker levels despite eGFR loss, supporting that eGFR decline is a consequence of haemodynamic changes [53]. Future studies will provide more robust information on the role of tubular markers in CKD follow-up.

15.6 Non-pharmacologic Treatment

15.6.1 Lifestyle Modifications

CKD is a progressive disease caused and/or aggravated by multiple conditions and therefore requires a holistic approach to improve BP control and delay progression to ESRD and mortality [54]. Lifestyle modifications may play an important role in management with or without an impact on BP control [55].

Lifestyle factors that may influence HTN include physical inactivity in obesity, anxiety, depression and sleep disturbance. Dietary weight loss and light daily exercise significantly reduce BP and albuminuria. Although it is controversial whether exercise slows the progression of GFR, it should continue to be recommended according to age [56].

Other changes, such as limiting alcohol intake and avoiding binge drinking, will not only help control HTN but will also reduce GFR decline [57]. Reducing stress [58] and improving sleep quality and sleep apnoea may reduce sympathetic overactivity and improve HTN control. Smoking cessation should be recommended to reduce CV risk, although it has no direct effect on HTN.

15.6.2 Disturbed Salt and Fluid Balance

The effect of dietary salt on HTN is well established at a population level, and the fact that CKD is a salt-sensitive condition leads to a general recommendation to reduce sodium intake in CKD patients to <2 g/day, with a beneficial effect in those with more advanced CKD [59]. However, few controlled studies have examined the association of dietary sodium with cardiovascular events and mortality in patients with CKD. The effect on blood pressure is more controversial, with a small number of randomised controlled trials [60]. While some find an effect of dietary salt on BP elevation [61], others conclude that there is no consistent association between dietary sodium and BP [62]. In this situation, dietary salt restriction should be recommended to reduce BP in patients with CKD.

Extracellular volume overload is common in patients with CKD, both asymptomatic and symptomatic, and contributes to renal damage. Interventions to reduce volume overload are limited because of reduced glomerular filtration and tubular salt sensitivity and are exacerbated in the presence of proteinuria. Maintaining a near-normal extracellular fluid volume is often necessary to treat hypertension and prevent progressive cardiovascular and renal damage [53]. Dietary sodium restriction and the use of diuretics are the main tools for preventing volume overload and lowering blood pressure.

15.7 Pharmacologic Treatment

Pharmacological treatment is the cornerstone of hypertension management. Its development since the 1950s has paralleled advances in the pathophysiological mechanisms of BP elevation and its consequences. The ability of the different classes of antihypertensive drugs to reduce BP in patients with CKD has been tested in a large number of studies, although difficulties have been encountered in assessing the individual effect of each class of drug. This is due to the fact that the drugs have usually been tested in combination with other drugs that also help to lower blood pressure before the test drug is administered. The lower the 'baseline' BP, the smaller is the magnitude of the BP reduction.

Treatment of HTN in CKD requires combination therapy due to the frequent presence of poorly controlled and/or resistant HTN. The European Society of Hypertension guidelines 2023 [64] recommend ACEi or ARBs plus CCB (dihydropyridine) and/or thiazide or thiazide/like diuretic. If GFR is <30 mL/min/1.73 m^2, a loop diuretic is recommended. Single pill administration is strongly recommended.

15.7.1 Diuretics

Diuretics play a relevant role in BP control in patients with CKD, despite doubts and controversy over many years due to their undervalued status compared with other classes of antihypertensive drugs, and they have been used in comparison or with combination therapy in clinical trials. Among the two classes of diuretics exists a belief that thiazide and thiazide-like agents lose efficacy as GFR decline, in reducing not only diuresis but also BP, and was not recommended to use in GFR <30 mL/min/1.73 m^2, switching them to loop diuretics. The mechanism to reduce BP with diuretics has a main component of extracellular volume overload reduction at the initiation of therapy, but after a few weeks, the volume overload resumes the presence due to RAAS activation, although BP control persists due to a reduction in peripheral resistance due to mechanisms not well determined. Among the possible activation mechanisms, vascular potassium channels, inhibition of calcium channels or release of nitric oxide and prostaglandins have been suggested [65].

Thiazides (hydrochlorothiazide) and thiazide-like agents (chlortalidone, metolazone, indapamide), despite their differences in chemical structure that determine different characteristics, exert the effect of blocking the Na^+-Cl^- cotransporter in the distal tubule where 5% of sodium handling occur. Chlortalidone is the member with longer duration of action and longer half-life elimination with a more prolonged effect in BP control. However, in the Diuretic Comparison Project, no differences were observed between chlortalidone and hydrochlorothiazide, and more side effects were observed with the use of chlortalidone [66]. Studies such as the Chlorthalidone in Chronic Kidney Disease (CLICK) trial [67] influence the recent KDIGO guideline "…appears to remain effective at GFR <30 mL/min/1.73 m^2", although the best thiazide or thiazide-like agent is not well defined [50].

Loop diuretics (furosemide, bumetanide, torsemide) are short-acting diuretics that act by inhibiting the Na^+–K^+–$2Cl^-$ cotransporter in the thick ascending limb, where 25% of sodium is reabsorbed, so the effect on volume reduction is greater than with thiazides. The mechanism of blood pressure control is twofold, as with thiazides, reduction of extracellular volume and reduction of vascular resistance [68]. Furosemide has a short duration of action, whereas torsemide has a long duration. Despite the recommendation to use thiazides or loop diuretics based on GFR, the combination of both classes is synergistic to facilitate control in subjects with volume overload refractory to treatment [69].

15.7.2 RAAS Blockers

Angiotensin-converting enzyme inhibitors (ACEi) and angiotensin AT2 receptor blockers (ARBs) are two groups of RAAS blockers with well-characterised reductions in angiotensin II activity using different approaches. Given the importance of angiotensin II in the mechanisms of BP elevation and renal damage, as well as CV risk, these are the first drugs recommended in CKD patients [70]. Treatment with RAAS blockers may cause a decrease in glomerular filtration rate (GFR) and hyperkalaemia. Although the former may be beneficial by reducing the risk of progression of kidney damage, the decline in GFR should be monitored at the time of initiation of treatment. Decreases of up to 20% in GFR are acceptable, larger decreases require a change in treatment dose, and 30% or more should lead to withdrawal of the drug and exclusion of renal artery stenosis. Hyperkalaemia can be reduced by the use of diuretics or, in unresponsive severe cases, potassium binders (patiromer and sodium zirconium cyclosilicate) [71]. The use of aldosterone antagonists with ACEi or ARBs in resistant HTN or heart failure in CKD patients' needs to be monitored for hyperkalaemia [72].

15.7.3 SGLT2i

A new class of drugs, the sodium-glucose cotransporter 2 inhibitors (SGLT2i), initially introduced for the treatment of diabetes, have additional benefits in reducing BP and albuminuria [73]. Office BP and 24-h BP are reduced by 4–5 mmHg and 3–4 mmHg, respectively. The mechanisms involved in BP control go beyond volume depletion and natriuresis, despite that the main action is in the proximal tubule where sodium reabsorption is up to 65%. The additive effect with other antihypertensive drugs, including RAAS blockers, allows their use in CKD patients with GFR >15 mL/min/1.73 m^2. Several studies in CKD patients, diabetic or not, the CREDENCE [74], DAPA-CDK [75], EMPA-KIDNEY [76], have demonstrated reductions in BP, albuminuria, and uric acid and long-term protection of renal function. As with RAAS blockers, a reduction in GFR was observed at the start of treatment, although the protective effect on renal function was demonstrated over time, with a synergistic effect with these agents.

Table 15.1 Recommendations for drug treatment of hypertension in CKD

DRUGS	BP threshold (mmHg)		BP Goal (mmHg)		GFR (ml/min/1.73m²)		Albuminuria (mg/g)		Potassium (mEq/L)	
	>140/90	>130/80	<130/80	<120/70	60-30	30-15	>30	<30	>5.5	<5.5
Monoterapia initial		Second line								
ARB	First line	First line	First line	First line	First line	First line	First line	First line	Second line	First line
ACEi	First line	First line	First line	First line	First line	First line	First line	First line	Second line	First line
CCB	Second line	Second line	Second line	Second line	Second line	Second line	Second line	First line	First line	Second line
Thiazide or Thiazide-like	Second line	Second line	Second line	Second line	Second line	Second line	Second line	Second line	First line	Second line
Loop diuretics						First line			First line	
Potassium sparing diuretics	Second line	Second line	Second line	Second line		Forbidden			Forbidden	
SGLT2i	Second line	Second line	Second line	Second line	First line		First line		First line	
Finerenone					First line	First line	First line			First line
Renal denervation					Second line		Second line	Second line		Second line

First line   Second line   Forbidden

15.7.4 Other Antihypertensive Drugs

The considered second-line class of drugs should be introduced in combination therapy with ACEi or ARBs, looking for an additive antihypertensive effect to help achieve the desired goal.

- Calcium channel blockers, mainly the dihydropyridines, have an additive effect to the RAAS blockers in lowering BP, mainly by acting on vascular resistance. Dilatation of the afferent arterioles to the glomerulus may increase albuminuria with the dihydropyridines that block the L calcium channel (nifedipine, amlodipine), but not with those that block the L and T calcium channels (azelnidipine) [77].
- Beta-blockers can be used if there is a specific indication.
- Other vasodilators such as minoxidil and hydralazine are not recommended because of side effects.
- Central agents such as clonidine, alpha-metil-DOPA and alpha-blockers are not recommended or may be used in specific indications.

Recommendations for drug treatment in CKD are summarised in Table 15.1.

15.8 Antihypertensive Medications in Proteinuric and Non-proteinuric CKD

Given the importance of RAAS overactivity in the development of HTN and in the progression of renal damage in patients with CKD, drugs that block the system, angiotensin converting enzyme inhibitors (ACEi) and angiotensin II receptor antagonists (ARBs), are the first class of antihypertensive treatment, mainly in patients with albuminuria or proteinuria, although they are formally indicated in patients without [70]. These drugs should be administered at high doses over 24 h, and while some can be administered once daily due to the long duration profile over 24 h, others require a 12-h dose. Nocturnal administration offers no advantage [78]. The introduction of SGLT2i also further reduces albuminuria/proteinuria and is recommended in these patients. The combination of ACEi and ARBs is not recommended as no beneficial effect is expected and the reduction in GFR may be exaggerated. Only patients with severe proteinuria and with careful follow-up can receive the combination of RAAS blockers.

The non-steroidal mineralocorticoid receptor blocker finerenone was introduced to reduce the metabolic side effects and hyperkalaemia induced by the previous molecules. Finerenone has been shown to reduce albuminuria and protect against the development of renal failure in the FIDELIO-DKD [79] and FIGARO-DKD [80] trials, but the reduction in BP is small (1–2 mmHg) [81]. The additive effect of finerenone with SGLT2i may result in synergies of renal protection and BP reduction, although more information is needed on the real effects and the order of administration to obtain the maximum benefit.

15.9 Resistant Hypertension

Resistant hypertension is common in patients with CKD, and a four-drug regimen is often chosen in addition to RAAS blockers, CCBs and diuretics. The use of the aldosterone antagonists, spironolactone or eplerenone, can increase serum potassium and is generally not recommended in patients with CKD stage 3b or higher, except in special circumstances such as low potassium levels or when BP control is not achieved with the addition of other agents [36]. In this case, additional potassium-binding agents are considered.

Renal denervation is becoming a relevant treatment option for hypertension as an important adjunct to pharmacological treatment by reducing sympathetic overactivity, an important mechanism in CKD patients [21, 82]. A meta-analysis, including 11 prospective studies with a total of 226 patients with CKD and treatment-resistant HTN receiving RDN, showed a significant reduction in office and ABPM and a small interruption in natural CKD progression [83]. One study stratified CKD patients into three groups according to GFR (46–90 mL/min, eGFR 15–45 mL/min and eGFR <15 mL/min group). RDN safely reduced SBP in CKD patients over 48 months, with the most pronounced reduction in the GFR 15–45 mL/min group [84]. Efficacy in reducing BP was seen in 475 patients with GFR between <60 and >15 mL/min/1.73 m^2 in the Global Simplicity Registry, with BP reduction similar to that seen in patients with normal GFR [85]. Protection against progression of renal damage remains to be proven, although a significant reduction was observed in albuminuric/proteinuric subjects. The rate of decline in GFR seems to decrease in the first year, but not thereafter. Finally, the risk of side effects appears to be similar to that in non-CKD patients, although more evidence is needed in patients with GFR <45 mL/min/1.73 m^2 [82]. Further studies will delineate the potential preventive role in these CKD patients.

Emerging agents are the dual endothelin blocker aprocitentan [86], the non-steroidal aldosterone mineralocorticoid receptor antagonist, ocedurenone, [87] and the aldosterone synthase inhibitor, baxdrostat [88], offers a new therapeutic approach, although before being recommended requires further studies in resistant HTN of CKD patients.

15.10 Conclusions

In recent years, a significant increase in the prevalence of chronic kidney disease (CKD) has been observed, affecting populations in all continents and demographic groups. Hypertension, a high prevalence condition in CKD, is the main factor in the progression to ESRD, and its treatment is a key issue not only to slow the progression of renal damage but also to reduce CV events and mortality. The best approach requires (1) the selection of more effective drugs and strategies, based on the knowledge of advances in the mechanisms underlying BP elevation and the results of randomised control trials and (2) the development of new drugs aimed at improving protection and tolerability. Although progress has been made in treatment in recent decades, the choice of target for BP reduction has been controversial for decades and an individualised approach with careful monitoring must be applied to a large number of patients. Finally, advances in the monitoring of tubular damage may help to assess therapeutic response and will take a place alongside the traditional markers of follow-up, GFR and albuminuria.

References

1. Tellez-Plaza M, Orozco-Beltran D, Gil-Guillen V, Pita-Fernandez S, Navarro-Pérez J, Pallares V, ; Escarval Study Group et al. Renal function and attributable risk of death and cardiovascular hospitalization in patients with cardiovascular risk factors from a registry-based cohort: the Cardiovascular Valencia-risk study. J Hypertens 2016;34:2266–2273. doi: https://doi.org/10.1097/HJH.0000000000001089.
2. Ku E, Lee BJ, Wei J, Weir MR. Hypertension in CKD: Core Curriculum 2019. Am J Kidney Dis. 2019;74:120–31. https://doi.org/10.1053/j.ajkd.2018.12.044.
3. Skalsky K, Shiyovich A, Steinmetz T, Kornowski R. Chronic renal failure and cardiovascular disease: a comprehensive appraisal. J Clin Med. 2022;11:1335. https://doi.org/10.3390/jcm11051335.
4. Simeoni M, Borrelli S, Garofalo C, Fuiano G, Esposito C, Comi A, Provenzano M. Atherosclerotic-nephropathy: an updated narrative review. J Nephrol. 2021;34:125–36. https://doi.org/10.1007/s40620-020-00733-0.
5. Savedchuk S, Phachu D, Shankar M, Sparks MA, Harrison-Bernard LM. Targeting glomerular hemodynamics for kidney protection. Adv Kidney Dis Health. 2023;30:71–84. https://doi.org/10.1053/j.akdh.2022.12.003.
6. Chagnac A, Zingerman B, Rozen-Zvi B, Herman-Edelstein M. Consequences of glomerular hyperfiltration: the role of physical forces in the pathogenesis of chronic kidney disease in diabetes and obesity. Nephron. 2019;143:38–42. https://doi.org/10.1159/000499486.
7. Sharma S, Smyth B. From proteinuria to fibrosis: an update on pathophysiology and treatment options. Kidney Blood Press Res. 2021;46:411–20. https://doi.org/10.1159/000516911.
8. Wiig H, Luft FC, Titze JM. The interstitium conducts extrarenal storage of sodium and represents a third compartment essential for extracellular volume and blood pressure homeostasis. Acta Physiol (Oxf). 2018;222(3):e13006. https://doi.org/10.1111/apha.13006.

9. Gburek J, Konopska B, Gołąb K. Renal handling of albumin-from early findings to current concepts. Int J Mol Sci. 2021;22:5809. https://doi.org/10.3390/ijms22115809.
10. Humphreys BD. Mechanisms of renal fibrosis. Annu Rev Physiol. 2018;80:309–26.
11. Sun HJ. Current opinion for hypertension in renal fibrosis. Adv Exp Med Biol. 2019;1165:37–47. https://doi.org/10.1007/978-981-13-8871-2_3.
12. Chen Y, Zou H, Lu H, Xiang H, Chen S. Research progress of endothelial-mesenchymal transition in diabetic kidney disease. J Cell Mol Med. 2022;26:3313–22.
13. Sánchez-Duffhues G, García de Vinuesa A, Ten Dijke P. Endothelial-to-mesenchymal transition in cardiovascular diseases: developmental signaling pathways gone awry. Dev Dyn. 2018;247:492–508.
14. Habas E Sr, Akbar RA, Alfitori G, Farfar KL, Habas E, Errayes N, et al. Effects of nondipping blood pressure changes: a nephrologist prospect. Cureus. 2023;15:e42681. https://doi.org/10.7759/cureus.42681.
15. Ameer OZ. Hypertension in chronic kidney disease: what lies behind the scene. Front Pharmacol. 2022;13:949260. https://doi.org/10.3389/fphar.2022.949260.
16. Hall JE. Renal dysfunction, rather than non-renal vascular dysfunction, mediates salt-induced hypertension. Circulation. 2016;133:894–906. https://doi.org/10.1161/CIRCULATIONAHA.115.018526.
17. Bovée DM, Cuevas CA, Zietse R, Danser AHJ, Mirabito Colafella KM, Hoorn EJ. Salt-sensitive hypertension in chronic kidney disease: distal tubular mechanisms. Am J Physiol Ren Physiol. 2020;319:F729–45. https://doi.org/10.1152/ajprenal.00407.2020.
18. Liang L, Shimosawa T. Molecular mechanisms of Na-Cl cotransporter in relation to hypertension in chronic kidney disease. Int J Mol Sci. 2022;24:286. https://doi.org/10.3390/ijms24010286.
19. Balafa O, Kalaitzidis RG. Salt sensitivity and hypertension. J Hum Hypertens. 2021;35:184–92. https://doi.org/10.1038/s41371-020-00407-1.
20. Jhee JH, Park HC, Choi HY. Skin sodium and blood pressure regulation. Electrolyte Blood Press. 2022;20:1–9. https://doi.org/10.5049/EBP.2022.20.1.1.
21. Grassi G, Biffi A, Seravalle G, Bertoli S, Airoldi F, Corrao G, Pisano A, Mallamaci F, Mancia G, Zoccali C. Sympathetic nerve traffic overactivity in chronic kidney disease: a systematic review and meta-analysis. J Hypertens. 2021;39:408–16. https://doi.org/10.1097/HJH.0000000000002661.
22. Tanaka S, Okusa MD. Crosstalk between the nervous system and the kidney. Kidney Int. 2020;97:466–76. https://doi.org/10.1016/j.kint.2019.10.032.
23. Kaur J, Young BE, Fadel PJ. Sympathetic overactivity in chronic kidney disease: consequences and mechanisms. Int J Mol Sci. 2017;18:1682.
24. Ewen S, Ukena C, Linz D, Schmieder RE, Böhm M, Mahfoud F. The sympathetic nervous system in chronic kidney disease. Curr Hypertens Rep. 2013;15:370–6. https://doi.org/10.1007/s11906-013-0365-0.
25. Jeong JH, Fonkoue IT, Quyyumi AA, DaCosta D, Park J. Nocturnal blood pressure is associated with sympathetic nerve activity in patients with chronic kidney disease. Physiol Rep. 2020;8:e14602. https://doi.org/10.14814/phy2.14602.
26. Gupta A, Nagaraju SP, Bhojaraja MV, Swaminathan SM, Mohan PB. Hypertension in chronic kidney disease: an update on diagnosis and management. S Med J. 2023;116(2):237–44. https://doi.org/10.14423/SMJ.0000000000001516.
27. Frąk W, Kućmierz J, Szlagor M, Młynarska E, Rysz J, Franczyk B. New insights into molecular mechanisms of chronic kidney disease. Biomedicines. 2022;10:2846. https://doi.org/10.3390/biomedicines10112846.
28. Yamada S, Nakano T. Role of chronic kidney disease (CKD)-mineral and bone disorder (MBD) in the pathogenesis of cardiovascular disease in CKD. J Atheroscler Thromb. 2023;30:835–50. https://doi.org/10.5551/jat.RV22006.
29. Aguilar A, Gifre L, Ureña-Torres P, Carrillo-López N, Rodriguez-García M, Massó E, et al. Pathophysiology of bone disease in chronic kidney disease: from basics to renal

osteodystrophy and osteoporosis. Front Physiol. 2023;14:1177829. https://doi.org/10.3389/fphys.2023.1177829.
30. Freundlich M, Gamba G, Rodriguez-Iturbe B. Fibroblast growth factor 23-klotho and hypertension: experimental and clinical mechanisms. Pediatr Nephrol. 2021;36:3007–22. https://doi.org/10.1007/s00467-020-04843-6.
31. Wang Q, Wang Y, Wang J, Zhang L, Zhao MH, Chinese Cohort Study of Chronic Kidney Disease (C-STRIDE); Chinese Cohort Study of Chronic Kidney Disease (C-STRIDE) Collaborators. Nocturnal systolic hypertension and adverse prognosis in patients with CKD. Clin J Am Soc Nephrol. 2021;16:356–64. https://doi.org/10.2215/CJN.14420920.
32. Lurbe E, Redon J, Kesani A, Pascual JM, Tacons J, Alvarez V, et al. Increase in nocturnal blood pressure and progression to microalbuminuria in type 1 diabetes. N Engl J Med. 2002;347:797–805. https://doi.org/10.1056/NEJMoa013410.
33. Minutolo R, Agarwal R, Borrelli S, Chiodini P, Bellizzi V, Nappi F, et al. Prognostic role of ambulatory blood pressure measurement in patients with nondialysis chronic kidney disease. Arch Intern Med. 2011;171:1090–8.
34. Katafuchi E, Nakayama M, Tanaka S, Sakoh T, Yoshitomi R, Fukui A, et al. Comparison of prognostic values of daytime and night-time systolic blood pressures on renal outcomes in patients with chronic kidney disease. Circ J. 2017;81:1454–62.
35. Redon J, Plancha E, Swift PA, Pons S, Muñoz J, Martinez F. Nocturnal blood pressure and progression to end-stage renal disease or death in nondiabetic chronic kidney disease stages 3 and 4. J Hypertens. 2010;28:602–7.
36. Fay KS, Cohen DL. Resistant hypertension in people with CKD: a review. Am J Kidney Dis. 2021;77:110–21. https://doi.org/10.1053/j.ajkd.2020.04.017.
37. Noubiap JJ, Nansseu JR, Nyaga UF, Sime PS, Francis I, Bigna JJ. Global prevalence of resistant hypertension: a meta-analysis of data from 3.2 million patients. Heart. 2019;105:98–105. https://doi.org/10.1136/heartjnl-2018-313599.
38. Thomas G, Xie D, Chen HY, Anderson AH, Appel LJ, Bodana S, CRIC Study Investigators, et al. Prevalence and prognostic significance of apparent treatment resistant hypertension in chronic kidney disease: report from the chronic renal insufficiency cohort study. Hypertension. 2016;67:387–96. https://doi.org/10.1161/HYPERTENSIONAHA.115.06487.
39. An J, Kurella Tamura M, Odden MC, Ni L, Thomas IC, et al. Prevalence of apparent treatment-resistant hypertension in chronic kidney disease in two large US health care systems. Clin J Am Soc Nephrol. 2022;17:1457–66. https://doi.org/10.2215/CJN.04110422.
40. Chang AR, Lóser M, Malhotra R, Appel LJ. Blood pressure goals in patients with CKD: a review of evidence and guidelines. Clin J Am Soc Nephrol. 2019;14:161–9. https://doi.org/10.2215/CJN.07440618.
41. Klahr S, Levey AS, Beck GJ, Caggiula AW, Hunsicker L, Kusek JW, Modification of Diet in Renal Disease Study Group, et al. The effects of dietary protein restriction and blood-pressure control on the progression of chronic renal disease. N Engl J Med. 1994;330:877–84.
42. Sarnak MJ, Greene T, Wang X, Beck G, Kusek JW, Collins AJ, et al. The effect of a lower target blood pressure on the progression of kidney disease: long-term follow-up of the modification of diet in renal disease study. Ann Intern Med. 2005;142:342–51. https://doi.org/10.7326/0003-4819-142-5-200503010-00009.
43. Wright JT Jr, Bakris G, Greene T, Agodoa LY, Appel LJ, Charleston J, African American Study of Kidney Disease and Hypertension Study Group, et al. Effect of blood pressure lowering and antihypertensive drug class on progression of hypertensive kidney disease: results from the AASK trial. JAMA. 2002;288:2421–31. https://doi.org/10.1001/jama.288.19.2421.
44. Appel LJ, Wright JT Jr, Greene T, Agodoa LY, Astor BC, Bakris GL, AASK Collaborative Research Group, et al. Intensive blood-pressure control in hypertensive chronic kidney disease. N Engl J Med. 2010;363:918–29. https://doi.org/10.1056/NEJMoa0910975.
45. Wright JT Jr, Williamson JD, Whelton PK, Snyder JK, Sink KM, Rocco MV, SPRINT Research Group, et al. A randomized trial of intensive versus standard blood-pressure control. N Engl J Med. 2015;373:2103–16.

46. Cheung AK, Rahman M, Reboussin DM, Craven TE, Greene T, Kimmel PL, SPRINT Research Group, et al. Effects of intensive BP control in CKD. J Am Soc Nephrol. 2017;28:2812–23. https://doi.org/10.1681/ASN.2017020148.
47. Beddhu S, Rocco MV, Toto R, Craven TE, Greene T, Bhatt U, ; SPRINT Research Group. et al Effects of intensive systolic blood pressure control on kidney and cardiovascular outcomes in persons without kidney disease: a secondary analysis of a randomized trial. Ann Intern Med 2017;167:375–383. doi: https://doi.org/10.7326/M16-2966.
48. Minutolo R, De Nicola L, Gallo C, Chiodini P, Provenzano M, Conte G, Collaborative Study Group on the Conservative Treatment of CKD of the Italian Society of Nephrology, et al. Generalizability of SPRINT-CKD cohort to CKD patients referred to renal clinics. J Nephrol. 2019;32:429–35. https://doi.org/10.1007/s40620-019-00588-0.
49. Malhotra R, Nguyen HA, Benavente O, Mete M, Howard BV, Mant J, et al. Association between more intensive vs less intensive blood pressure lowering and risk of mortality in chronic kidney disease stages 3–5: a systematic review and meta analysis. JAMA Intern Med. 2017;177:1498–505. https://doi.org/10.1001/jamainternmed.2017.4377.
50. Cheung AK, Chang TI, Cushman WC, Furth SL, Hou FF, Ix JH, et al. Executive summary of the KDIGO 2021 clinical practice guideline for the management of blood pressure in chronic kidney disease. Kidney Int. 2021;99:559–69. https://doi.org/10.1016/j.kint.2020.10.026.
51. Bullen AL, Katz R, Jotwani V, Garimella PS, Lee AK, Estrella MM, et al. Biomarkers of kidney tubule health, CKD progression, and acute kidney injury in SPRINT (Systolic Blood Pressure Intervention Trial) participants. Am J Kidney Dis. 2021;78:361–8.e1. https://doi.org/10.1053/j.ajkd.2021.01.021.
52. Bullen AL, Ascher SB, Scherzer R, Garimella PS, Katz R, Hallan SI, et al. Markers of kidney tubular secretion and risk of adverse events in SPRINT participants with CKD. J Am Soc Nephrol. 2022;33:1915–26. https://doi.org/10.1681/ASN.2022010117.
53. Malhotra R, Craven T, Ambrosius WT, Killeen AA, Haley WE, Cheung AK, ; SPRINT Research Group et al. Effects of intensive blood pressure lowering on kidney tubule injury in CKD: a longitudinal subgroup analysis in SPRINT. Am J Kidney Dis 2019;73:21–30. doi: https://doi.org/10.1053/j.ajkd.2018.07.015.
54. Nagata D, Hishida E, Masuda T. Practical strategy for treating chronic kidney disease (CKD)-associated with hypertension. Int J Nephrol Renovasc Dis. 2020;13:171–8. https://doi.org/10.2147/IJNRD.S259931.
55. Alkhatib L, Velez Diaz LA, Varma S, Chowdhary A, Bapat P, Pan H, et al. Lifestyle modifications and nutritional and therapeutic interventions in delaying the progression of chronic kidney disease: a review. Cureus. 2023;15:e34572. https://doi.org/10.7759/cureus.34572.
56. Nakamura K, Sasaki T, Yamamoto S, Hayashi H, Ako S, Tanaka Y. Effects of exercise on kidney and physical function in patients with non-dialysis chronic kidney disease: a systematic review and meta-analysis. Sci Rep. 2020;10:18195. https://doi.org/10.1038/s41598-020-75405-x.
57. Bundy JD, Bazzano LA, Xie D, Cohan J, Dolata J, Finket JC, et al. Self-reported tobacco, alcohol, and illicit drug use and progression of chronic kidney disease. Clin J Am Soc Nephrol. 2018;13:993–1001. https://doi.org/10.2215/CJN.11121017.
58. Bruce MA, Griffith DM, Thorpe RJ Jr. Stress and the kidney. Adv Chronic Kidney Dis. 2015;22:46–53. https://doi.org/10.1053/j.ackd.2014.06.008.
59. KDIGO CKD Work Group. KDIGO 2012 clinical practice guideline for the evaluation and management of chronic kidney disease. Kidney Int Suppl. 2013;3:1–150
60. Aljuraiban GS, Gibson R, Chan DS, Van Horn L, Chan Q. The role of diet in the prevention of hypertension and management of blood pressure: an umbrella review of meta-analyses of interventional and observational studies. Adv Nutr. 2023;15:100123. https://doi.org/10.1016/j.advnut.2023.09.011.
61. Slagman MC, Waanders F, Hemmelder MH, Woittiez AJ, Janssen WM, Lambers Heerspink HJ, HOlland NEphrology STudy Group, et al. Moderate dietary sodium restriction added to angiotensin converting enzyme inhibition compared with dual blockade in lowering proteinuria and blood pressure: randomised controlled trial. BMJ. 2011;343:d4366. https://doi.org/10.1136/bmj.d4366.

62. Pathak CM, Ix JH, Anderson CAM, Woodell TB, Smits G, Persky MS, et al. Variation in sodium intake and intra-individual change in blood pressure in chronic kidney disease. J Ren Nutr. 2018;28:125–8. https://doi.org/10.1053/j.jrn.2017.07.002.
63. Ellison DH. Treatment of disorders of sodium balance in chronic kidney disease. Adv Chronic Kidney Dis. 2017;24:332–41. https://doi.org/10.1053/j.ackd.2017.07.003.
64. Mancia G, Kreutz R, Brunström M, Burnier M, Grassi G, Januszewicz A, et al. 2023 ESH guidelines for the management of arterial hypertension the task force for the management of arterial hypertension of the European Society of Hypertension: Endorsed by the International Society of Hypertension (ISH) and the European Renal Association (ERA). Hypertension. 2023;41:1874–2071. https://doi.org/10.1097/HJH.0000000000003480.
65. Jo W, Koh ES, Chung S. Therapeutic roles of thiazides and loop diuretics in blood pressure control and renal protection against chronic kidney disease. Clin Hypertens. 2023;29:14. https://doi.org/10.1186/s40885-023-00238-5.
66. Ishani A, Cushman WC, Leatherman SM, Lew RA, Woods P, Glassmanet PA, Diuretic Comparison Project Writing Group, et al. Chlorthalidone vs. hydrochlorothiazide for hypertension-cardiovascular events. N Engl J Med. 2022;387:2401–10. https://doi.org/10.1056/NEJMoa2212270.
67. Agarwal R, Sinha AD, Cramer AE, Balmes-Fenwick M, Dickinson JH, Ouyang F, et al. Chlorthalidone for hypertension in advanced chronic kidney disease. N Engl J Med. 2021;385:2507–19. https://doi.org/10.1056/NEJMoa2110730.
68. Novak JE, Ellison DH. Diuretics in states of volume overload: Core Curriculum 2022. Am J Kidney Dis. 2022;80:264–76. https://doi.org/10.1053/j.ajkd.2021.09.029.
69. Ali S, Navaneethan SD, Virani SS, Gregg LP. Revisiting diuretic choice in chronic kidney disease. Curr Opin Nephrol Hypertens. 2022;31:406–13. https://doi.org/10.1097/MNH.0000000000000814.
70. Georgianos PI, Agarwal R. Hypertension in chronic kidney disease—treatment standard 2023. Nephrol Dial Transplant. 2023;38:2694–703. https://doi.org/10.1093/ndt/gfad118.
71. Dong L, Xu W, Deng Y, Tan J, Qin W. Efficacy and safety of potassium binders in the treatment of patients with chronic kidney disease and hyperkalemia. Eur J Pharmacol. 2022;931:175174. https://doi.org/10.1016/j.ejphar.2022.175174.
72. Costa D, Patella G, Provenzano M, Ielapi N, Faga T, Zicarelli M, et al. Hyperkalemia in CKD: an overview of available therapeutic strategies. Front Med (Lausanne). 2023;10:1178140. https://doi.org/10.3389/fmed.2023.1178140.
73. Mende CW. Chronic kidney disease and SGLT2 inhibitors: a review of the evolving treatment landscape. Adv Ther. 2022;39:148–64. https://doi.org/10.1007/s12325-021-01994-2.
74. Perkovic V, Jardine MJ, Neal B, Bompoint S, Heerspink HJL, Charytan DM, CREDENCE Trial Investigators, et al. Canagliflozin and renal outcomes in type 2 diabetes and nephropathy. N Engl J Med. 2019;380:2295–306. https://doi.org/10.1056/NEJMoa1811744.
75. Heerspink HJL, Stefánsson BV, Correa-Rotter R, Chertow GM, Greene T, Hou FF, DAPA-CKD Trial Committees and Investigators, et al. Dapagliflozin in patients with chronic kidney disease. N Engl J Med. 2020;383:1436–46. https://doi.org/10.1056/NEJMoa2024816.
76. The EMPA-KIDNEY Collaborative Group, Herrington WG, Staplin N, Wanner C, Green JB, Hauske SJ, Emberson JR, et al. Empagliflozin in patients with chronic kidney disease. N Engl J Med. 2023;388:117–27. https://doi.org/10.1056/NEJMoa2204233.
77. Ram CVS. Therapeutic usefulness of a novel calcium channel blocker azelnidipine in the treatment of hypertension: a narrative review. Cardiol Ther. 2022;11:473–89. https://doi.org/10.1007/s40119-022-00276-4.
78. Mackenzie IS, Rogers A, Poulter NR, Williams B, Brown MJ, Webb DJ, ; TIME Study Group. et al Cardiovascular outcomes in adults with hypertension with evening versus morning dosing of usual antihypertensives in the UK (TIME study): a prospective, randomised, open-label, blinded-endpoint clinical trial. Lancet 2022;400:1417–1425. doi: https://doi.org/10.1016/S0140-6736(22)01786-X.

79. Bakris GL, Agarwal R, Anker SD, Pitt B, Ruilope LM, Rossing P, FIDELIO-DKD Investigators, et al. Effect of finerenone on chronic kidney disease outcomes in type 2 diabetes. N Engl J Med. 2020;383:2219–29. https://doi.org/10.1056/NEJMoa2025845.
80. Pitt B, Filippatos G, Agarwal R, Anker SD, Bakris GL, Rossing P, FIGARO-DKD Investigators, et al. Cardiovascular events with finerenone in kidney disease and type 2 diabetes. N Engl J Med. 2021;385:2252–63. https://doi.org/10.1056/NEJMoa2110956.
81. Redon J. New insights of cardiovascular and renal protection in diabetic chronic kidney disease with finerenone. Cardiovasc Res. 2022;118:e36–7. https://doi.org/10.1093/cvr/cvac024.
82. Schmieder RE. Renal denervation in patients with chronic kidney disease: current evidence and future perspectives. Nephrol Dial Transplant. 2023;38:1089–96. https://doi.org/10.1093/ndt/gfac189.
83. Mohammad AA, Nawar K, Binks O, Abdulla MH. Effects of renal denervation on kidney function in patients with chronic kidney disease: a systematic review and meta-analysis. J Hum Hypertens. 2023;38:29–44. https://doi.org/10.1038/s41371-023-00857-3.
84. Cai H, Fang Z, Lin R, Cai W, Han Y, Su J. Insight on efficacy of renal artery denervation for refractory hypertension with chronic kidney diseases: a long-term follow-up of 24-hour ambulatory blood pressure. J Interv Cardiol. 2022;2022:6895993. https://doi.org/10.1155/2022/6895993.
85. Ott C, Mahfoud F, Mancia G, Narkiewicz K, Ruilope LM, Fahy M, et al. Renal denervation in patients with versus without chronic kidney disease: results from the global SYMPLICITY registry with follow-up data of 3 years. Nephrol Dial Transplant. 2022;37:304–10. https://doi.org/10.1093/ndt/gfab154.
86. Mahfooz K, Najeed S, Tun HN, Khamosh M, Grewal D, Hussain A, et al. New dual endothelin receptor antagonist aprocitentan in hypertension: a systematic review and meta-analysis. Curr Probl Cardiol. 2023;48:101686. https://doi.org/10.1016/j.cpcardiol.2023.101686.
87. Bakris GL, Yang YF, McCabe JM, Liu JR, Tan XJ, Benn VJ, et al. Efficacy and safety of ocedurenone: subgroup analysis of the BLOCK-CKD study. Am J Hypertens. 2023;36:612–3. https://doi.org/10.1093/ajh/hpad066.
88. Freeman MW, Halvorsen YD, Marshall W, Pater M, Isaacsohn J, Pearce C, BrigHTN Investigators, et al. Phase 2 trial of baxdrostat for treatment-resistant hypertension. N Engl J Med. 2023;388:395–405. https://doi.org/10.1056/NEJMoa2213169.

16 Approach to the Diagnosis and Management of Hypertension in Patients on Dialysis

Rajiv Agarwal

16.1 Introduction

Hypertension is a pervasive and often undertreated condition among patients with end-stage renal disease (ESRD) or kidney failure requiring dialysis. This complex health issue is characterized by numerous challenges, including difficulties in accurate diagnosis, treatment complexities, and a limited understanding of optimal blood pressure targets. Despite its significant impact on cardiovascular morbidity and mortality, hypertension in dialysis patients remains a persistent clinical challenge. This review delves into the epidemiology, diagnostic challenges, treatment strategies, and the evolving landscape of managing hypertension in this vulnerable population.

16.2 Epidemiology

Due to varying definitions and techniques of diagnosing hypertension especially among patients on hemodialysis, the prevalence of hypertension can differ from one study to the next. However, most studies show that hypertension remains poorly controlled in patients on hemodialysis. For example, in a 2003 report of 2535 patients on hemodialysis at 69 centers in the United States, the prevalence of hypertension, defined by 1-week average predialysis blood pressure (BP) of ≥150/85 mmHg or the use of antihypertensive medications was 86%; 88% were

Supported by National Heart Lung and Blood Institute: R01 HL126903 and the Department of Veterans Affairs: 5I01CX001753.

R. Agarwal (✉)
Richard L. Roudebush Veterans Administration Medical Center, Indianapolis, IN, USA
e-mail: ragarwal@iu.edu

A. E. Berbari et al. (eds.), *Blood Pressure Disorders in Acute and Chronic Kidney Diseases*, Updates in Hypertension and Cardiovascular Protection,
https://doi.org/10.1007/978-3-031-81292-7_16

treated, but only 30% were controlled [1]. In a 2011 report of 369 patients on hemodialysis at a single center who underwent 44-h ambulatory BP monitoring (ABPM) over an interdialytic interval—the gold standard for BP control—the prevalence of hypertension defined as 44-interdialytic average of ≥135/85 mmHg was 82%; 89% were treated, but only 38% were controlled [2]. The prevalence of hypertension in the latter study was associated with fewer years on dialysis, a lower body mass index, and epoetin use. Poor control was associated with a greater use of antihypertensive medications and a wider inferior vena diameter suggesting volume overload [2]. In a 1999, multicenter study of 504 peritoneal dialysis patients in Italy, 88% of the patients had hypertension of which 79% of the patients treated with antihypertensive drugs remained poorly controlled [3]. Ambulatory BP monitoring in the same cohort also revealed that 77% of the patients had poorly controlled hypertension [3].

16.3 Blood Pressure Measurement in Dialysis Patients, Including Timing and Location

The timing of blood pressure in hemodialysis patient depends on the intention or the intended purpose for its measurement [4]. If our intention is to monitor hemodynamic stability, then we must measure the blood pressure during dialysis, or the intradialytic measurement. This is the usual practice in every dialysis unit. If our intention is to diagnose or manage hypertension, the optimal timing of the blood pressure measurement is more complicated.

This question was addressed in a 2009 study of 150 dialysis patients who had blood pressure measured in the dialysis unit, at home, and by 44-h interdialytic ambulatory monitoring [5]. Home BP was measured three times a day for the whole week which allowed the estimation of mean systolic and diastolic BP. The BP change was not linear; systolic BP gradually increased over the first 2 days and flattened out after 2 days over the long intradialytic interval. Diastolic blood pressure showed a similar trend, although it was not as remarkable. Thus, pulse pressure amplified during the intradialytic interval.

The systolic BP change is dependent on both the time elapsed since the last dialysis and the amount of weight gained [5]. For a typical patient on dialysis (with a median weight gain of 2.35 kg over the intradialytic interval), the systolic BP increased on average 9.6 mmHg over a 24-h period for the first 48 h. In a patient who gained more weight, systolic BP starts at a lower level and amplifies even more over the interdialytic interval. In contrast, if the patient gains less weight, systolic BP starts higher and amplifies less. At 24-h after the end of dialysis, the time trends for systolic BP intersect for the categories of weight gains. Thus, one might be tempted to think that the measurement of blood pressure at 24 h would be the most opportune because it would neutralize the effect of the intradialytic weight gain. While true, this would not give us an accurate picture of the interdialytic diastolic BP. Diastolic BP time trends intersect at about 40 h, not 24 h. Thus, sampling BP over a wide variety of times might be more practical than fixing the most opportune time. Empirical evidence shows that measuring BP twice a day for 4 days after the midweek dialysis gives the best test performance [5]. For example, if the patient is on Monday, Wednesday, Friday, dialysis, Wednesday would be the midweek dialysis. BP measured twice dialysis from Thursday through Sunday would be sufficient and we validated this in a cohort of patients. As a practical matter, keeping a BP monitor in the bedroom, measuring BP before bed and on waking up would provide eight recordings, and this would be sufficient to manage hypertension. Specifically, this recording method would be superior to diagnose and manage hypertension compared to recordings in the dialysis unit [6].

16.4 Out of Clinic Blood Pressure Monitoring in Dialysis

16.4.1 Prognostic Value

Whether BP measurements obtained outside of dialysis units such as through home BP or interdialytic ambulatory blood pressure measurements are of greater value than BP measurements obtained in the dialysis unit has been subject to several investigations. A 2007 study measured blood pressure in three different locations: the dialysis unit, at home where blood pressure was self-measured by the patients, and by using an ambulatory blood pressure monitor where blood pressure was automatically measured over the entire intradialytic period without direct patient intervention [7]. Furthermore, blood pressure measured in the dialysis unit was recorded using a routine method, which is whatever the method the dialysis unit used, or a standardized measurement which required 5 min of seated rest, an appropriate cuff size, and an oscillometric technique [7]. Home BP was measured over a week, three times daily. The quartiles of each of these four BP methods which were dialysis unit (routine or standardized), home, and ambulatory were associated with mortality. The results of the study revealed that when we measure BP in the dialysis unit using the routine method or standardized method, it was not predictive of all-cause mortality. On the other hand, systolic home BP monitoring was directly associated with mortality. Furthermore, interdialytic ambulatory blood pressure monitoring demonstrated the strongest association with all-cause mortality. The systolic home and ambulatory BP associated with the lowest mortality were different; the optimal home systolic BP was between 125 and 145 mmHg, whereas the optimal systolic interdialytic ambulatory blood pressure was between 115 and 125 mmHg [7].

A 2010 study with a longer follow up revealed that dialysis unit BP recordings obtained either prior to or following the end of dialysis revealed no association with all-cause mortality [8]. Home blood pressure and ambulatory blood pressure demonstrated a U-shaped relationship; higher systolic ambulatory or home BP was associated with a higher mortality [5].

The next question that emerges is whether the value of out-of-office BP is simply because of a greater number of measurements or a better quality of recordings. In a 2007 study, BP was recorded by each of the three methods: in the dialysis unit before dialysis at each treatment for 2 weeks, at home thrice daily for a week, and over an interdialytic interval over 44 h [9]. The number of recordings from home or ambulatory BP was matched to the dialysis unit BP. In other words, six recordings from ambulatory BP measurements or home BP measurements were randomly selected. This revealed that despite fewer number of home or ambulatory recordings, they still retained the prognostic information over and above the recordings obtained in the dialysis unit. In other words, it doesn't appear that there's a greater number of recordings, but a better quality of out-of-dialysis unit BP recordings that leads to a stronger relationship between all-cause mortality and BP [9].

One multicenter study—the Chronic Renal Insufficiency Cohort (CRIC) study—also reveals that out of dialysis unit blood pressure is superior to pre- or postdialysis blood pressure measurements in predicting mortality [10]. The dialysis unit systolic BP had a U-shaped relationship with mortality. In contrast, systolic BP measured outside the dialysis unit during an interdialytic day was directly associated with all-cause mortality [10].

16.4.2 Therapeutic Value

Does targeting home or dialysis unit BP matter with respect to outcomes? A 2009 randomized trial in approximately 65 long-term hemodialysis patients guided BP management to either where the treatment was guided by predialysis systolic BP or one where treatment was guided by home systolic BP [11]. At the end of 6 months, the success of the intervention was measured by the change from baseline in interdialytic ambulatory systolic BP. Home blood pressure-guided therapy resulted in systolic ambulatory BP reduction over and above home systolic BP by 7 mmHg that was clinically and statistically significant.

16.4.3 Peritoneal Dialysis Patients

In a 2019 diagnostic test study from Greece ascertained the value of home or clinic BP measurement for the diagnosis of hypertension among 81 patients on peritoneal dialysis [12]. BP in the clinic was measured in a standardized manner and patients self-measure home BP. The reference standard was 24-h ambulatory systolic BP. The area under the curve of the receiver operating characteristic curve, which is a measure of diagnostic test performance was similar for home BP (0.90) or clinic BP (0.86). It should be noted that clinic BP was measured using a standardized method, not just a routine technique without attention to detail.

Two systematic reviews ask the question whether dialysis unit or out of dialysis unit BP measurement should be the measurement technique to diagnose and manage hypertension in dialysis patients. The Canadian review found that both the home blood pressure and ambulatory blood pressures are superior to the routine or standardized measurement of blood pressures obtained during dialysis [13]. The US review noted that home blood pressure may lead to more active participation in health care by patients, and similar benefits are accrued by ambulatory BP

Table 16.1 Benefits of home BP monitoring

Compared to ambulatory BP monitoring, easier and less expensive
Provides readings over a longer time span say over weeks or months and therefore more suitable to assessing response to treatment
May better evaluate antihypertensive effect compared to predialysis or postdialysis BP recordings
Reduces white coat effect and masked hypertension
May improve adherence to therapy because of greater involvement of the patient in self-management
Better predicts target organ damage such as left ventricular mass
Better predicts all-cause mortality compared to dialysis unit recordings

monitoring [14]. The various benefits of home BP monitoring are listed in Table 16.1. However, some issues with home BP monitoring should be noted. Home BP monitoring provokes anxiety in some people and does not rule out white coat hypertension or masked hypertension. For these conditions, 24-h ambulatory BP monitoring is needed. Patients may modify the drug regimen, and occasionally, the readings may be confabulated. The lack of BP measurement during sleep with home BP monitoring is circumvented by ambulatory blood pressure monitoring.

In summary, home BP monitoring is especially important for patients with end-stage kidney disease for diagnosing and managing hypertension. On a monthly basis, 4 days of measurement performed twice daily following the midweek dialysis appears to be the minimum necessary to manage hypertension in these patients. The target for treatment in dialysis patients remains unknown. We target systolic home BP between 120 and 140 mmHg. The interdialytic 44-h ambulatory systolic BP is the gold standard; the best mortality outcomes are seen in the range of 110–120 mmHg systolic. However, whether 110–120 mmHg systolic BP should be the treatment target remains unknown because randomized trials to establish this goal are absent.

16.4.4 Dialysis Unit BP Monitoring to Diagnose and Treat Hypertension

When home or ambulatory BP measurements are not available or the patient is unwilling to perform, one might still find value in dialysis unit BP recordings. It is not the predialysis blood pressure or postdialysis blood pressure, and it's not the average of the two, but the median midweek dialysis unit blood pressure that best associates with interdialytic ambulatory BP recordings. A 2008 diagnostic test study found the median intradialytic systolic BP to be more valuable than BP measurements obtained on other occasions [15]. The threshold median dialysis unit BP on a Wednesday, on a Monday, Wednesday, Friday patient was ≥140 mmHg to diagnose hypertension. For Monday, the threshold was ≥145 and for Friday ≥130 mmHg. A subsequent 2010 study revealed that median interdialytic BP can track changes evoked by probing dry weight [16]. A summary of diagnosis of hypertension in hemodialysis appears in Table 16.2.

Table 16.2 Diagnosis of hypertension in hemodialysis

Interdialytic 44-h ambulatory BP monitoring is the reference standard for the diagnosis of hypertension
BP increases approximately linearly over the first 2 days following dialysis and then tends to plateau. Measurements at home after the midweek dialysis taken twice daily for 4 days are sufficient for clinical decision making in the management of hypertension in hemodialysis patients
If home or ambulatory BP are not available, predialysis or postdialysis BP by themselves should be avoided in diagnosing hypertension
Median intradialytic systolic BP during a midweek dialysis of 140 mmHg or more is sufficient to make a diagnosis of hypertension when out of dialysis unit measurements are not available

16.5 Importance of Treating Hypertension in Hypertensive Dialysis Patients

16.5.1 Associations of BP and Cardiovascular and Mortality Outcomes in Epidemiological Surveys

In a 1999 study from the United States Renal Data System (USRDS) reported the association of the systolic BP in the predialysis period and cardiovascular death [17]. Compared to patients who had a blood pressure between 110 and 119 mmHg, predialysis systolic BP <109 mmHg was associated with a higher cardiovascular mortality; the risk ratio for cardiovascular death was 1.86. High predialysis BP measurements were not associated with a higher mortality. A 1998 study from a non-profit dialysis chain showed that there is a U-shaped association between blood pressure and mortality in dialysis patients [18]. A 2005 study revealed a similar U-shaped association between predialysis systolic BP and cardiovascular death [19]. A similar U-shaped association emerged between postdialysis systolic BP and cardiovascular death [19]. Another 2006 study from a for-profit dialysis chain revealed that changes in blood pressure also were associated with mortality in a U-shaped manner [20]. But before we embrace therapeutic nihilism, let us consider that correlation is not a causation. This is illustrated by a secondary analysis of the African American Study of Kidney (AASK) Disease [21]. In the AASK randomized trial, among Blacks with hypertension, BP was lowered to two different goals. There was no difference in the primary kidney outcome whether patients were targeted to a lower blood pressure or to the usual blood pressure. The cumulative incidence of hard kidney endpoints, such as a decline in GFR ≥50% or decline by ≥25 mL/min/1.73 m^2 or ESRD or death, was again no different by the randomized group. These data analyzed in an observational way illustrated that a higher BP associates with a greater decline in eGFR and a greater likelihood of hard renal endpoints [21]. Thus, target blood pressure, not achieved blood pressure, should inform clinical goals. When analyses are based on achieved blood pressure, they can lead to markedly different inferences than the intention to treat and this may be because of confounding achieved blood pressure with comorbidities, disease severity, adherence to medications, so clinicians and policymakers should exercise caution when making frequent recommendations based on analyses relating outcomes to achieve blood pressure. Thus, deliberate lowering of blood pressure is not a spontaneously lower blood pressure.

16.5.2 Randomized Trials of Antihypertensive Drugs and Outcomes in Dialysis

Meta-analysis of randomized trials of antihypertensive drugs and hemodialysis patients suggests that there is a benefit to blood pressure lowering. A 2009 meta-analysis revealed that a lower blood pressure lowered the risk of CVD events by 29% [22]. Excluding studies that were not published, produced 36% relative risk reduction in CVD events [22]. An independent 2009 meta-analysis noted that excluding normotensives from the pool of patients on dialysis, produced even a higher relative risk reduction [23]. In other words, lowering blood pressure in patients with hypertension appeared to afford a benefit that was greater than lowering BP in those with normotension. In summary, deliberate lowering of blood pressure in people with hypertension might lower CVD risk. Thus, controlling hypertension among dialysis patients might be worthwhile.

16.6 Strategies to Control Hypertension

The treatment of hypertension in dialysis patients is both simultaneously simple and difficult. Getting the BP down rests on removing sodium from diet, dialysate, and the patient [24]. Occasionally patients would have the kidney removed in the hopes of controlling hypertension, but this should almost never be performed [25]. Some physicians believe that they have failed because they haven't taken out the kidney in the patient on dialysis and they perform bilateral nephrectomies but removing sodium to lower BP is more evidence based [26].

Dietary sodium restriction requires a team effort. A dialysis center in Tassin, France, provides free bread with no sodium, and this center has been successful in limiting interdialytic weight gain for a long period of time [27]. Lowering dialysate sodium is a double-edged sword. Sometimes patients can get quite symptomatic from having low dialysate sodium, because dialysate sodium in individual patients is important for affording hemodynamic stability [28]. On the other hand, lowering dialysate sodium in some individuals can drastically limit interdialytic weight gain, and therefore, blood pressure control might be easier [29].

Dietary sodium restriction and dialysate sodium restriction are important ancillary measures but only when sodium is truly removed from the body by targeting a lower dry weight will the BP be lowered. Volume reduction is the most important way to treat hypertension [30]. In a 1999 editorial, Dr. Belding Scribner was asked the question whether antihypertensive medications could control blood pressure among hemodialysis patients [31]. He concludes that, "in the case of dialysis patient, this low normal level of extracellular fluid volume is maintained by the powerful tool of ultrafiltration which if properly used, along with a moderate dietary sodium restriction is the only proven method of controlling blood pressure" [31].

This opinion was tested in a randomized trial and which asked whether among hypertensive hemodialysis patients volume reduction, probing dry-weight can improve blood pressure [32]. Probing dry weight is the act of lowering post dialysis weight by a small amount, say 0.2–0.3 kg, per treatment till the patient experiences symptoms of intradialytic hypotension such as cramps, need for saline, termination of dialysis, dizziness or lightheadedness or fatigue. In the 2009 study, dry-weight reduction in hypertensive hemodialysis patients (DRIP) patients were randomized to two groups [32]. The intervention group had dry weight probed ($n = 100$), and the control group ($n = 50$) had visits by the researchers every dialysis treatment for 8 weeks. Dry weight was reduced ever so slightly by clinical assessment in the intervention group over 8 weeks. At the beginning, 4 weeks and at the end of the trial at 8 weeks we measured 44-h ambulatory BP monitoring. A validated kidney disease quality of life questionnaire was also administered at baseline and at 8 weeks. On average, at 8 weeks, compared to controls, there was approximately 1 kg reduction in postdialysis weight with the intervention.

At 4 weeks, in the control group, there was a 3.8 mmHg reduction in systolic BP. In the group treated with incremental ultrafiltration, 10.7 mmHg reduction in systolic BP was seen (Fig. 16.1). The difference between the systolic BP reduction of the control group and the ultrafiltration group was 6.9 mmHg [95% confidence interval (CI), −12.4 to −1.3 mmHg, $p = 0.018$). The benefit was sustained at

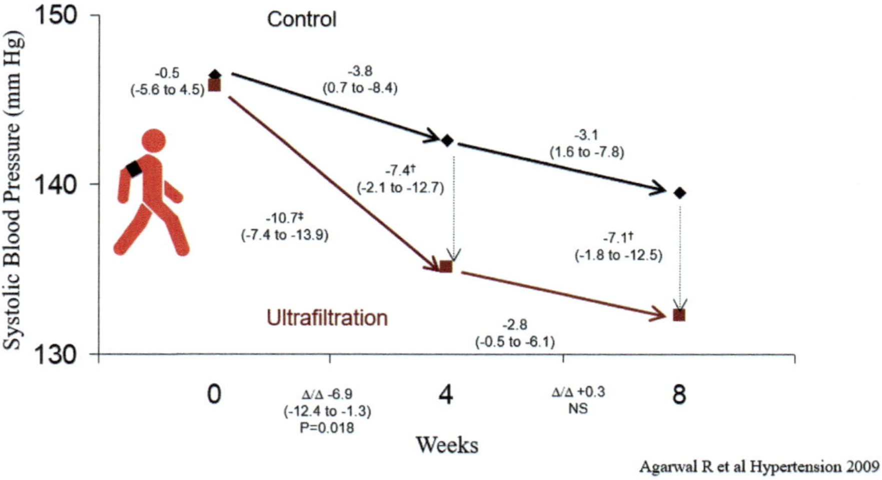

Fig. 16.1 Key results of the dry weight reduction in hypertensive hemodialysis patients (DRIP) trial. The trial probed dry weight in 100 hypertensive hemodialysis patients and 50 patients who were also hypertensive served as controls. Changes in baseline to 4 weeks in systolic 44-h interdialytic ambulatory BP were clinically and statistically significant, and the effects were sustained over 8 weeks

8 weeks. Compared to the control group, with ultrafiltration diastolic BP, likewise improved 3.1 mmHg (95% CI −6.2 to −0.02, $p = 0.048$).

When dry weight was reduced, patients experienced more cramping, hypotension, dizziness, lightheadedness, lack of energy, or fatigue. However, compared to baseline, at 8 weeks there was no difference in any of the domains of the kidney disease quality of life between the control group and the ultrafiltration group.

Despite the short duration of the trial, 10% of patients in the control group had to be removed because their BP became too high to safely participate in the study [32]. There were two patients who had clotted accesses in the control group and six patients in the ultrafiltration group. While these events are not statistically significant, it is possible that ultrafiltration can provoke hypotension or clotted accesses, and this should be carefully monitored especially when probing dry weight. One patient in the trial had chest pain and hypotension. He was administered sublingual nitroglycerin resulting in further drop in systolic BP, syncope and seizures and the need for intravenous saline. The patient illustrates the dangers of giving sublingual nitroglycerin to volume depleted patients.

In a 2021 report, Lung Water by Ultrasound Guided Treatment in Hemodialysis Patients (LUST) randomized trial (NCT02310061) a treatment policy that was guided by extravascular lung water measurements by ultrasound was tested to usual care [33]. The cumulative incidence of composite endpoint was death, myocardial infarction, or heart failure. The original goal was to randomize 500 patients, but the trial enrolled 367 (73% of intended) patients, 183 in the active arm, and 180 in the control arm [33]. In the active arm, the predialysis lung scan was used to titrate ultrafiltration during dialysis and drug treatment. In total, 307 (83.7%) of the patients completed the study. During a mean follow-up of 1.49 years, lung congestion was significantly more frequently relieved in the active (78%) than in the control (56%) arm. However, the postdialysis weight in the lung scan group was 74 kg and remained unchanged at the last visit. Similarly, the postdialysis weight in the control group was 72 kg and remained unchanged at the last visit. The primary composite end point did not significantly differ between the two study arms (Hazard Ratio 0.88; 95% CI: 0.63–1.24). The risk for all-cause and cardiovascular hospitalization and the changes of left ventricular mass and function also did not differ among the two groups. Thus, a treatment strategy guided by lung ultrasound was not more effective than usual care in improving the primary or secondary end points of the trial. The results are not surprising because the control group received clinical intervention that reduced lung congestion among 56% of patients. Although lung congestion was relieved more often (78%) in the ultrasound group, the 22% greater effectiveness in addition to reduced trial recruitment was underpowered in demonstrating a cardiovascular benefit. However, the results of the trial reveal that the lung scans might improve tolerability to dialysis. For example, in the control group 1292 dialysis treatments were complicated by hypotension compared to 858 in the lung scan group ($p < 0.001$).

16.7 Pharmacological Approach to the Treatment of Hypertension in Dialysis

A few studies have rigorously examined the role of antihypertensive drugs in patients on long term dialysis. We consider one trial in detail to illustrate the challenges when studying these drugs in this high-risk population.

16.7.1 Comparison of Atenolol to Lisinopril

The hypertensive hemodialysis patients randomized to atenolol or lisinopril (HDPAL) trial, compared the effects of atenolol or lisinopril each administered three times weekly [34]. The primary endpoint was the difference between groups in the change of left ventricular mass index from baseline to end of the trial.

In this open-label trial, patients were randomized to either the lisinopril group or the atenolol group [34]. Echocardiograms and interdialytic 44-h ambulatory BP monitoring were measured at baseline and then repeated at 6 months and 12 months. Additionally, ambulatory BP monitoring was repeated at 3 months. The goal BP for the trial was <140/90 by using home BP recording. Patients were asked to record home BP for a week before they came in for their monthly visit. Medications were titrated to response. For example, lisinopril was titrated from 10 mg three times a week to 20 mg three times a week to finally 40 mg three times a week. The corresponding doses of atenolol were 25 mg, 50 mg, and 100 mg three times a week. We then added felodipine 10 mg along with other antihypertensive therapies. However, we paid particular attention to managing dry weight and dialysate sodium. At 3 months, using this strategy, systolic 44-h ambulatory BP dropped 19.8 mmHg in the atenolol group and 14.2 mmHg in the lisinopril group. Compared with lisinopril, systolic 44-h ambulatory BP with atenolol was 5.6 mmHg lower at 3 months, 4.9 mmHg lower at 6 months, and 3.6 mmHg lower at 12 months. Home systolic BP between 3 and 12 months was between 5 and 10 mmHg lower with atenolol.

The higher BP experienced with lisinopril was not because of differential medication or dry weight goals achieved. In fact, compared to atenolol, between 3 and 12 months, postdialysis weight was between 1.7 and 3.1 kg lower with lisinopril. In fact, at 12 months, patients treated with lisinopril had postdialysis weight that was 2.9 kg lower compared to atenolol. The need for antihypertensive medications increased in both groups. Between 3 and 12 months, the group treated with atenolol had 0.4–0.7 more antihypertensive medications. In contrast, the group treated with lisinopril had 0.8–1.1 more antihypertensive medications. In fact, compared with atenolol, at the end of 12 months, there were 0.4 more BP medications taken by the lisinopril group. Thus, despite greater reductions in dry weight and a greater need for antihypertensive agents, lisinopril was not able to achieve a similar systolic BP compared to atenolol.

A signal for cardiovascular safety emerged on an interim analysis after complete randomization and an independent data safety monitoring board recommended termination of the trial. We found 14 patients had 18 serious cardiovascular events in the atenolol group (24.6 events/100 patient years), and 26 patients had 40 events in the lisinopril group (58 events/100 patient years). The incidence rate ratio (IRR) was 2.36 (95% CI 1.36–4.23, $p = 0.001$). IRR for the combined endpoint of myocardial infarction, stroke, heart failure hospitalization, and cardiovascular death was 2.29 (95% CI 1.07–5.21, $p = 0.02$). Compared to atenolol, with lisinopril the IRR for hospitalization for heart failure was 3.13 ($p = 0.02$), all-cause hospitalization was 1.61 ($p < 0.01$), all-cause serious adverse events were 1.47 ($p < 0.001$), hypertensive crisis was 3.81 ($p = 0.03$), and hyperkalemia was 3.38 ($p = 0.05$). Echocardiographic findings were similar between the two groups.

These data point to the superiority of atenolol over lisinopril in long-term hemodialysis patients.

16.7.2 Angiotensin-Converting Enzyme (ACE) Inhibitors and Angiotensin Receptor Blockers

Studies using ACE inhibitors and ARBs in dialysis patients in general have also been disappointing. For example, the largest among them was the Fosinopril in Dialysis (FOSIDIAL) study, which randomized 397 patients with left ventricular hypertrophy on long-term hemodialysis to either fosinopril (5–20 mg/day) or matching placebo with the primary endpoint of fatal and non-fatal cardiovascular events [35]. Cardiovascular events included cardiovascular death, nonfatal myocardial infarction, unstable angina, stroke, percutaneous or surgical coronary revascularization, hospitalization for heart failure, and resuscitated cardiac arrest. No significant benefit for fosinopril was observed (relative risk reduction 0.93, 95% CI 0.68–1.26, $P = 0.35$) [36]. Finally, a 2023 meta-analysis of five drug trials of either ACE inhibitors or angiotensin receptor blockers (ARBs) in 1582 patients on dialysis also shows lack of cardiovascular protection or the lowering of all-cause mortality when compared with placebo or no add-on treatment [37].

16.7.3 Mineralocorticoid Receptor Antagonists

The story with spironolactone has vacillated between exuberance and apathy but remains incomplete. In a 2014 study from Japan, randomized long-term hemodialysis patients to 25 mg spironolactone ($n = 157$) or to a control group ($n = 152$) where no additional treatment was given [38]. During the 3-year follow-up, the primary outcome comprised of cardiovascular death or hospitalization due to cardiovascular causes occurred in 5.7% of patients in the treatment group and in 12.5% of patients in the control group. Hazard ratios (HRs) for the primary outcome for treatment were 0.404 (95% confidence interval [CI]: 0.202–0.809; $p = 0.017$). Thus, the risk of cardiovascular death or hospitalization for cardiovascular causes was reduced nearly 60%. All-cause mortality was reduced by nearly 55%. Only 1.9% of the participants required treatment discontinuation due to hyperkalemia and gynecomastia was seen in 10% of the patients. This was an open-label trial; the controls received no placebo. Furthermore, only 309 patients were randomized, whereas the intended sample size was 600. Therefore, the study lacked power, and the likelihood of false discovery rate is high.

In a 2019 randomized trial of long-term hemodialysis patients, 50 were randomized to spironolactone 50 mg/day and 47 to placebo and followed for 9 months with the primary endpoint of a change in left ventricular mass index by cardiac magnetic resonance imaging [39]. Spironolactone group had −2.9 g/m^2 change in left ventricular mass index; the placebo group had +0.4 g/m^2 change. The between-group difference was not significant ($p = 0.337$). A 24-h ambulatory systolic BP was similarly changed at 9 months ($p = 0.433$). Serum potassium was between 6.0 and 6.5 mEq/L in 150 occasions in spironolactone group and 80 occasions in the placebo group ($p = 0.034$). A similar study done in the USA shows that 50 mg of spironolactone is associated with much more hyperkalemia.

In a 2019 report of spironolactone in dialysis-dependent ESRD (SPin-D), a randomized, placebo-controlled, double-blind, multiple dosage trial, 129 maintenance hemodialysis patients were assigned to placebo ($n = 51$) or spironolactone 12.5 mg ($n = 27$), 25 mg ($n = 26$), or 50 mg ($n = 25$) daily for 36 weeks to assess safety, tolerability, and feasibility and to explore cardiovascular efficacy [40]. The lowest dose of spironolactone was similar to placebo with respect to hyperkalemia. However, 50 mg dose was associated with significant hyperkalemia. Gynecomastia was reported rarely.

Finally, a 2022 meta-analysis of 15 drug trials of MRAs in 1258 patients on dialysis shows promising results [41]. Spironolactone treatment significantly decreased all-cause mortality (RR = 0.42, $P < 0.0001$), cardiovascular events (RR = 0.54, $P = 0.008$) and left ventricular mass index (MD = −6.28, $P = 0.002$). After spironolactone supplementation, serum potassium concentration was increased (MD = 0.22, $P < 0.0001$), but the risk of hyperkalemia remained unchanged (RR = 1.21, $P = 0.31$). As expected, spironolactone increased the occurrence of gynecomastia (RR = 4.36, $P = 0.0005$). No changes were seen in left ventricular ejection fraction (MD = 2.63, $P = 0.05$), systolic BP (MD = −4.61, $P = 0.14$), and diastolic BP (MD = −0.12, $P = 0.94$). Compared to Whites, both advantages and disadvantages of spironolactone were magnified in those of Asian ancestry [41].

Report of a reasonably sized trial casts a shadow of doubt on the meta-analysis [41]. A multicenter European trial—ALCHEMIST—compared spironolactone to placebo in long-term dialysis patients on its potential to prevent cardiovascular outcomes (NCT01848639). This trial, yet to be published, was reported by Dr. Patrick Rossignol at the ASN meeting in November 2023. Cardiovascular outcomes were as follows: nonfatal myocardial infarction, acute coronary syndrome, hospitalization for heart failure, nonfatal stroke, or cardiovascular mortality. The intended sample size was 825 patients, but the trial reportedly randomized 644 patients. Spironolactone did not affect the primary outcome: (hazard ratio [HR], 0.996; 95% CI, 0.729–1.362; $P = 0.9819$). The full results are awaiting publication.

The Aldosterone bloCkade for Health Improvement EValuation in End-stage Renal Disease trial (ACHIEVE) trial is ongoing (NCT03020303). It is the largest trial planned to date and intends to recruit 2750 long-term hemodialysis or peritoneal dialysis patients (aged ≥45 years, or ≥18 years with a history of diabetes). The primary endpoint is death or hospitalization for heart failure.

16.7.4 Diuretic Use

A 2011 review suggested the use of loop diuretics among non-oliguric PD patients to maintain sodium balance [42]. However, evidence for this practice is sparse. For example, using 2000 mg furosemide, a 7-patient peritoneal dialysis cross-over study demonstrated a median increase in urinary sodium of 54 mmol/day and a median increase in urine volume of 400 mL/day [43]. In an open-label randomized trial of 61 incident peritoneal dialysis patients who made about a liter of urine at baseline, 250 mg of furosemide was administered to the intervention group with an additional treatment with 5 mg metolazone if urine output was not at least 500 mL/day [44]. In the diuretic group 9/31 (29%) withdrew and in the control group 5/30 (17%). At the end of 12 months, there was approximately 350 mL greater urine output in the treated group. However, there was no preservation of residual kidney function, and more important, the change in body weight from baseline to 12 months was not different between groups. In a pilot study of 39 patients with hemodialysis-dependent kidney failure at three North Carolina clinics, the efficacy, safety, and tolerability of furosemide over 18 weeks was assessed. Patients were recruited if they reported ≥1 cup urine output per day. Doses of oral furosemide were escalated to a maximum dose of 320 mg/day. No change in between-group interdialytic weight gain was seen, making the clinical significance of furosemide in hemodialysis patients untenable [45].

Given the existing high pill burden, limited data to support their use, and potential toxicity, we do not prescribe diuretics or recommend their use in patients with ESKD.

16.7.5 A Step-Care Approach to Pharmacological Management

Thus, when sequencing antihypertensive medications, for the control of hypertension, we prefer to use atenolol, followed by long-acting dihydropyridine calcium channel blockers such as amlodipine and felodipine, and only then ACE inhibitors or ARBs. In our practice, we do not prescribe MRAs or diuretics to dialysis patients. We also avoid the use of alpha blockers due to the risk of orthostatic hypotension and falls in the hypovolemic state. We also do not recommend the use of short-acting hydralazine due to rapid and potent falls in systolic BP we have observed with the use of this drug with interdialytic ambulatory BP monitoring. Centrally acting agents such as clonidine or vasodilators such as minoxidil are used as agents of last resort.

Table 16.3 Key points

The diagnosis of hypertension in dialysis patients is best made by measurements outside the dialysis unit such as by home or 44-h interdialytic ambulatory BP monitoring
Predialysis and postdialysis BP recordings in isolation should not be used to made diagnostic decisions regarding hypertension. Median intradialytic BP recordings are more suitable
Although the exact targets of BP remain unknown in dialysis patients, home BP range of 120–140 mmHg systolic appear reasonable
Dietary and dialysate sodium restriction but more important attention to dry weight remains the key strategy to control hypertension in dialysis patients
When using antihypertensives, we recommend atenolol administered three times a week following dialysis, followed by long acting dihydropyridines such as amlodipine and felodipine, and then ACE inhibitors or angiotensin receptor blockers. We do not recommend spironolactone or loop diuretics

16.8 Conclusions

In conclusion, hypervolemia is a major cause of hypertension in dialysis patients. Among chronic dialysis patients, blood pressure should be lowered. Blood pressure lowering does not increase mortality. An accurate diagnosis can be made with home blood pressure monitoring. Ambulatory blood pressure monitoring is the gold standard but is not required for day-to-day management. Dry weight should be continuously assessed and managed. This is particularly important if the patient is hospitalized and, upon discharge, comes back hypertensive. A lot of uncertainty exists on blood pressure goals and strategies to treat hypertension in dialysis patients, so better outcome trials are needed in this difficult-to-treat patients. The key points of this chapter are summarized in Table 16.3.

References

1. Agarwal R, Nissenson AR, Batlle D, Coyne DW, Trout JR, Warnock DG. Prevalence, treatment, and control of hypertension in chronic hemodialysis patients in the United States. Am J Med. 2003;115:291–7. https://doi.org/10.1016/s0002-9343(03)00366-8.
2. Agarwal R. Epidemiology of interdialytic ambulatory hypertension and the role of volume excess. Am J Nephrol. 2011;34:381–90. https://doi.org/10.1159/000331067.
3. Cocchi R, Esposti ED, Fabbri A, Lucatello A, Sturani A, Quarello F, et al. Prevalence of hypertension in patients on peritoneal dialysis: results of an Italian multicentre study. Nephrol Dial Transplant. 1999;14:1536–40.
4. Agarwal R. How should hypertension be assessed and managed in hemodialysis patients? Home BP, not dialysis unit BP, should be used for managing hypertension. Semin Dial. 2007;20:402–5.
5. Agarwal R, Light RP. Chronobiology of arterial hypertension in hemodialysis patients: implications for home blood pressure monitoring. Am J Kidney Dis. 2009;54:693–701. https://doi.org/10.1053/j.ajkd.2009.03.018.
6. Agarwal R, Peixoto AJ, Santos SF, Zoccali C. Pre- and postdialysis blood pressures are imprecise estimates of interdialytic ambulatory blood pressure. Clin J Am Soc Nephrol. 2006;1:389–98. https://doi.org/10.2215/CJN.01891105.

7. Alborzi P, Patel N, Agarwal R. Home blood pressures are of greater prognostic value than hemodialysis unit recordings. Clin J Am Soc Nephrol. 2007;2:1228–34. https://doi.org/10.2215/Cjn.02250507.
8. Agarwal R. Blood pressure and mortality among hemodialysis patients. Hypertension. 2010;55:762–8. https://doi.org/10.1161/Hypertensionaha.109.144899.
9. Agarwal R, Andersen MJ, Light RP. Location not quantity of blood pressure measurements predicts mortality in hemodialysis patients. Am J Nephrol. 2007;28:210–7.
10. Bansal N, McCulloch CE, Rahman M, Kusek JW, Anderson AH, Xie D, et al. Blood pressure and risk of all-cause mortality in advanced chronic kidney disease and hemodialysis: the chronic renal insufficiency cohort study. Hypertension. 2015;65:93–100. https://doi.org/10.1161/HYPERTENSIONAHA.114.04334.
11. da Silva GV, de Barros S, Abensur H, Ortega KC, Mion D Jr. Home blood pressure monitoring in blood pressure control among haemodialysis patients: an open randomized clinical trial. Nephrol Dial Transplant. 2009;24:3805–11.
12. Vaios V, Georgianos PI, Vareta G, Dounousi E, Dimitriadis C, Eleftheriadis T, et al. Clinic and home blood pressure monitoring for the detection of ambulatory hypertension among patients on peritoneal dialysis. Hypertension. 2019;74:998–1004. https://doi.org/10.1161/HYPERTENSIONAHA.119.13443.
13. Roberts MA, Pilmore HL, Tonkin AM, Garg AX, Pascoe EM, Badve SV, et al. Challenges in blood pressure measurement in patients treated with maintenance hemodialysis. Am J Kidney Dis. 2012;60:463–72. https://doi.org/10.1053/j.ajkd.2012.04.025.
14. Drawz PE, Abdalla M, Rahman M. Blood pressure measurement: clinic, home, ambulatory, and beyond. Am J Kidney Dis. 2012;60:449–62. https://doi.org/10.1053/j.ajkd.2012.01.026
15. Agarwal R, Metiku T, Tegegne GG, Light RP, Bunaye Z, Bekele DM, et al. Diagnosing hypertension by intradialytic blood pressure recordings. Clin J Am Soc Nephrol. 2008;3:1364–72. https://doi.org/10.2215/CJN.01510308.
16. Agarwal R, Light RP. Median intradialytic blood pressure can track changes evoked by probing dry-weight. Clin J Am Soc Nephrol. 2010;5:897–904. https://doi.org/10.2215/Cjn 08341109.
17. Port FK, Hulbert-Shearon TE, Wolfe RA, Bloembergen WE, Golper TA, Agodoa LY, et al. Predialysis blood pressure and mortality risk in a national sample of maintenance hemodialysis patients. Am J Kidney Dis. 1999;33:507–17.
18. Zager PG, Nikolic J, Brown RH, Campbell MA, Hunt WC, Peterson D, et al. "U" curve association of blood pressure and mortality in hemodialysis patients. Medical directors of dialysis clinic, Inc. Kidney Int. 1998;54:561–9.
19. Kalantar-Zadeh K, Kilpatrick RD, McAllister CJ, Greenland S, Kopple JD. Reverse epidemiology of hypertension and cardiovascular death in the hemodialysis population: the 58th annual fall conference and scientific sessions. Hypertension. 2005;45:811–7.
20. Li Z, Lacson E Jr, Lowrie EG, Ofsthun NJ, Kuhlmann MK, Lazarus JM, et al. The epidemiology of systolic blood pressure and death risk in hemodialysis patients. Am J Kidney Dis. 2006;48:606–15.
21. Davis EM, Appel LJ, Wang X, Greene T, Astor BC, Rahman M, et al. Limitations of analyses based on achieved blood pressure: lessons from the African American study of kidney disease and hypertension trial. Hypertension. 2011;57:1061–8.
22. Heerspink HJ, Ninomiya T, Zoungas S, de Zeeuw D, Grobbee DE, Jardine MJ, et al. Effect of lowering blood pressure on cardiovascular events and mortality in patients on dialysis: a systematic review and meta-analysis of randomised controlled trials. Lancet. 2009;373:1009–15.
23. Agarwal R, Sinha AD. Cardiovascular protection with antihypertensive drugs in dialysis patients: systematic review and meta-analysis. Hypertension. 2009;53:860–6. https://doi.org/10.1161/HYPERTENSIONAHA.108.128116.
24. Agarwal R, Weir MR. Dry-weight: a concept revisited in an effort to avoid medication-directed approaches for blood pressure control in hemodialysis patients. Clin J Am Soc Nephrol. 2010;5:1255–60. https://doi.org/10.2215/CJN.01760210.

25. Zazgornik J, Biesenbach G, Janko O, Gross C, Mair R, Brucke P, et al. Bilateral nephrectomy: the best, but often overlooked, treatment for refractory hypertension in hemodialysis patients. Am J Hypertens. 1998;11:1364–70.
26. Vertes V. Management of hypertension associated with chronic renal failure. Including the role of bilateral nephrectomy. Postgrad Med. 1972;52:123–6.
27. Charra B, Calemard E, Ruffet M, Chazot C, Terrat J-C, Vanel T, et al. Survival as an index of adequacy of dialysis. Kidney Int. 1992;41:1286–91.
28. Henrich WL, Woodard TD, McPhaul JJ Jr. The chronic efficacy and safety of high sodium dialysate: double-blind, crossover study. Am J Kidney Dis. 1982;2:349–53.
29. Santos SF, Peixoto AJ. Revisiting the dialysate sodium prescription as a tool for better blood pressure and interdialytic weight gain management in hemodialysis patients. Clin J Am Soc Nephrol. 2008;3:522–30.
30. Sinha AD, Agarwal R. Can chronic volume overload be recognized and prevented in hemodialysis patients? The pitfalls of the clinical examination in assessing volume status. Semin Dial. 2009;22:480–2.
31. Scribner BH. Can antihypertensive medications control BP in haemodialysis patients: yes or no? Nephrol Dial Transplant. 1999;14:2599–601.
32. Agarwal R, Alborzi P, Satyan S, Light RP. Dry-weight reduction in hypertensive hemodialysis patients (DRIP): a randomized, controlled trial. Hypertension. 2009;53:500–7. https://doi.org/10.1161/HYPERTENSIONAHA.108.125674.
33. Zoccali C, Torino C, Mallamaci F, Sarafidis P, Papagianni A, Ekart R, et al. A randomized multicenter trial on a lung ultrasound-guided treatment strategy in patients on chronic hemodialysis with high cardiovascular risk. Kidney Int. 2021;100:1325–33. https://doi.org/10.1016/j.kint.2021.07.024.
34. Agarwal R, Sinha AD, Pappas MK, Abraham TN, Tegegne GG. Hypertension in hemodialysis patients treated with atenolol or lisinopril: a randomized controlled trial. Nephrol Dial Transplant. 2014;29:672–81. https://doi.org/10.1093/ndt/gft515.
35. Zannad F, Kessler M, Grunfeld JP, Thuilliez C. FOSIDIAL: a randomised placebo controlled trial of the effects of fosinopril on cardiovascular morbidity and mortality in haemodialysis patients. Study design and patients' baseline characteristics. Fundam Clin Pharmacol. 2002;16:353–60.
36. Zannad F, Kessler M, Lehert P, Grunfeld JP, Thuilliez C, Leizorovicz A, et al. Prevention of cardiovascular events in end-stage renal disease: results of a randomized trial of fosinopril and implications for future studies. Kidney Int. 2006;70:1318–24.
37. Georgianos PI, Tziatzios G, Roumeliotis S, Vaios V, Sgouropoulou V, Tsalikakis DG, et al. Effect of angiotensin-converting enzyme inhibitors or angiotensin receptor blockers on cardiovascular outcomes in dialysis patients: a systematic review and meta-analysis. Nephrol Dial Transplant. 2023;38:203–11. https://doi.org/10.1093/ndt/gfac253.
38. Matsumoto Y, Mori Y, Kageyama S, Arihara K, Sugiyama T, Ohmura H, et al. Spironolactone reduces cardiovascular and cerebrovascular morbidity and mortality in hemodialysis patients. J Am Coll Cardiol. 2014;63:528–36. https://doi.org/10.1016/j.jacc.2013.09.056.
39. Hammer F, Malzahn U, Donhauser J, Betz C, Schneider MP, Grupp C, et al. A randomized controlled trial of the effect of spironolactone on left ventricular mass in hemodialysis patients. Kidney Int. 2019;95:983–91. https://doi.org/10.1016/j.kint.2018.11.025.
40. Charytan DM, Himmelfarb J, Ikizler TA, Raj DS, Hsu JY, Landis JR, et al. Safety and cardiovascular efficacy of spironolactone in dialysis-dependent ESRD (SPin-D): a randomized, placebo-controlled, multiple dosage trial. Kidney Int. 2019;95:973–82. https://doi.org/10.1016/j.kint.2018.08.034.
41. Liu J, Jia W, Yu C. Safety and efficacy of spironolactone in dialysis-dependent patients: meta-analysis of randomized controlled trials. Front Med (Lausanne). 2022;9:828189. https://doi.org/10.3389/fmed.2022.828189.
42. Ortega LM, Materson BJ. Hypertension in peritoneal dialysis patients: epidemiology, pathogenesis, and treatment. J Am Soc Hypertens. 2011;5:128–36.

43. van Olden RW, Guchelaar HJ, Struijk DG, Krediet RT, Arisz L. Acute effects of high-dose furosemide on residual renal function in CAPD patients. Perit Dial Int. 2003;23:339–47.
44. Medcalf JF, Harris KP, Walls J. Role of diuretics in the preservation of residual renal function in patients on continuous ambulatory peritoneal dialysis. Kidney Int. 2001;59:1128–33. https://doi.org/10.1046/j.1523-1755.2001.0590031128.x.
45. Flythe JE, Assimon MM, Tugman MJ, Narendra JH, Singh SK, Jin W, et al. Efficacy, safety, and tolerability of oral furosemide among patients receiving hemodialysis: a pilot study. Kidney Int Rep. 2022;7:2186–95. https://doi.org/10.1016/j.ekir.2022.07.003.

Renal Denervation

17

Fosca Quarti-Trevano and Guido Grassi

17.1 Rationale

Arterial hypertension (HT) is the most prevalent and major modifiable contributor to cardiovascular (CV) morbidity and mortality [1, 2]. Although several antihypertensive drug classes are available, blood pressure (BP) remains uncontrolled in many patients who are not achieving the target values recommend by the guidelines [3, 4]. Approximately 10% of patients display resistant hypertension despite using a diuretic and two or more additional antihypertensive drugs with different mechanisms of action at maximal tolerated doses [4, 5]. Moreover, medication adherence is often poor (<50% after 1 year of treatment) [4, 6, 7]. Hence, a significant number of patients remains at risk of adverse CV events, justifying the development of novel therapies. Although minimally invasive renal denervation (RDN) technologies have been available in Europe since several years, some conflicting results of earlier studies and the perceived low benefit versus potential risks have long partially limited their application. However, with an aging population and in the absence of new antihypertensive therapies, it may be worthwhile to reconsider these non-pharmacological methods in particular selected cases.

RDN is a device-based procedure historically studied in the treatment of resistant hypertension. RND is an invasive treatment modality for resistant hypertension that employs catheter-based techniques to ablate the afferent and efferent sympathetic nervous fibers coursing along the renal arteries implicated in driving hypertension, modulating the overactive signaling between the kidney and central nervous system.

The kidney plays a central role in regulating cardiovascular function and blood pressure homeostasis. Two main functions of the kidney are involved in cardiovascular control: (1) production and the release of renin resulting in the production of

F. Quarti-Trevano (✉) · G. Grassi
Clinica Medica, Department of Medicine and Surgery, University Milan-Bicocca, Milan, Italy
e-mail: fosca.quarti@unimib.it; guido.grassi@unimib.it

A. E. Berbari et al. (eds.), *Blood Pressure Disorders in Acute and Chronic Kidney Diseases*, Updates in Hypertension and Cardiovascular Protection,
https://doi.org/10.1007/978-3-031-81292-7_17

angiotensin II, a potent vasoconstrictor agent, and (2) the urinary excretion of sodium which affects the fluid balance. Both of these effects are under the influence of adrenergic nerve factors, which exert a key role in controlling renin release and balancing saline through both direct and indirect mechanisms [8, 9].

The sympathetic innervation of the renal parenchyma includes both afferent and efferent fibers, both of crucial importance for pressure homeostasis. Direct afferent sympathetic fibers to the kidney regulate renal vascular resistance, blood flow to the kidney, and the release of renin from the juxtaglomerular cells, while sympathetic efferent fibers directed to the central nervous system are involved in the activation of the main hypothalamic nerve centers and bulbar, which are in turn also stimulated by signals from excitatory conduits through the carotid sinus and nerve fibers aortic (Fig. 17.1). In addition to the afferent and efferent renal nerve fibers, a contribution to the nervous control of renal function is also provided from the so-called renal-renal reflexes [8]. The renal innervation and its interactions with other neurohumoral systems play an important role in the pathophysiology of arterial hypertension in the development and progression of organ damage.

The interest of devices-based treatment in the hypertensive state comes from the evidence of a marked increase in the sympathetic activity associated with all forms of essential hypertension (systolic, systolic isolated, masked, white coat) [10]. This last aspect carries important implications, because in hypertension the adrenergic tone is increased in different districts, including the renal one. This makes the RDN a rational procedure for interrupting the vicious circle between the sympathetic nervous system, renin-angiotensin axis, and increased blood pressure. Previous data collected by using the microneurographic technique have shown that sympathetic activation is markedly sustained in patients with resistant hypertension, given an additional pathophysiological background to the use of this invasive technique in this phenotype of patient.

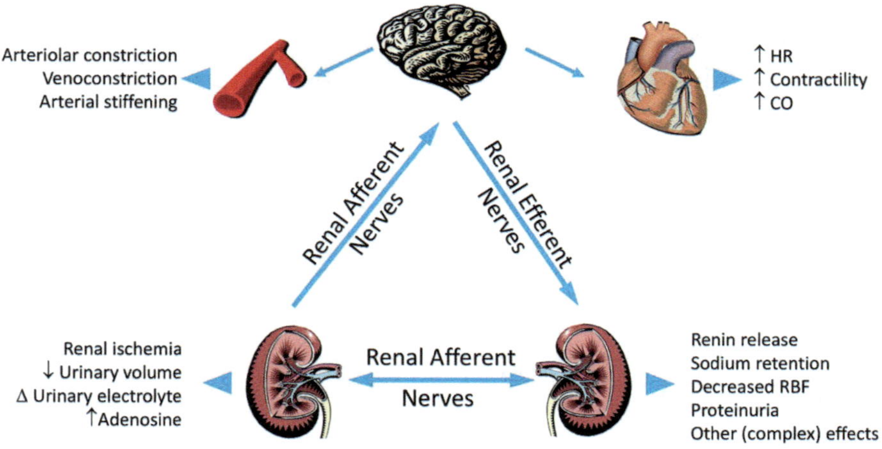

Fig. 17.1 Effects of afferent and efferent sympathetic innervation on renal parenchyma. *HR* heart rate; *CO* cardiac output; *RBF* renal blood flow

Currently, technologies used for RDN in patients with hypertension, as well as other conditions characterized by similar sympathetic imbalance, are essentially based on different methods: radiofrequency energy (RF), high-focused ultrasound energy (US), and perivascular injection of alcohol.

17.2 Blood Pressure Effects

Catheter-based renal denervation (RDN) has been introduced in the first decade of the new millennium as a new interventional approach targeting sympathetic activity in hypertensive subjects. RDN offered a safer approach to reducing localized renal sympathetic activity by using catheter-based ablation techniques. In preclinical translational studies, afferent sensory and sympathetic efferent renal denervation were correlated with decreased renal norepinephrine spillover and increased renal plasma flow; afferent denervation was also correlated with decreased central sympathetic nervous system activity [11]. Disruption of renal nerve activity specifically has been shown to prevent, delay, or reduce the magnitude of hypertension in a wide variety of animal models [12].

Proof-of-concept human studies on RDN applying radiofrequency energy, high-focused ultrasound energy, or perivascular injection of alcohol found substantial decreases in BP in patients with resistant uncontrolled hypertension [13, 14]. The first non-randomized, proof-of-concept study (Symplicity HTN-1) [15] on resistant hypertensives allowed to observe a BP reduction of 27/17 mmHg at 6 months from the RDN procedure supporting the development of devices with different energy sources. The second randomized controlled study (Symplicity HTN-2) [16] was performed in subjects with office BP ≥160 mmHg after 2 weeks of an observation period. The active group showed a BP reduction of 32/12 mmHg. This BP reduction was also maintained at 36 months from the RDN procedure, suggesting that along this period of follow-up a reinnervation did not occur [17, 18]. To overcome the limitations of these studies (lack of 24 h BP monitoring, unblinded design, white coat effect not excluded), a new prospective, single-blind, randomized sham-controlled study (Symplicity HTN-3) was performed [19]. This study confirmed the safety of the procedure but did not reach the end point of BP reduction. BP was significantly reduced from baseline, but active and sham groups did not show significant differences at 6 months of follow-up [19]. A possible interpretation of this negative result could be due to the reduced number of patients with a complete four-quadrant ablation [20]. There were also differences in the population enrolled with a great amount of African Americans in this third study. It is well known the difference in the response to BP treatment according to race suggesting different antihypertensive drug strategies in African Americans versus other racial groups [21]. Other possible reasons for the failure of Symplicity HTN-3 include frequent medication changes during the study period, lack of experience of many operators, procedure variability, and inadequate follow-up duration. After this trial several changes in terms of concomitant therapy, study population, and procedural aspects have been adopted.

Studies carried out more recently with different catheters capable to reduce the catheter manipulation and decrease procedure time obtained similar BP effects. Five sham-controlled randomized trials showed the safety and efficacy of second-generation RF or US systems in patients with or without concomitant medical therapy [22–26]. The reduction in office SBP ranged from −9.0 to −10.8 mmHg and in the diastolic blood pressure (DBP) from −5.0 to −5.5 mmHg, whereas the decrease in ambulatory BP ranges from −4.7 to −9.0 mmHg for SBP and −3.7 to −6.0 mmHg for DBP [13]. Also, the RADIANCE II trial demonstrated a significant reduction in daytime ambulatory SBP at 2 months with US-RDN (mean −7.9 mmHg) vs the sham procedure (mean −1.8 mmHg) in the absence of antihypertensive medications [27].

The duration of BP reduction after the RDN procedure was sustained at 3 years, as shown in the SPYRAL HTN-ON MED, RADIANCE HTN-SOLO trial, and the Global SIMPLICITY Registry [28–30]. In the Global SYMPLICITY Registry, SBP reduction after RDN was sustained over 3 years, including decreases in both office (−16.5 ± 28.6 mmHg, $P < 0.001$) and 24-h ambulatory SBP (−8.0 ± 20.0 mmHg; $P < 0.001$) [31]. A significant BP reduction was also confirmed in high-risk patients, including elderly patients (age ≥ 65 years) and patients with atrial fibrillation, diabetes mellitus type II, severe treatment resistant hypertension, chronic kidney disease (eGFR <60 mL/min/1.73 m^2), and isolated systolic hypertension [31]. More recently, the final analysis of the SYMPLICITY HTN-3 trial showed that patients in the RDN group had significantly larger reductions from baseline to 36-month follow-up in both office and 24 h ambulatory SBP compared with the sham control group [32]. Two single-arm studies, including patients undergoing RF-based RDN, have shown longer-term efficacy up to 10 years after the procedure [33, 34]. Durable BP reduction is also supported by preclinical data that showed a lack of nerve function 180 days after RDN with sustained reduction of axon density and nerve atrophy in a normotensive swine model [35].

Furthermore, RDN has been shown to reduce whole-body and renal sympathetic activity in humans with a considerable reduction of systemic norepinephrine spillover (42%) and reduction in renal noradrenaline spillover and plasma renin activity [36–39]. Indeed, RDN targets sympathetic nerves at the renal artery level, reducing sympathetic overactivity and lowering BP. However, a recent meta-analysis of available studies has reported a limited relationship between the RDN-dependent reduction of sympathetic activity as measured by microneurography and the BP reduction [40]. In fact, BP-lowering effects of RDN, although being associated with a significant muscle sympathetic nerve activity (MSNA) reduction and thus with a reduction in central sympathetic neural outflow, do not necessarily depend only on a central sympathoinhibition. It is possible that mechanisms besides the neuroadrenergic inhibition may also be involved in the development of the BP-lowering effects of RDN. A potential candidate is represented by the renin-angiotensin system because angiotensin II may exert direct and indirect pressor effects and a reduction in plasma renin activity levels, displaying a significant relationship with the BP decrease [41, 42]. This humoral mechanism may also be responsible, together with the baroreflex improvement, for the MSNA reduction. It should be noted that studies meta-analyzed were all based on the microneurographic technique, which provides information on the potential central sympathoinhibitory effects of RDN but not on the sympathetic neural effects at the level of the renal district, which are more sensitive to the procedure as documented by renal norepinephrine spillover data.

17.3 Open Questions

Several questions regarding the RDN need to be addressed. First, considering the large variability in BP response after RDN treatment, the identification of clinical predictors represents major unresolved challenges. A solid predictor of future BP reduction has not yet been identified, except for pre-treatment baseline BP, which is, however, not specific for RDN and applies to antihypertensive treatment in general [13]. Other predictors of response to RDN have been suggested, such as the number and type of medications at baseline, resting heart rate, presence of abdominal obesity, plasma renin activity, aldosterone levels, and detection of obstructive sleep apnoea [43, 44]. In the SPYRAL-HTN OFF MED study, the reduction in the 24-h average SBP and DBP, as well as heart rate, was significantly greater in patients with a median heart rate >73.5 bpm, than those <73.5 bpm, possibly identifying a subgroup of hypertensive patients, that could benefit more from RDN [45]. It has also been showed that higher baseline PRA levels (>0.65 ng/mL/h) were associated with a significantly greater reduction in office and 24-h SBP [42] after RDN. Nevertheless, none of the predictors of BP response to RDN reported so far is sensitive and specific enough to allow an individualized patient selection [45].

Second, despite the efficacy in reducing BP, until now there are no available randomized controlled trials that have analyzed the direct effect of RDN on clinical outcomes. A continuous linear relationship between elevated BP and adverse CV events has been described [46]. A reduction of 5 and 10 mmHg of office SBP was associated with a decrease in major cardiovascular events respectively of 10 and 20% and of stroke by 13–26%, regardless of how this reduction has been obtained [46, 47]. Based on BP reduction observed in high-risk patients from the Global SIMPLICITY registry and event reductions from a published meta-regression analysis, it was estimated a significant absolute reduction in major adverse cardiovascular events over 3 years compared with the projected control (8.6% observed vs. 11.7% for projected control; $p < 0.01$), primarily due to reduced stroke incidence. In addition, an analysis of Global Simplicity Registry showed that Time in Target Range (TTR) of BP after RDN through 6 months was 30.6% and a 10% increase in TTR after RDN through 6 months was associated with significant risk reductions from 6 to 36 months of 15% for major adverse CV events ($P < 0.001$) [48].

Another important question relates to whether the various technologies to conduct RDN have a different benefit-risk ratio, that is, BP-lowering efficacy and safety. In all sham-controlled randomized trials, the rate of major adverse events in the RDN group was comparable to the sham group [22–26]. Femoral vascular access site-related complications (e.g., hematoma, pseudoaneurysm, fistula, bleeding, etc.) were the most reported complications [22–26]. Vascular access site complications may be reduced by designing RDN systems suitable for radial access, but no dedicated catheter system is yet commercially available for transradial RDN.

Complications related to renal artery ablation (e.g., renal artery dissection, spasm, post-procedural stenosis) have been infrequently reported [22]. No significant decrease in kidney function has been reported after the RDN procedure. In a meta-analysis of 48 studies, no differences have been found in the estimated glomerular filtration rate (eGFR) after an average follow-up of 9.1 months [49]. Renal safety was also confirmed at 3 years follow-up in the Global Simplicity Registry, with observed eGFR decrease within the bounds of the expected decline in patients with severe hypertension [30]. Renal safety data are not valid for patients with an eGFR <40 mL/min/1.73 m^2, and further randomized studies will be investigated this question in patients with eGFR <40 mL/min/1.73 m^2. Finally, the value of sympathetic denervation of organs besides the kidney is unclear and remains to be investigated. We must also remember that to date there is no simple and reliable method to confirm the success of RDN at an intraprocedural level and that the usefulness of repeating RDN among patients with persistent uncontrolled hypertension has not been studied.

17.4 Conclusions

RDN can be considered a third-line option for treatment of individuals with uncontrolled BP despite the use of antihypertensive drug combination therapy and eGFR >40 mL/min/1.73 m^2. RND might also be used in selected patients intolerant to drug treatment following an expert review. Several sham-controlled trials have shown the BP-lowering efficacy and safety of RDN in subjects with and without antihypertensive therapy. A multidisciplinary team is of primary importance for patient's selection and follow-up. RDN should only be performed in experienced specialized centers involving experts on hypertension and percutaneous CV interventions. Proceduralists require expertise in renal interventions and specific training in RDN procedures, and centers performing RDN should be able to treat any potential complications. Ongoing studies and future research might answer open questions and are needed to investigate RDN for indications other than hypertension.

References

1. Virani SS, Alonso A, Benjamin EJ, Bittencourt MS, Callaway CW, Carson AP, et al. Heart disease and stroke Statistics-2020 update: a report from the American Heart Association. Circulation. 2020;141:e139–596. https://doi.org/10.1161/CIR.0000000000000757.
2. Mills KT, Stefanescu A, He J. The global epidemiology of hypertension. Nat Rev Nephrol. 2020;16:223–37. https://doi.org/10.1038/s41581-019-0244-2.
3. Mancia G, Kreutz R, Brunström M, Burnier M, Grassi G, Januszewicz A, et al. 2023 ESH guidelines for the management of arterial hypertension the task force for the management of arterial hypertension of the European Society of Hypertension Endorsed by the International

Society of Hypertension (ISH) and the European renal association (ERA). J Hypertens. 2023;41:1874–2071. https://doi.org/10.1097/HJH.0000000000003480.
4. Whelton PK, Carey RM, Aronow WS, Casey DE, Collins KJ, Dennison Himmelfarb C, et al. 2017 ACC/AHA/AAPA/ABC/ACPM/AGS/APhA/ASH/ASPC/NMA/PCNA guideline for the prevention, detection, evaluation, and management of high blood pressure in adults: executive summary: a report of the American College of Cardiology/American Heart Association Task Force on Clinical Practice Guidelines. Hypertension. 2018;7:1269–324. https://doi.org/10.1161/HYP.0000000000000066.
5. Nazarzadeh M, Pinho-Gomes AC, Rahimi K. Resistant hypertension in times of changing definitions and treatment recommendations. Heart. 2019;105:96–7. https://doi.org/10.1136/heartjnl-2018-313786.
6. Vrijens B, Vincze G, Kristanto P, Urquhart J, Burnier M. Adherence to prescribed antihypertensive drug treatments: longitudinal study of electronically compiled dosing histories. BMJ. 2008;336:1114–7. https://doi.org/10.1136/bmj.39553.670231.25.
7. Hill MN, Miller NH, Degeest S, American Society of Hypertension Writing Group, Materson BJ, Black HR, Izzo JL, Oparil S, Weber MA. Adherence and persistence with taking medication to control high blood pressure. J Am Soc Hypertens. 2011;5:56–63. https://doi.org/10.1016/j.jash.2011.01.001.
8. Stella A, Zanchetti A. Functional role of renal afferents. Physiol Rev. 1991;71:659–82. https://doi.org/10.1152/physrev.1991.71.3.659.
9. DiBona GF, Kopp UC. Neural control of renal function. Physiol Rev. 1997;77:75–197. https://doi.org/10.1152/physrev.1997.77.1.75.
10. Grassi G. Sympathetic neural activity in hypertension and related diseases. Am J Hypertens. 2010;23:1052–60.
11. DiBona GF, Esler M. Translational medicine: the antihypertensive effect of renal denervation. Am J Physiol-Regul Integr Comp Physiol. 2010;298:R245–53. https://doi.org/10.1152/ajpregu.00647.2009.
12. Rippy MK, Zarins D, Barman NC, Wu A, Duncan KL, Zarins CK. Catheter-based renal sympathetic denervation: chronic preclinical evidence for renal artery safety. Clin Res Cardiol Off J Ger Card Soc. 2011;100:1095–101. https://doi.org/10.1007/s00392-011-0346-8.
13. Schmieder RE, Mahfoud F, Mancia G, Azizi M, Böhm M, Dimitriadis K, et al. European Society of Hypertension position paper on renal denervation 2021. J Hypertens. 2021;39:1733–41. https://doi.org/10.1097/HJH.0000000000002933.
14. Lauder L, Azizi M, Kirtane AJ, Böhm M, Mahfoud F. Device-based therapies for arterial hypertension. Nat Rev Cardiol. 2020;17:614–28. https://doi.org/10.1038/s41569-020-0364-1.
15. Krum H, Schlaich M, Withbourn R, Sobotka PA, Sadowski J, Bartu K, et al. Catheter-based renal sympathetic denervation for resistant hypertension: a multicentre safety and proof-of-principle cohort study. Lancet. 2009;373:1275–81. https://doi.org/10.1016/S0140-6736(09)60566-3.
16. Esler MD, Krum H, Sobotka PA, Schlaich M, Shimieder ME, Bohm M, et al. Renal sympathetic denervation in patients with treatment resistant hypertension: a randomized controlled trial. Lancet. 2010;376:1903–9. https://doi.org/10.1016/S0140-6736(10)62039-9.
17. Krum H, Schlaich MP, Sobotka PA, Böhm M, Mahfoud F, Rocha-Singh K, et al. Percutaneous renal denervation in patients with treatment-resistant hypertension: final 3-year report of the Symplicity HTN-1 study. Lancet. 2014;383:622–9. https://doi.org/10.1016/S0140-6736(13)62192-3.
18. Esler MD, Bohm M, Sievert H, Rump CL, Schmieder RE, Krum H, et al. Catheter-based renal denervation for treatment of patients with treatment-resistant hypertension: 36 months results from the Symplicity HTN-2 randomized clinical trial. Eur Heart J. 2014;35:1752–9. https://doi.org/10.1093/eurheartj/ehu209.
19. Bhatt DL, Kandzari DE, O'Neill WW, D'Agostino R, Flack JM, Katzen BT, et al. A controlled trial of renal denervation for resistant hypertension. N Engl J Med. 2014;370:1393–401. https://doi.org/10.1056/NEJMoa1402670.
20. Bhatt DL, Bakris GL. Renal denervation for resistant hypertension. N Engl J Med. 2014;371:184. https://doi.org/10.1056/NEJMc1405677.

21. Weber MA, Schiffrin EL, White WB, Mann S, Lindholm LH, Kenerson JG, et al. Clinical practice guidelines for the management of hypertension in the community: a statement by the American Society of Hypertension and the International Society of Hypertension. J Clin Hypertens. 2014;16:14–26. https://doi.org/10.1111/jch.12237.
22. Townsend RR, Mahfoud F, Kandzari DE, Kario K, Pocock S, Weber MA, et al. Catheter-based renal denervation in patients with uncontrolled hypertension in the absence of antihypertensive medications (SPYRAL HTN-OFF MED): a randomised, sham-controlled, proof-of-concept trial. Lancet. 2017;390:2160–70. https://doi.org/10.1016/S0140-6736(17)32281-X.
23. Kandzari DE, Böhm M, Mahfoud F, Townsend RR, Weber MA, Pocock S, et al. Effect of renal denervation on blood pressure in the presence of antihypertensive drugs: 6-month efficacy and safety results from the SPYRAL HTN-ON MED proof-of-concept randomised trial. Lancet. 2018;391:2346–55. https://doi.org/10.1016/S0140-6736(18)30951-6.
24. Azizi M, Schmieder RE, Mahfoud F, Weber MA, Daemen J, Davies J, et al. Endovascular ultrasound renal denervation to treat hypertension (RADIANCE-HTN SOLO): a multicentre, international, single-blind, randomised, sham-controlled trial. Lancet. 2018;391:2335–45. https://doi.org/10.1016/S0140-6736(18)31082-1.
25. Böhm M, Kario K, Kandzari DE, Mahfoud F, Weber MA, Schmieder RE, et al. Efficacy of catheter-based renal denervation in the absence of antihypertensive medications (SPYRAL HTN-OFF MED pivotal): a multicentre, randomised, sham-controlled trial. Lancet. 2020;395:1444–51. https://doi.org/10.1016/S0140-6736(20)30554-7.
26. Azizi M, Sanghvi K, Saxena M, Gosse P, Reilly JP, Levy T, et al. Ultrasound renal denervation for hypertension resistant to a triple medication pill (RADIANCE-HTN TRIO): a randomised, multicentre, single-blind, sham-controlled trial. Lancet. 2021;397:2476–86. https://doi.org/10.1016/S0140-6736(21)00788-1.
27. Azizi M, Saxena M, Wang Y, Jenkins JS, Devireddy C, Rader F, et al. Endovascular ultrasound renal denervation to treat hypertension: the RADIANCE II randomized clinical trial. JAMA. 2023;329:651–61. https://doi.org/10.1001/jama.2023.0713.
28. Mahfoud F, Kandzari DE, Kario K, Townsend RR, Weber MA, Schmieder RE, et al. Long-term efficacy and safety of renal denervation in the presence of antihypertensive drugs (SPYRAL HTN-ON MED): a randomised, sham-controlled trial. Lancet. 2022;399:1401–10. https://doi.org/10.1016/S0140-6736(22)00455-X.
29. Rader F, Kirtane AJ, Wang Y, Daemen J, Lurz P, Sayer J, et al. Durability of blood pressure reduction after ultrasound renal denervation: three-year follow-up of the treatment arm of the randomised RADIANCE-HTN SOLO trial. EuroIntervention. 2022;18:e677–85. https://doi.org/10.4244/EIJ-D-22-00305.
30. Mahfoud F, Böhm M, Schmieder R, Narkiewicz K, Ewen S, Ruilope L, et al. Effects of renal denervation on kidney function and long-term outcomes: 3-year follow-up from the global SYMPLICITY registry. Eur Heart J. 2019;40:3474–82. https://doi.org/10.1093/eurheartj/ehz118.
31. Mahfoud F, Mancia G, Schmieder R, Narkiewicz K, Ruilope L, Schlaich M, et al. Renal denervation in high-risk patients with hypertension. J Am Coll Cardiol. 2020;75:2879–88. https://doi.org/10.1016/j.jacc.2020.04.036.
32. Bhatt DL, Vaduganathan M, Kandzari DE, Leon MB, Rocha-Singh K, Townsend RR, et al. Long-term outcomes after catheter-based renal artery denervation for resistant hypertension: final follow-up of the randomised SYMPLICITY HTN-3 trial. Lancet. 2022;400:1405–16. https://doi.org/10.1016/S0140-6736(22)01787-1.
33. Sesa-Ashton G, Nolde JM, Muente I, Carnagarin R, Lee R, Macefield VG, et al. Catheter-based renal denervation: 9-year follow-up data on safety and blood pressure reduction in patients with resistant hypertension. Hypertension. 2023;80:811–9. https://doi.org/10.1161/HYPERTENSIONAHA.122.20853.
34. Al Ghorani H, Kulenthiran S, Recktenwald MJM, Lauder L, Kunz M, Götzinger F, et al. 10-year outcomes of catheter-based renal denervation in patients with resistant hypertension. J Am Coll Cardiol. 2023;81:517–9. https://doi.org/10.1016/j.jacc.2022.11.038.

35. Sharp ASP, Tunev S, Schlaich M, Lee DP, Finn AV, Trudel J, et al. Histological evidence supporting the durability of successful radiofrequency renal denervation in a normotensive porcine model. J Hypertens. 2022;40:2068–75. https://doi.org/10.1097/HJH.0000000000003236.
36. Schlaich MP, Sobotka PA, Krum H, Whitbourn R, Walton A, Esler MD. Renal denervation as a therapeutic approach for hypertension: novel implications for an old concept. Hypertension. 2009;54:1195–201. https://doi.org/10.1161/HYPERTENSIONAHA.109.138610.
37. Grassi G, Seravalle G, Brambilla G, Trabattoni D, Cuspidi C, Corso R, et al. Blood pressure responses to renal denervation precede and are independent of the sympathetic and Baroreflex effects. Hypertension. 2015;65:1209–16. https://doi.org/10.1161/HYPERTENSIONAHA.114.04823.
38. Hering D, Lambert EA, Marusic P, Walton AS, Krum H, Lambert GW, et al. Substantial reduction in single sympathetic nerve firing after renal denervation in patients with resistant hypertension. Hypertension. 2013;61:457–64. https://doi.org/10.1161/HYPERTENSIONAHA.111.00194.
39. Esler M. Illusions of truths in the Symplicity HTN-3 trial: generic design strengths but neuroscience failings. J Am Soc Hypertens. 2014;8:593–8. https://doi.org/10.1016/j.jash.2014.06.001.
40. Biffi A, Dell'Oro R, Quarti-Trevano F, Cuspidi C, Corrao G, Mancia G, et al. Effects of renal denervation on sympathetic nerve traffic and correlates in drug-resistant and uncontrolled hypertension: a systematic review and meta-analysis. Hypertension. 2023;80:659–67. https://doi.org/10.1161/HYPERTENSIONAHA.122.20503.
41. Laragh JH, Sealey JE. The plasma renin test reveals the contribution of body sodium-volume content (V) and renin-angiotensin (R) vasoconstriction to long-term blood pressure. Am J Hypertens. 2011;24:1164–80. https://doi.org/10.1038/ajh.2011.171.
42. Mahfoud F, Townsend RR, Kandzari DE, Kario K, Schmieder RE, Tsioufis K, et al. Changes in plasma renin activity after renal artery sympathetic denervation. J Am Coll Cardiol. 2021;77:2909–19. https://doi.org/10.1016/j.jacc.2021.04.044.
43. Fink GD, Phelps JT. Can we predict the blood pressure response to renal denervation? Auton Neurosci. 2017;204:112–8. https://doi.org/10.1016/j.autneu.2016.07.011.
44. Böhm M, Mahfoud F, Townsend RR, Kandzari DE, Pocock S, Ukena C, et al. Ambulatory heart rate reduction after catheter-based renal denervation in hypertensive patients not receiving anti-hypertensive medications: data from SPYRAL HTN-OFF MED, a randomized, sham-controlled, proof-of-concept trial. Eur Heart J. 2019;40:743–51. https://doi.org/10.1093/eurheartj/ehy871.
45. Barbato E, Azizi M, Schmieder RE, Lauder L, Böhm M, Brouwers S, et al. Renal denervation in the management of hypertension in adults. A clinical consensus statement of the ESC Council on Hypertension and the European Association of Percutaneous Cardiovascular Interventions (EAPCI). Eur Heart J. 2023;44:1313–30. https://doi.org/10.1093/eurheartj/ehad054.
46. Nazarzadeh M, Bidel Z, Canoy D, Copland E, Wamil M, Majert J, et al. Pharmacological blood pressure lowering for primary and secondary prevention of cardiovascular disease across different levels of blood pressure: an individual participant-level data meta-analysis. Lancet. 2021;397:1625–36. https://doi.org/10.1016/S0140-6736(21)00920-6.
47. Thomopoulos C, Parati G, Zanchetti A. Effects of blood pressure lowering on outcome incidence in hypertension. 1. Overview, meta-analyses, and meta-regression analyses of randomized trials. J Hypertens. 2014;32:2285–95. https://doi.org/10.1097/HJH.0000000000000378.
48. Mahfoud F, Mancia G, Schmieder RE, Ruilope L, Narkiewicz K, Schlaich M, et al. Cardiovascular risk reduction after renal denervation according to time in therapeutic systolic blood pressure range. J Am Coll Cardiol. 2022;80:1871–80. https://doi.org/10.1016/j.jacc.2022.08.802.
49. Sanders MF, Reitsma JB, Morpey M, Gremmels H, Bots ML, Pisano A, et al. Renal safety of catheter-based renal denervation: systematic review and meta-analysis. Nephrol Dial Transplant. 2017;32:1440–7. https://doi.org/10.1093/ndt/gfx088.

18 Interaction of Renal Disease and Blood Pressure Control

Adel E. Berbari and Najla A. Daouk

18.1 Introduction

The clinical triad of hypertension (HT), chronic kidney disease (CKD), and cardiovascular disease (CVD) portends a state of an ominous cardiorenal risk profile, which results from the impact of each of its components and their interactions [1, 2]. Further, the concomitant presence of classical risk factors (diabetes, dyslipidemia, and smoking) magnifies the clinical impact of the cardiorenal risk profile [3].

The cardiorenal risk profile predisposes to the development of a wide spectrum of renovascular disorders associated with increased morbidity and mortality [4].

The aims of this chapter are (1) to define the relationships between components of the clinical triad and (2) to assess the impact of BP control on renovascular disorders.

18.2 Blood Pressure and Renovascular Interactions

Hypertension remains a major risk for a wide spectrum of renovascular disorders, including chronic kidney disease, coronary artery disease, and stroke [1]. This is due to an increasing prevalence of hypertension associated with aging of the population and sub-optimal BP control despite the availability of potent antihypertensive medications [3].

Data from 1999 to 2004 National Health and Nutrition Examination Study (NHANES) revealed that the prevalence of hypertension in the USA increased from 27% in 1999 to 29% in 2004 [5, 6]. Further, the increase in occurrence in

A. E. Berbari (✉) · N. A. Daouk
Department of Internal Medicine, American University of Beirut Medical Center, Beirut, Lebanon
e-mail: ab01@aub.edu.lb; nd00@aub.edu.lb

A. E. Berbari et al. (eds.), *Blood Pressure Disorders in Acute and Chronic Kidney Diseases*, Updates in Hypertension and Cardiovascular Protection,
https://doi.org/10.1007/978-3-031-81292-7_18

hypertension involved older subjects. Hypertension was reported in 47% of participants aged 55 years or older, and in 56% of those 75–84 years old [7, 8].

Similarly, the data of the NHANES surveys reported an increase in CKD in hypertensive subjects [2]. The prevalence of stage 1 CKD rose from 4.9% in 2003–2006 to 7% in 2015–2018 [2]. In contrast, the severity of CKD in hypertensive population decreased. The prevalence of stages 3–5 CKD declined from 10.9% in 2011–2014 to 8.9% in 2015–2018, suggesting that progression of renal disease in hypertension was slower [2].

Epidemiologic and observational studies demonstrate that primary hypertension is a major risk factor for CKD [9].

Data from the United States Renal Data System (USRDS) listed hypertension as a cause of end-stage renal disease (ESRD) in 25–30% of patients starting renal replacement therapy, after diabetes mellitus [10–12].

Whether mild-to-moderate primary (essential) hypertension can produce renal insufficiency remains questionable [13].

The percentage of patients with mild-to-moderate primary (essential) hypertension who develop progression of renal impairment appears to be low [14]. In the Multiple Risk Factor Intervention Trial, only 0.15% of patients developed a doubling of serum creatinine concentration >2 mg/dL over 7 years [14]. On the other hand, other studies revealed an increasing relationship between baseline BP from the high normal range and the risk of ESRD 16–17 years later [13]. In an analysis of 316,675 subjects with baseline estimated glomerular filtration rate >60 mL/min/1.73 m^2 and negative proteinuria and/or hematuria by dipstick urinalysis, Hsu et al. reported that even relatively modest BP elevation from optimal levels were independently related to the incidence of ESRD [15].

The clinical syndrome which characterizes hypertension-attributed CKD/ESRD has been termed hypertensive nephrosclerosis, hypertensive nephropathy, or nephroangiosclerosis [13, 16].

The term nephrosclerosis was coined by the German nephrologist Fahr in 1919 [17]. The term nephrosclerosis derived from the Greek (nephros → kidney, sklerosis → hardening) means literary kidney hardening [18].

Two clinicopathologic patterns have been described, namely, malignant nephrosclerosis and benign nephrosclerosis [13]. Malignant nephrosclerosis, associated with accelerated or malignant hypertension, is characterized by fibroid necrosis and myointimal hyperplasia [13]. If untreated, malignant hypertension leads to renal insufficiency [13]. The second pattern, namely benign nephrosclerosis, is characterized by histopathologic lesions, which include arteriosclerosis, arteriolosclerosis, glomerulosclerosis, tubulointerstitial fibrous, and, less commonly, focal segmental glomerulosclerosis in the absence of immune deposits [19, 20]. The degree of proteinuria is variable [4, 19].

In patients with primary (essential) hypertension and normal GFR, renal histopathologic changes are often absent in the early course of the disease [19]. However, in these patients, renal blood flow is reduced and filtration fraction is increased, suggesting impairment of renal vascular function [19, 21]. Further, in studies of renal biopsies, Smithovick and Heptinstall reported that about 10–20% subjects with mild-to-moderate primary (essential) hypertension have little or no intrarenal vascular disease and minimal or nonsignificant changes in 50% [22–26].

Benign hypertensive nephrosclerosis is the pathohistologic pattern observed in patients with uncomplicated primary (essential) hypertension [19, 20]. Though focal glomerular obsolescence and nephron loss over time, renal function is not seriously compromised except in susceptible individuals, such as those with concurrent disease such as diabetes or in blacks [27–29].

Nephrosclerosis is a common cause of CKD in Afro-Americans but is less common in European (white) Americans, in whom it progresses less frequently to renal insufficiency, suggesting that nephrosclerosis progression has a genetic basis [19].

Benign hypertensive nephrosclerosis accounts for 40% of ESRD in Afro-Americans and about 25% of US whites, occurring in patients older than 65 years old [28].

Hypertensive nephrosclerosis is reported to be a less common risk factor for end-stage renal disease (ESRD) [30]. Observational studies indicate that the rates of severe renal dysfunction related to uncomplicated primary (essential) hypertension are low with ESRD of 0.2% during a follow-up of 10–25 years [30]. However, they are strongly influenced by BP levels in a dose-dependent relation, especially in Afro-Americans [30].

NHANES data from 1996 to 2006 involving 12,240 adults from the general US population revealed an interaction between hypertension and albuminuria as predictors of CKD defined as estimated glomerular filtration rate <60 mL/min/1.73 m^2 [31, 32]. Among subjects with urine albumin/creatinine ratio greater than 30 mg/g, the prevalence of CKD increased with BP levels (95% confidence intervals): normotension 1.4% (1.3–1.6%), pre-hypertension 3.4% (3.2–3.7%), undiagnosed hypertension 11% (10.3–11.7%), and diagnosed hypertension 11.7% (11.1–12.4%) [31, 32]. Further, a meta-analysis of 16 observational cohorts which include 315,321 patients with a mean age of 40–65 years, with baseline BP in the pre-hypertensive (BP = 120–139/80–89 mmHg) and hypertensive (BP > 140/90 mmHg) ranges and normal renal function at baseline (eGFR >60 mL/min/1.73 m^2) revealed a dose-dependent risk of incident CKD (defined as an eGFR <60 mL/min/1.73 m^2) with increasing BP [33]. During a mean follow-up of 6.5 years, the presence of pre-hypertension and hypertension increased renal risk by RR of 1.19 (95% CI 1.07–1.33) and RR of 1.76 (95% CI 1.58–1.97), respectively. Every 10 mmHg increase in systolic and diastolic BP was associated with higher risk for reduced eGFR RR of 1.08 (95% CI 1.04–1.11) and RR of 1.12 (95% CI 1.04–1.20), respectively, with the effects being more pronounced in the elderly [33]. Further, nonmalignant hypertension is an etiologic factor in many patients with stages ¾ CKD [30].

Based on clinical and observational studies performed in a systematic screening of kidney disease (renal function and urinalysis), it appears that nonmalignant hypertension may play a major role as a cause of progressive CKD and ESRD [33]

Despite significant geographic differences in countries and continents, nonmalignant hypertension (hypertensive nephropathy) is listed as the primary diagnosis in about 10–30% of patients with advanced ESRD requiring dialysis [12, 30]. In the USA, the prevalence of hypertensive nephropathy is over expressed among

Afro-Americans [30]. Although Afro-Americans represent one-third of all US patients receiving dialysis for ESRD, they account for over 40% of those whose primary diagnosis is hypertensive nephropathy [12, 30].

Afro-Americans are more likely to develop progressive kidney disease compared to European Americans, and this risk involves the leading causes of end-stage kidney disease (ESRD), such as diabetes, hypertensive-associated kidney disease, and glomerulonephritis [34, 35]. Further, the hypertension attributed nephropathy is associated with a threefold increase in incidence of ESRD in Afro-Americans, especially in younger subjects [35].

Black-white differences in hypertensive ESRD are not limited to the United States but have been reported in other countries [29]. In a study in South Africa, Seedat et al. reported that hypertension was the cause of ESRD in 32% of black as opposed to only 10% of white patients referred for evaluation of end-stage renal failure [36]. However, the prevalence of hypertension in Afro-Americans remains twice as frequent as that of Blacks born outside the United States (42.8% vs. 27.4%), which is unrelated to the length of US residency [37].

Recent studies have demonstrated that genetic factors contribute to the increased prevalence of hypertension-attributed ESRD in Afro-Americans [38]. A region in chromosome 22 associated with renal disease was identified in Afro-Americans [38]. The region contains apolipoprotein LI (APOLI) and the non-muscle myosin heavy chain type 2 (MYH9) genes [38].

Genetic variants in APOLI are strongly associated with renal disease [38]. To be pathogenic and confer risk of renal disease, 2 APOLI genetic variants, termed G1 and G2, are present [31]. In the AASK study, about 23% of participants have 2 APOLI risk variants compared to 12% of controls [31, 38]. The presence of 2 APOLI risk alleles is associated with development and progression of renal disease as manifested by more proteinuria at baseline (urine protein/creatinine ratio greater than 0.6 g/g in 48% of participants) and greater risk of progression of renal disease (progression of serum creatinine to greater than 3 mg/dL or ESRD during follow-up) [31, 38]. The presence of APOLI risk alleles defines a subgroup of hypertensive Afro-Americans characterized by more severe proteinuria at presentations and more rapid progression of renal disease [31].

Among Afro-Americans, ESRD-attributed to hypertension has a peak incidence at ages 30–59 years [31]. Further, there is a strong association of the APOLI gene with FSGS [38].

In contrast, a single APOLI gene does not appear to confer any risk of hypertension-related renal disease [31].

Although it is well established that hypertensive nephrosclerosis is a potent cause of ESRD in the black population, the mechanisms that link hypertension to renal disease remains poorly clarified [12, 30, 39].

APOLI risk variants, which involve about 25% of the AASK study population, tend to have more proteinuria at presentation and tend to progress more rapidly to more advanced stages of CKD despite the use of effective antihypertensive therapies and optimal BP control [30, 31]. The mechanisms by which APOLI disease associated variants disrupt cellular metabolism remain poorly clarified [31]. The

APOLI protein, a lipid-binding protein which is expressed in several sites in the kidney and the circulation, could be pathogenic and contribute to renal disease [31]

Over three quarters of Afro-Americans in the AASK study lack 2 APOLI risk alleles [30, 31]. In this population, several factors have been postulated to account for the pathogenesis of hypertension-attributed renal disease. These factors which induce microvascular pathology include hypertension, diabetes, obesity, smoking, and oxidative stress [30, 31].

18.3 Chronic Kidney Disease - Renovascular Connections

CKD represents a major public health burden [40]. It is an important cause of hypertension and is associated with a high risk of cardiovascular disease [9, 40]. Most patients with CKD die before reaching ESRD, with cardiovascular disease being the most important cause of death [41].

CKD is defined as the presence of markers of kidney damage (albuminuria, abnormal urinary sediments, imaging tests, and/or kidney biopsy) and impaired renal function (increasing serum creatinine, decreased glomerular filtration rate—eGFR <60 mL/min/1.73 m^2, and low urine volume) persisting for over 3 months [42, 43].

CKD and hypertension frequently coexist [42, 43]. Prevalence of hypertension is markedly elevated among non-dialysis CKD patients with rates up to 95% [5, 8].

Several studies indicate that the prevalence of hypertension increases with declining renal function. The 2010 URSDS report which summarizes the NHANES 1999–2006 data demonstrated that, in comparison to individuals without CKD, the presence of any CKD stage (stages CKD 1–5) was associated with higher rates of hypertension [8]. The rates of occurrence of hypertension increased from 23% (without CKD) to 36% in stage 1 CKD and 84% in stages 4–5 CKD [9]. Similar findings were reported in another study. The prevalence of hypertension increased progressively from 65% to 95% as GFR fell from 85 to 15 mL/min/1.73 m^2 [44].

Hypertension is very common in patients on renal replacement therapy, with rates of 85% in hemodialysis and peritoneal dialysis and 70% in renal transplant recipients [9].

The application of out-office BP monitoring (24 h ambulatory BP monitoring—ABPM—and home BP measuring devices) in association with BP measurements in the office has led to the characterization of hypertension phenotypes and classification of hypertension severity in CKD patients [45]. Several hypertension phenotypes and 24 h BP patterns have been identified, namely white-coat hypertension (WCH), masked hypertension (MH), resistant/refractory hypertension, and nocturnal BP alterations [45–47].

The prevalence of hypertension phenotype varies markedly and appears to depend upon several factors, including the method of BP measurement, definition of hypertension, ethnicity, and presence of cardiovascular risk factors [48].

White coat hypertension is defined as high office BP and normal home or ambulatory BP, while masked hypertension represents normal office BP associated with high home or ambulatory BP [45, 48]. Recent studies indicate that, in CKD, the prevalence of WCH ranges between 5 and 29% while MH occurs in 5–31% of patients [49]. This large variability has been attributed to the ethnicity of the cohorts. The prevalence of WCH is higher than that of MH in Caucasians while Africo-American and Asian patients have a higher occurrence of MH than WCH [48, 50]. In the AASK cohort, 43% of patients have MH, and in the Chronic Kidney Disease Japan cohort, the prevalence is 31% [50, 51]. Further, in kidney transplant recipients, two pooled analysis of 11 and 10 studies revealed an average prevalence of MH of 26% [46, 52].

Most cases of MH in CKD are due to an elevated nighttime BP [50]. In a retrospective evaluation of a cohort of patients with non-dialysis CKD and hypertension, 0.8% had isolated daytime uncontrolled hypertension (MUCH), 63% had isolated nighttime MUCH, and 36% in day-night MUCH [46, 53].

The application of out-of-office BP monitoring associated with office BP measurements has been used to evaluate hypertension phenotypes and classification of hypertension severity using a threshold BP <140/80 mmHg for office BP and <130/80 mmHg for 24 h BP monitoring, the classification of hypertension severity was explored among 7518 patients with CKD, provided by the International Database of Ambulatory BP in Renal Patients (I-DARP) collaborative group [45, 54]. This study revealed the following estimates of hypertension severity: well-controlled hypertension (CH) in 25%, masked uncontrolled hypertension (MUCH) in 16%, sustained uncontrolled hypertension (SUCH) in 39%, and WCH in 20% of patients [54].

Severity of hypertension appears to be related to proteinuria and increments in BP [45]. In a cross-sectional analysis of 232 veterans with CKD, the strongest relationship of SBP was reported with log of urinary protein-to-creatinine ratio (UPCR), irrespective of how SBP is measured [45, 55]. In contrast, eGFR was not an independent determinant of SBP [45, 55]. Further observational studies indicate that increments of daytime/nighttime 24 h ambulatory BP are associated with increased risk of cardiovascular and renal outcomes [45, 56]. In contrast, office BP increments alone are not prognostically significant [45, 56, 57].

Resistant hypertension and refractory hypertension are common hypertension phenotypes in CKD [45].

Resistant (apparent) hypertension is defined as uncontrolled BP with concomitant administration of three antihypertensive drug classes, which include a long-acting calcium channel blocker, a blocker of the renin-angiotensin system, and a diuretic, each one administered at maximum or maximally tolerated doses [45]. Patients whose BP is well controlled with more than four antihypertensive drugs are also classified as having resistant (apparent) hypertension [45].

The prevalence of resistant hypertension is twofold higher in CKD compared to the general population (28.8% vs. 14.7%) [45, 57, 58]. Further, the prevalence of resistant hypertension increases both with decreasing GFR and rising proteinuria [45, 59]. Several factors have been reported to increase the risk of resistant (apparent) hypertension, including poor adherence to therapy, older age, male sex, black race, diabetes, and higher body mass index [46].

Patients with resistant hypertension are at increased risk of developing ESRD [46] over a median follow-up of 6.4 years, compared with patients without apparent resistant hypertension at baseline. Those with apparent resistant hypertension have been shown to have 6.32 fold likelihood of developing ESRD [46, 60].

Refractory hypertension represents a rare but severe hypertension phenotype characterized by complete failure to control BP above goal when receiving more than five antihypertensive medications including a diuretic [46, 61]. The 2017 AHA/ACC guidelines define refractory hypertension as a failure to control BP despite administration of antihypertensive medications of different classes, including a long-acting thiazide-like diuretic such as chlorothalidone and a mineralocorticoid receptor antagonist such as spironolactone [46]. Among patients with apparent resistance hypertension, the prevalence of refractory hypertension is reported to be 6.2% [46, 62]. Patients with refractory hypertension appear more likely to have diabetes, cardiovascular disease, and kidney disease compared to drug-treated hypertensives with or without resistant hypertension [46]. Further, the long-term prognostic significance of refractory hypertension remains unclear [46].

Variations in circadian BP profiles are commonly disrupted in CKD and are characterized by isolated nocturnal hypertension, non-dipping, and reverse dipping patterns [45].

Nighttime BP elevation was an exclusive abnormality in 50% of a cohort of CKD patients [45]. Further, the absence of nocturnal dipping was significantly more prevalent in patients with CKD than in age, sex, and race matched controls with essential hypertension (53% vs. 30%) [46].

In the CRIC study (Chronic Renal Insufficiency Cohort) that enrolled participants aged 21–74 years with an eGFR 20–70 mL/min/1.73 m^2, reverse and non-dippers were reported in 54.8% of the 1492 participants [46, 54]. Similarly, in the AASK (African American Study of Kidney Disease Cohort Study), the non-dipping and reverse dipping patterns were present in over 80% of non-dialyzed patients [50].

In patients with CKD on chronic hemodialysis, non-dipping pattern was reported in more than 80% of patients [45, 63].

Several mechanisms have been postulated to explain the lack of dipping in CKD, among them overactivity of neurohormonal systems [45]; further, a reverse relationship between renal functional impairment and nocturnal BP for the maintenance of sodium balance [45, 64]. Patients with reduced renal function require a high BP throughout the night to remain in sodium balance [64]. Fukuda et al. demonstrated that a small group of CKD patients require a longer time until BP falls during the night [65]. In addition, the time to dipping was strongly associated with the degree of renal impairment [65].

Several studies have demonstrated that altered circadian BP profiles and nocturnal hypertension are strongly associated with adverse cardiovascular events in CKD [51, 56].

Several causes of primary nephropathy which more frequently comprise patients starting dialysis include diabetic nephropathy (40%), hypertensive nephrosclerosis and vascular disease (20%), primary glomerulopathy (18%), tubulointerstitial nephropathy (7%), and cystic disease (5%) [66].

18.4 Hypertension–Chronic Kidney Disease–Cardiovascular Disease Interactions

HT, CKD, and CVD represent major public health challenges due to their association with cardiorenal complications and premature death [9].

HT and CKD are closely interlinked pathologic disorders. Sustained HT is a major risk for worsening kidney function, while progressive decline in kidney function can lead to rising BP and worsening BP control [46].

Primary HT is a major risk for CVD, while CKD, the most common form of secondary HT, is an independent risk for cardiovascular morbidity and mortality [9].

Several studies have demonstrated that elevated BP is a leading cause for cardiovascular disorders, such as coronary artery disease, heart failure, atrial fibrillation, peripheral artery disease, stroke, impaired cognitive function, and dementia [46, 67]. Further, mortality from coronary disease and stroke increases exponentially from BP levels as low as 115/75 mmHg upward, with the risk involving all age-groups 40–80 years [46, 68].

Recent work has provided insights about the relationship between CKD and cardiovascular risk. A large community-based cohort of 1,120,275 adults from Kaiser Permanente of Northern California with outpatient measures of serum creatinine were followed up from 1996 through 2000 for longitudinal changes in kidney function using the MDRD estimated GFR (>60, 45–59, 30–44, 15–29, <15 mL/min/1.73 m^2) [69, 70]. Outcomes evaluated included CV events and death [69, 70]. Patients with lower baseline GFR had a higher prevalence of traditional risk factors [69, 70]. The age-adjusted rate of CV events (coronary artery disease, heart failure, stroke, and peripheral artery disease) increased markedly below an estimated GFR of 60 mL/min/1.73 m^2 and especially below 45 mL/min/1.73 m^2 [69, 70]. Statistical adjustments for a variety of confounding factors found that lower estimated GFR remained an independent predictor of adverse outcomes [69, 70]. The relationship was even stronger for all-cause mortality [69, 70].

This study suggests that the relationship between CKD and CVD is not linearly associated with the level of GFR, especially in stage 3 CKD (GFR = 30–55 mL/min/1.73 m^2) [69, 70]. It also demonstrated that CV events occur much more commonly than the development of ESRD among patients with CKD [69, 70].

Primary HT and CKD are associated with a heightened cardiovascular risk profile and often interact [71]. They display a wide spectrum of vascular pathologies, which involve both the macrocirculation and microcirculation [72].

18.5 Macrocirculatory Vascular Diseases

18.5.1 Atherosclerosis

Atherosclerosis reflects an intimal vascular disease characterized by the presence of plaques, occlusive lesions, and occasionally by intimal calcification [72].

Atherosclerotic vascular lesions are initiated by traditional risk factors (diabetes, hypertension, obesity, dyslipidemia, and smoking) [72]. Clinical presentation includes ischemic heart disease, heart failure, and cerebrovascular disorders [72].

18.5.2 Arteriosclerosis

Arteriosclerosis is defined as stiffening of the arteries, especially the elastic arteries (aorta/major branches, common carotid artery), and is characterized by increased luminal diameter, media thickness, destruction of the elastic lamellae, and extensive medial calcification [72]. These structural alterations reduce elasticity, increase stiffness of elastic arteries, and impair cushion function of the large arterial system [72].

Arterial aging, impaired renal function, and hypertension are the major determinants of arterial stiffness [72]. Disturbed mineral metabolism also may contribute to stiffness of the arterial system in CKD.

Ejection of left ventricular stroke into the stiff arterial system results in increased SBP, reduced DBP, wide pulse pressure, and increased pulse wave velocity [72]. Clinical manifestations include coronary heart disease, heart failure, impaired renal function, and cognitive dysfunction [72].

18.6 Microcirculatory Vascular Diseases

Microvascular diseases occur frequently in HT and CKD/ESRD [72]. They are characterized by impaired endothelial function, remodeling of the resistance arteries and capillary rarefactions [72].

Several factors have been implicated in the pathogenesis of microvascular disease in HT, CKD/ESRD: (1) impaired nitric oxide release or bioavailability due to accumulation of asymmetric dimethyl arginine; (2) oxidative stress; (3) activation of the renin-angiotensin system; (4) dyslipidemia; (5) impaired calcium-phosphorous metabolism, hyperparathyroidism, reduced vitamin D1,25 levels; and (6) chronic inflammation [72].

18.7 Cardiac Diseases as a Promoter of Renal Impairment

Several studies have demonstrated a bidirectional relationship between CKD and CVD [70]. Although it is well established that CKD can initiate CVD, heart disease has been shown to promote the development of renal dysfunction in patients without overt CKD [73, 74].

In patients with severe acute myocardial infarction, systemic hemodynamics are altered [73, 74]. The low cardiac output associated with under filling of the systemic and renal circulations triggers a series of compensatory vascular responses characterized by increased systemic and renal resistances and activation of neurohumoral mechanisms, which tend to maintain systemic BP but impair renal hemodynamics [74]. These factors initiate the onset of acute kidney injury (AKI) [74, 75]. The incidence and severity of AKI correlate with the severity of acute cardiac decompensation [74].

In chronic heart failure, the pathophysiologic mechanisms linking CVD and CKD have not been well delineated [19]. In uncomplicated heart failure, the low cardiac output does not appear to contribute to worsening renal function [74]. No correlation has been reported between GFR and LV ejection [74]. On the other hand, old age, diabetes, hypertension, and macrovascular and microvascular diseases are associated with worsening renal function in chronic heart failure [74].

Cardiac diseases have been linked to CKD by other undefined mechanisms. In autopsy studies of individuals without clinically overt coronary artery disease dying from violent or natural causes, coronary atherosclerosis was strongly associated with nephrosclerosis, suggesting similar mechanisms underlying the pathophysiology of coronary atherosclerosis and nephrosclerosis [74, 75].

18.8 Interaction Between Blood Pressure Control and Cardiorenal Outcomes

Uncontrolled hypertension can lead to a significant cardiovascular morbidity and mortality and acceleration to end-stage renal disease in CKD patients [76].

Several large randomized controlled trials of patients with CKD evaluated the relationship of BP control and CKD progression [46].

In the SPRINT trial, 9361 participants including 2600 participants with stage 3 CKD older than 50 years were assigned to a systolic BP <120 mmHg versus <140 mmHg [77, 78]. Participants assigned to lower BP treatment target had lower risk for cardiovascular events (myocardial infarction, other acute coronary syndromes, stroke, heart failure, or death from cardiovascular causes) and all-cause mortality [77, 78]. However, no difference in CKD progression was noted [77, 78]. Further, in a subset of SPRINT trial participants, those assigned to lower BP targets were also reported to have a lower risk of mild cognitive impairment and dementia [76–78].

In contrast, in three large controlled trials of patients with non-diabetic kidney disease (MDRD—Modification of Diet in Renal Disease study; AASK—African American Study of Kidney Disease in Hypertension; REIN-2—Ramipril Efficacy in Nephropathy 2) that assigned BP target <130/80 mmHg failed to demonstrate a benefit for renal (eGFR decline or ESRD risk) or cardiovascular outcomes compared with BP targets in the range <140/90 mmHg [76]. Further, in the STEP (Strategy of Blood Pressure Intervention in the Elderly Hypertensive Patients) trial, a randomized control trial that enrolled 8511 patients aged 60–80 years with a high BP and a high cardiovascular risk, reducing BP to a mean of 127 or 135 mmHg did not alter the rate of GFR decline or the number of patients reaching eGFR <30 mL/min/1.73 m^2 [46].

Even in the presence of adequate BP control, the residual cardiorenal risk remains high [46, 79]. However, novel agents such as sodium glucose transporter 2 ($SGLT_2$) inhibitors and the new non-steroidal mineralocorticoid antagonist Finerenone can delay the progression of CKD and reduce cardiovascular complications [46, 79].

Results of two large phase III trials demonstrated that Finerenone, a selective non-steroidal MR antagonist with greater selectivity than Spironolactone, reduced CV events by 14% and CKD progression by 18% in diabetic patients CKD stages 3/4 with moderately severe albuminuria and in CKD stage 2 with severe proteinuria [79–82]. The cardiorenal benefits appear to be independent of BP changes [79–82].

Several very large randomized placebo-controlled trials have demonstrated favorable effects of $SGLT_2$ inhibitors on cardiovascular and renal outcomes in CKD patients [79]. The Nuffield Department of Population Health Renal Studies Group and $SGLT_2$ inhibitor Meta-analysis Cardiorenal Trialists Consortium revealed that, compared to placebo, being on $SGHLT_2$ inhibitor reduced the risk of CKD progression by 37% irrespective of the presence or absence of diabetes, cardiovascular mortality by 14% and other cardiovascular events by 23% [46, 79, 83–85]. Further, $SGLT_2$ inhibitors have shown to reduce diurnal and nocturnal BP by ABPM [84].

Several mechanisms have been postulated to account for the cardiorenal protection independent of BP control, afforded by Finerenone and $SGLT_2$ inhibitors in CKD hypertensives [46].

18.9 Conclusion

The renovascular triad of hypertension (HT), chronic kidney disease (CKD), and cardiovascular disease (CVD), a major public health burden, is associated with heightened risk of cardiorenal complications.

HT is very common in CKD and represents the most common form of secondary HT. Its prevalence increases with worsening renal function, representing the second leading cause of ESRD in patients starting renal replacement therapy.

Hypertensive CKD is a major cause of cardiorenal complications and is associated with a wide spectrum of histopathologic lesions characterized by nephrosclerosis and macro–microvascular changes.

Apoli variant HT phenotype occurs in 25% of Afro-Americans in AASK study. It is characterized by decreased GFR, and albuminuria at baseline and risk of progression to ESRD.

Although CKD predisposes to the development of cardiorenal disorders, CVD can be a promoter of CKD in patients without renal disease at baseline.

The introduction of Finerenone, a novel selective MR antagonist and SGLT2 inhibitors, has been associated with improved BP control and reduction/prevention of cardiorenal complications and progression to ESRD in hypertensive CKD.

References

1. Jones DW, Clark DC. Hypertension (blood pressure) and lifetime risk of target organ damage. Curr Hypertens Rep. 2020;22:75.
2. Zeng X, Zeng O, Zhou L, Zhu H, Luo J. Prevalence of chronic kidney disease among US adults with hypertension, 1999 to 2018. Hypertension. 2023;80:2149–58.
3. Bakris GL, Texter SC. Hypertension. The American Society of Nephrology: nephrology self-assessment program. J Am Soc Nephrol. 2005;Suppl 4:75–109.
4. Wiederkehr M, Toto R, Fenves AZ, Ram CVS. Hypertension and the kidney. Sem Nephrol. 2005;25:236–45.
5. Coresh J, Selvin E, Stevens LA, Manzi J, Kusek JW, Eggers P, et al. Prevalence of chronic kidney disease in the United States. JAMA. 2007;298:2038–47.
6. Ong KL, Cheung BMY, Man YW, Lau CP, Lam KSL. Prevalence, awareness, treatment, and control of hypertension among United States adults 1999-2004. Hypertension. 2007;49:69–75.
7. Schoenborn CA, Heyman KM. Health characteristics of adults aged 55 years and over: United States, 2004-2007. Natl Health Stat Report. 2009;16:1–31.
8. Udani S, Lazich I, Bakris GL. Epidemiology of hypertensive kidney disease. Nat Rev Nephrol. 2011;7:11–21.
9. Tedla FM, Brar A, Browne R, Brown C. Hypertension in chronic kidney disease: navigating the evidence. Int J Hypertens. 2011;2011:132405.
10. USRDS 1997 annual data report: executive summary. Am J Kidney Dis. 1997;30(suppl 1):S10–20.
11. US Renal Data System. USRDS 2010 annual data report: atlas of chronic kidney disease and end-stage renal disease in the United States. Bethesda, MD: National Institutes of Health, National Institute of Diabetes and Digestive and Kidney Diseases; 2010.
12. US Renal Data System. USRDS 2012 annual data report: atlas of chronic kidney disease and end-stage renal disease in the United States. Bethesda, MD: National Institutes of Health, National Institute of Diabetes and Digestive and Kidney Diseases; 2012.
13. Marín R, Gorostidi M, Fernández-Vega F, Alvarez-Navascués R. Systemic and glomerular hypertension and progression of chronic renal disease: the dilemma of nephrosclerosis. Kidney Int. 2005;68(Suppl 99):S52–6.
14. Multiple Risk Factor Intervention Trial Research Group. Coronary heart disease death, nonfatal acute myocardial infarction and other clinical outcomes in the multiple risk factor intervention trial. Am J Cardiol. 1986;58:1–13.
15. Hsu CY, McCulloch CE, Darbinian J, Go AS, Iribarren C. Elevated blood pressure and risk of end-stage renal disease in subjects without baseline kidney disease. Arch Intern Med. 2005;165:923–8.
16. Bleyer AJ, Appel RG. Risk factors associated with hypertensive nephrosclerosis. Nephron. 1999;82:193–8.
17. Fahr T. Uber nephroskleroses. Virchowis Archa. 1919;26:119–78.
18. Freedman BI, Iskandar SS, Appel RG. The link between hypertension and nephrosclerosis. Am J Kidney Dis. 1995;25:207–21.
19. Rosario RF, Wesson DE. Primary hypertension and nephropathy. Curr Opin Nephrol Hypertens. 2006;15:130–4.
20. Fogo AB. Mechanisms in nephrosclerosis and hypertension-beyond hemodynamics. J Nephrol. 2001;14(Suppl 4):S63–9.
21. Perry HM Jr, Miller JP, Fornoff JR, Baty JD, Sambhi M, Rutan G, et al. Early predictors of 15-year end-stage renal disease in hypertensive patients. Hypertension. 1995;25:587–94.
22. Castleman B, Smithwick RH. The relation of vascular disease to the hypertensive state; the adequacy of the renal biopsy as determined from a study of 500 patients. N Engl J Med. 1948;239:729–32.
23. Castleman B, Smithwick RH. The relation of vascular disease to the hypertensive state based on a study of renal biopsies from one hundred hypertensive patients. JAMA. 1943;121:1256–61.

24. Sommers SC, Relman AS, Smithwick RH. Histologic studies of kidney biopsy specimens from patients with hypertension. Am J Pathol. 1958;34:685–715.
25. Helmchen U, Wenzel UO. Benign and malignant nephrosclerosis and renovascular disease. In Tisher CC, Brenner B, editors. Renal pathology with clinical and functional correlations. 2nd ed. JB Lippincott Co; 1991. p. 1201–36.
26. Heptinstall RH. Renal biopsies in hypertension. Br Heart J. 1954;16:133–41.
27. Goldman JM. Hypertensive kidney disease. In: McCauley J, Maarouf OH, Hamrahian SM, editors. Approaches to chronic kidney disease. Springer Nature Switzerland; 2022. p. 103–29.
28. Laskow DA, Curtis J, Luke R, Jones P, Barber H, Deierhoi M, et al. Cyclosporine impairs the renal response to volume depletion. Transplant Proc. 1988;20(Suppl 3):568–71.
29. Whelton PK, Klag MJ. Hypertension as a risk factor for renal disease. Review of clinical and epidemiological evidence. Hypertension. 1989;13(Suppl I):I19–27.
30. Peixoto AJ, Bakris GL. Approach to the patient with hypertensive nephrosclerosis. In: Kimmel PL, Rosenberg ME, editors. Chronic renal disease. Academic Press; 2020. p. 737–52.
31. Kopp JB. Rethinking hypertensive kidney disease: arterionephrosclerosis as a genetic, metabolic, and inflammatory disorder. Curr Opin Nephrol Hypertens. 2013;22:266–72.
32. Yan P, Zhu X, Li H, Shrubsole MJ, Shi H, Zhang MZ, et al. Association of high blood pressure with renal insufficiency: role of albuminuria, from NHANES, 1999-2006. PLoS One. 2012;7:e37837.
33. Garofalo C, Borrelli S, Pacilio M, Minutolo R, Chiodini P, De Nicola L, et al. Hypertension and prehypertension and prediction of development of decreased estimated GFR in the general population: a meta-analysis of cohort studies. Am J Kidney Dis. 2016;67:89–97.
34. Kiberd BA, Clase CM. Cumulative risk for developing end-stage renal disease in the US population. J Am Soc Nephrol. 2002;13:1635–44.
35. Collins AJ, Foley RN, Chavers B, Gilbertson D, Herzog C, Johansen K, et al. United States renal data system 2011 annual data report: atlas of chronic kidney disease & end-stage renal disease in the United States. Am J Kidney Dis. 2012;59(1 Suppl 1):e1–420.
36. Seedat YK, Naicker S, Rawat R, Parsoo I. Racial differences in the causes of end-stage renal failure in Natal. S Afr Med J. 1984;65:956–8.
37. Brown AGM, Houser RF, Mattei J, Mozaffarian D, Lichtenstein AH, Folta SC. Hypertension among US-born and foreignborn non-Hispanic blacks: National Health and Nutrition Examination Survey 2003-2014 data. J Hypertens. 2017;35:2380–7.
38. Lipkowitz MS, Freedman BI, Langefeld CD, Comeau ME, Bowden DW, Kao WHL, et al. Apolipoprotein L1 gene variants associate with hypertension-attributed nephropathy and the rate of kidney function decline in African Americans. Kidney Int. 2013;83:114–20.
39. Marcantoni C, Ma LJ, Federspiel C, Fogo AB. Hypertensive nephrosclerosis in African Americans versus Caucasians. Kidney Int. 2002;62:172–80.
40. Castro AF, Coresh J. CKD surveillance using laboratory data from the population-based National Health and Nutrition Examination Survey (NHANES). Am J Kidney Dis. 2009;53(3 Suppl 3):S46–55.
41. Gansevoort RT, Correa-Rotter R, Hemmelgarn BR, Jafar TH, Heerspink HJL, Mann JF, et al. Chronic kidney disease and cardiovascular risk: epidemiology, mechanisms, and prevention. Lancet. 2013;382:339–52.
42. Levey AS, Levin A, Kellum JA. Definition and classification of kidney diseases. Am J Kidney Dis. 2013;61:686–8.
43. National Kidney Foundation. K/DOQI clinical practice guidelines for chronic kidney disease: evaluation, classification, and stratification. Am J Kidney Dis. 2002;39(2 Suppl 1):S1–266.
44. Buckalew VM Jr, Berg RL, Wang SR, Porush JG, Rauch S, Schulman G. Prevalence of hypertension in 1,795 subjects with chronic renal disease: the modification of diet in renal disease study baseline cohort. Modification of Diet in Renal Disease Study Group. Am J Kidney Dis. 1996;28:811–21.
45. Georgianos PI, Agarwal R. Hypertension in Chronic Kidney Disease (CKD): diagnosis, classification, and therapeutic targets. Am J Hypertens. 2021;34:318–26.

46. Burnier M, Damianaki A. Hypertension as cardiovascular risk factor in chronic kidney disease. Circ Res. 2023;132:1050–63.
47. Burnier M, Wuerzner G. What is the hypertension "phenotype"? Curr Cardiovasc Risk Rep. 2015;9:9. https://doi.org/10.1007/s12170-015-0438-5.
48. Bangash F, Agarwal R. Masked hypertension and white-coat hypertension in chronic kidney disease: a meta-analysis. Clin J Am Soc Nephrol. 2009;4:656–64.
49. Minutolo R, Gabbai FB, Agarwal R, Chiodini P, Borrelli S, Bellizzi V, et al. Assessment of achieved clinic and ambulatory blood pressure recordings and outcomes during treatment in hypertensive patients with CKD: a multicenter prospective cohort study. Am J Kidney Dis. 2014;64:744–52.
50. Pogue V, Rahman M, Lipkowitz M, Toto R, Miller E, Faulkner M, et al. Disparate estimates of hypertension control from ambulatory and clinic blood pressure measurements in hypertensive kidney disease. Hypertension. 2009;53:20–7.
51. Iimuro S, Imai E, Watanabe T, Nitta K, Akizawa T, Matsuo S, et al. Clinical correlates of ambulatory BP monitoring among patients with CKD. Clin J Am Soc Nephrol. 2013;8:721–30.
52. Pisano A, Mallamaci F, D'Arrigo G, Bolignano D, Wuerzner G, Ortiz A, et al. Assessment of hypertension in kidney transplantation by ambulatory blood pressure monitoring: a systematic review and meta-analysis. Clin Kidney J. 2021;15:31–42.
53. Fu X, Ren H, Xie J, Wang W, Li Y, Gao P, et al. Association of nighttime masked uncontrolled hypertension with left ventricular hypertrophy and kidney function among patients with chronic kidney disease not receiving dialysis. JAMA Netw Open. 2022;5:e2214460.
54. Drawz PE, Brown R, De Nicola L, Fujii N, Gabbai FB, Gassman J, et al. Variations in 24-hour BP profiles in cohorts of patients with kidney disease around the world: the I-DARE study. Clin J Am Soc Nephrol. 2018;13:1348–57.
55. Agarwal R, Andersen MJ. Correlates of systolic hypertension in patients with chronic kidney disease. Hypertension. 2005;46:514–20.
56. Agarwal R, Andersen MJ. Blood pressure recordings within and outside the clinic and cardiovascular events in chronic kidney disease. Am J Nephrol. 2006;26:503–10.
57. Minutolo R, Agarwal R, Borrelli S, Chiodini P, Bellizzi V, Nappi F, et al. Prognostic role of ambulatory blood pressure measurement in patients with nondialysis chronic kidney disease. Arch Intern Med. 2011;171:1090–8.
58. Noubiap JJ, Nansseu JR, Nyaga UF, Sime PS, Francis I, Bigna JJ. Global prevalence of resistant hypertension: a metaanalysis of data from 3.2 million patients. Heart. 2019;105:98–105.
59. Tanner RM, Calhoun DA, Bell EK, Bowling CB, Gutiérrez OM, Irvin MR, et al. Prevalence of apparent treatment-resistant hypertension among individuals with CKD. Clin J Am Soc Nephrol. 2013;8:1583–90.
60. Tanner RM, Calhoun DA, Bell EK, Bowling CB, Gutiérrez OM, Irvin MR, et al. Incident ESRD and treatment-resistant hypertension: the reasons for geographic and racial differences in stroke (REGARDS) study. Am J Kidney Dis. 2014;63:781–8.
61. Acelajado MC, Pisoni R, Dudenbostel T, Dell'Italia LJ, Cartmill F, Zhang B, et al. Refractory hypertension: definition, prevalence, and patient characteristics. J Clin Hypertens (Greenwich). 2012;14:7–12.
62. Buhnerkempe MG, Botchway A, Prakash V, Al-Akchar M, Nolasco Morales CE, Calhoun DA, et al. Prevalence of refractory hypertension in the United States from 1999 to 2014. J Hypertens. 2019;37:1797–804.
63. Farmer CK, Goldsmith DJ, Cox J, Dallyn P, Kingswood JC, Sharpstone P. An investigation of the effect of advancing uraemia, renal replacement therapy and renal transplantation on blood pressure diurnal variability. Nephrol Dial Transplant. 1997;12:2301–7.
64. Burnier M, Coltamai L, Maillard M, Bochud M. Renal sodium handling and nighttime blood pressure. Semin Nephrol. 2007;27:565–71.
65. Fukuda M, Mizuno M, Yamanaka T, Motokawa M, Shirasawa Y, Nishio T, et al. Patients with renal dysfunction require a longer duration until blood pressure dips during the night. Hypertension. 2008;52:1155–60.

66. Whaley-Connell AT, Sowers JR, Stevens LA, McFarlane SI, Shlipak MG, Norris KC, et al. CKD in the United States: Kidney Early Evaluation Program (KEEP) and National Health and Nutrition Examination Survey (NHANES) 1999-2004. Am J Kidney Dis. 2008;51(4 Suppl 2):S13–20.
67. van den Hoogen PC, Feskens EJ, Nagelkerke NJ, Menotti A, Nissinen A, Kromhout D. The relation between blood pressure and mortality due to coronary heart disease among men in different parts of the world. Seven Countries Study Research Group. N Engl J Med. 2000;342:1–8.
68. Lewington S, Clarke R, Qizilbash N, Peto R, Collins R, Prospective Studies Collaboration. Age-specific relevance of usual blood pressure to vascular mortality: a meta-analysis of individual data for one million adults in 61 prospective studies. Lancet. 2002;360:1903–13.
69. Go AS, Chertow GM, Fan D, McCulloch CE, Hsu C-y. Chronic kidney disease and the risks of death, cardiovascular events, and hospitalization. N Engl J Med. 2004;351:1296–305.
70. Go AS, Lo JC. Epidemiology of non-dialysis-requiring chronic kidney disease and cardiovascular disease. Curr Opin Nephrol Hypertens. 2006;15:296–302.
71. Berbari A, Daouk N. Hypertension-chronic kidney disease relationships. Nephrol Open J. 2017;3:e18–21. https://doi.org/10.17140/NPOJ-3-e009.
72. Berbari AE, Daouk NA, Daouk MM. Chronic kidney disease and renovascular interactions. In: Berbari A, Mancia G, editors. Arterial disorders: definition, clinical manifestations, mechanisms and therapeutic approaches. Cham: Springer; 2015. p. 299–312.
73. Laskar SR, Dries DL. The prognostic significance of renal dysfunction in patients with chronic systolic heart failure. Curr Cardiol Rep. 2003;5:205–10.
74. Berbari AE. Links between chronic kidney disease and cardiovascular disease: a bidirectional relationship. In: Berbari AE, Mancia G, editors. Cardiorenal syndrome. Milano: Springer; 2010. p. 3–14.
75. Tracy RE, Strong JP, Newman WP 3rd, Malcom GT, Oalmann MC, Guzman MA. Renovasculopathies of nephrosclerosis in relation to atherosclerosis at ages 25 to 54 years. Kidney Int. 1996;49:564–70.
76. Ku E, Lee BJ, Wei J, Weir MR. Hypertension in CKD: core curriculum 2019. Am J Kidney Dis. 2019;74:120–31.
77. Lucas B, Taal MW. Blood pressure targets in chronic kidney disease: still no consensus. Curr Opin Nephrol Hypertens. 2023;32:497–501.
78. Wright JT Jr, Williamson JD, Whelton PK, Snyder JK, Sink KM, Rocco MV, et al. A randomized trial of intensive versus standard blood-pressure control. N Engl J Med. 2015;373:2103–16.
79. Damianaki A, Polychronopoulou E, Wuerzner G, Burnier M. New aspects in the management of hypertension in patients with chronic kidney disease not on renal replacement therapy. High Blood Press Cardiovasc Prev. 2022;29:125–35.
80. Bakris GL, Agarwal R, Anker SD, Pitt BP, Ruilope LM, Rossing P, et al. Effect of Finerenone on chronic kidney disease outcomes in type 2 diabetes. N Engl J Med. 2020;383:2219–29.
81. Pitt B, Filippatos G, Agarwal R, Anker SD, Bakris GL, Rossing P, et al. Cardiovascular events with Finerenone in kidney disease and type 2 diabetes. N Engl J Med. 2021;385:2252–63.
82. Filippatos G, Anker SD, Agarwal R, Pitt B, Ruilope LM, Rossing P, et al. Finerenone and cardiovascular outcomes in patients with chronic kidney disease and type 2 diabetes. Circulation. 2021;143:540–52.
83. Mancia G, Cannon CP, Tikkanen I, Zeller C, Ley L, Woerle HJ, et al. Impact of Empagliflozin on blood pressure in patients with type 2 diabetes mellitus and hypertension by background antihypertensive medication. Hypertension. 2016;68:1355–64.
84. Georgianos PI, Agarwal R. Ambulatory blood pressure reduction with SGLT-2 inhibitors: dose-response meta-analysis and comparative evaluation with low-dose hydrochlorothiazide. Diabetes Care. 2019;42:693–700.
85. Nuffield Department of Population Health Renal Studies Group; SGLT2 Inhibitor Meta-Analysis Cardio-Renal Trialists' Consortium. Impact of diabetes on the effects of sodium glucose co-transporter-2 inhibitors on kidney outcomes: collaborative meta-analysis of large placebo-controlled trials. Lancet. 2022;400:1788–801.

GPSR Compliance

The European Union's (EU) General Product Safety Regulation (GPSR) is a set of rules that requires consumer products to be safe and our obligations to ensure this.

If you have any concerns about our products, you can contact us on ProductSafety@springernature.com

In case Publisher is established outside the EU, the EU authorized representative is:

Springer Nature Customer Service Center GmbH
Europaplatz 3
69115 Heidelberg, Germany

Batch number: 10593240

Printed by Printforce, the Netherlands